Grashey
(1876-1950)

Dandy
(1886-1946)

Sweet
(1860-1926)

Law
(1875-1947)

Caldwell
(1870-1918)

Béclère, A.
(1856-1939)

Graham
(1883-1957)

Scholten B. Jones

Volume Three

MERRILL'S ATLAS *of*

RADIOGRAPHIC POSITIONING & PROCEDURES

MASTER ANATOMY & POSITIONING WITH THESE GREAT RESOURCES!

Mosby's Radiography Online: Anatomy & Positioning to Accompany *Merrill's Atlas of Radiographic Positioning & Procedures, 11th Edition*

Supplementing the 11th edition of *Merrill's Atlas*, this online course helps you develop skills that are essential in the clinical setting. It enhances your understanding of anatomy and positioning by providing interactive activities and self-assessment reviews. *Special Situations* sections highlight the imaging challenges presented by specific injuries and diseases. Each module also includes a section on film evaluation that demonstrates positioning and technical errors.

(User guide and access code only) **ISBN: 0-323-04491-3 • ISBN-13: 978-0-323-04491-2**

Workbook for *Merrill's Atlas of Radiographic Positioning & Procedures, 11th Edition*

Practice and review the concepts presented in *Merrill's Atlas*! This popular workbook includes exercises on anatomy labeling and positioning, illustrations to help you understand concepts, self-tests, and an answer key. Exercises include matching, labeling and identifying, short-answer and multiple-choice questions, crosswords, and true/false and fill-in-the-blank questions. With a thorough review of anatomy and radiographic procedures plus terminology, this workbook set is a must-have!

2-volume set • **ISBN: 0-323-04216-3 • ISBN-13: 978-0-323-04216-1**

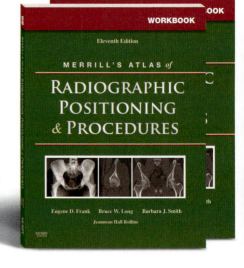

Merrill's Pocket Guide to Radiography, 6th Edition

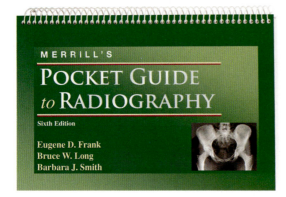

This handy pocket companion presents radiographic essentials in a quick-reference format ideal for the clinical setting. Bulleted, step-by-step explanations illustrate how to position the patient for more than 150 of the most common radiographic projections, including mobile and neonatal procedures. Unique to this guide is coverage of digital radiography and reference radiographs with each positioning presentation.

376 pp., 347 illus. • **ISBN: 0-323-04209-0 • ISBN-13: 978-0-323-04209-3**

Get your copies today!

 Online at www.elsevierhealth.com

 Call 1-800-545-2522

 Visit your local bookstore

MOSBY

ELSEVIE

HP-06251

Eleventh Edition
Volume Three

MERRILL'S ATLAS *of*

RADIOGRAPHIC POSITIONING & PROCEDURES

Eugene D. Frank, MA, RT(R), FASRT, FAERS

Director, Radiography Program
Riverland Community College
Austin, Minnesota;
Retired, Assistant Professor of Radiology
Mayo Clinic College of Medicine
Rochester, Minnesota

Bruce W. Long, MS, RT(R)(CV), FASRT

Director and Associate Professor
Radiologic Sciences Programs
Indiana University School of Medicine
Indianapolis, Indiana

Barbara J. Smith, MS, RT(R)(QM), FASRT

Instructor, Radiologic Technology
Medical Imaging Department
Portland Community College
Portland, Oregon

MOSBY

ELSEVIER

MOSBY
ELSEVIER

11830 Westline Industrial Drive
St. Louis, Missouri 63146

MERRILL'S ATLAS OF RADIOGRAPHIC POSITIONING AND PROCEDURES, EDITION 11
Volume Three

Three-Volume Set

ISBN-13: 978-0-323-04212-3
ISBN-10: 0-323-04212-0
ISBN-13: 978-0-323-03317-6
ISBN-10: 0-323-03317-2

Notice

Knowledge and best practice in this field are constantly changing. As new research and experience broaden our knowledge, changes in practice, treatment, and drug therapy may become necessary or appropriate. Readers are advised to check the most current information provided (i) on procedures featured or (ii) by the manufacturer of each product to be administered, to verify the recommended dose or formula, the method and duration of administration, and contraindications. It is the responsibility of the practitioner, relying on his or her own experience and knowledge of the patient, to make diagnoses, to determine dosages and the best treatment for each individual patient, and to take all appropriate safety precautions. To the fullest extent of the law, neither the Publisher nor the Authors assume any liability for any injury and/or damage to persons or property arising out or related to any use of the material contained in this book.

The Publisher

ISBN-13: 978-0-323-04212-3 (Volume Three)
ISBN-13: 978-0-323-03317-6 (Three-Volume Set)
ISBN-10: 0-323-04212-0 (Volume Three)
ISBN-10: 0-323-03317-2 (Three-Volume Set)

Publisher: Andrew Allen
Executive Editor: Jeanne Wilke
Senior Developmental Editor: Linda Woodard
Publishing Services Manager: Patricia Tannian
Project Manager: Kristine Feeherty
Cover Designer: Paula Ruckenford
Text Designer: Paula Ruckenford
Medical Illustrator: Jeanne Robertson

Printed in the United States of America

Last digit is the print number: 9 8 7 6 5 4 3 2 1

PREVIOUS AUTHORS

Vinita Merrill
1905-1977

Vinita Merrill had the foresight, talent, and knowledge to write the first
edition of this atlas in 1949. The text she wrote became known
as *Merrill's Atlas* in honor of the significant contribution she made
to the profession of radiography and in acknowledgment of the benefit
of her work to generations of students and practitioners.

Philip Ballinger became the author of *Merrill's Atlas* in its fifth edition,
which published in 1982. He served as author through the tenth edition, helping to launch successful careers for thousands of students
who have learned radiographic positioning from *Merrill's*. Phil is now
Assistant Professor Emeritus in the Radiologic Technology Division of
the School of Allied Medical Professions at The Ohio State University.
In 1995, he retired after a 25-year career as Radiography Program
Director, and after ably guiding *Merrill's Atlas* through six editions, he
retired as *Merrill's* author. Phil continues to be involved in professional
activities, such as speaking engagements at state, national, and international meetings.

AUTHORS

Eugene D. Frank, MA, RT(R), FASRT, FAERS, retired from the Mayo Clinic/Foundation in 2001 after 31 years of employment. He was Assistant Professor of Radiology in the College of Medicine and Director of the Radiography Program. He continues to work in radiography education as Director of the Radiography Program at Riverland Community College, Austin, Minnesota. He frequently presents at professional gatherings throughout the world and has held leadership positions in state, national, and international organizations. He is the coauthor of two radiography textbooks (*Quality Control in Diagnostic Imaging* and *Radiography Essentials for Limited Practice),* two radiography workbooks, and two book chapters, in addition to being coauthor of the atlas. The eleventh edition is Gene's third edition as coauthor.

Bruce W. Long, MS, RT(R)(CV), FASRT, is Director and Associate Professor of the Indiana University Radiologic Sciences Programs, where he has taught for 20 years. A life member of the Indiana Society of Radiologic Technologists, he frequently presents at state and national professional meetings. His publication activities include 28 articles in national professional journals and two books, *Orthopaedic Radiography* and *Radiography Essentials for Limited Practice.* The eleventh edition is Bruce's first as coauthor of the atlas.

Barbara J. Smith, MS, RT(R)(QM), FASRT, is an instructor in the Radiologic Technology program at Portland Community College, where she has taught for 22 years. The Oregon Society of Radiologic Technologists inducted her as a life member in 2003. She presents at state, regional, and national meetings and is involved in professional activities at these levels. Her publication activities include articles, book reviews, and chapter contributions. The eleventh edition is Barb's first as coauthor of the atlas.

ADVISORY BOARD

This edition of *Merrill's Atlas* benefits from the expertise of a special advisory board. The following board members have provided professional input and advice and have helped the authors make decisions about atlas content throughout the preparation of the eleventh edition:

Valerie J. Palm, RT(R), ACR, ID, MEd, FCAMRT

Instructor, Medical Radiography Program
School of Health
British Columbia Institute of Technology
Burnaby, British Columbia

Roger A. Preston, MSRS, RT(R)

Program Director, Reid Hospital &
Health Care Services
School of Radiologic Technology
Richmond, Indiana

Ms. Johnnie B. Moore, MEd, RT(R)

Chair, Radiography Program
Barnes-Jewish College of Nursing and
Allied Health
St. Louis, Missouri

Diedre Costic, MPS, RT(R)(M)

Associate Professor and Department
Chair, Diagnostic Imaging Program
Orange County Community College
Middletown, New York

Joe A. Garza, MS, RT(R)

Associate Professor, Radiography
Program
Montgomery College
Conroe, Texas

Andrea J. Cornuelle, MS, RT(R)

Associate Professor, Radiologic
Technology Program
Northern Kentucky University
Highland Heights, Kentucky

CONTRIBUTORS

Valerie F. Andolina, RT(R)(M)
Imaging Technology Manager
Elizabeth Wende Breast Clinic
Rochester, New York

Albert Aziza, BHA, BSc, MRT(R)
Manager, Imaging Guided Therapy
The Hospital for Sick Children
Toronto, Canada

Peter J. Barger, MS, RT(R)(CT)
Radiography Program Director
College of Nursing and Health Sciences
Cape Girardeau, Missouri

Terri Bruckner, MA, RT(R)(CV)
Clinical Instructor and Clinical
    Coordinator
The Ohio State University
Columbus, Ohio

Thomas H. Burke, RT(R)(CV), FAVIR
Clinical Manager
Microvention, Inc.
Grosse Pointe Woods, Michigan

Leila A. Bussman-Yeakel, BS, RT(R)(T)
Director, Radiation Therapy Program
Mayo School of Health Sciences
Mayo Clinic College of Medicine
Rochester, Minnesota

JoAnn P. Caudill, RT(R)(M)(BD),CDT
Bone Health Program Manager
Erickson Retirement Communities
Catonsville, Maryland

Ellen Charkot, MRT(R)
Chief Technologist, Diagnostic Imaging
    Department
The Hospital for Sick Children
Toronto, Ontario

Sharon A. Coffey, MS, RT(R)
Instructor in Medical Radiography
Houston Community College
Coleman College of Health Sciences
Houston, Texas

**Luann J. Culbreth, MEd,
RT(R)(MR)(QM), CRA, FSMRT**
Director of Imaging Services
Baylor Regional Medical Center at Plano
Plano, Texas

**Sandra L. Hagen-Ansert, MS, RDMS,
RDCS, FSDMS**
Scripps Clinic, Torrey Pines
Cardiac Sonographer
San Diego, California

Nancy L. Hockert, BS, ASCP, CNMT
Program Director, Nuclear Medicine
    Technology
Assistant Professor
Mayo Clinic College of Medicine
Rochester, Minnesota

Steven C. Jensen, PhD, RT(R)
Director, Radiologic Sciences Program
Southern Illinois University
Carbondale, Illinois

Timothy J. Joyce, RT(R)(CV)
Clinical Group Manager
Microvention, Inc.
Dearborn, Michigan

Sara A. Kaderlik, RT(R)
Special Procedures Radiographer
Providence St. Vincent Cardiovascular Lab
Beaverton, Oregon

**Eric P. Matthews, MSEd,
RT(R)(CV)(MR), EMT**
Visiting Assistant Professor, Radiologic
    Sciences Program
Southern Illinois University
Carbondale, Illinois

Elton A. Mosman, MBA, CNMT
Clinical Coordinator, Nuclear Medicine
    Program
Mayo Clinic College of Medicine
Rochester, Minnesota

Sandra J. Nauman, BS, RT(R)(M)
Clinical Coordinator, Radiography
    Program
Riverland Community College
Austin, Minnesota

**Paula Pate-Schloder, MS,
RT(R)(CV)(CT)(VI)**
Associate Professor, Medical Imaging
    Department
College Misericordia
Dallas, Pennsylvania

Joel A. Permar, RT(R)
Surgical Radiographer
University of Alabama Hospital
Birmingham, Alabama

**Jeannean Hall Rollins, MRC,
BSRT(R)(CV)**
Associate Professor, Radiologic Sciences
Arkansas State University
Jonesboro, Arkansas

Kari J. Wetterlin, MA, RT(R)
Unit Supervisor, Surgical Radiology
Mayo Clinic/Foundation
Rochester, Minnesota

Gayle K. Wright, BS, RT(R)(MR)(CT)
Instructor, Radiologic Technology Program
Portland Community College
Portland, Oregon

PREFACE

Welcome to the eleventh edition of *Merrill's Atlas of Radiographic Positioning and Procedures*. The eleventh edition continues the tradition of excellence begun in 1949, when Vinita Merrill wrote the first edition of what has become a classic text. Over the last 58 years, *Merrill's Atlas* has provided a strong foundation in anatomy and positioning for thousands of students around the world who have gone on to successful careers as imaging technologists. *Merrill's Atlas* is also a mainstay for everyday reference in imaging departments all over the world. As the coauthors of the eleventh edition, we are honored to follow in Vinita Merrill's footsteps.

Learning and Perfecting Positioning Skills

Merrill's Atlas has an established tradition of helping students learn and perfect their positioning skills. After covering preliminary steps in radiography, radiation protection, and terminology in introductory chapters, *Merrill's* then teaches anatomy and positioning in separate chapters for each bone group or organ system. The student learns to position the patient properly so that the resulting radiograph provides the information the physician needs to correctly diagnose the patient's problem. The atlas presents this information for commonly requested projections, as well as those less commonly requested, making it the most comprehensive text and reference available.

The third volume of the atlas provides basic information about a variety of special imaging modalities, such as mobile, surgical, geriatrics, computed tomography, cardiac catheterization, magnetic resonance imaging, ultrasound, nuclear medicine technology, and radiation therapy.

Merrill's Atlas is not only a sound resource for students to learn from but also an indispensable reference as they move into the clinical environment and ultimately into their practice as imaging professionals.

New to This Edition

Since the first edition of *Merrill's Atlas* in 1949, many changes have occurred. This new edition incorporates many significant changes designed not only to reflect the technologic progress and advancements in the profession but also to meet the needs of today's radiography students. The major changes in this edition are highlighted as follows.

NEW ORTHOPEDIC PROJECTION

One new projection, the Coyle Method for demonstrating the elbow after trauma, has been added to this edition. Also added is a modification of the Judet Method of demonstrating the acetabulum on trauma patients.

NEW ABBREVIATIONS BOXES AND ADDENDUM

Each chapter in this edition contains all the essential abbreviations used in the chapter that have not been introduced in previous chapters. Students become familiar with the common abbreviations, which are then used throughout the chapter. All the abbreviations used in Volumes 1 and 2 are summarized in addendums at the end of the volume.

NEW CHAPTER AND REVISED CHAPTERS

A new chapter on the theory and use of compensating filters is included in this edition. The compensating filters chapter contains high-quality radiographs made with and without filters to demonstrate the positive effect of the filter. In addition, projections that benefit from the use of a filter are identified in the text with the use of a special icon and heading titled "Compensating Filter." The new filter icon is shown here:

◤ COMPENSATING FILTER

The Sectional Anatomy chapter in Volume 3 had been entirely revised with new high-resolution CT and MRI images and correlating art. This chapter will provide instructors and students with information needed for the proposed ASRT curriculum updates.

The Geriatrics chapter has been updated to include patient positioning photographs and radiographs with common pathology.

DIGITAL RADIOGRAPHY UPDATED

Because of the rapid expansion and acceptance of computed radiography (CR) and direct digital radiography (DR), either selected positioning considerations and modifications or special instructions are indicated where necessary. A special icon alerts the reader to digital notes. The icon is shown here:

DIGITAL RADIOGRAPHY 💻

ESSENTIAL PROJECTIONS

Essential projections are identified with the special icon shown here: 🔺

One new projection has been designated essential for this edition: the Coyle Method for demonstrating the elbow for trauma. Essential projections are those most frequently performed and determined to be necessary for competency of entry-level practitioners. Of the more than 375 projections described in this atlas, 184 have been identified as essential based on the results of two extensive surveys performed in the United States and Canada.[1]

OBSOLETE PROJECTIONS DELETED

Projections identified as obsolete by the authors and the advisory board have been deleted. A summary is provided at the beginning of any chapter containing deleted projections so that the reader may refer to previous editions for information. Several projections have been deleted in this edition, most of them in the cranial chapters.

CHAPTERS DELETED OR MERGED

The chapters "Radiation Protection" and "Computed Radiography" have been eliminated from this edition of the atlas because these chapters are more closely aligned to physics and exposure and are best studied in comprehensive texts devoted to these topics. The Temporal Bone chapter of the skull has been merged with the general Skull chapter. The Digital Angiography chapter had been merged with the Circulatory System chapter. The Positron Emission Tomography chapter has been merged with the Nuclear Medicine chapter. These merges will enable students to more easily learn the concepts presented in these chapters.

[1]Ballinger PW, Glassner JL: Positioning competencies for radiography graduates, *Radiol Technol* 70:181, 1998.

NEW 3D LINE ART

Many new line illustrations have been added to this edition. Each is designed to clarify anatomy or projections that are difficult to visualize. More than 24 new line art figures appear throughout the three volumes, including the Compensating Filters chapter of Volume 1.

NEW RADIOGRAPHS

Nearly every chapter contains new and additional optimum radiographs, including many that demonstrate pathology. With the addition of more than 30 new radiographic images, the eleventh edition has the most comprehensive collection of high-quality radiographs available to students and practitioners.

NEW MRI AND CT IMAGES INTEGRATED INTO THE TEXT

Nearly every chapter in Volumes 1 and 2 contains new MRI or CT images in the anatomy section to aid the reader in learning radiographic anatomy. These 40 images not only help the student to learn the exact size, shape, and placement of anatomical parts, but also help the reader become familiar with images produced by these commonly used modalities.

NEW PATIENT PHOTOGRAPHY

More than 35 new color anatomy, patient positioning, or procedure-related photographs have been added. These added or replacement photographs aid students in learning radiography positioning concepts.

Learning Aids for the Student

POCKET GUIDE TO RADIOGRAPHY

A new edition of *Merrill's Pocket Guide to Radiography* complements the revision of *Merrill's Atlas*. In addition to instructions for positioning the patient and the body part for all the essential projections, the new pocket guide includes information on digital radiography and automatic exposure control (AEC). kVp information has been added. Tabs have been added to help the user locate the beginning of each section. Space is provided for writing department techniques specific to the user.

RADIOGRAPHIC ANATOMY, POSITIONING, AND PROCEDURES WORKBOOK

The new edition of this two-volume workbook retains most of the features of the previous editions: anatomy labeling exer-

cises, positioning exercises, self-tests, and an answer key. The exercises include labeling of anatomy on drawings and radiographs, crossword puzzles, matching, short answers, and true/false. At the end of each chapter is a multiple-choice test to help students assess their comprehension of the whole chapter. New to this edition are exercises for the Pediatrics, Geriatrics, Mobile, Surgical, and Computed Tomography chapters in Volume 3. Also new to this edition are more image evaluations to give students additional opportunities to evaluate radiographs for proper positioning and more positioning questions to complement the workbook's strong anatomy review. Exercises in these chapters will help students learn the theory and concepts of these special techniques with greater ease.

Teaching Aids for the Instructor

INSTRUCTOR'S ELECTRONIC RESOURCE (IER)

This comprehensive resource provides valuable tools, such as teaching strategies, power point slides, and an electronic test bank, for teaching an anatomy and positioning class. The test bank includes more than 1500 questions, each coded by category and level of difficulty. Four exams are already compiled within the test bank to be used "as is" at the instructor's discretion. The instructor also has the option of building new tests as often as desired by pulling questions from the pool or using a combination of questions from the test bank and questions that the instructor adds.

All the images, photographs, and line illustrations in *Merrill's Atlas* are also available on the Electronic Image Collection on the IER CD-ROM.

More information about the IER is available from an Elsevier sales representative.

MOSBY'S RADIOGRAPHY ONLINE

Mosby's Radiography Online: Anatomy and Positioning is a well-developed online course companion that includes animations with narration and interactive activities and exercises to assist in the understanding of anatomy and positioning. Used in conjunction with the *Merrill's Atlas* textbook, it offers greater learning opportunities while accommodating diverse learning styles and circumstances. This unique program promotes problem-based learning with the goal of developing critical thinking skills that will be needed in the clinical setting.

EVOLVE—ONLINE COURSE MANAGEMENT

Evolve is an interactive learning environment designed to work in coordination with *Merrill's Atlas*. Instructors may use Evolve to provide an Internet-based course component that reinforces and expands on the concepts delivered in class.

Evolve may be used to publish the class syllabus, outlines, and lecture notes; set up "virtual office hours" and e-mail communication; share important dates and information through the online class Calendar; and encourage student participation through Chat Rooms and Discussion Boards. Evolve allows instructors to post exams and manage their grade books online. For more information, visit http://www.evolve.elsevier.com or contact an Elsevier sales representative.

We hope you will find this edition of *Merrill's Atlas of Radiographic Positioning and Procedures* the best ever. Input from generations of readers has helped to keep the atlas strong through ten editions, and we welcome your comments and suggestions. We are constantly striving to build on Vinita Merrill's work, and we trust that she would be proud and pleased to know that the work she began 58 years ago is still so appreciated and valued by the imaging sciences community.

Eugene D. Frank
Bruce W. Long
Barbara J. Smith

ACKNOWLEDGMENTS

In preparing for the eleventh edition, our advisory board continually provided professional expertise and aid in decision making on the revision of this edition. The advisory board members are listed on p. vii. We are most grateful for their input and contributions to this edition of the atlas.

The new Coyle Method for demonstrating the elbow for trauma was written by **Tammy Curtis, MS, RT(R),** from Northwestern State University, Shreveport, Louisiana. Ms. Curtis also performed the research and wrote all of the abbreviations for this edition of the atlas.

Special thanks goes out to a former student and 3D reconstruction specialist, **J. Louis Rankin, BS, RT(R)(MR),** from Indiana University Hospital, Indianapolis, Indiana, for the significant amount of time he spent assisting in acquiring new CT and MRI images used in the non–Sectional Anatomy chapters in the atlas.

Reviewers

The group of radiography professionals listed below reviewed aspects of this edition of the atlas and made many insightful suggestions for strengthening the atlas. We are most appreciative of their willingness to lend their expertise.

Kenneth Bontrager, MA, RT(R)
Radiography Author
Sun City West, Arizona

Kari Buchanan, BS, RT(R)
Mayo Clinic Foundation
Rochester, Minnesota

Barry Burns, MS, RT(R), DABR
University of North Carolina
Chapel Hill, North Carolina

Linda Cox, MS, RT(R)(MR)CT)
Indiana University School of Medicine
Indianapolis, Indiana

Tammy Curtis, MS, RT(R)
Northwestern State University
Shreveport, Louisiana

Timothy Daly, BS, RT(R)
Mayo Clinic Foundation
Rochester, Minnesota

Dan Ferlic, RT(R)
Ferlic Filters
White Bear Lake, Minnesota

Ginger Griffin, RT(R), FASRT
Baptist Medical Center
Jacksonville, Florida

Henrique da Guia Costa, MBA, RT(R)
Radiographer
Radiography Consultant
Lisbon, Portugal

Dimitris Koumoranos, MSc, RT(R)(CT)(MR)
Radiographer, General Hospital Elpis
Athens, Greece

Seiji Nishio, BA, RT(R)
Radiographer, Komazawa University
Tokyo, Japan

Rosanne Paschal, PhD, RT(R)
College of DuPage
Glen Ellyn, Illinois

Susan Robinson, MS, RT(R)
Indiana University School of Medicine
Indianapolis, Indiana

Lavonne Rohn, RT(R)
Mankato Clinic
Mankato, Minnesota

Jeannean Hall Rollins, MRC, BSRT(R)(CV)
Associate Professor, Radiologic Sciences
Arkansas State University
Jonesboro, Arkansas

Carole South-Winter, MEd, RT(R), CNMT
Reclaiming Youth International
Lennox, South Dakota

Richard Terrass, MEd, RT(R)
Massachusetts General Hospital
Boston, Massachusetts

Beth Vealé, MEd, RT(R)(QM)
Midwestern State University
Wichita Falls, Texas

CONTENTS

Volume Three

MERRILL'S ATLAS *of*

RADIOGRAPHIC POSITIONING & PROCEDURES

24

CENTRAL NERVOUS SYSTEM

PAULA PATE-SCHLODER

Myelogram: lateral projection showing subarachnoid space narrowing *(arrow)*.

For descriptive purposes, the central nervous system (CNS) is divided into two parts: (1) the *brain,** which occupies the cranial cavity, and (2) the *spinal cord,* which is suspended within the vertebral canal.

---

*Many italicized words are defined at the end of the chapter.

Brain

The brain is composed of an outer portion of gray matter called the *cortex* and an inner portion of *white matter.* The brain consists of the *cerebrum; cerebellum;* and *brainstem,* which is continuous with the spinal cord (Fig. 24-1). The brainstem consists of the *midbrain, pons,* and *medulla oblongata.*

The cerebrum is the largest part of the brain and is referred to as the *forebrain.* Its surface is convoluted by sulci and grooves that divide it into lobes and lobules. The stemlike portion that connects the cerebrum to the pons and cerebellum is termed the *midbrain.* The cerebellum, pons, and medulla oblongata make up the *hindbrain.*

A deep cleft, called the *longitudinal sulcus* (interhemispheric fissure), separates the cerebrum into *right* and *left hemispheres,* which are closely connected by bands of nerve fibers, or commissures. The largest commissure between the cerebral hemispheres is the *corpus callosum.* The corpus callosum is a midline structure inferior to the longitudinal sulcus. Each cerebral hemisphere contains a fluid-filled cavity called a *lateral ventricle.* At the diencephalon, or second portion of the brain, the thalami surround the *third ventricle.* Inferior to the diencephalon is the *pituitary gland,* the master endocrine gland of the body. The pituitary gland resides in the hypophyseal fossa of the sella turcica.

The cerebellum, the largest part of the hindbrain, is separated from the cerebrum by a deep transverse cleft. The hemispheres of the cerebellum are connected by a median constricted area called the *vermis.* The surface of the cerebellum contains numerous transverse sulci that account for its cauliflower-like appearance. The tissues between the curved sulci are called *folia.* The pons, which forms the upper part of the hindbrain, is the commissure or bridge between the cerebrum, cerebellum, and medulla oblongata. The medulla oblongata, which extends between the pons and spinal cord, forms the lower portion of the hindbrain. All the fiber tracts between the brain and spinal cord pass through the medulla.

Fig. 24-1 Lateral surface and midsection of brain.

Spinal Cord

The *spinal cord* is a slender, elongated structure consisting of an inner, gray, cellular substance, which has an H shape on transverse section, and an outer, white, fibrous substance (Figs. 24-2 and 24-3). The cord extends from the brain, where it is connected to the medulla oblongata at the level of the foramen magnum, to the approximate level of the space between the first and second lumbar vertebrae. The spinal cord ends in a pointed extremity called the *conus medullaris.* The *filum terminale* is a delicate fibrous strand that extends from the terminal tip and attaches the cord to the upper coccygeal segment.

In an adult the spinal cord is between 18″ and 20″ long and is connected to 31 pairs of spinal nerves. Each pair of spinal nerves arises from two roots at the sides of the spinal cord. The nerves are transmitted through the intervertebral and sacral foramina. Spinal nerves below the termination of the spinal cord extend inferiorly through the vertebral canal. These nerves resemble a horse's tail and are referred to as the *cauda equina.* The spinal cord and nerves work together to transmit and receive sensory, motor, and reflex messages to and from the brain.

Meninges

The brain and spinal cord are enclosed in three continuous protective membranes called *meninges.* The inner sheath, called the *pia mater* (Latin, "tender mother"), is highly vascular and closely adherent to the underlying brain and cord structure.

The delicate central sheath is called the *arachnoid.* This membrane is separated from the pia mater by a comparatively wide space called the *subarachnoid space,* which is widened in certain areas. These areas of increased width are called *subarachnoid cisterns.* The widest area is the cisterna magna (cisterna cerebellomedullaris). This triangular cavity is situated in the lower posterior fossa between the base of the cerebellum and the dorsal surface of the medulla oblongata. The subarachnoid space is continuous with the ventricular system of the brain and communicates with it through the foramina of the fourth ventricle. The ventricles of the brain and the subarachnoid space contain *cerebrospinal fluid* (CSF). CSF is the tissue fluid of the brain and spinal cord; it surrounds and cushions the structures of the CNS.

The outermost sheath, called the *dura mater* (Latin, "hard mother"), forms the strong fibrous covering of the brain and spinal cord. The dura is separated from the arachnoid by the *subdural space* and from the vertebral periosteum by the *epidural space.* These spaces do not communicate with the ventricular system. The dura mater is composed of two layers throughout its cranial portion. The outer layer lines the cranial bones, thus serving as periosteum to their inner surface. The inner layer protects the brain and supports the blood vessels. The layer also has four partitions that provide support and protection for the various parts of the brain. One of these partitions, the *falx cerebri,* runs through the interhemispheric fissure and provides support for the cerebral hemispheres. The *tentorium* is a tent-shaped fold of dura that separates the cerebrum and cerebellum. Changes in the normal positions of these structures often indicate pathology. The dura mater extends below the spinal cord (to the level of the second sacral segment) to enclose the spinal nerves, which are prolonged inferiorly from the cord to their respective exits. The lower portion of the dura mater is called the *dural sac.* The cauda equina is enclosed by the dural sac.

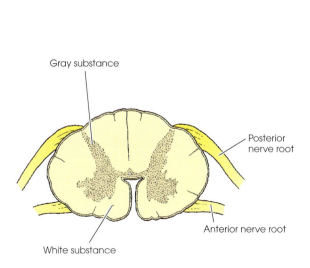

Fig. 24-2 Transverse section of spinal cord.

Fig. 24-3 Sagittal section showing spinal cord.

3

Ventricular System

The ventricular system of the brain consists of four irregular, fluid-containing cavities that communicate with one another through connecting channels (Figs. 24-4 to 24-6). The two upper cavities are an identical pair and are simply called the *right* and *left lateral ventricles.* They are situated, one on each side of the midsagittal plane, in the inferior medial part of the corresponding hemisphere of the cerebrum.

Each lateral ventricle consists of a central portion called the *body* of the cavity. The body is prolonged anteriorly, posteriorly, and inferiorly into hornlike portions that give the ventricle an approximate U shape. The prolonged portions are known as the *anterior, posterior,* and *inferior horns.* Each lateral ventricle is connected to the third ventricle by a channel called the *interventricular foramen* or foramen of Monroe, through which it communicates directly with the third ventricle and indirectly with the opposite lateral ventricle.

The *third ventricle* is a slitlike cavity with a somewhat quadrilateral shape. It is situated in the midsagittal plane just inferior to the level of the bodies of the lateral ventricles. This cavity extends antero-inferiorly from the pineal gland, which produces a recess in its posterior wall, to the optic chiasm, which produces a recess in its anteroinferior wall.

The interventricular foramina, one from each lateral ventricle, open into the anterosuperior portion of the third ventricle. The cavity is continuous posteroinferiorly with the fourth ventricle by a passage known as the *cerebral aqueduct* or aqueduct of Sylvius.

The *fourth ventricle* is diamond shaped and is located in the area of the hindbrain. The fourth ventricle is anterior to the cerebellum and posterior to the pons and the upper portion of the medulla oblongata. The distal, pointed end of the fourth ventricle is continuous with the central canal of the medulla oblongata. CSF exits the fourth ventricle into the subarachnoid space via the *median aperture* (foramen of Magendie) and the *lateral apertures* (foramen of Luschka).

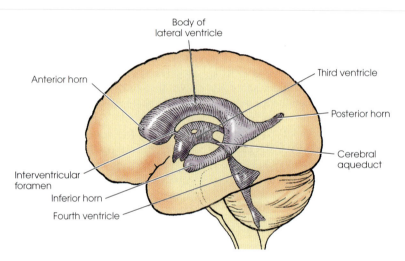

Fig. 24-4 Lateral aspect of cerebral ventricles in relation to surface of brain.

Fig. 24-5 Anterior aspect of lateral cerebral ventricles in relation to surface of brain.

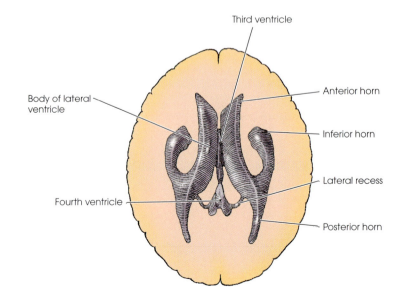

Fig. 24-6 Superior aspect of cerebral ventricles in relation to surface of brain.

Plain Radiographic Examination

Neuroradiologic assessment should begin with noninvasive imaging procedures. Radiographs of the cerebral and visceral cranium and the vertebral column may be employed to demonstrate bony anatomy. In traumatized patients (see Chapter 8) radiographs are obtained to detect bony injury, subluxation, or dislocation of the vertebral column and to determine the extent and stability of the bony injury.

For a traumatized patient with possible CNS involvement, a cross-table lateral cervical spine radiograph should be obtained first to rule out fracture or misalignment of the cervical spine. Approximately two thirds of significant pathologic conditions affecting the spine can be detected on this initial image. Care must be taken to demonstrate the entire cervical spine adequately including the C7-T1 articulation. Employing the Twining (Swimmers) method (see Chapter 8) may be necessary to demonstrate this anatomic region radiographically.

After the cross-table lateral radiograph has been checked and cleared by a physician, the following cervical spine projections should be obtained: an anteroposterior (AP), bilateral AP oblique (trauma technique may be necessary), and an AP to demonstrate the dens. A vertebral arch, or pillar image, of the cervical spine may provide additional information about the posterior portions of the cervical vertebrae (see Chapter 8). An upright lateral cervical spine radiograph may also be requested to better demonstrate alignment of the vertebrae and to assess the normal lordotic curvature of the spine.

Tomography may be used to supplement images of the spine for initial screening purposes (see Chapter 32). However, tomography has been largely replaced by computed tomography (CT) in many institutions (see Chapter 31). Tomography may be employed to demonstrate long continuous areas of the spine. Disadvantages of tomography include the lack of soft tissue detail and the difficulty in positioning a traumatized patient for lateral tomographic radiographs.

Radiographs of the spine should always be obtained before myelography. Routine images of the vertebral column are helpful in assessing narrowed disk spaces because of degeneration of the disk, osteoarthritis, postoperative changes in the spine, and other pathologies of the vertebral column. Because the contrast agents used in myelography may obscure some anomalies, noncontrast spinal images complement the myelographic examination and often provide additional information.

Routine skull images should be obtained when the possibility of a skull fracture exists. In trauma patients a cross-table lateral or upright lateral skull radiograph must be obtained to demonstrate air-fluid levels in the sphenoid sinus. In many instances these air-fluid levels may be the initial indication of a basilar skull fracture. In addition, skull images are helpful in diagnosing reactive bone formation and general alterations in the skull resulting from a variety of pathologic conditions including Paget's disease, fibrous dysplasia, hemangiomas, and changes in the sella turcica.

Myelography

Myelography (Greek, *myelos,* "marrow; the spinal cord") is the general term applied to radiologic examination of the CNS structures situated within the vertebral canal. This examination is performed by introducing a nonionic, water-soluble contrast medium into the subarachnoid space by spinal puncture, most commonly at the L2-L3 or L3-L4 interspace or at the cisterna magna between C1 and the occipital bone. Injections into the subarachnoid space are termed *intrathecal injections.*

Most myelograms are performed on an outpatient basis, with patients recovering for approximately 4 to 8 hours after the procedure before being released to return home. In many parts of the country, however, magnetic resonance imaging (MRI) (see Chapter 33) has largely replaced myelography. Myelography continues to be the preferred examination method for assessing disk disease in patients with contraindications to MRI, such as pacemakers or metallic posterior spinal fusion rods.

Myelography is employed to demonstrate extrinsic spinal cord compression caused by a herniated disk, bone fragments, or tumors, as well as spinal cord swelling resulting from traumatic injury. These encroachments appear radiographically as a deformity in the subarachnoid space or an obstruction of the passage of the column of contrast medium within the subarachnoid space. Myelography is also useful in identifying narrowing of the subarachnoid space by evaluating the dynamic flow patterns of the CSF.

CONTRAST MEDIA

A non–water-soluble, iodinated ester (iophendylate [Pantopaque]) was introduced in 1942. Because it could not be absorbed by the body, this lipid-based contrast medium required removal after the procedure. Frequently some contrast remained in the canal and could be seen on noncontrast radiographs of patients who had the myelography procedure before the introduction of the newer medium. Iophendylate was used in myelography for many years but is no longer commercially available. The first water-soluble, nonionic, iodinated contrast agent, metrizamide, was introduced in the late 1970s. Thereafter, water-soluble contrast media quickly became the agents of choice. Nonionic, water-soluble contrast media provide good visualization of nerve roots (Fig. 24-7) and good enhancement for follow-up CT of the spine. In addition, these agents are readily absorbed by the body. Over the past 2 decades, nonionic, water-soluble agents including iopamidol (Isovue) and iohexol (Omnipaque) have become the most commonly used agents for myelography. Improvements in nonionic contrast agents have resulted in fewer side effects.

Fig. 24-7 Myelogram using nonionic, water-soluble contrast medium (iopamidol) on a postsurgical patient.

Technologists who perform myelography should be educated regarding the use of contrast media. Intrathecal administration of ionic contrast media may cause severe and fatal neurotoxic reactions. Because vials of ionic and nonionic agents may look similar, departments are encouraged to store contrast media for myelography separately from other agents. Importantly, proper medication guidelines must be followed when administering intrathecal agents. Contrast vials should be checked three times, checked with the physician performing the examination, and kept until the procedure is completed. All appropriate documentation should be completed.

PREPARATION OF EXAMINING ROOM

One of the radiographer's responsibilities is to prepare the examining room before the patient's arrival. The radiographic equipment should be checked. Because the procedure involves aseptic technique, the table and overhead equipment must be cleaned. The footboard should be attached to the table, and the padded shoulder supports should be placed and ready for adjustment to the patient's height. The image intensifier should be locked so that it cannot accidentally come in contact with the spinal needle, sterile field, or both (Fig. 24-8).

The spinal puncture and contrast medium injection are performed in the radiology department. Under fluoroscopic observation, placement of the 20- to 22-gauge spinal needle in the subarachnoid space is verified and the contrast medium is injected. The sterile tray and the nonsterile items required for this initial procedure should be ready for convenient placement.

EXAMINATION PROCEDURE

Premedication of the patient for myelography is rarely necessary. The patient should be well hydrated, however, because a nonionic, water-soluble contrast medium is used. To reduce apprehension and prevent alarm at unexpected maneuvers during the procedure, the radiographer should explain the details of myelography to the patient before the examination begins. The patient should be informed that the angulation of the examining table will repeatedly and acutely change. The patient should also be told why the head must be maintained in a fully extended position when the table is tilted to the Trendelenburg position. The radiographer must provide assurance that the patient will be safe when the table is acutely angled and that everything possible will be done to avoid causing unnecessary discomfort.

Scout images including a cross-table lateral lumbar spine prone (Fig. 24-9) are often requested. Some physicians prefer to have the patient placed on the table in the prone position for the spinal puncture. Many physicians, however, have the patient adjusted in the lateral position with the spine flexed to widen the interspinous spaces for easier introduction of the needle.

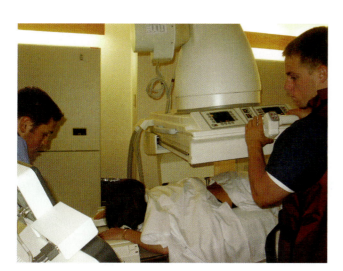

Fig. 24-8 Patient set up with shoulder supports and image intensifier in locked position.

Fig. 24-9 Lateral scout projection of cross-table lumbar spine myelogram.

The physician usually withdraws CSF for laboratory analysis and slowly injects approximately 9 to 12 mL of nonionic contrast medium. After completing the injection, the physician removes the spinal needle. Travel of the contrast medium column is observed and controlled fluoroscopically. Angulation of the table allows gravity to direct the contrast to the area of interest. Spot images are taken throughout the procedure. The radiographer obtains images at the level of any blockage or distortion in the outline of the contrast column. Conventional radiographic studies, with the central ray directed verti-cally or horizontally, may be performed as requested by the radiologist. The *conus projection* is used to demonstrate the *conus medullaris.* For this the patient is placed in the AP position with the central ray centered to T12-L1. A 24 × 30 cm (10 × 12 inch) cassette is used. Cross-table lateral radiographs are obtained with grid-front cassettes or a stationary grid; they must be closely collimated (Figs. 24-10 to 24-14).

The position of the patient's head must be guarded as the contrast column nears the cervical area to prevent the medium from passing into the cerebral ventricles. Acute extension of the head compresses the cisterna magna and thus prevents further ascent of the medium. Because the cisterna magna is situated posteriorly, neither forward nor lateral flexion of the head compresses the cisternal cavity.

After completion of the procedure, the patient must be monitored in an appropriate recovery area. Most physicians recommend that the patient's head and shoulders be elevated 30 to 45 degrees during recovery. Bedrest for several hours is recommended, and fluids are encouraged. The puncture site must be examined before the patient is released from the recovery area.

Fig. 24-10 A, Lumbar myelogram: cross-table lateral demonstrating needle tip in subarachnoid space. **B,** Lumbar myelogram: cross-table lateral demonstrating contrast enhancement.

Fig. 24-12 Myelogram: prone cross-table lateral projection showing dentate ligament and posterior nerve roots (*arrow*).

Fig. 24-11 Cervical myelogram: AP projection showing symmetric nerve roots (*arrows*) and axillary pouches (*a*) on both sides, as well as spinal cord.

Fig. 24-13 Myelogram: prone, cross-table lateral projection showing contrast medium passing through foramen magnum and lying against lower clivus (*arrows*).

Fig. 24-14 Myelogram: lateral projection showing subarachnoid space narrowing (*arrow*).

Fig. 24-15 Postinfusion (C1) CT scan of the brain, demonstrating a cystic mass "highlighted" by the intravenous contrast material *(arrows).*

Fig. 24-16 CT angiography of the brain demonstrating an aneurysm *(arrows),* later confirmed by vascular imaging.

Computed Tomography

CT is a rapid, noninvasive imaging technique that was first introduced for clinical use in the early 1970s. It produces sectional images of the brain called *slices.* CT imaging of the head and spine expanded rapidly because of improvements in computer technology and this imaging modality's ability to demonstrate abnormalities with a precision never before possible. Digital image processing techniques in CT allow for changes in the density and contrast of an image, called *windowing.* The use of different windows allows for visualization of both soft tissue and bony structures. (See Chapter 31 for more detail.)

A CT examination of the brain is commonly performed in an axial orientation with the gantry placed at an angle of 20 to 25 degrees to the orbitomeatal line, which allows the lowest slice to provide an image of both the upper cervical/foramen magnum and the roof of the orbit. Normally 12 to 14 slices are obtained, depending on the size of the patient's head and the thickness of the CT image slices. Imaging continues superiorly until the entire head has been examined. A slice thickness of 8 to 10 mm is often used, but most institutions use 3- to 5-mm slices through the area of the posterior fossa. Coronal images may also be obtained and are quite helpful in evaluating abnormalities of the pituitary gland and sella turcica, as well as facial bones and sinuses. The computer may be used to reconstruct and display the images in a variety of imaging planes.

CT scans of the brain are often obtained before and after intravenous (IV) injection of a nonionic, water-soluble contrast agent. These are often referred to as *preinfusion* (C−) and *postinfusion* (C+) scans (Fig. 24-15). Common indications for scans with and without contrast agents include suspected primary neoplasms; suspected metastatic disease; suspected arteriovenous malformation (AVM); demyelinating disease, such as multiple sclerosis; seizure disorders; and bilateral, isodense hematomas. Common indications for CT of the brain without an IV infusion of contrast material include assessment of dementia, craniocerebral trauma, hydrocephalus, and acute infarcts. In addition, CT is often used for postevacuation follow-up examinations of hematomas.

CT of the brain is particularly useful in demonstrating the size, location, and configuration of mass lesions, as well as surrounding edema. CT is also quite helpful in assessing cerebral ventricle or cortical sulcus enlargement. Shifting of midline structures resulting from the encroachment of a mass lesion, cerebral edema, or a hematoma can be visualized without contrast media. CT of the head is also the imaging modality of choice in evaluating hematomas, suspected aneurysms (Fig. 24-16), ischemic or hemorrhagic strokes, and acute infarcts within the brain. CT of the brain is the initial diagnostic procedure performed to assess craniocerebral trauma because it provides an accurate diagnosis of acute intracranial injuries, such as brain contusions and subarachnoid hemorrhage. Bone windows are used for fracture evaluation of trauma patients (Fig. 25-17).

CT of the spine is helpful in diagnosing vertebral column hemangiomas and lumbar spinal stenosis. CT of the cervical spine following trauma is performed frequently to rule out fractures of the axis and atlas and to better demonstrate the lower cervical and upper thoracic vertebrae. This examination can clearly demonstrate the size, number, and location of fracture fragments in the cervical, thoracic, and lumbar spine. The information gained from the CT scans can greatly assist the surgeon in distinguishing neural compression by soft tissue from compression by bone (Fig. 24-18). Postoperatively, CT is used to assess the outcome of the surgical procedure. Multiplanar reconstructions are often performed (Fig. 24-19).

A   B

Fig. 24-17 A, Normal CT scan of the brain using brain windows. **B,** Normal CT scan of the brain using bone windows for fracture evaluation.

Fig. 24-18 Axial CT of the cervical spine demonstrating multiple fractures *(arrows).*

Fig. 24-19 Sagittal CT lumbar spine: reconstruction of axial images showing a compression fracture of T12 and L1 subsequent to osteoporosis *(arrows).*

Computed tomography myelography (CTM) involves CT examination of the vertebral column after the *intrathecal* injection of a water-soluble contrast agent. The examination may be performed at any level of the vertebral column. Today most conventional myelograms are followed by CTM. Multiple thin sections (1.5 to 3 mm) are obtained with the gantry tilted to permit imaging parallel to the plane of the intervertebral disk. Because CT has the ability to distinguish among relatively small differences in contrast, the contrast agent may be visualized up to 4 hours following the conventional myelogram. CTM demonstrates the size, shape, and position of the spinal cord and nerve roots (Fig. 24-20). CTM is extremely useful in patients with compressive injuries or in determining the extent of dural tears resulting in extravasation of the CSF. (CT is discussed further in Chapter 31.)

Magnetic Resonance Imaging

MRI was approved for clinical use in the early 1980s and quickly became the modality of choice for evaluating many anomalies of the brain and spinal cord. MRI is a noninvasive procedure that provides excellent anatomic detail of the brain, spinal cord, intervertebral disks, and CSF within the subarachnoid space. Furthermore, unlike conventional myelography, MRI of the spinal cord and subarachnoid space does not require intrathecal injection of a contrast agent. (MRI is discussed in Chapter 33.)

Because magnetic resonance images are created primarily by the response of loosely bound hydrogen atoms to the magnetic field, this modality is basically "blind" to bone, unlike other conventional radiologic imaging modalities.

Therefore MRI allows clear visualization of areas of the CNS normally obscured by bone, such as the vertebral column and structures in the base of the skull. The exact relationship between soft tissue structures and surrounding bony structures can be seen. This makes MRI the preferred modality in evaluating the middle cranial fossa and posterior fossa of the brain. When these structures are imaged with CT, they are often obscured by artifacts. MRI is also the preferred modality for evaluating the spinal cord because it allows direct visualization of the cord, nerve roots, and surrounding CSF. In addition, MRI may be performed in a variety of planes (sagittal, axial, and coronal) after acquisition to aid in the diagnosis and treatment of neurologic disorders. A variety of imaging protocols including T1- and T2-weighted images may be obtained to assist in the diagnosis, with a head coil used for the brain and cervical spine images and a body coil used in combination with a surface coil for the remainder of the spine. Paramagnetic IV contrast agents such as gadolinium are used to enhance tumor visualization (Fig. 24-21).

Fig. 24-20 CT myelogram of the lumbar spine demonstrating subarachnoid space narrowing *(arrows)*.

MRI is helpful in assessing demyelinating disease, such as multiple sclerosis, spinal cord compression, paraspinal masses, postradiation therapy changes in spinal cord tumors, metastatic disease, herniated disks, and congenital anomalies of the vertebral column (Fig. 24-22). In the brain, MRI is excellent for evaluating middle and posterior fossa abnormalities, acoustic neuromas, pituitary tumors, primary and metastatic neoplasms, hydrocephalus, AVMs, and brain atrophy.

Contraindications to MRI are primarily related to the use of a magnetic field. MRI should not be used in patients with pacemakers, ferromagnetic aneurysm clips, or metallic spinal fusion rods. In addition, MRI is of little value in assessing osseous bone abnormalities of the skull, intracerebral hematomas, and subarachnoid hemorrhage. CT provides better visualization of these pathologies.

A

Fig. 24-22 Sagittal MRI of the lumbar spine demonstrating distal spinal cord and cauda equina (arrows).

B

Fig. 24-21 Sagittal MRI section through the brain demonstrating an occipital lobe mass without contrast (A) and after gadolinium injection (B) (arrows).

Cardiovascular and Interventional Procedures

In general, cardiovascular and interventional procedures are performed after non-invasive evaluation techniques when it is necessary to obtain information about the vascular system or to perform an interventional technique. *Angiography* may be used to assess vascular supply to tumors; demonstrate the relationship between a mass lesion and intracerebral vessels; or illustrate anomalies of a vessel, such as an aneurysm or a vascular occlusion. An angiographic procedure is performed in a specialized imaging suite under sterile conditions. (Cardiovascular and interventional radiology of the cerebral circulation is discussed in more detail in Chapter 25.)

Cardiovascular and interventional imaging equipment requires multiplanar imaging and digital subtraction capabilities. Angiographic x-ray tubes should have a minimum focal spot size of 1.3 mm for routine imaging and a magnification focal spot size of 0.3 mm. The procedure requires the introduction of a catheter into the vascular system under fluoroscopic guidance. The image intensifier must be designed to move around the patient so that various tube angles may be obtained without moving the patient. The catheter is most commonly placed in the femoral artery; however, access may be gained using other arteries or veins, depending on the patient's clinical history and the area of interest. After the catheter is placed in the appropriate vessel, a nonionic water-soluble contrast agent is injected into the vessels and rapid-sequence images are obtained for evaluation.

Fig. 24-23 Digital subtraction angiographic image demonstrating stenosis of the internal carotid artery at the bifurcation *(arrow)*.

Angiography is helpful in assessing vascular abnormalities within the CNS, such as arteriosclerosis (Fig. 24-23), arteriovenous malformations, aneurysms, subarachnoid hemorrhage, transient ischemic attacks, certain intracerebral hematomas, and cerebral venous thrombosis. Cerebral angiography provides a presurgical road map (Fig. 24-24) and is also performed in combination with interventional techniques to assess the placement of devices before and after the procedures.

Interventional radiology involves the placement of various coils, medications, filters, stents, or other devices to treat a particular problem or provide therapy. One type of interventional technique involves the introduction of small spheres, coils, or other materials into vessels to occlude blood flow. Embolization techniques are often performed to treat AVMs and aneurysms as well as to decrease blood supply to various vascular tumors (Fig. 24-25). Other interventional tech-

niques are used to open occluded vessels by the injection of specialized anticoagulant medications or by the inflation of small balloons within the vessel, as in the case of percutaneous angioplasty. In addition, therapeutic devices such as filters, stents, and shunts may be placed in the cardiovascular and interventional area, thereby eliminating the need for a more invasive surgical procedure.

Fig. 24-24 Digital subtraction angiography demonstrating anterior and middle cerebral arteries.

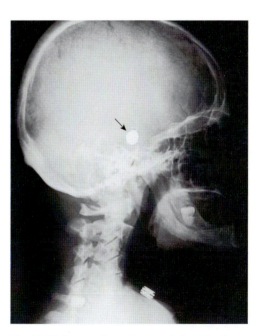

Fig. 24-25 Conventional lateral skull projection demonstrating an embolization coil placed just posterior and superior to the sella turcica (*arrow*).

Other Neuroradiographic Procedures

Diskography and *nucleography* are terms used to denote the radiologic examination of individual intervertebral disks. The examination is performed with a small quantity of one of the water-soluble, iodinated media injected into the center of the disk by way of a double-needle entry. This procedure was introduced by Lindblom[1] in 1950, and it has been further detailed by Cloward and Buzaid,[2] Cloward,[3] and Butt.[4]

---

[1]Lindblom K: Technique and results in myelography and disc puncture, *Acta Radiol* 34:321, 1950.
[2]Cloward RB, Buzaid LL: Discography, *AJR* 68:552, 1952.
[3]Cloward RB: Cervical discography: a contribution to the etiology and mechanism of neck, shoulder, and arm pain, *Ann Surg* 150:1052, 1959.
[4]Butt WP: Discography—some interesting cases, *J Can Assoc Radiol* 17:167, 1966.

Diskography is used in the investigation of internal disk lesions, such as rupture of the nucleus pulposus, which cannot be demonstrated by myelographic examination (Fig. 24-26). Diskography may be performed separately, or it may be combined with myelography. Patients are given only a local anesthetic so that they remain fully conscious and therefore able to inform the physician about pain when the needles are inserted and the injection is made. MRI and CTM have largely replaced diskography. (More information on diskography is presented in Chapter 29 of the seventh edition of this atlas.)

Fig. 24-26 Lumbar diskogram demonstrating normal nucleus pulposus of round contour type.

VERTEBROPLASTY AND KYPHOPLASTY

Vertebroplasty and kyphoplasty are interventional radiology procedures used to treat spinal compression fractures and other pathologies of the vertebral bodies that do not respond to conservative treatment. Vertebral fractures are common, especially in older patients with a history of osteoporosis. Estimates indicate that osteoporosis causes more than 700,000 vertebral fractures per year in the United States. About half of these fractures occur silently without any pain. Some fractures, however, are extremely painful and severely limit the patient's quality of life. Vertebroplasty and kyphoplasty are used in cases of severe pain that does not improve over a number of weeks of treatment.

Percutaneous vertebroplasty is defined as the injection of a radiopaque bone cement (e.g., polymethyl methacrylate) into a painful compression fracture under fluoroscopic guidance. This procedure is typically performed in the special procedures suite or the operating room with the patient sedated but awake. A specialized trocar needle is advanced into the fractured vertebral body under fluoroscopy (Fig. 24-27). Intraosseous venography using nonionic contrast media is performed to confirm needle placement. When the physician is satisfied with the needle placement, the cement is injected (Fig. 24-28). The cement stabilizes fracture fragments and leads to reduction in pain. Postprocedural imaging includes AP and lateral projections of the spine to confirm cement position (Fig. 24-29, *A* and *B*). A CT scan may also be performed.

Percutaneous kyphoplasty differs from vertebroplasty in that a balloon catheter is used to expand the compressed vertebral body to near its original height before injection of the bone cement. Inflation of the balloon creates a pocket for the placement of the cement. Kyphoplasty can help restore the spine to a more normal curvature and reduce hunchback deformities.

The success of these procedures is measured by reduction of pain reported by the patient. With proper patient selection and technique, success rates have been reported between 80% and 90%. However, both vertebroplasty and kyphoplasty have risks of serious complications. The most common complication is leakage of the cement before it hardens.

Pulmonary embolism and death, although rare, have been reported. Patients should be encouraged to discuss risks, benefits, and alternatives with their physicians. Technologists who perform these procedures need to be properly educated and ensure that informed consent has been documented.

Fig. 24-27 Lateral projection of compressed vertebral body with bone needle in place.

Fig 24-28 Bone cement injected during vertebroplasty under image guidance.

A

B

Fig. 24-29 A and **B,** AP and lateral projections demonstrate bone cement in L1.

Definition of Terms

angiography Radiographic examination of the blood vessels after the injection of contrast medium.

arachnoid A thin delicate membrane surrounding the brain and spinal cord.

brain The portion of the central nervous system contained within the cranium.

cauda equina A collection of nerves located in the spinal canal inferior to the spinal cord.

cerebellum The part of the brain located in the posterior cranial fossa behind the brainstem.

cerebral aqueduct An opening between the third and fourth ventricles.

cerebrospinal fluid The fluid that flows through and protects the ventricles, subarachnoid space, brain, and spinal cord.

cerebrum The largest uppermost portion of the brain.

conus medullaris The most inferior portion of the spinal cord.

cortex The outer surface layer of the brain.

dura mater The tough outer layer of the meninges, which lines the cranial cavity and spinal canal.

epidural space Outside or above the dura mater.

falx cerebri A fold of dura mater that separates the cerebral hemispheres.

filum terminale A threadlike structure that extends from the distal end of the spinal cord.

gadolinium An IV contrast medium used in MRI.

hindbrain The portion of the brain within the posterior fossa; it includes the pons, medulla oblongata, and cerebellum.

interventional radiology A branch of radiology that uses catheters to perform therapeutic procedures.

intrathecal injection An injection into the subarachnoid space of the spinal canal.

kyphoplasty An interventional radiology procedure used to treat vertebral body compression fractures using a specialized balloon and bone cement.

pons An oval-shaped area of the brain anterior to the medulla oblongata.

slices Sectional images of the body produced with either CT or MRI.

spinal cord An extension of the medulla oblongata that runs through the spinal canal to the upper lumbar vertebrae.

stereotactic surgery A radiographic procedure performed during neurosurgery to guide needle placement into the brain.

tentorium The layer of dura that separates the cerebrum and cerebellum.

vermis A wormlike structure that connects the two cerebellar hemispheres.

vertebroplasty An interventional radiology procedure used to treat vertebral body compression fractures by stabilizing bone fragments with cement.

Selected bibliography

Brown DB et al: Treatment of chronic symptomatic vertebral compression fractures with percutaneous vertebroplasty, *AJR* 182:319, 2004.

Kelly LL, Petersen CM: *Sectional anatomy for imaging professionals,* St Louis, 1997, Mosby.

Linger L: Percutaneous polymethacrylate vertebroplasty, *Radiol Technol* 76:109, 2004.

Martin JB et al: Vertebroplasty: clinical experience and follow-up results, *Bone* 25:11, 1999.

Osborn A: *Diagnostic neuroradiology,* St Louis, 1994, Mosby.

Ramsey R: *Neuroradiology,* ed 3, Philadelphia, 1994, Saunders.

Seeram E: *Computed tomography physical principles, clinical applications and quality control,* Philadelphia, 2001, Saunders.

Spivak JM: Vertebroplasty and kyphoplasty: percutaneous injection procedures for vertebral fractures: http://www.spine-health.com. Accessed May 2004.

Stark D, Bradley W: *Magnetic resonance imaging,* ed 2, vols 1 and 2, St Louis, 1992, Mosby.

Tortorici MR, Apfel PJ: *Advanced radiographic and angiographic procedures,* Philadelphia, 1995, FA Davis.

Wojtowycz M: *Handbook of radiology and angiography,* St Louis, 1995, Mosby.

Woodruff W: *Fundamentals of neuroimaging,* Philadelphia, 1993, Saunders.

Zoarski GH et al: Percutaneous vertebroplasty for osteoporotic compression fractures: quantitative prospective evaluation of long-term outcomes, *J Vasc Interv Radiol* 13:139, 2002

25

CIRCULATORY SYSTEM AND CARDIAC CATHETERIZATION

THOMAS H. BURKE

TIMOTHY J. JOYCE

SARA A. KADERLIK

Portal venogram. *m,* Main portal v.; *s,* superior mesenteric v.; *i,* inferior mesenteric v.; *sp,* splenic v.; *c,* coronary varices.

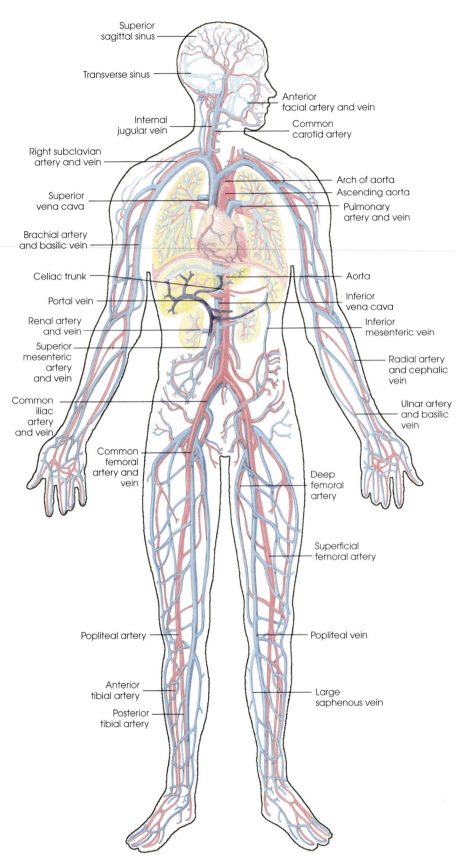

Superior sagittal sinus

Transverse sinus

Internal jugular vein

Right subclavian artery and vein

Superior vena cava

Brachial artery and basilic vein

Celiac trunk

Portal vein

Renal artery and vein

Superior mesenteric artery and vein

Common iliac artery and vein

Common femoral artery and vein

Popliteal artery

Anterior tibial artery

Posterior tibial artery

Anterior facial artery and vein

Common carotid artery

Arch of aorta
Ascending aorta
Pulmonary artery and vein

Aorta

Inferior vena cava

Inferior mesenteric vein

Radial artery and cephalic vein

Ulnar artery and basilic vein

Deep femoral artery

Superficial femoral artery

Popliteal vein

Large saphenous vein

Fig. 25-1 Major arteries and veins: *red,* arterial; *blue,* venous; *purple,* portal.

Circulatory System

The *circulatory system** has two complex systems of intimately associated vessels. Through these vessels, fluid is transported throughout the body in a continuous, unidirectional flow. The major portion of the circulatory system transports blood and is called the *blood-vascular system* (Fig. 25-1). The minor portion, called the *lymphatic system,* collects fluid from the tissue spaces. This fluid is filtered throughout the lymphatic system, which then conveys it back to the blood-vascular system. The fluid conveyed by the lymphatic system is called *lymph.* Together the blood-vascular and lymphatic systems carry oxygen and nutritive material to the tissues. They also collect and transport carbon dioxide and other waste products of metabolism from the tissues to the organs of excretion: the skin, lungs, liver, and kidneys.

---

*Almost all italicized words on the succeeding pages are defined at the end of the chapter.

Blood-Vascular System

The blood-vascular system consists basically of the *heart, arteries, capillaries,* and *veins.* The *heart* serves as a pumping mechanism to keep the blood in constant circulation throughout the vast system of blood vessels. *Arteries* convey the blood *away* from the heart. *Veins* convey the blood *back* toward the heart.

There are two circuits of blood vessels that branch out of the heart (Fig. 25-2). The first circuit is the arterial circuit or the *systemic circulation,* which carries oxygenated blood to the organs and tissues. Every organ has its own vascular circuit that arises from the trunk artery and leads back to the trunk vein for return to the heart. The systemic arteries branch out, treelike, from the aorta to all parts of the body. The arteries are usually named according to their location. The systemic veins usually lie parallel to their respective arteries and are given the same names.

The second circuit is the *pulmonary circulation* which takes blood to the lungs for carbon dioxide exchange and for the re-oxygenation of the blood, which is then carried back to the arterial systemic circulation. The pulmonary trunk arises from the right ventricle of the heart, passes superiorly and posteriorly for a distance of about 2 inches (5 cm), and then divides into two branches, the right and left pulmonary arteries. These vessels enter the root of the respective lung and, following the course of the bronchi, divide and subdivide to form a dense network of capillaries surrounding the alveoli of the lungs. Through the thin walls of the capillaries, the blood discharges carbon dioxide and absorbs oxygen from the air contained in the alveoli. The oxygenated blood passes onward through the pulmonary veins for return to the heart. In the pulmonary circulation, the deoxygenated blood is transported by the pulmonary arteries and the oxygenated blood is transported by the pulmonary veins.

There are two main trunk vessels that arise from the heart. The first is the aorta for the systemic circulation—the arteries progressively diminish in size as they divide and subdivide along their course, finally ending in minute branches called *arterioles.* The arterioles divide to form the capillary vessels, and the branching process is then reversed: The *capillaries* unite to form *venules,* the beginning branches of the veins, which in turn unite and reunite to form larger and larger vessels as they approach the heart. These venous structures empty into the right atrium, then into the right ventricle, and then into the second main trunk that arises from the heart—the pulmonary trunk, or the pulmonary circulation. The process of oxygen exchange is carried out in small venous structures, and then in larger and larger pulmonary veins. The pulmonary veins join to form four large veins (two from each lung), which then empty into the left atrium, then into the left ventricle, and then into the aorta, which starts the circulation again throughout the body.

The pathway of venous drainage from the abdominal viscera to the liver is called the *portal system.* Unlike the systemic and pulmonary circuits, which begin and end at the heart, the portal system begins in the capillaries of the abdominal viscera and ends in the capillaries and sinusoids of the liver. The blood is filtered and then exits the liver via the hepatic venous system, which then empties into the inferior vena cava just proximal to the right atrium.

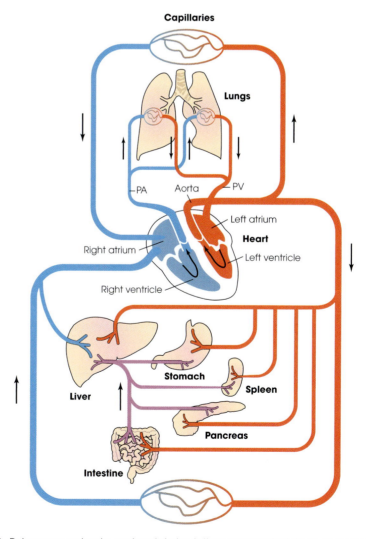

Fig. 25-2 Pulmonary, systemic, and portal circulation: oxygenated *(red),* deoxygenated *(blue),* and nutrient-rich *(purple)* blood.

21

The systemic veins are arranged in a superficial set and in a deep set with which the superficial veins communicate; both sets converge at a common trunk vein. The systemic veins end in two large vessels opening into the heart: The *superior vena cava* leads from the portion of the body above the diaphragm, and the *inferior vena cava* leads from below the level of the diaphragm.

The capillaries connect the arterioles and venules to form networks that pervade most organs and all other tissues supplied with blood. The capillary vessels have exceedingly thin walls through which the essential functions of the blood-vascular system take place—the blood constituents are filtered out and the waste products of cell activity are absorbed. The exchange takes place through the medium of tissue fluid, which is derived from the blood plasma and is drained off by the lymphatic system for return to the blood-vascular system. The tissue fluid undergoes modification in the lymphatic system. As soon as this tissue fluid enters the lymphatic capillaries, it is called *lymph.*

The *heart* is the central organ of the blood-vascular system and functions solely as a pump to keep the blood in circulation. It is shaped somewhat like a cone and measures approximately 4¾ inches (12 cm) in length, 3½ inches (9 cm) in width, and 2½ inches (6 cm) in depth. The heart is situated obliquely in the central mediastinum, largely to the left of the midsagittal plane. The base of the heart is directed superiorly, posteriorly, and to the right. The apex of the heart rests on the diaphragm against the anterior chest wall and is directed anteriorly, inferiorly, and to the left.

The muscular wall of the heart is called the *myocardium.* Because of the force required to drive blood through the extensive systemic vessels, the myocardium is about three times as thick on the left side (the arterial side) as on the right (the venous side). The membrane that lines the interior of the heart is called the *endocardium.* The heart is enclosed in the double-walled *pericardial sac.* The exterior wall of this sac is fibrous. The thin, closely adherent membrane that covers the heart is referred to as the *epicardium* or, because it also serves as the serous inner wall of the pericardial sac, the *visceral pericardium.* The narrow, fluid-containing space between the two walls of the sac is called the *pericardial cavity.*

The heart is divided by a septa into right and left halves, with each half subdivided by a constriction into two cavities, or chambers. The two upper chambers are called *atria,* and each atrium consists of a principal cavity and a lesser cavity called the *auricle.* The two lower chambers of the heart are called *ventricles.* The opening between the right atrium and right ventricle is controlled by the right atrioventricular (tricuspid) valve, and the opening between the left atrium and left ventricle is controlled by the left atrioventricular (mitral or bicuspid) valve.

The atria and ventricles separately contract (systole) in pumping blood and relax or dilate (diastole) in receiving blood. The atria precede the ventricles in contraction; therefore while the atria are in systole, the ventricles are in diastole. One phase of contraction (referred to as the heartbeat) and one phase of dilation are called the *cardiac cycle.* In the average adult, one cardiac cycle lasts 0.8 second. However, the heart rate, or number of pulsations per minute, varies with size, age, and gender. Heart rate is faster in small persons, young individuals, and females. The heart rate is also increased with exercise, food, and emotional disturbances.

The atria function as receiving chambers; the superior and inferior venae cavae empty into the right atrium (Fig. 25-3). The two right and left pulmonary veins empty into the left atrium. The ventricles function as distributing chambers. The right side of the heart handles the venous, or deoxygenated blood, and the left side handles the arterial, or oxygenated, blood. The left ventricle pumps oxygenated blood through the aortic valve into the aorta and the systemic circulation. The three major portions of the aorta are the ascending aorta, the aortic arch, and the descending aorta. The right ventricle pumps deoxygenated blood through the pulmonary valve into the pulmonary trunk and the pulmonary circulation.

Blood is supplied to the myocardium by the right and left coronary arteries. These vessels arise in the aortic sinus immediately superior to the aortic valve (Fig. 25-4). Most of the cardiac veins drain into the coronary sinus on the posterior aspect of the heart, and this sinus drains into the right atrium (Fig. 25-5).

The ascending aorta arises from the superior portion of the left ventricle and passes superiorly and to the right for a short distance. It then arches posteriorly and to the left and descends along the left side of the vertebral column to the level of L4, where it divides into the right and left common iliac arteries. The common iliac arteries pass to the level of the lumbosacral junction, where each ends by dividing into the internal iliac, or hypogastric, artery and the external iliac artery. The internal iliac artery passes into the pelvis. The external iliac artery passes to a point about midway between the anterior superior iliac spine and pubic symphysis and then enters the upper thigh to become the common femoral artery.

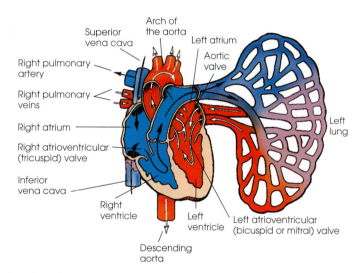

Fig. 25-3 Heart and great vessels: deoxygenated blood flow (black arrows); oxygenated blood flow (white arrows).

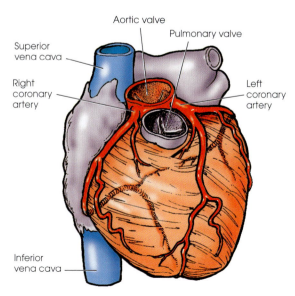

Fig. 25-4 Anterior view of coronary arteries.

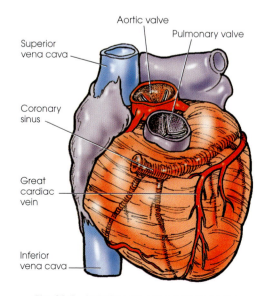

Fig. 25-5 Anterior view of coronary veins.

The velocity of blood circulation varies with the rate and intensity of the heartbeat. Velocity also varies in the different portions of the circulatory system based on distance from the heart. Therefore the speed of blood flow is highest in the large arteries arising at or near the heart because these vessels receive the full force of each wave of blood pumped out of the heart. The arterial walls expand with the pressure from each wave. The walls then rhythmically recoil, gradually diminishing the pressure of the advancing wave from point to point, until the flow of blood is normally reduced to a steady, nonpulsating stream through the capillaries and veins. The beat, or contraction and expansion of an artery, may be felt with the fingers at a number of points and is called the *pulse.*

Complete circulation of the blood through both the systemic and pulmonary circuits, from a given point and back again, requires about 23 seconds and an average of 27 heartbeats. In certain contrast examinations of the cardiovascular system, tests are conducted to determine the circulation time from the point of contrast medium injection to the site of interest.

Lymphatic System

The lymphatic system consists of an elaborate arrangement of closed vessels that collect fluid from the tissue spaces and transport it to the blood-vascular system. Almost all lymphatic vessels are arranged in two sets: (1) a superficial set that lies immediately under the skin and accompanies the superficial veins and (2) a deep set that accompanies the deep blood vessels and with which the superficial lymphatics communicate (Fig. 25-6). The lymphatic system lacks a pumping mechanism such as the heart of the blood-vascular system. The lymphatic vessels are richly supplied with valves to prevent backflow, and the movement of the lymph through the system is believed to be maintained largely by extrinsic pressure from the surrounding organs and muscles.

The lymphatic system begins in complex networks of thin-walled, absorbent capillaries situated in the various organs and tissues. The capillaries unite to form larger vessels, which in turn form networks and unite to become still larger vessels as they approach the terminal collecting trunks. The terminal trunks communicate with the blood-vascular system.

The lymphatic vessels are small in caliber and have delicate, transparent walls. Along their course the collecting vessels pass through one or more nodular structures called *lymph nodes.* The nodes occur singly but are usually arranged in chains or groups of 2 to 20. The nodes are situated so that they form strategically placed centers toward which the conducting vessels converge. The nodes vary from the size of a pinhead to the size of an almond or larger. They may be spherical, oval, or kidney shaped. Each node has a hilum through which the arteries enter and veins and efferent lymph vessels emerge; the afferent lymph vessels do not enter at the hilum. In addition to the lymphatic capillaries, blood vessels, and supporting structures, each lymph node contains masses, or follicles, of lymphocytes that are arranged around its circumference and from which cords of cells extend through the medullary portion of the node.

A number of conducting channels, here called *afferent lymph vessels,* enter the node opposite the hilum and break into wide capillaries that surround the lymph follicles and form a canal known as the *peripheral* or *marginal lymph sinus.*

The network of capillaries continues into the medullary portion of the node, widens to form medullary sinuses, and then collects into several *efferent lymph vessels* that leave the node at the hilum. The conducting vessels may pass through several nodes along their course, each time undergoing the process of widening into sinuses. Lymphocytes, a variety of white blood cells formed in the lymph nodes, are added to the lymph while it is in the nodes. It is thought that a majority of the lymph is absorbed by the venous system from these nodes and only a small portion of the lymph is passed on through the conducting vessels.

The absorption and interchange of tissue fluids and cells take place through the thin walls of the capillaries. The lymph passes from the beginning capillaries through the conducting vessels, which eventually empty their contents into terminal lymph trunks for conveyance to the blood-vascular system. The main terminal trunk of the lymphatic system is called the *thoracic duct.* The lower, dilated portion of the duct is known as the *cisterna chyli.* The thoracic duct receives lymphatic drainage from all parts of the body below the diaphragm and from the left half of the body above the diaphragm. The thoracic duct extends from the level of L2 to the base of the neck, where it ends by opening into the venous system at the junction of the left subclavian and internal jugular veins.

Three terminal collecting trunks—the right jugular, the subclavian, and the bronchomediastinal trunks—receive the lymphatic drainage from the right half of the body above the diaphragm. These vessels open into the right subclavian vein separately or occasionally after uniting to form a common trunk called the *right lymphatic duct.*

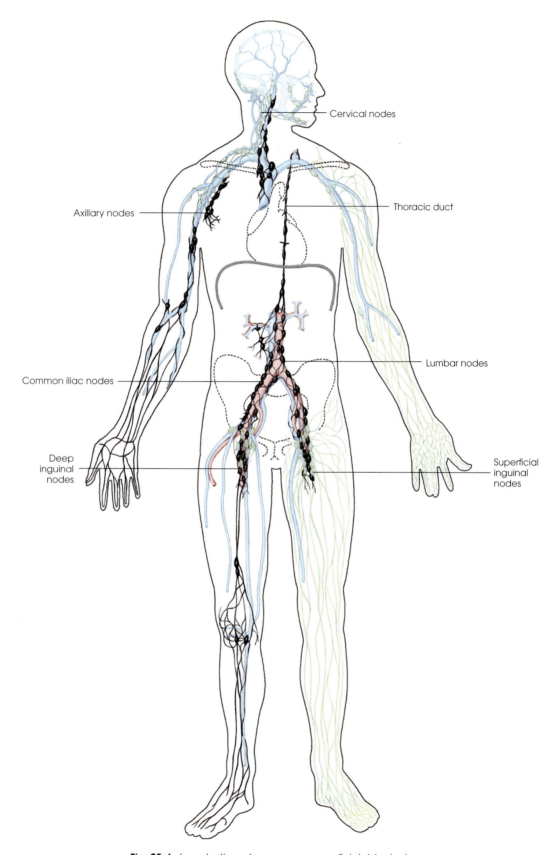

Cervical nodes

Thoracic duct

Axillary nodes

Lumbar nodes

Common iliac nodes

Deep
inguinal
nodes

Superficial
inguinal
nodes

Fig. 25-6 Lymphatic system: *green,* superficial; *black,* deep.

Definitions and Indications

Blood vessels are not normally visible in conventional radiography because no natural contrast exists between them and other soft tissues of the body. Therefore these vessels must be filled with a radiopaque contrast medium to delineate them for radiography. *Angiography* is a general term that describes the radiologic examination of vascular structures within the body after the introduction of an iodinated contrast medium or gas.

The visceral and peripheral angiography procedures identified in this chapter can be categorized generally as either *arteriography* or *venography*. Examinations are more precisely named for the specific blood vessel opacified and the method of injection.

Angiography is primarily used to identify the anatomy or pathologic process of blood vessels. Chronic cramping leg pain following physical exertion, a condition known as *claudication,* may prompt a physician to order an arteriogram of the lower limbs to determine whether atherosclerosis is diminishing the blood supply to the leg muscles. A *stenosis* or *occlusion* is commonly caused by *atherosclerosis* and is an indication for an arteriogram. Cerebral angiography is performed to detect and verify the existence and exact position of an intracranial vascular lesion such as an *aneurysm*. Although most angiographic examinations are performed to investigate anatomic variances, some evaluate the motion of the part. Other vascular examinations evaluate suspected tumors by opacifying the organ of concern; once diagnosed, these lesions may be amendable to some type of intervention. Interventional radiology diagnoses lesions and then treats these lesions through an endovascular approach.

Historical Development

In January 1896, just 10 weeks after the announcement of Roentgen's discovery, Haschek and Lindenthal announced that they had produced a radiograph demonstrating the blood vessels of an amputated hand using Teichman's mixture, a thick emulsion of chalk, as the contrast agent. This work heralded the beginning of angiography. The potential for this new type of examination to delineate vascular anatomy was immediately recognized. However, the advancement of angiography was hindered by the lack of suitable contrast media and low-risk techniques to deliver the media to the desired location. By the 1920s researchers were using sodium iodide as a contrast medium to produce lower limb studies comparable in quality to studies seen in modern angiography.

Yet limitations still existed. Until the 1950s, contrast medium was most commonly injected through a needle that punctured the vessel or through a ureteral catheter that passed into the body through a surgically exposed peripheral vessel. Then in 1952, shortly after the development of a flexible thin-walled catheter, Seldinger announced a *percutaneous* method of catheter introduction. The Seldinger technique eliminated the surgical risk, which exposed the vessel and tissues (see Fig. 25-15).

Early angiograms consisted of single radiographs or the visualization of vessels by fluoroscopy. Because the advantage of *serial imaging* was recognized, cassette changers, roll film changers, cut film changers, and cine and serial spot-filming/digital devices were developed. Pumps to inject contrast media were also developed to allow more rapid and precise control of injection rates and volumes than were possible by hand. Early mechanical injectors were powered by pressurized gas, and the injection rate was a function of the pressure setting. Electrically powered automatic injectors were subsequently developed that allowed the injection rate to be precisely set.

Angiographic Studies
CONTRAST MEDIA

Opaque contrast medium containing organic iodine solutions is used in angiographic studies. Although usually tolerated, the injection of iodinated contrast medium may cause undesirable consequences. The contrast is subsequently filtered out of the bloodstream by the kidneys. It causes physiologic cardiovascular side effects, including peripheral vasodilation, blood pressure decrease, and cardiotoxicity. It may also produce nausea and an uncomfortable burning sensation in about 1 of 10 patients. Most significantly, the injection of iodinated contrast medium may invoke allergic reactions. These reactions may be minor (hives or slight difficulty in breathing) and not require any treatment, or they may be severe and require immediate medical intervention. Severe reactions are characterized by a state of shock in which the patient exhibits shallow breathing and a high pulse rate and may lose consciousness. Historically, 1 of every 14,000 patients suffers a severe allergic reaction. The administration of contrast medium is clearly one of the significant risks in angiography.

At the kilovolt (peak) (kVp) used in angiography, iodine is slightly more radiopaque, atom for atom, than lead. The iodine is incorporated into water-soluble molecules formed as triiodinated benzene rings. These molecules vary in exact composition. Some forms are organic salts that dissociate in solution and are therefore ionic. The iodinated anion is diatrizoate iothalamate or ioxaglate. The radiolucent cation is meglumine, sodium, or a combination of both. These ionic forms yield two particles in solution for every three iodine atoms (a 3:2 ratio) and are six to eight times as osmolar as plasma.

Other triiodinated benzene rings are created as nonionic molecules. These forms have three iodine atoms on each particle in solution (a 3:1 ratio) because they do not dissociate and are only two to three times as osmolar as plasma. Studies indicate that these properties of nonionic contrast media result in decreased nephrotoxicity to the kidneys. Nonionic contrast media also cause fewer physiologic cardiovascular side effects, less intense sensations, and fewer allergic reactions.

Another form of contrast medium is a dimer whose two benzene rings are bonded together as the anion. Ionic contrast with a dimer results in six iodine atoms for every two particles in solution, which yields the same 3:1 ratio as a nonionic contrast medium. The ionic dimer has advantages over the ionic monomeric molecule, primarily by reducing osmolality, but it lacks some of the properties of the nonionic molecule. Nonionic contrast can also be found as a dimer, which yields a ratio of 6:1 because it will not dissociate into two particles, producing an osmolality similar to blood.

All forms of iodinated contrast media are available in a variety of iodine concentrations. The agents of higher concentration are more opaque. Typically, 30% iodine concentrations are used for cerebral and limb arteriography, whereas 35% concentrations are used for visceral angiography. Peripheral venography may be performed with 30% or lower concentrations. The ionic agents of higher concentration and the nonionic agents are more viscous and produce greater resistance in the catheter during injection.

Patients with a predisposition to allergic reaction may be pretreated with a regimen of antihistamines and steroids to help prevent anaphylactic reactions to contrast media. Patients who exhibit a history of severe reaction to iodinated contrast or with compromised renal function may undergo procedures in which CO_2 is used as a contrast agent. CO_2 is less radiopaque than blood and appears as a negative or void in angiographic imaging. CO_2 is only approved for use below the diaphragm because the possibility of emboli is too great near the brain. CO_2 imaging is only possible in the digital subtraction angiography (DSA) environment because it requires a narrow contrast window and the ability to stack or combine multiple images to provide a single image free of bubbles or fragmented vascular opacification. Specific kVp values should be employed to optimally display the CO_2 in contrast to the rest of the body.

Another alternative to iodinated contrast is the use of gadolinium. Gadolinium is primarily used as a contrast agent in magnetic resonance imaging (MRI) studies. However, it can be substituted for iodine contrast when the patient has a history of contrast reactions or compromised renal function. Gadolinium is less radiopaque than iodine; therefore narrow windows must be used in DSA imaging.

INJECTION TECHNIQUES

Selective injection through a catheter involves placing the catheter within a vessel so that the vessel and its major branches are opacified. In a selective injection, the catheter tip is positioned into the orifice of a specific artery so that only that specific vessel is injected. This has the advantage of more densely opacifying the vessel and limiting the superimposition of other vessels.

A contrast medium may be injected by hand with a syringe but ideally should be injected by an automatic injector. The major advantage of automatic injectors is that a specific quantity of contrast medium can be injected during a predetermined period of time. Automatic injectors have controls to set the injection rate, injection volume, and maximum pressure. Another useful feature is a control to set a time interval during which the injector gradually achieves the set injection rate, which is the linear rise. This may prevent a catheter from being dislodged by whiplash.

Because the opacifying contrast medium is often carried away from the area of interest by blood flow, the injection and demonstration of opacified vessels usually occur simultaneously. Therefore the injector is often electronically connected to the rapid imaging equipment to coordinate the timing between the injector and the onset of imaging.

EQUIPMENT

Until the early 1990s, most angiograms recorded flowing contrast medium in a series of images that required *rapid film changers* or cinefluorography devices; however, now DSA systems are used almost exclusively. Although some institutions may still have rapid film changers, most often the filming technique is by DSA. The newer imaging equipment has much better image quality and produces images at a rate of up to 30 frames per second. In addition, digital imaging is cost effective in that images are stored electronically, thus reducing the need for expensive film and film storage. Digital images can be archived and retrieved in seconds from within the institution or any network connection. DSA imaging provides the interventionalist with a variety of tools for image manipulation analysis and measurement.

Lower limb angiograms are now performed using specialized DSA imaging techniques such as bolus chasing or stepping DSA. These techniques involve motorized movement of the table or C-arm to follow contrast media as it flows distally into the lower extremities.

Digital Subtraction Angiographic Procedures

A DSA study begins with catheter placement performed in the same manner as for conventional angiography. Injection techniques vary, but typically similar rates and volumes are used as in cut film. An automatic pressure injector is used to ensure consistency of injection and to facilitate computer control of injection timing and image acquisition.

The intravascular catheter is positioned using conventional fluoroscopic apparatus and technique, and a suitable imaging position is selected. At this point an image that does not have a large dynamic range should be established; no part of the image should be significantly brighter than the rest of the image. This can be accomplished by proper positioning, but it often requires the use of compensating filters. The filters can be bags of saline or thin pieces of metal inserted in the imaging field to reduce the intensity of bright regions. Metal filters are often part of the collimator, and water or saline bags are placed directly on or adjacent to the patient.

If proper placement of compensating filters is not performed, image quality is reduced significantly. The reason is that the video camera operates most effectively with video signals that are at a fixed level. Automatic controls in the system adjust the exposure factors so that the brightest part of the image is at that level. An unusually bright spot satisfies the automatic controls and causes the rest of the image to lie at significantly reduced levels, where the camera performance is worse. An alternative to proper filter placement is to adjust the automatic sensing region, similar to automatic exposure control (AEC) for conventional radiography, to exclude the bright region. This solution is less desirable than the use of compensating filters, and it is not always effective for some positions of the bright spot on the image. One should not rely on digital and video compensation. Proper positioning and technique are essential for high-quality imaging.

As the imaging sequence begins, an image that will be used as a subtraction mask (without contrast medium) is acquired, digitized, and stored in the digital memory. This mask image and those that follow are produced when the x-ray tube is energized and x-rays are produced, usually 1 to 30 exposures per second at 65 to 95 kVp and between 5 and 1000 mAs. The radiation dose received by the patient for each image can be adjusted during installation. The dose may be reduced or the same as that used for a conventional radiograph. Images can be acquired at variable rates, from one image every 2 to 3 seconds up to 30 images per second.

The *acquisition rate* can also be varied during a run. Most commonly, images are acquired at a faster rate during the passage of iodine contrast medium through the arteries and then at a reduced rate in the venous phase, during which the blood flow is much slower. This procedure minimizes the radiation exposure to the patient but provides a sufficient number of images to demonstrate the clinical information. Each of these digitized images is electronically *subtracted* from the mask, and the subtraction image is amplified (contrast enhanced) and displayed in real time so that the subtraction images appear essentially instantaneously during the imaging procedure (Fig. 25-7). The images are simultaneously stored on a *digital disk* or *videotape recorder.*

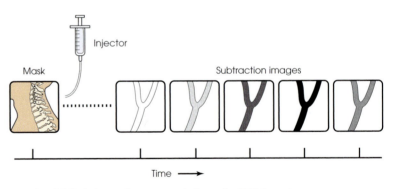

Fig. 25-7 Schematic representation of a DSA imaging sequence.

Some DSA equipment allows the table or the image intensifier (II)/TV system to be moved during acquisition. The movement is permitted to "follow" the flow of iodine contrast material as it passes through the arteries. Sometimes called the "bolus chase" or "DSA stepping" method, this technique is particularly useful for evaluating the arteries in the pelvis and lower limb. Previously, several separate imaging sequences would be performed with the II/TV positioned in a different location for each sequence, but this method required an injection of iodine contrast material for each sequence. The bolus chase method requires only one injection of iodine, and the imaging sequence follows (or "chases") the iodine as it flows down the limb. The imaging sequence may be preceded or followed by a duplicate sequence without iodine injection to enable subtraction. Occasionally, this method may need to be repeated as the contrast in one leg may flow faster than in the other.

Misregistration, a major problem in DSA, occurs when the mask and the images displaying the vessels filled with contrast medium do not exactly coincide. Misregistration is sometimes caused by voluntary movements of the patient, but it is also caused by involuntary movements such as bowel peristalsis or heart contractions. Preparing the patient by describing the sensations associated with contrast-medium injection and the importance of holding still can help eliminate voluntary movements. It is also important to have the patient suspend respiration during the procedure. Compression bands, glucagon, and cardiac gating can be effective in reducing misregistration caused by involuntary movement.

During the imaging procedure the subtraction images appear on the display monitor (Fig. 25-8). Often a preliminary diagnosis can be made at this point or as the images are reviewed immediately after each exposure sequence. However, a formal reading session occurs after the patient study has been completed; at that time the final diagnosis is made.

Some *postprocessing* is performed after each exposure sequence to improve visualization of the anatomy of interest or to correct misregistration. More involved postprocessing, including quantitative analysis, is performed after the patient study has been completed. The processed images are available on the computer monitor for review by the radiologist. Because the images are digital, it is possible to store them in a *picture archive and communication system* (PACS). PACS allows images to be archived in digital format on various computer devices, including magnetic tape and optical disk. The images also can be transmitted via a computer network throughout the hospital or to remote locations for consultation with an expert or the referring physician. As an alternative to digital storage and reading, hard copy images may be produced using a *laser printer* or *multiformat camera,* with several images appearing on each radiograph. When produced, they are normally used for the formal reading session and are also kept for archival purposes.

Fluoroscopy, cine, and DSA systems consist essentially of a camera that photographs the output phosphor of an image intensification system. Fluoroscopy and DSA employ a video camera. In DSA, the fluoroscopic image is digitized into serial images that are stored by a computer. The computer subtracts an early image, the mask image (before contrast medium enters the vessel), from a later image (after the vessel opacifies) and displays the difference, or subtraction image, on the fluoroscopy monitor. Almost all image intensification devices used for vascular procedures include television monitoring. Such equipment allows angiographic examinations to be viewed on a television screen in real time and be simultaneously recorded.

Fig. 25-8 DSA image of common carotid artery demonstrating stenosis *(arrow)* of internal carotid artery.

A cine camera is rarely used because digital techniques have surpassed the usefulness of cine film. Cine uses 16- or 35-mm roll film and usually can achieve sequential exposure rates of up to 60 frames or more per second. The result is true motion picture radiography. The photographic resolution achieved with cine units is not as great as that seen with rapid film changers. However, many more events can be photographed with the cine attachment, and dynamic function can be more satisfactorily evaluated with cinefluorography. Therefore cine is typically found in the cardiac catheter laboratory.

Imaging systems may be used either singly or in combination at right angles to obtain simultaneous frontal and lateral images of the vascular system under investigation with one injection of contrast medium. This arrangement of units is called a *biplane* imaging system.

Rapid serial radiographic imaging requires large focal-spot x-ray tubes capable of withstanding a high heat load. Magnification studies, however, require fractional focus tubes with focal spot sizes of between 0.1 and 0.3 mm. X-ray tubes may have to be specialized to satisfy these extreme demands. Rapid serial imaging also necessitates radiographic generators with high-power output. Because short exposure times are needed to compensate for all patient motion, the generators must be capable of producing high-milliampere output. The combination of high kilowatt-rated generators and rare earth film-screen technology significantly aids in decreasing the radiation dose to the patient while producing radiographs of improved quality, with the added advantage of prolonging the life of the high-powered generators and x-ray tubes.

A comprehensive angiographic room contains a great amount of equipment other than radiologic devices. Monitoring systems record patient electrocardiographic data and blood pressure readings, as well as pulse oximetry. Emergency equipment may include resuscitation equipment (e.g., a defibrillator for the heart) and anesthesia apparatus. The cardiovascular and interventional technologist (CIT) must be familiar with the use of each piece of equipment (Fig. 25-9).

Fig. 25-9 Modern biplane digital angiographic suite.

MAGNIFICATION

Magnification occurs both intentionally and unintentionally in angiographic imaging sequences. DSA imaging allows different magnification levels by employing different focusing filters inside the image intensifier. This type of magnification can be increased by varying the distance of the image receptor. Intentional use of magnification can result in a significant increase in resolution of fine vessel recorded detail. Fractional focal spot tubes of 0.3 mm or less are necessary for direct radiographic magnification techniques. The selection of a fractional focal spot necessitates the use of low milliamperage. Short exposure time (1 to 200 ms) is necessary due to the size and load capacity of the smaller focal spot.

The formula for manual magnification is:

$$M = \frac{SID}{SOD} \; or \; \frac{SID}{SID - OID}$$

The SID is the *source–to–image-receptor distance,* the SOD is the *source-to-object distance,* and the OID is the *object–to–image-receptor distance.* For a 2:1 magnification study using an SID of 40 inches (101 cm), both the focal spot and the image receptor are positioned 20 inches (50 cm) from the area of interest. A 3:1 magnification study using a 40-inch (101-cm) SID is accomplished by placing the focal spot 13 inches (33 cm) from the area of interest and the image receptor 27 inches (68 cm) from the area of interest.

Unintentional magnification occurs when the area of interest cannot be placed in direct contact with the image receptor. This is particularly a problem in the biplane imaging sequence, in which the need to center the area of interest in the first plane may create some unavoidable distance of the body part to the image receptor in the second plane. Even in single plane imaging, vascular structures are separated from the image receptor by some distance. The magnification that occurs as a result of these circumstances is frequently 20% to 25%. For example, a 25% magnification occurs when a vessel within the body is 8 inches (20 cm) from the image receptor—an OID of 8 inches (20 cm)—and the SID is 40 inches (101 cm).

Angiographic images therefore do not represent vessels at their actual size. This must be taken into account when direct measurements are made from angiographic images. Increasing the SID while maintaining the OID can reduce unintentional magnification. Increasing the SID may not be an option, however, if the increase in technical factors would exceed tube output capacity or exposure time maximum. When any measurement is necessary, the DSA postprocessing quantitative analysis programs will require the angiographer to calibrate the system by measuring an object in the imaging field of known value. Some systems will calibrate by using the known position of the table, the II and x-ray tube, and the tube angulation.

DIGITAL SUBTRACTION ANGIOGRAPHY PROGRAMMING

DSA programming is the task of controlling the rate and number of serial exposures made with an imaging system. Programming is accomplished by either selecting a predetermined imaging sequence from the DSA system or by manually inputting a sequence based on patient flow dynamics and anatomy. When two image receptors operate together for simultaneous biplane imaging, exposures in both planes cannot be made at the same moment because scatter radiation would fog the opposite plane image. Yet biplane imagers must cycle exactly together so that synchronization can be electronically controlled. Therefore it is necessary to alternate the exposures in the two planes. The x-ray tubes in a biplane system must fire alternately to prevent exposure of the opposite II. In addition, the II that is not being exposed is "blanked" or is powered off for an instant so as not to receive any input from the opposite exposure. The difference in the alternating exposures is about 3 ms.

THREE-DIMENSIONAL INTRAARTERIAL ANGIOGRAPHY

The latest diagnostic tool is three-dimensional (3D) angiography. To acquire a 3D model of a vascular structure, a C-arm is rotated around the region of interest (ROI) at speeds up to 60 degrees per second. The C-arm makes a preliminary sweep while mask images are acquired. Images are acquired at 7.5 to 30 frames per second. The C-arm returns to its initial position and a second sweep is initiated. Just before the second sweep, contrast is injected to opacify the vascular anatomy. The second sweep matches mask images from the first sweep, producing a rotational subtracted DSA sequence. The DSA sequence is sent to a 3D rendering computer where a 3D model is constructed. This model provides an image that can be manipulated and analyzed. It has proved to be a valuable tool for interventional approaches as well as for evaluation before surgery. Various methods of vessel analysis are available with 3D models. Aneurysm volume calculation, interior wall analysis, bone fusion, and device display are all possible (Figs. 25-10 and 25-11).

Fig. 25-10 3D angiography provides for reconstruction of the vessels as well as the skeletal anatomy.

Fig. 25-11 3D reconstruction of left internal carotid artery. Note the anterior communicating artery aneurysm (*arrow*).

ANGIOGRAPHIC SUPPLIES AND EQUIPMENT

Needles

Vascular access needles are necessary when performing percutaneous procedures. Needle size is based on the external diameter of the needle and is assigned a gauge size. However, to allow for appropriate guidewire matching, the internal diameter of the needle must be known. Vascular access needles come in different types, sizes, and lengths. The most commonly used access needle for adult cardiovascular procedures is an 18-gauge needle that is 2.75 inches long. This particular needle is compatible with a 0.035 guidewire, which is the most frequently used guidewire in cardiovascular procedures. Appropriate needle size is predicated on the type or size of guidewire needed, the size of the patient, and the targeted entry vessel. To decrease the chances of vascular complications, the smallest gauge needle that meets the above criteria is used for vascular access. Access needles for the pediatric patient come in smaller gauge sizes with shorter lengths (Fig. 25-12).

Guidewires

Guidewires, also commonly referred to as a spring guide or wire guide, are used in angiography and other special procedures as a platform over which the catheter is to be advanced. To decrease the possibilities of complications, the guidewire should be advanced into the vasculature ahead of the catheter. Once positioned in the area of interest, the position of the guidewire is fixed and the catheter advanced until it meets the tip of the guidewire. Similar to needles, guidewires come in a variety of sizes, shapes, and lengths, and care must be taken to match the proper guidewire to the selected access needle and catheter.

The majority of guidewires are constructed of stainless steel, with a core or mandrel encased circumferentially within a tightly wound spiral outer core of spring wire. The mandrel gives the guidewire its stiffness and body. The length of the mandrel within the wire determines the flexibility of the wire. The shorter the mandrel, the more flexible the wire and the more likely it is to traverse tortuous anatomy. A safety ribbon is built into the tip of the guidewire to prevent wire dislodgment in case the wire fractures. Many of the stainless steel guidewires are coated with Teflon to provide lubricity and to decrease the friction between the catheter and wire. Similarly, it is thought that the Teflon coating helps decrease the thrombogenicity of the guidewire.

More recently, plastic alloy guidewires consisting of a hydrophilic plastic polymer coating have been introduced. These new wires provide a very smooth outer coating, with a pliable tip, and exhibit a high degree of torque or maneuverability (Fig. 25-13).

Fig. 25-12 Various needles used during catheterization.

Fig. 25-13 The hydrophilic guidewire is a special type of guidewire that allows the user a high degree of torque and maneuverability. Like other guidewires, it is offered in various lengths and has various shaped tips.

Introducer sheaths

Introducer sheaths are frequently used on angiographic procedures when multiple catheters will be used. A variation of the previously described Seldinger technique allows the introducer sheath to be placed in lieu of the catheter during percutaneous entry of the vascular system. Once the sheath has been placed, controlled access of the vasculature is assured while at the same time reducing vessel trauma by limiting numerous catheter passages through the vessel itself.

Introducer sheaths are short catheters consisting of a slotted, rubberized backbleed valve and a sidearm extension port. The backbleed valve prevents the loss of blood volume during catheter exchanges or guidewire manipulations. The sidearm extension port may be used to infuse medications or monitor blood pressure.

Similar to vascular catheters, introducer sheaths come in various sizes and lengths. Typically, most introducer sheaths range in length from 10 to 90 cm. While catheters are measured by their outside diameters and expressed in units of French size (Fr), introducer sheaths are named according to the French size catheter they can accommodate. To accomplish this, the outer diameters of introducer sheaths are 1.5 to 2 Fr sizes larger than the catheter they can accept. Therefore a 5-Fr introducer has an outer diameter of nearly 7 Fr and accepts a 5-Fr catheter (Fig. 25-14).

CATHETERIZATION

Catheterization for filling vessels with contrast media is a technique that is preferred to needle injection of the media. The advantages of catheterization are as follows:

1. The risk of *extravasation* is reduced.
2. Most body parts can be reached for selective injection.
3. The patient can be positioned as needed.
4. The catheter can be safely left in the body while radiographs are being examined.

The femoral, axillary, and brachial arteries are the most commonly punctured vessels. The transfemoral site is preferred because it is associated with the fewest risks.

The most widely used catheterization method is the Seldinger technique.[1] Seldinger described the method as puncture of both walls of the vessel (the anterior and posterior walls). However, the modified Seldinger technique allows for puncture of the anterior wall only. The steps of the technique are described in Fig. 25-15. The procedure is performed under sterile conditions. The catheterization site is suitably cleaned and then surgically draped. The patient is given local anesthesia at the catheterization site.

[1]Seldinger SF: Percutaneous selective angiography of the aorta: preliminary report, *Acta Radiol* (Stockh) 45:15, 1956.

With this percutaneous technique, the arteriotomy or venotomy is no larger than the catheter itself. Therefore hemorrhage is minimized. Patients can usually resume normal activity within 24 hours after the examination. In some diagnostic angiograms, the procedure can be performed in the early morning and the patient may be discharged later that same day. Most often an uncomplicated interventional procedure may be performed and the patient will recover in an ambulatory care area and then be discharged home, usually within 24 hours. The risk of infection is lower than in surgical procedures because the vessel and tissues are not exposed.

After a catheter is introduced into the blood-vascular system, it can be maneuvered by pushing, pulling, and turning the part of the catheter still outside the patient so that the part of the catheter inside the patient travels to a specific location. A wire is sometimes positioned inside the catheter to help manipulate and guide the catheter to the desired location. When the wire is removed from the catheter, the catheter is infused with sterile solution, most commonly heparinized saline, to help prevent clot formation. Infusing the catheter and assisting the physician in the catheterization process may be the CIT's responsibility.

When the examination is complete, the catheter is removed. Pressure is applied to the site until complete hemostasis is achieved, but blood flow through the vessel is maintained. The patient is placed on complete bedrest and observed for the development of bleeding or *hematoma.* Newer closure devices, which close the vessel percutaneously, can also be used to close the puncture site.

When peripheral artery sites are unavailable, a catheter may sometimes be introduced into the aorta using the translumbar aortic approach. For this technique the patient is positioned prone, and a special catheter introducer system is inserted percutaneously through the posterolateral aspect of the back and directed superiorly so that the catheter enters the aorta around the T11-T12 level.

Fig. 25-14 Various types of introducer sheaths used during catheterization.

Fig. 25-15 Seldinger technique. **A,** The ideal puncture occurs in the femoral artery just below the inguinal ligament. **B,** A beveled compound needle containing an inner cannula pierces through the artery. **C,** The needle is withdrawn slowly until there is blood flow. **D,** The needle's inner cannula is removed, and a flexible guidewire is inserted. **E,** The needle is removed; pressure fixes the wire and reduces hemorrhage. **F,** The catheter is slipped over the wire and into the artery. **G,** The guidewire is removed, leaving the catheter in the artery.

Digital subtraction angiographic procedures

Catheters are produced in various forms, each with a particular advantage in shape, maneuverability or torque, and maximum injection rate (Fig. 25-16). Angiographic catheters are made of pliable plastic that allows them to straighten for insertion over the guidewire, also called a *wire guide*. They normally resume their original shape after the guidewire is withdrawn. However, it usually requires manipulation from the angiographer to resume its original shape. Catheters with a predetermined design or shape are maneuvered into the origins of vessels for selective injections. They may have only an end hole, or they may have multiple side holes. Some catheters have multiple side holes to facilitate high injection rates but are used only in large vascular structures for flush injections. A "pigtail" catheter is a special multiple side hole catheter that allows higher volumes of contrast to be injected with less whiplash effect, thus causing less damage to the vessel being injected.

Common angiographic catheters range in size from 4 Fr (0.05 in) to 7 Fr (0.09 in), although even smaller or larger sizes may be used. Most have inner lumens that allow them to be inserted over guidewires ranging from 0.032 to 0.038 inch in diameter.

PATIENT CARE

Before the initiation of an angiographic procedure, it is appropriate to explain the process and the potential complications to the patient. Written consent is often obtained after an explanation. Potential complications include a vasovagal reaction; stroke; heart attack; death; bleeding at the puncture site; nerve, blood vessel, or tissue damage; and an allergic reaction to the contrast medium. Bleeding at the puncture site is usually easily controlled with pressure to the site. Blood vessel and tissue damage may require a surgical procedure. A vasovagal reaction is characterized by sweating and nausea caused by a drop in blood pressure. The patient's legs should be elevated, and intravenous (IV) fluids may be administered to help restore blood pressure. Minor allergic reactions to iodinated contrast media, such as hives and congestion, are usually controlled with medications and may not require treatment. Severe allergic reactions may result in shock, which is characterized by shallow breathing, high pulse rate, and possibly loss of consciousness. Of course, angiography is performed only if the benefits of the examination outweigh the risks.

Patients are usually restricted to clear liquid intake and routine medications before undergoing angiography. Adequate hydration from liquid intake may minimize kidney damage caused by iodinated contrast media. Solid food intake is restricted to reduce the risk of aspiration related to nausea. Contraindications to angiography are determined by physicians and include previous severe allergic reaction to iodinated contrast media, severely impaired renal function, impaired blood clotting factors, and inability to undergo a surgical procedure or general anesthesia.

Because the risks of general anesthesia are greater than those associated with most angiographic procedures, conscious sedation may be used for the procedure. Thoughtful communication from the CIT and physician also calms and reassures the patient. The CIT or physician should warn the patient about the sensations caused by the contrast medium and the noise produced by the imaging equipment. This information also reduces the patient's anxiety and helps ensure a good radiographic series with no patient motion.

Fig. 25-16 Selected catheter shapes used for angiography.

(Courtesy Cook, Inc., Bloomington, Ind.)

PREPARATION OF EXAMINING ROOM

It cannot be stated too often that the angiographic suite and every item in it should be scrupulously clean. The room should be fully prepared, with every item needed or likely to be needed on hand before the patient is admitted. Cleanliness and advance preparation are of vital importance in procedures that must be carried out under aseptic conditions. The CIT should observe the following guidelines in preparing the room:

- Check the angiographic equipment and all working parts of the equipment, and adjust the controls for the exposure technique to be employed.
- Place identification markers and all accessories in a convenient location.
- Have restraining bands available for application in combative patients.
- Adapt immobilization of the head (by suitable strapping) to the type of equipment employed.
- Make arrangements for immediate image processing as the procedure proceeds.

The sterile and nonsterile items required for introduction of the contrast medium vary according to the method of injection. The supplies specified by the interventionalist for each procedure should be listed in the angiographic procedure book. Sterile trays or packs, set up to specifications, can usually be obtained from the central sterile supply room. Otherwise, it is the responsibility of a qualified member of the interventional team to prepare them. Extra sterile supplies should always be on hand in case of a complication. Preparation of the room includes having life-support and emergency equipment immediately available.

RADIATION PROTECTION

As in all radiographic examinations, the patient is protected by filtration totaling not less than 2.5 mm of aluminum, by sharp restriction of the beam of radiation to the area being examined, and by avoidance of repeat exposures. In angiography, each repeated exposure necessitates repeated injection of the contrast material. For this reason, only skilled and specifically educated CITs should be assigned to take part in these examinations.

Angiography suites should be designed to allow observation of the patient at all times as well as to provide adequate protection to the physician and radiology personnel. These goals are usually accomplished with leaded glass observation windows.

ANGIOGRAPHIC TEAM

The angiographic team consists of the physician (usually an interventional radiologist), the CIT, and other specialists, such as an anesthetist and a nurse.

The CIT often assists in performing procedures that require sterile technique and may be responsible for operating monitoring devices and emergency equipment, as well as the radiographic equipment. When required to operate the supporting apparatus, the CIT must receive adequate training for proper use of the equipment. Instruction in patient care techniques and sterile procedure is included in the basic preparation of the CIT.

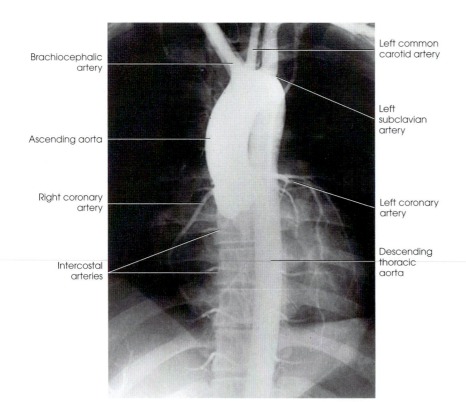

Fig. 25-17 AP thoracic aorta that also demonstrates right and left coronary arteries.

Brachiocephalic artery

Left common carotid artery

Ascending aorta

Left subclavian artery

Right coronary artery

Left coronary artery

Intercostal arteries

Descending thoracic aorta

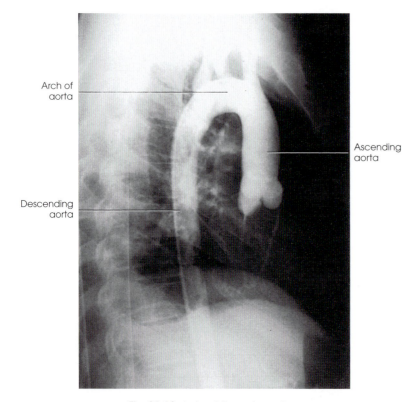

Fig. 25-18 Lateral thoracic aorta.

Arch of aorta

Ascending aorta

Descending aorta

The most satisfactory visualization of the aorta is achieved by placing a multihole catheter into the aorta at the desired level, using the Seldinger technique. *Aortography* is usually performed with the patient in the supine position for simultaneous frontal and lateral imaging, with the central ray perpendicular to the imaging system. For translumbar aortic catheter introduction, the patient must be in the prone position.

Thoracic Aortography

Thoracic aortography may be performed to rule out an aortic aneurysm or to evaluate congenital or postsurgical conditions. The examination is also used in patients with *aortic dissection.* Biplane imaging is recommended so that anteroposterior (AP) or posteroanterior (PA) and lateral projections can be obtained with one contrast medium injection. The CIT observes the following guidelines:

- For lateral projections, move the patient's arms superiorly so they do not appear in the image.
- For best results, increase the lateral SID, usually to 60 inches (152 cm), so that magnification is reduced.
- If biplane equipment is not available, use a single-plane 45-degree right posterior oblique (RPO) or left anterior oblique (LAO) body position, which often produces an adequate study of the aorta.
- For all projections, direct the perpendicular central ray to the center of the chest at the level of T7. This should allow visualization of the entire thoracic aorta, including the proximal brachiocephalic, carotid, and subclavian vessels.

The contrast medium is injected at rates ranging from 25 to 35 mL/sec for a total volume of 50 to 70 mL. The CIT then performs the following steps:

- Begin imaging simultaneously with injection of the contrast material.
- Make exposures in each plane at rates ranging from 1½ to 3 exposures per second for 3 to 4 seconds; exposures may then slow to one image or less per second for an additional 3 to 5 seconds.
- Make the exposures at the end of suspended inspiration (Figs. 25-17 and 25-18).

Abdominal Aortography

Abdominal aortography may be performed to evaluate abdominal aortic aneurysm, occlusion, or atherosclerotic disease. Simultaneous AP and lateral projections are recommended. The CIT observes the following guidelines:

- For the lateral projection, move the patient's arms superiorly so that they are out of the image field.
- Usually, collimate the field in the AP aspect of the lateral projection.
- Direct the perpendicular central ray at the level of L2 so that the aorta is visualized from the diaphragm to the aortic bifurcation. The AP projection best demonstrates the renal artery origins, the aortic bifurcation, and the course and general condition of all abdominal visceral branches. The lateral projection best demonstrates the origins of the celiac and superior mesenteric arteries because these vessels arise from the anterior abdominal aorta.
- Make the exposures. Representative injection and imaging programs are 25 mL/sec for a 60-mL total volume of contrast medium and two images per second for 4 seconds followed by one image per second for 4 seconds in each plane.
- Begin making the exposures simultaneously with the beginning of the injection and the end of suspended expiration (Figs. 25-19 and 25-20).

Hepatic artery

Right renal artery

Right common iliac artery

Splenic artery

Left renal artery

Abdominal aorta

Fig. 25-19 AP abdominal aorta.

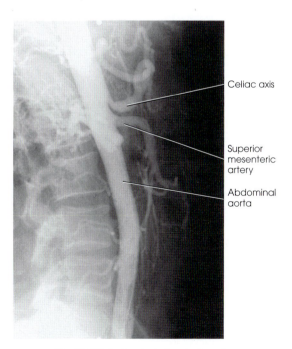

Celiac axis

Superior mesenteric artery

Abdominal aorta

Fig. 25-20 Lateral abdominal aorta.

Fig. 25-21 Right pulmonary artery during early phase of injection.

Fig. 25-22 Left pulmonary artery during early phase of injection; note the pulmonary outflow tract *(arrow)*.

Pulmonary Arteriography

Under fluoroscopic control, a catheter is passed from a peripheral vein through the vena cava and right side of the heart and into the pulmonary arteries. This technique is usually employed for a selective injection, and the examination is primarily performed for the evaluation of pulmonary embolic disease.

Simultaneous AP and oblique projections (Figs. 25-21 and 25-22) of the supine patient are recommended for this procedure. The suggested SID for the lateral projection is 60 inches (152 cm). The CIT observes the following guidelines:

- Move the patient's arms superiorly so they are out of the field of view.
- When biplane projections are not possible, use a single-plane 25- to 35- degree right anterior oblique (RAO) and LAO or left posterior oblique (LPO) and RPO position.
- Direct the central ray perpendicular to the image receptor for all exposures.
- A compensating (trough) filter can be used to obtain a radiograph with more uniform density between the vertebrae and the lungs if needed.
- In studies of the pulmonary arteries, lengthen the time of the imaging program to reveal the opacified left atrium, left ventricle, and thoracic aorta (Figs. 25-23 and 25-24).
- Make the exposures. Representative injection and imaging programs are 25 mL/sec for a 50-mL total volume of contrast medium and two to four images per second for 4 seconds followed by one image per second for an additional 4 seconds in each plane.

Ⅰ. PULMONARY VENOUS SYSTEM WITH LEFT HEART

Fig. 25-23 Late-phase right pulmonary artery injection demonstrating left atrium, left ventricle, and thoracic aorta.

LT. PULMONARY VENOUS SYSTEM WITH LEFT HEART

Fig. 25-24 Late-phase left pulmonary artery injection demonstrating left atrium, left ventricle, and thoracic aorta.

Fig. 25-25 Abdominal aortogram demonstrating the visceral arteries.

Selective Abdominal Visceral Arteriography

Abdominal visceral arteriographic studies (Fig. 25-25) are usually performed to visualize tumor vascularity or to rule out atherosclerotic disease, thrombosis, occlusion, and bleeding. An appropriately shaped catheter is introduced, usually from a transfemoral artery puncture, and advanced into the orifice of the desired artery. The CIT observes the following steps:

- Perform all selective studies initially with the patient in the supine position for single-plane frontal images.
- Direct the central ray perpendicular to the image receptor.
- In most patients, obtain a preliminary radiograph to establish optimum exposure and positioning and to check for retained contrast material.
- If necessary, use oblique projections to improve visualization or avoid superimposition of vessels.
- For all abdominal visceral studies, obtain radiographs during suspended expiration.

Selective abdominal visceral arteriograms are described in the following sections.

CELIAC ARTERIOGRAM

The celiac artery normally arises from the aorta at the level of T12 and carries blood to the stomach and the proximal duodenum, liver, spleen, and pancreas. These steps are followed:

- For the angiographic examination, center the patient to the image receptor.
- Direct the central ray to L1 (Fig. 25-26).
- Make the exposures. Representative injection and image programs are 10 mL/sec for a 40-mL total volume of contrast medium and two images per second for 5 seconds followed by one image per second for 5 seconds.

Fig. 25-26 Superselective celiac artery injection.

HEPATIC ARTERIOGRAM

The common hepatic artery branches from the right side of the celiac artery and supplies circulation to the liver, stomach and proximal duodenum, and pancreas. The CIT follows these steps:

- Position the patient so that the upper and right margins of the liver are at the respective margins of the image receptor (Fig. 25-27).
- Make the exposures. Representative injection and imaging programs are 8 mL/sec for a 40-mL total volume of contrast medium and two images per second for 5 seconds followed by one image per second for 5 seconds.

SPLENIC ARTERIOGRAM

The splenic artery branches from the left side of the celiac artery and supplies blood to the spleen and pancreas. The steps are as follows:

- Position the patient to place the left and upper margins of the spleen at the respective margins of the image receptor (Fig. 25-28).
- Splenic artery injection can demonstrate the portal venous system on the late venous images.
- For demonstration of the portal vein, center the patient to the image receptor.
- Make the exposures. Representative injection and imaging programs for a standard splenic arteriogram are 8 mL/sec for a 40-mL total volume of contrast medium and two images per second for 5 seconds followed by one image per second for 5 seconds. Representative programs for portal vein visualization are 8 mL/sec for a 40-mL total volume and one image per second for 20 seconds.

Fig. 25-27 Superselective hepatic artery injection.

Fig. 25-28 Superselective splenic artery injection.

Fig. 25-29 Selective SMA injection.

Fig. 25-30 Selective IMA injection.

SUPERIOR MESENTERIC ARTERIOGRAM

The superior mesenteric artery (SMA) supplies blood to the small intestine and the ascending and transverse colon. It arises at about the level of L1 and descends to L5-S1. The CIT follows these steps:

- To demonstrate the SMA, center the patient to the midline of the image receptor.
- Direct the central ray to the level of L3 (Fig. 25-29).
- Make the exposures. Representative injection and imaging programs are 8 mL/sec for a 50-mL total volume of contrast medium and two images per second for 5 seconds followed by one image per second for 5 seconds.
- When attempting to visualize bleeding sites, conduct the imaging at one image per second for 18 seconds.
- Use an increased injection volume and an extended imaging sequence to optimize visualization of the mesenteric and portal veins.

INFERIOR MESENTERIC ARTERIOGRAM

The inferior mesenteric artery (IMA) supplies blood to the splenic flexure, descending colon, and rectosigmoid area. It arises from the left side of the aorta at about the level of L3 and descends into the pelvis. The steps are as follows:

- To best visualize the IMA, use a 15-degree RAO or LPO position that places the descending colon and rectum at the left and inferior margins of the image (Fig. 25-30).
- Make the exposures. A representative injection program is 3 mL/sec for a 15-mL total volume of contrast medium. The imaging is the same as that for the SMA.

RENAL ARTERIOGRAM

The renal arteries arise from the right and left side of the aorta between L1 and L2 and supply blood to the respective kidney. The following steps are observed:

- Before performing this selective study, check the patient's IV urogram or renal flush arteriogram for the exact size and location of the kidneys. This step enables precise collimation to the kidney being studied and ensures exact centering of the patient and central ray.
- A renal flush aortogram may be accomplished by injecting 25 mL/sec for a 40-mL total volume of contrast medium through a multiple side hole catheter positioned in the aorta at the level of the renal arteries. A representative selective injection is 8 mL/sec for a 12-mL total volume. Imaging for both methods of injections is commonly three to six images per second for 2 to 3 seconds followed by perhaps only one or two nephrogram images made 5 to 10 seconds after the beginning of the injection.
- For a right renal arteriogram, position the patient so that the central ray enters at the level of L2 midway between the center of the spine and the patient's right side.
- For a selective left renal arteriogram, position the patient so that the central ray usually enters at the level of L1 midway between the center of the spine and the patient's left side (Fig. 25-31).

OTHER ABDOMINAL ARTERIOGRAMS

Other arteries branching from the aorta may be selectively studied to demonstrate anatomy and possible pathologic condition. The positioning for these procedures depends on the area to be studied and the surrounding structures. (These may include spinal, lumbar, adrenal, and phrenic.)

Fig. 25-31 Selective left renal artery injection in early arterial phase.

Selective abdominal visceral arteriography

Central Venography

Venous blood in veins flows proximally toward the heart. Injection into a central venous structure may not opacify the peripheral veins that *anastomose* to it. However, the position of peripheral veins can be indirectly documented by the filling defect from unopacified blood in the opacified central vein. The CIT observes the following guidelines:

- Place the patient in the supine position for either a single-plane AP or PA projection or biplane projections. Move the patient's arms out of the field of view.
- Obtain lateral projections at increased SID, if possible, to reduce magnification.
- Remember that collimation to the long axis of the vena cava improves image quality but may prevent visualization of peripheral or *collateral veins.*

SUPERIOR VENACAVOGRAM

Venography of the superior vena cava is performed primarily to rule out the existence of thrombus or the occlusion of the superior vena cava. The contrast medium may be injected through a needle or an angiographic catheter introduced into a vein in an antecubital fossa, although superior opacification results from injection through a catheter positioned in the axillary or subclavian vein. Radiographs should include the opacified subclavian vein, brachiocephalic vein, the superior vena cava, and the right atrium (Fig. 25-32). The injection program depends mostly on whether a needle, an angiographic catheter, or a regular catheter is used. A representative program for a catheter injection is 10 to 15 mL/sec for a 30- to 50-mL total volume of contrast medium. Images are produced in both planes, if desired, at a rate of one or two images per second for 5 to 10 seconds and are made at the end of suspended inspiration.

INFERIOR VENACAVOGRAM

Venography of the inferior vena cava is performed primarily to rule out the existence of thrombus or the occlusion of the inferior vena cava. The contrast medium is injected through a multiple side hole catheter inserted through the femoral vein and positioned in the common iliac vein or the inferior aspect of the inferior vena cava. Radiographs may need to include the opacified vasculature from the catheter tip to the right atrium (Figs. 25-33 and 25-34). Representative injection and imaging programs are 20 mL/sec for a 40-mL total volume of contrast medium and two images per second for 4 to 8 seconds in both planes. Imaging begins at the end of suspended expiration.

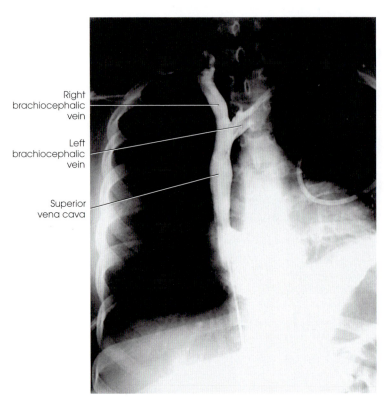

Right brachiocephalic vein

Left brachiocephalic vein

Superior vena cava

Fig. 25-32 AP superior vena cava.

Inferior
vena cava

Right common
iliac vein

Fig. 25-33 AP inferior vena cava.

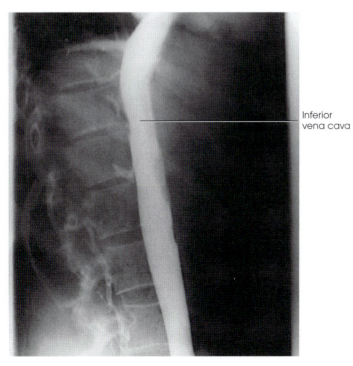

Inferior
vena cava

Fig. 25-34 Lateral inferior vena cava.

Fig. 25-35 Portal venogram. *m,* Main portal v.; *s,* superior mesenteric v.; *i,* inferior mesenteric v.; *sp,* splenic v.; *c,* coronary varices.

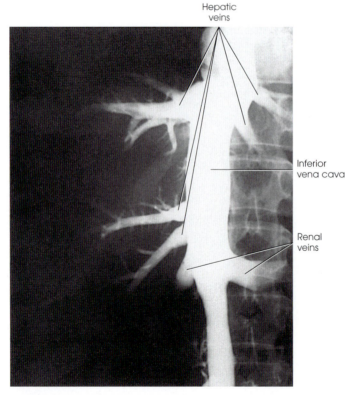

Fig. 25-36 Hepatic vein visualization from reflux from an inferior vena cava injection. (Note reflux into bilateral renal veins.)

Selective Visceral Venography

The visceral veins are often visualized by extending the imaging program of the corresponding visceral artery injection. For example, the veins that drain the small bowel are normally visualized by extending the imaging program of a superior mesenteric arteriogram. Portal venography (Fig. 25-35) can be performed by injecting the portal vein directly from a percutaneous approach, but it is usually accomplished by late-phase imaging of a splenic artery injection or an SMA injection.

HEPATIC VENOGRAM

Hepatic venography is usually performed to rule out stenosis or thrombosis of the hepatic veins. These veins are also catheterized to obtain pressure measurements from the interior of the liver. The hepatic veins carry blood from the liver to the inferior vena cava. (The portal vein carries nutrient-rich blood from the viscera to the liver.) The hepatic veins are most easily catheterized from a jugular vein or an upper limb vein approach, but a femoral vein approach may also be used. The CIT follows these steps:

- Place the patient in the supine position for AP or PA projections that include the liver tissue and the extreme upper inferior vena cava (Fig. 25-36).
- Make the exposures. Representative injection and imaging programs are 10 mL/sec for a 30-mL total volume of contrast medium and one image per second for 8 seconds.
- Make exposures at the end of suspended expiration.

RENAL VENOGRAM

Renal venography is usually performed to rule out thrombosis of the renal vein. The renal vein is also catheterized for blood sampling, usually to measure the production of renin, an enzyme produced by the kidney when it lacks adequate blood supply. The renal vein is most easily catheterized from a femoral vein approach. The following steps are observed:

- Place the patient in the supine position for a single-plane AP or PA projection.
- Center the selected kidney to the image receptor, and collimate the field to include the kidney and area of the inferior vena cava (Fig. 25-37).
- Make the exposures. Representative injection and imaging programs are 8 mL/sec for a 16-mL total volume of contrast medium and two images per second for 4 seconds.
- Make exposures at the end of suspended expiration.

Left renal veins

Fig. 25-37 Selective left renal venogram. AP projection.

Peripheral Angiography
UPPER LIMB ARTERIOGRAMS

Upper limb arteriography is most often performed to evaluate traumatic injury, atherosclerotic disease, or other vascular lesions. The arteriograms are usually obtained by using the Seldinger technique to introduce a catheter, most often at a femoral artery site for selective injection into the subclavian or axillary artery. The contrast medium may also be injected at a more distal site through a catheter. The area to be radiographed may therefore be just a hand or another selected part of the arm, or it may include the entire upper limb and thorax.

The recommended projection is a true AP projection with the arm extended and the hand supinated. Hand arteriograms may be obtained in the supine or prone arm position (Figs. 25-38 and 25-39). The injection and imaging programs depend on the equipment used. The injection varies from 3 or 4 mL/sec through a catheter positioned distally to 10 mL/sec through a proximally positioned catheter. Images are obtained by using a bolus chase technique or by performing serial runs over each segment of the extremity.

Fig. 25-38 Right hand arteriogram (2:1 magnification) showing severe arteriooclusive disease *(arrows)* affecting digits after cold-temperature injury.

UPPER LIMB VENOGRAMS

Upper limb venography is most often performed to look for thrombosis or occlusions. The contrast medium is injected through a needle or catheter into a superficial vein at the elbow or wrist. The radiographs should cover the vasculature from the wrist or elbow to the superior vena cava.

The projection and imaging sequence depend on the location of the injection site (Fig. 25-40). If the injection and filling of veins are observed with a fluoroscopic spot-film device, radiographs or digital spot films can be exposed as the vessels opacify. Injections may be made by hand, or an automatic injector may be set to deliver a total of 40 to 80 mL at a rate of 1 to 4 mL/sec, depending on whether a needle or catheter is used. If the study is performed with the patient supine, tourniquets positioned proximal to the wrist and elbow will force the contrast medium into the deep veins.

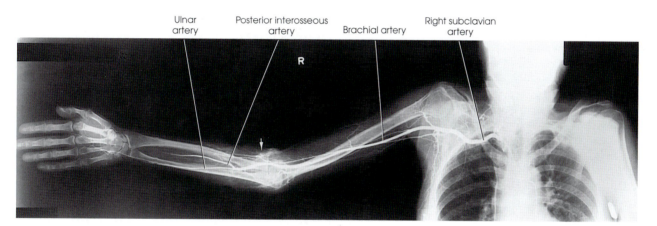

Fig. 25-39 Right subclavian artery injection demonstrating iatrogenic occlusion of radial artery *(arrow)*.

Fig. 25-40 Normal right upper limb venogram.

Aortofemoral arteriograms

Aortofemoral arteriography is usually performed to determine whether atherosclerotic disease is the cause of *claudication*. A catheter is usually introduced into a femoral artery using the Seldinger technique. The catheter tip is positioned superior to the aortic bifurcation so that bilateral arteriograms are obtained simultaneously. When only one leg is to be examined, the catheter tip is placed below the bifurcation, or the contrast medium is injected through a needle placed in the femoral artery. The CIT then observes the following guidelines:

- For a bilateral examination, place the patient in the supine position for single-plane AP projections and center the patient to the midline of the image receptor to include the area from the renal arteries to the ankles.
- Place the patient in the prone position for a translumbar aortic catheterization if needed.
- For either patient position, internally rotate the legs 30 degrees.
- For best results, use a cassette changer with a length of 48 inches (122 cm).
- If the cassette changer is not available, have the cassettes overlap to ensure coverage of all vasculature. Overlapping cassettes can be produced automatically by "stepping" systems with moving tables or C-arms.
- Make exposures of the opacified lower abdominal aorta and aortic bifurcation with the patient in suspended expiration.

Imaging programs vary and are set based on the predicted rate of flow through the long arterial course of the lower limb. Flow through normal arteries may take as little as 10 seconds, whereas flow through severely diseased arteries may take 30 seconds or more. A representative injection program designed to create a long bolus of contrast medium is 10 mL/sec for a 100-mL total volume (Fig. 25-41).

Examinations of a specific area of the leg such as the popliteal fossa or foot are occasionally performed. For these procedures the preferred injection site is usually the femoral artery. AP, lateral, or both projections may be obtained with the patient centered to the designated area.

LOWER LIMB VENOGRAMS

Lower limb venography is common and is usually performed to rule out thrombosis of the deep veins of the leg. Venograms are usually obtained with contrast medium injected through a needle placed directly into a superficial vein in the foot. The CIT then observes the following guidelines:

- Obtain radiographs with the patient on a tilt table in a semiupright position at a minimum angle of 45 degrees if possible.
- Begin imaging at the patient's ankle, and proceed superiorly to include the inferior vena cava as the injection continues.
- Without fluoroscopy, usually obtain AP projections with the leg internally rotated 30 degrees to include the entire area of interest (Fig. 25-42). Exact positioning is often determined with fluoroscopic direction.
- Perform lateral projections if needed.
- If imaging is performed with the patient supine, apply tourniquets just proximal to the ankle and knee to force filling of the deep veins in the leg.
- Usually, expose serial radiographs 5 to 10 seconds apart. Injections may be made by hand, or an automatic injector may be set to deliver 1 or 2 mL/sec for a total of 50 to 100 mL.

Angiography in the Future

Visceral and peripheral angiography is a dynamic area that challenges angiographers to keep abreast of new techniques and equipment. New diagnostic modalities that reduce or eliminate irradiation may be developed and may replace a number of current angiographic procedures. Some diagnostic information, however, can be obtained only through conventional angiographic methods. Consequently, angiography will continue to be used to examine vasculature and, through therapeutic procedures, to provide beneficial treatment. However, noninvasive imaging techniques, such as MR angiography and computed tomography (CT) angiography, are being used more often. These less invasive procedures may eliminate some diagnostic angiographic procedures, but at this point, therapeutic procedures continue.

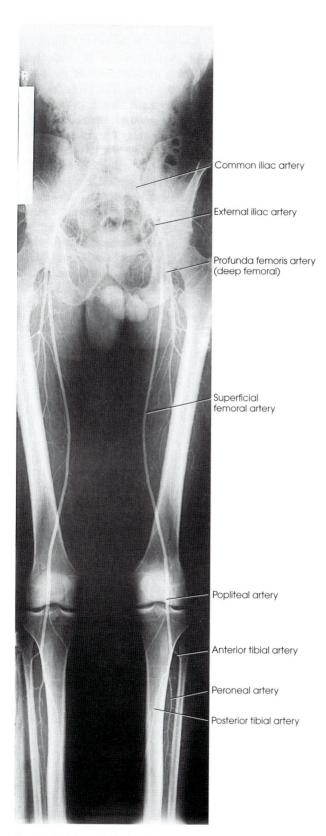

Common iliac artery

External iliac artery

Profunda femoris artery
(deep femoral)

Superficial
femoral artery

Popliteal artery

Anterior tibial artery

Peroneal artery

Posterior tibial artery

Fig. 25-41 Normal abdominal aortogram and bilateral femoral arteriogram in late arterial phase.

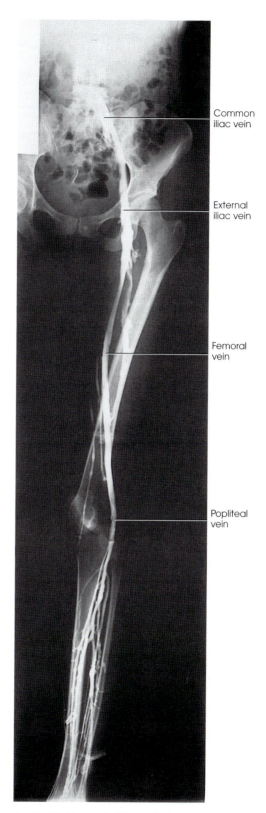

Common
iliac vein

External
iliac vein

Femoral
vein

Popliteal
vein

Fig. 25-42 Normal left lower limb venogram.

Circulatory system and cardiac catheterization

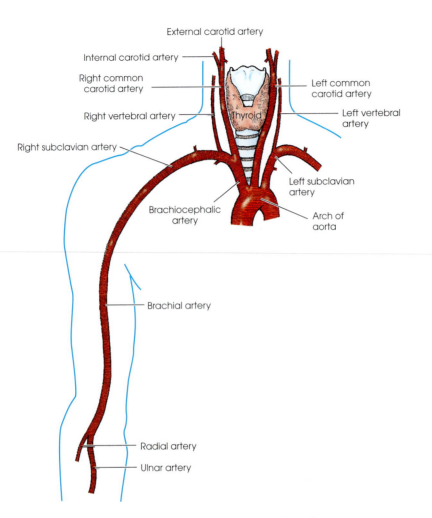

External carotid artery

Internal carotid artery

Right common
carotid artery

Right vertebral artery

Thyroid

Left common
carotid artery

Left vertebral
artery

Right subclavian artery

Left subclavian
artery

Brachiocephalic
artery

Arch of
aorta

Brachial artery

Radial artery

Ulnar artery

Fig. 25-43 Major arteries of upper chest, neck, and arm.

Cerebral Anatomy

Cerebral angiography is the radiologic/angiographic examinations of the blood vessels of the brain. The procedure was introduced by Egas Moniz[1] in 1927. It is performed to investigate intracranial vascular lesions such as aneurysms, arteriovenous malformations (AVMs), tumors, and atherosclerotic or stenotic lesions.

The brain is supplied by four trunk vessels or great vessels (Fig. 25-43): the right and left common carotid arteries, which supply the anterior circulation; and the right and left vertebral arteries, which supply the posterior circulation. These paired arteries branch from the arch of the aorta and ascend through the neck.

[1]Egas Moniz AC: L'encéphalographie artérielle, son importance dans la localisation des tumeurs cérébrales, *Rev Neurol* 2:72, 1927.

The first branch of the aortic arch is the *innominate artery* or the *brachiocephalic artery*. It then bifurcates into the right common carotid and the right subclavian artery. The second branch of the aortic arch is the left common carotid, followed by the left subclavian artery. Each of the vessels originate directly from the aortic arch. Both vertebral arteries most commonly take their origins from the subclavian arteries. Although this branching pattern is common in most patients, there can be some *anomalous* origins of these great vessels. Each common carotid artery passes superiorly and somewhat laterally alongside the trachea and larynx to the level of C4. There each divides into internal and external carotid arteries. The external carotid artery contributes blood supply to the extracranial and extraaxial circulation. There can be some collateral circulation into the internal carotid circulation in some situations. The internal carotid artery enters the cranium through the carotid foramen of the temporal bone and then bifurcates into the anterior and middle cerebral arteries (Fig. 25-44). These vessels in turn branch and rebranch to supply the anterior circulation of the respective hemisphere of the brain.

Fig. 25-44 Right common carotid artery injection demonstrating right internal carotid artery *(arrows)* and anterior cerebral blood circulation, including reflux across the anterior communication artery *(small arrow)*.

The vertebral arteries ascend through the cervical transverse foramina and then pass medially to enter the cranium through the foramen magnum. The vertebral arteries unite to form the basilar artery, which, after a short superior course along the posterior surface of the dorsum sellae, bifurcates into the right and left posterior cerebral arteries. The blood supply to the posterior fossa (cerebellum) originates from the vertebral and basilar arteries (Fig. 25-45).

The anterior and posterior cerebral arteries are connected by communicating arteries at the level of the midbrain to form the *circle of Willis*. The anterior communicating artery forms an anastomosis between the anterior cerebral arteries, which communicate between the right and left hemispheres. The right and left posterior communicating arteries each form an anastomosis between the internal carotid artery and the posterior cerebral artery connecting the anterior and posterior circulation. A chart detailing intracerebral circulation is provided in Fig. 25-46.

Fig. 25-45 Left vertebral artery injection demonstrating the posterior cerebral blood circulation, including reflux into the posterior communicating artery *(arrows)*.

LATERAL PROJECTION   ANTEROPOSTERIOR PROJECTION

Carotid artery

Carotid artery

Internal carotid arteriogram

Vertebral artery

Vertebral artery

Vertebral arteriogram

Superior sagittal sinus

Superior sagittal sinus

Transverse sinus

Transverse sinus

Internal carotid venogram

Fig. 25-46 Diagram of the intracranial circulation: arterial and venous phase.

(From Bean BC: A chart of the intracerebral circulation, ed 2, *Med Radiogr Photogr* 34:25, 1958; courtesy Dr. Berton C. Bean and Eastman Kodak Co.)

Cerebral Angiographic Studies

TECHNIQUE

Cerebral angiography should be performed only in facilities equipped to produce studies of high technical quality with minimal risk to the patient. The ability to obtain rapid-sequence biplane images with automatic injection represents the minimum standard. This equipment is available in all major medical centers and in most large hospitals (see Fig. 25-9).

Cerebral angiography is most commonly performed from a transfemoral approach; however, a brachial or axillary artery approach can be employed. Selective catheterization techniques also allow the internal and external carotid circulation to be studied separately, which is useful in delineating the blood supply of some forms of cerebral tumors and vascular malformations.

The final position of the catheter depends on the information sought from the angiographic study. When atherosclerotic disease of the extracranial carotid, subclavian, and vertebral arteries is being evaluated, injection of the aortic arch with imaging of the extracranial portion of these vessels is an appropriate way to begin.

Fig. 25-47 Right internal carotid injection, lateral projection, demonstrates arterial phase of circulation. Note the posterior communicating artery *(arrow)*.

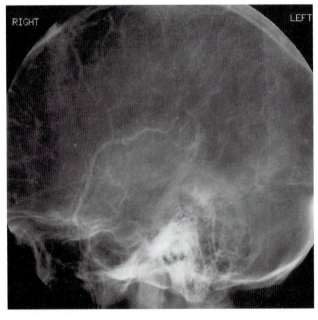

Fig. 25-48 Right internal carotid injection, lateral projection, demonstrates capillary phase of carotid circulation.

CIRCULATION TIME AND IMAGING PROGRAM

Egas Moniz[1] stated that the transit time of the cerebral circulation is only 3 seconds for the blood to circulate from the internal carotid artery to the jugular vein, with the circulation time being slightly prolonged by the injected contrast solution. Greitz,[2] who measured the cerebral circulation time as "the time between the points of maximum concentration (of contrast medium) in the carotid siphon and in the parietal veins," found a normal mean value of 4.13 seconds. This time is a highly important factor in cerebral angiography.

Certain pathologic conditions significantly alter the cerebral circulation time. AVMs shorten the transit time, or arterial vasospasm may cause a considerable delay.

A standard radiographic program should include a radiograph taken before the arrival of contrast material to serve as a subtraction mask and rapid-sequence images at 1½ to 3 images per second in the AP and lateral projections during the early, or arterial, phase (first 1½ to 2½ seconds) of the arteriogram (Fig. 25-47). After the arterial phase, imaging may be slowed to one image per second for the capillary, or parenchymal, phase (Fig. 25-48) and maintained at one image per second or every other second for the venous phase (Fig. 25-49) of the angiogram. The entire program should cover 7 to 10 seconds, depending on the preference of the angiographer. The imaging program must be tailored to demonstrate the suspected pathologic condition.

Injection rates and volumes through the catheter are coupled with the imaging program, usually by automatic means. Injections at rates of 5 to 9 mL/sec for 1 to 2 seconds are most often employed in the cerebral vessels, with variations dependent on vessel size and the patient's circulatory status.

[1]Egas Moniz AC: *L'angiographie cérébrale,* Paris, 1934, Masson & Cie.
[2]Greitz T: A radiologic study of the brain circulation by rapid serial angiography of the carotid artery, *Acta Radiol* 46(Suppl 140):1, 1956.

EQUIPMENT

Rapid-sequence biplane imaging with either film or DSA electronically coupled with an automatic injector is employed almost universally in cerebral angiography.

Collimating to the area of the head and neck is essential for improving image quality in the nonmagnified study. The standard tube collimator may be used for this purpose, or lead cutout diaphragms may also be positioned on the collimator. These diaphragms may have openings in the shape of a circle or a "keyhole." The keyhole diaphragm openings are rounded in the area of the cranium and taper inward in the area of the neck. The frontal and lateral keyhole diaphragms are each designed to resemble the shape of the head and neck in their respective images.

PREPARATION OF PATIENT

Other than withholding the preceding meal, preliminary preparation depends on the patient's condition and is accordingly determined by the radiologist and the referring physician. Whenever possible, adult patients are examined under local anesthesia in conjunction with conscious sedation. Adequate sedation minimizes the intensity of the burning pain felt along the course of the vessel and the areas supplied by it during the rapid injections of iodinated medium. It is imperative that conscious patients receive a careful explanation of what to expect during the procedure and what is expected of them. This explanation is essential for the successful completion of the procedure.

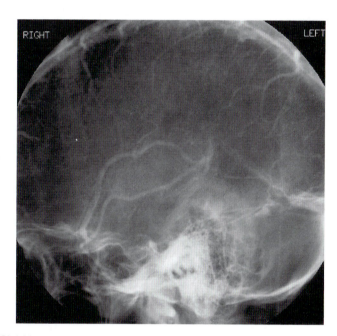

Fig. 25-49 Right internal carotid injection, lateral projection, demonstrates venous phase of circulation.

POSITIONING FOR EXAMINATION
Position of patient

In positioning the patient, the CIT observes the following steps:

- Place the patient in the supine position.
- Regardless of whether the patient is awake, place suitable supports under points of strain (small of the back, knees, and ankles).
- Apply wrist restraints and compression bands across the body as indicated by the patient's condition.
- Although the catheter is unlikely to be unseated during positioning, exercise care to prevent excessive patient motion, especially with extremely selective studies. General anesthesia may be required for certain procedures to help prevent any movement of the patient.

Position of head

The centering and angulation of the central ray required for demonstration of the anterior circulation differ from those required for demonstration of the posterior circulation. The same head position is used for the basic AP and lateral projections of both regions. The following steps are observed:

- For the initial right-angle studies, center the head to both the AP and lateral image receptors.
- Adjust the patient's head to place its midsagittal plane exactly perpendicular to the headrest and consequently exactly parallel with the laterally placed image receptor.
- Place the infraorbitomeatal line (IOML) perpendicular to the horizontal plane when positioning is manually accomplished.
- Angle the central ray for caudally inclined AP and AP oblique projections from the vertically placed IOML, or adjust the central ray so that it is parallel to the floor of the anterior fossa, as indicated by a line extending from the supraorbital margin to a point ¾ inch (1.9 cm) superior to the external acoustic meatus (EAM).

In this chapter, head positioning is presented as if the image receptors were fixed in the horizontal and vertical planes. This necessitates the use of facial landmarks for precise positioning of the head in relation to the central ray to achieve certain projections. However, in some angiographic suites, fluoroscopy can be used to determine the final position of the head and the angulation of the central ray required to achieve the desired image.

Frontal projections are described in this section as AP projections, but equivalent PA projections also exist. Many angiographic imaging systems place the image receptor above the tabletop and the x-ray tube below. Because patients usually lie supine for cerebral angiography, the central ray, coming from below, enters the posterior cranium and exits the anterior cranium on its course to the image receptor. The position of the central ray results in PA projections equivalent to the AP projections described.

The literature on cerebral angiography contains numerous position variations concerning the degree of central ray angulation, the base from which the central ray should be angled or the line that it should parallel, and the degree of part rotation for oblique studies. This chapter discusses the most frequently employed images and reasonably standard specifications for obtaining them.

The number of radiographs required for satisfactory delineation of a lesion depends on the nature and location of the lesion. Oblique projections and/or variations in central ray angulation are used to separate the vessels that overlap in the basic positions and to evaluate any existing abnormality.

Aortic Arch Angiogram (for Cranial Vessels)

An aortic arch angiogram is most commonly obtained to visualize atherosclerotic or occlusive disease of the extracranial carotid, vertebral, and subclavian arteries. A multiple side hole catheter is positioned in the ascending thoracic aorta so that the subsequent injection fills all of the vessels simultaneously.

SIMULTANEOUS BIPLANE OBLIQUE PROJECTIONS

For best results, simultaneous biplane oblique projections are produced so that superimposition of vessels is minimized (Fig. 25-50).

The CIT observes the following steps:

- Place the patient in a 35-degree RPO position on the tabletop, with the midsagittal plane of the head either perpendicular to the AP image receptor or in an RPO position. This patient position opens the aortic arch and the origins of the great vessels for the AP oblique projection frees the carotid and vertebral arteries from superimposition.
- Raise the patient's chin to superimpose the inferior margin of the mandible onto the occiput so that as much of the neck as possible is exposed in the frontal radiograph.
- Move the patient's shoulders inferiorly so that they are removed as much as possible from the lateral image.
- If possible, use offset biplane imaging systems for this procedure.
- Position the lateral image receptor similarly to the AP projection to get another image of the origins of the great vessels.

- For the AP and lateral projection, direct the central ray perpendicular to the center of the image receptor to enter the patient at a level 1¼ inch (3 cm) superior to the sternal angle.

A representative injection program for an aortic arch examination is 15 to 20 mL/sec for a total volume of 35 to 40 mL. A representative imaging program is two to three images per second in each plane for 4 seconds. Because subtraction images are frequently produced from aortic arch angiograms, the initial images should be exposed before the injection begins. An alternative imaging program exposes one image in each plane, pauses 1 second as the injection begins, and then continues with two to three images per second for 3 seconds.

Fig. 25-50 Digital subtracted images of the thoracic aortogram demonstrating the origins of the great vessels.

Fig. 25-51 Cerebral angiogram: lateral projection as part of a biplane setup.

Anterior Circulation
LATERAL PROJECTION

The CIT observes the following steps:

- Center the patient's head to the vertically placed image receptor.
- Extend the patient's head enough to place the IOML perpendicular to the horizontal.
- Adjust the patient's head to place the midsagittal plane vertical and thereby parallel with the plane of the image receptor.
- Adapt immobilization to the type of equipment being employed.
- Perform lateral projections of the anterior, or carotid, circulation with the central ray directed horizontally to a point slightly cranial to the auricle and midway between the forehead and the occiput. This centering allows for patient variation (Figs. 25-51 to 25-53).

NOTE: See Fig. 25-46 for assistance in identifying the cerebral vessels in the image.

Fig. 25-52 Lateral projection.

Fig. 25-53 Left internal carotid artery injection. Cerebral angiogram: lateral projection demonstrating anterior circulation. Note the posterior communicating artery *(arrow)*.

AP AXIAL PROJECTION (SUPRAORBITAL)

The CIT observes the following steps:

- Adjust the patient's head so that its midsagittal plane is centered over and perpendicular to the midline of the grid and so that it is extended enough to place the IOML vertically.
- Immobilize the patient's head.
- Keep in mind that achieving the goal in this angiogram requires superimposition of the supraorbital margins on the superior margin of the petrous ridges so that the vessels are projected above the floor of the anterior cranial fossa.
- To obtain this result in most patients, direct the central ray 20 degrees caudally for the AP axial or 20 degrees cephalad for the PA axial projection along a line passing ¾ inch (1.9 cm) superior to and parallel with a line extending from the supraorbital margin to a point ¾ inch (1.9 cm) superior to the EAM; the latter line coincides with the floor of the anterior fossa (Figs. 25-54 to 25-56).

Fig. 25-54 Carotid angiogram: PA axial (supraorbital) projection.

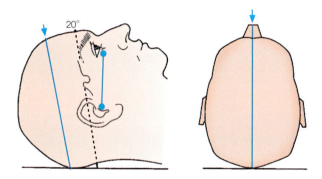

Fig. 25-55 AP axial (supraorbital).

Fig. 25-56 Left common carotid artery injection demonstrating AP axial (supraorbital) projection. Arterial phase of circulation.

AP AXIAL OBLIQUE PROJECTION (SUPRAORBITAL)

The following steps are observed:
- Maintain the preceding position for the patient's head, but rotate the head approximately 30 degrees away from the injected side, or angle the central ray 30 degrees toward the injected side.
- Direct the central ray 20 degrees caudal (Figs. 25-57 and 25-58).

AP AXIAL PROJECTION (TRANSORBITAL)

The CIT observes the following steps:
- Adjust the patient's head for the basic AP projection.

- Direct the central ray through the mid-orbits at an average angle of 20 degrees cephalad. The central ray should coincide with a line passing through the center of the orbit and a point about ¾ inch (1.9 cm) superior to the auricle of the ear (Figs. 25-59 and 25-60).

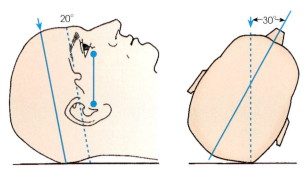

Fig. 25-57 AP axial oblique (supraorbital) projection.

Fig. 25-58 Right common carotid artery injection demonstrating AP axial oblique (supraorbital) projection.

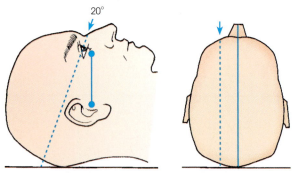

Fig. 25-59 AP axial (transorbital) projection.

Fig. 25-60 Right internal carotid artery injection demonstrating AP axial (transorbital) projection. Note the middle cerebral artery aneurysm (arrow).

AP AXIAL OBLIQUE PROJECTION (TRANSORBITAL)

The oblique transorbital projection demonstrates the internal carotid bifurcation and the anterior communicating and middle cerebral arteries within the orbital shadow. The steps are as follows:

- From the position for the basic AP transorbital projection, rotate the patient's head approximately 30 degrees away from the injected side, or angle the central ray 30 degrees toward the injected side.
- Angle the central ray 20 degrees cephalad and center it to the midorbit of the uppermost side (Figs. 25-61 and 25-62).

AP AXIAL AND AP OBLIQUE PROJECTIONS

AP axial and/or AP axial oblique projections are used in carotid angiography, when indicated, for further evaluation of vessel displacement or of aneurysms.

For an AP axial projection, the following steps are observed:

- Adjust the patient's head in the basic AP position.
- Direct the central ray to the region approximately 1½ inches (3.8 cm) superior to the glabella at an average angle of 30 degrees caudad for the AP axial projection or 30 degrees cephalad for the PA axial projection. The central ray exits at the level of the EAM (Figs. 25-63 to 25-65).

For an AP axial oblique projection, the following steps are observed:

- Rotate the patient's head 35 to 45 degrees away from the injected side, or angle the central ray 35 to 45 degrees toward the injected side.
- Angle the central ray 30 degrees caudad (Figs. 25-66 and 25-67).

Fig. 25-61 AP axial oblique (transorbital) projection.

Fig. 25-62 Right internal carotid artery injection demonstrating AP axial oblique (transorbital) projection.

Fig. 25-63 PA axial projection.

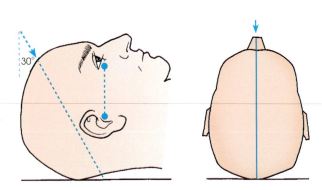

Fig. 25-64 AP axial projection.

Fig. 25-65 Right internal carotid artery injection demonstrating AP axial projection.

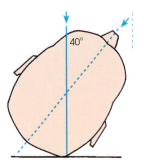

Fig. 25-66 AP axial oblique projection.

Fig. 25-67 Left internal carotid artery injection demonstrating AP axial oblique projection.

Posterior Circulation
LATERAL PROJECTION

The CIT observes the following steps:

- Center the patient's head to the vertically placed image receptor.
- Extend the patient's head enough to place the IOML perpendicular to the horizontal plane, and then adjust the head to place the midsagittal plane vertically and thereby parallel with the plane of the image receptor.
- Rigidly immobilize the patient's head.
- Perform lateral projections of the posterior, or vertebral, circulation with the central ray directed horizontally to the mastoid process at a point about ⅜ inch (1 cm) superior to and ¾ inch (1.9 cm) posterior to the EAM.
- Restrict the exposure field to the middle and posterior fossae for lateral studies of the posterior circulation (Figs. 25-68 and 25-69). Inclusion of the entire skull is neither necessary nor, from the standpoint of optimal technique, desirable.

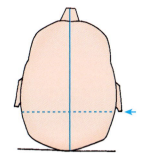

Fig. 25-68 Lateral projection for posterior circulation.

Fig. 25-69 Right vertebral artery injection demonstrating lateral projection and showing vertebrobasilar system.

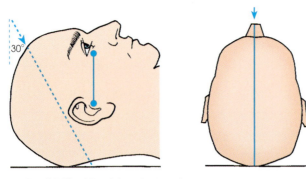

Fig. 25-70 AP axial projection for posterior circulation.

AP AXIAL PROJECTION

The following steps are observed:

• Adjust the patient's head so that the midsagittal plane is centered over and perpendicular to the midline of the grid, and extend the head enough so that the IOML is vertical.

• Immobilize the patient's head.

• Direct the central ray to the region approximately 1½ inches (3.8 cm) superior to the glabella at an angle of 30 to 35 degrees caudad. The central ray exits at the level of the EAM. For this projection, the supraorbital margins are positioned approximately ¾ inch (1.9 cm) below the superior margins of the petrous ridges (Figs. 25-70 and 25-71).

Fig. 25-71 Right vertebral artery injection demonstrating AP axial projection, showing vertebrobasilar system.

Circulatory system and cardiac catheterization

SUBMENTOVERTICAL PROJECTION

A modified submentovertical (SMV) projection is sometimes employed for the investigation of the posterior circulation. It is also used for the examination of the anterior circulation when a middle cranial fossa lesion is suspected.

The success of this projection depends on the patient's ability to hyperextend the neck and maintain this hyperextension for the time required for an imaging sequence (Figs. 25-72 and 25-73). This body position may not be possible for elderly patients with cervical degenerative arthritis.

Fig. 25-72 SMV projection.

Fig. 25-73 Right internal carotid artery injection demonstrating SMV projection. Note the multiple aneurysm clips.

Interventional radiology has a therapeutic rather than diagnostic purpose in that it intervenes in, or interferes with, the course of a disease process or other medical condition. Since the conception of this form of radiology in the early 1960s, its realm has become so vast and sophisticated that publishers of periodicals struggle to keep abreast of this rapidly advancing specialty.

Interventional radiology allows the angiographer to assume an important role in the management and treatment of disease in many patients. Interventional radiologic procedures reduce hospital stays in many patients and help some patients avoid surgery, with consequent reductions in medical costs.

Every interventional radiologic procedure must include two integral processes. The first is the interventional or medical side of the procedure, in which the highly skilled radiologist uses needles, catheters, and special medical devices (e.g., occluding coils, guidewires) to produce an improvement in the patient's status or condition. The second process involves the use of fluoroscopy and radiography to guide and document the progress of the steps taken during the first process. The CIT must receive special education in the angiographic and interventional suite. This skilled CIT has a very important role in assisting the angiographer in the interventional procedures.

The more frequently performed interventional procedures are described in the succeeding pages. Resources containing more detailed information are cited in the selected bibliography at the end of the chapter.

Percutaneous Transluminal Angioplasty and Stenting

Percutaneous transluminal angioplasty (PTA) is a therapeutic radiologic procedure designed to dilate or reopen stenotic or occluded areas within a vessel using a catheter introduced by the Seldinger technique. PTA using a coaxial catheter method was first described by Dotter and Judkins[1] in 1964. First, a guidewire is passed through the narrowed area of a vessel. Then, a smaller catheter is passed over the guidewire through the stenosis to begin the dilation process. Finally, a larger catheter is passed over the smaller catheter to cause further dilation. This method is referred to as the "Dotter method" (Fig. 25-74). Although this method can achieve dilation of stenosis, it has the significant disadvantage of creating an arteriotomy as large as the dilating catheters.

[1] Dotter CT, Judkins MP: Transluminal treatment of arteriosclerotic obstruction: description of a new technique and preliminary report of its application, *Circulation* 30:654, 1964.

Fig. 25-74 Coaxial angioplasty of atherosclerotic stenosis, the "Dotter method": **A,** Guidewire advanced through stenosis. **B,** Small catheter advanced through stenosis. **C,** Large catheter advanced through stenosis. **D,** Postangioplasty stenotic area.

In 1974, Gruntzig and Hopff[1] introduced the double-lumen, balloon-tipped catheter. One lumen allows the passage of a guidewire and fluids through the catheter. The other lumen communicates with a balloon at the distal end of the catheter. When inflated, the balloon expands to a size much larger than the catheter. Double-lumen, angioplasty balloon catheters are available in sizes ranging from 3 to 9 Fr, with attached balloons varying in length and expanding to diameters of 2 to 20 mm or more (Fig. 25-75).

Fig. 25-76 illustrates the process of *balloon angioplasty*. The stenosis is initially identified on a previously obtained angiogram. The balloon diameter used for a procedure is often the measured diameter of the normal artery adjacent to the stenosis. The angioplasty procedure is often performed at the same time and through the same catheterization site as the initial diagnostic examination.

[1]Gruntzig A, Hopff H: Perkutane rekanalisation chronischer arterieller Verschlusse mit einem neuen dilatationskatheter; modifikation der Dotter-Technik, *Deutsch Med Wochenschr* 99:2502, 1974.

Fig. 25-75 Balloon angioplasty catheters with varied diameters and lengths.

(Courtesy Bard Radiology.)

Fig. 25-76 Balloon angioplasty of atherosclerotic stenosis. **A,** Guidewire advanced through stenosis. **B,** Balloon across stenosis. **C,** Balloon inflated. **D,** Postangioplasty stenotic area.

After the guidewire is positioned across the stenosis, the angiographic catheter is removed over the wire. The angioplasty balloon catheter is then introduced and directed through the stenosis over the guidewire. The balloon is usually inflated with a diluted contrast medium mixture for 15 to 45 seconds, depending on the degree of stenosis and the vessel being treated. The balloon is then deflated and repositioned or withdrawn from the lesion. Contrast medium can be injected through the angioplasty catheter for a repeat angiogram to determine whether or not the procedure was successful. The success of the angioplasty procedure may also be determined by comparing transcatheter blood pressure measurements from a location distal and a location proximal to the lesion site. Nearly equal pressures indicate a reopened stenosis.

Transluminal angioplasty can be performed in virtually any vessel that can be reached percutaneously with a catheter (Figs. 25-77 and 25-78). In 1978, however, Molnar and Stockum[1] described the use of balloon angioplasty for dilation of strictures within the biliary system (Fig. 25-79). Balloon angioplasty is also conducted in venous structures, ureters, and the gastrointestinal tract.

[1]Molnar W, Stockum AE: Transhepatic dilatation of choledochoenterostomy strictures, *Radiology* 129:59, 1978.

Fig. 25-77 Digital subtracted images of the abdominal aortogram/bilateral iliac arteries. **A,** High-grade stenosis of the right common iliac artery *(arrow)*. **B,** Abdominal aortogram/bilateral iliac arteries, postangioplasty, demonstrating widely patent iliac system.

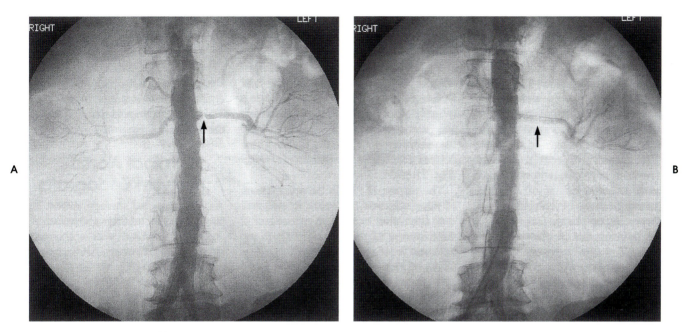

Fig. 25-78 Abdominal aortogram before and after angioplasty of the left renal artery. **A,** High-grade stenosis of the left renal artery *(arrow).* **B,** Postangioplasty and stent placement within the left renal artery *(arrow).*

Fig. 25-79 Biliary duct injection with balloon angioplasty of two separate ducts. **A,** Balloon wasting in an inferior duct *(arrow).* **B,** Balloon wasting in a superior duct *(arrow).*

Balloon angioplasty has been successfully to manage various diseases that cause arterial narrowing. The most common form of arterial stenosis treated by transluminal angioplasty is caused by atherosclerosis. Dotter and Judkins[1] speculated that this atheromatous material was soft and inelastic and therefore could be compressed against the artery wall. The success of coaxial and balloon method angioplasty was initially attributed to enlargement of the arterial lumen because of compression of the atherosclerotic plaque. Later research showed, however, that the plaque does not compress. If plaque surrounds the inner diameter of the artery, the plaque cracks at its thinnest portion as the arterial lumen is expanded. Continued expansion cracks the arterial wall's inner layer, the *intima*, then stretches and tears the middle layer, the *media*, and finally stretches the outer layer, the *adventitia*. The arterial lumen is increased by permanently enlarging the artery's outer diameter. Restenosis, when it occurs, is usually caused by deposits of new plaque, not arterial wall collapse.

A final possibility for percutaneous treatment of vessel stenoses is the placement of vascular stents. A vascular *stent* is made up of a metal material, stainless steel or nitinol, and can be covered or uncovered with a biologic material that is introduced through a catheter system and positioned across a stenosis to keep the narrowed area spread apart. These devices permanently remain in the vessel (Fig. 25-80).

The success of PTA in the management of atherosclerosis has made it a significant alternative to surgical procedures in the treatment of this disease. PTA is not indicated in all cases, however. Long segments of occlusion, for example, may be best treated by surgery. PTA has a lower risk than surgery but is not totally without risk. Generally patients must be able to tolerate the surgical procedure that may be required to repair vessel damage, which can be caused by PTA. Unsuccessful transluminal angioplasty procedures rarely prevent or complicate necessary subsequent surgery. In selected cases the procedure is effective and almost painless and can be repeated as often as necessary with no apparent increase in risk to the patient. The recovery time is often no longer than the time required to stabilize the arteriotomy site, usually a matter of hours, and general anesthesia is normally not required. Therefore the hospital stay and the cost to the patient are reduced.

Abdominal Aortic Aneurysm Endografts

An interventional therapy started in the late 1990s is treating abdominal aortic aneurysms (AAAs) with a transcatheter approach and stenting. AAAs have been historically treated with an open repair of the aneurysm by a vascular surgeon. This approach has its risks associated with abdominal surgery and a long hospital stay for recovery of the incision. The stent graft or endograft is a nitinol-covered stent that comes in pieces or one intact device depending on the manufacturer (Fig. 25-81). A cut-down approach to bilateral femoral arteries is done and sheaths and delivery catheters are advanced to deliver the

[1]Dotter CT, Judkins MP: Transluminal treatment of arteriosclerotic obstruction: description of a new technique and preliminary report of its application, *Circulation* 30:654, 1964.

Fig. 25-80 Intravascular stents. **A,** Gianturco Rosch biliary Zstent. **B,** Memotherm. **C,** Palmez; unexpanded and expanded. **D,** Symphony. **E,** Wallstent.

Fig. 25-81 A stent graft or endograft used to repair aneurysm in the aorta and iliac region.

device. A large amount of planning is done before a patient can undergo this approach to treating an AAA. Patients must have an aneurysm that is infrarenal or occurring below the renal arteries. The stent is a covered device and would occlude the renals. Preliminary abdominal and iliac arteriograms are obtained using a calibrated catheter that the radiologist or vascular surgeon can use for measuring the vasculature (Fig. 25-82). CT is a standard of care for imaging and will be used as the primary source for measurements. This procedure is done either in the catheterization laboratory or in the operating room depending on the hospital. If done in the operating room, a portable C-arm is needed with DSA capabilities to reproduce the function of the catheterization laboratory DSA.

Although most PTA procedures are conducted in the radiology angiographic suite, angioplasty involving the arteries of the heart is generally performed in a more specialized laboratory. *Percutaneous transluminal coronary angioplasty* (PTCA) takes place in the cardiac catheterization laboratory because of the possibility of potentially serious cardiac complications. Further information on PTCA is provided later in this chapter.

A

B

C

Fig. 25-82 **A,** Abdominal aortagram. **B,** Placement of endograft. **C,** Follow-up aortogram demonstrating repair.

Transcatheter Embolization

Transcatheter embolization was first described by Brooks[1,2] in 1930. He described vessel occlusion for closure of arteriovenous fistula. Transcatheter embolization involves the therapeutic introduction of various substances to occlude or drastically reduce blood flow within a vessel (Box 25-1). The three main purposes for embolization are (1) to stop active bleeding sites, (2) to control blood flow to diseased or malformed vessels (e.g., tumors or AVMs), and (3) to stop or reduce blood flow to a particular area of the body before surgery.

[1]Brooks B: The treatment of traumatic arteriovenous fistula, *South Med J* 23:100, 1930.
[2]Brooks B: Discussion. In Nolan L, Taylor AS: Pulsating exophthalmos, *Trans South Surg Assoc* 43:176, 1931.

The patient's condition and the situation must be considered when choosing an embolic agent. The interventionalist usually identifies the appropriate agent to be used. Embolic agents must be administered with care to ensure that they flow to the predetermined vessel or target. Embolization is a permanent treatment; the effects on the lesion are irreversible. Many embolic agents are available (Box 25-2), and the choice of agent depends on whether the occlusion is to be temporary or permanent (Table 25-1).

Temporary agents such as Gelfoam* or Avitene may be used as a means to reduce the pressure head of blood to a specific site. These temporary agents reduce flow

*Gelfoam is the trademark for a sterile, absorbable, water-insoluble gelatin-base sponge.

into a bleeding site so that hemostasis may be achieved. Temporary agents can also be used to protect normal vessels from being inadvertently embolized.

Vasoconstricting drugs can be used to temporarily reduce blood flow. Vasoconstrictors such as vasopressin (Pitressin) drastically constrict vessels, resulting in hemostasis.

When permanent occlusion is desired, as in trauma to the pelvis that causes hemorrhage or when vascular tumors are supplied by large vessels, the Gianturco stainless steel coil may be used. This coil (Fig. 25-83), which functions to produce thrombogenesis, is simply a looped segment of guidewire with Dacron fibers attached to it. The coil is initially straight and is easily introduced into a catheter that has been placed into the desired vessel. The coil is then pushed out of the catheter tip with a guidewire. The coil assumes its

BOX 25-1
Lesions amendable to embolization

a. Aneurysm
b. Pseudoaneurysm
c. Hemorrhage
d. Neoplasms
   • Malignant
   • Benign
e. Arteriovenous malformations
f. Arteriovenous fistula
g. Infertility (varicocele)
h. Impotence due to venous leakage
i. Redistribution of blood flow

BOX 25-2
Particulate agents

• Polyvinyl alcohol
• Embosphere
• Avitene
• Gelfoam
• Suture material

Metal coils
• Gianturco coils
• Metal coils
• Detachable coils
   • Platinum
   • Coated

Liquid agents (occluding, sclerosing)
• Ethanol
• Thrombin
• Boiling contrast
• Hypertonic glucose
• Sodium tetradecyl sulfate
• Ethibloc
• EVAL
• Onyx

Detachable balloons
• Latex—Debrun
• Silicone—Heishima

Liquid adhesives
• N-butyl 2-cyanoacrylate

Autologous material

TABLE 25-1
Particulate agent sizes

Agent	Size
Gelfoam powder	40-60 microns
Gelfoam sponges	Pledgets-torpedoes
Avitene	100-150 microns
Polyvinyl alcohol	100-1200 microns
Embosphere	100-1200 microns

looping shape immediately as it enters the bloodstream. It is important that the catheter tip be specifically placed in the vessel so that the coil springs precisely into the desired area. Numerous coils can be placed as needed to occlude the vessel. A new generation of coils promises to deliver more effective closure of vascular structures by using various coatings on the outside of the coil. One such coil uses a coating that initiates a foreign body/ scarring response. Another type of coil is coated with an expansile gel that swells in the presence of blood, thus occluding the vessel. Tissue will grow inside and around the gel to provide healing.

Fig. 25-84 shows a hypervascular uterine fibroid that was causing significant symptoms. This uterine fibroid was successfully embolized with total occlusion of the lesion.

Fig. 25-83 Fibered Gianturco stainless steel occluding coil (magnified).

A

B

Fig. 25-84 Hypervascular uterine fibroid. **A,** Bilateral uterine artery injections using coaxial microcatheters, demonstrating hypervascular uterine fibroid. **B,** Bilateral iliac artery injections, postembolization, demonstrating total occlusion of both uterine arteries *(arrows)*.

Transcatheter embolization has also been used in the cerebral vasculature of the brain. Vascular lesions within the cerebral vasculature, such as aneurysms, AVMs, and tumors, can be managed using multiple embolic agents, PVA, or tissue adhesive. Very small catheters (2 or 3 Fr) are passed through a larger catheter, a coaxial system that is positioned in the cerebral vessels. The smaller catheter is then manipulated into the appropriate cerebral vessel, and lesions such as an aneurysm and the embolic material are delivered through it until the appropriate embolization is achieved (Fig. 25-85).

Percutaneous Nephrostomy Tube Placement and Related Procedures

Nephrostomy tube drainage is indicated in the patient who has some type of ureteral or bladder blockage that causes *hydrone-phrosis*. If urine is not eliminated from the kidney, renal failure with necrosis to the kidney may occur, as may sepsis.

A nephrostomy tube is a catheter that has multiple side holes at the distal end through which urine can enter. The urine drains into a bag connected to the proximal end of the drainage catheter outside the patient's body. These catheters range in size from 8 to 12 Fr and are usually about 12 inches (30 cm) in length. Nephrostomy tubes are also placed in patients with kidney stones to facilitate subsequent passage of ultrasonic lithotripsy catheters.

The renal pelvis must be opacified to provide a target for percutaneous nephrostomy tube placement. Percutaneous nephrogram may be performed to accomplish this. For this procedure, the patient is positioned prone or in an anterior oblique position on the tabletop. The patient's back and posterolateral aspect of the affected side are prepared and surgically draped. Following the administration of a local anesthetic, a 7-inch (17-cm) thin-wall cannula needle is passed through the back under fluoroscopic control and the cannula is removed. The needle is examined for drainage of urine. When urine returns through the needle, contrast medium is injected to opacify the renal pelvis.

A posterior calyx of the opacified renal pelvis is often selected as the target for the nephrostomy tube placement. After a local anesthetic is administered, a 7-inch (17-cm) cannula needle is inserted through the posterolateral aspect of the back and directed toward the renal pelvis. A fluoroscopic C-arm offers a distinct advantage for this process. The C-arm can be obliqued to match the angle between the needle insertion site and the target. The needle can then be advanced directly toward the target visualized on the fluoroscopic monitor. The C-arm is then angled obliquely 90 degrees to determine whether the needle tip has reached the renal pelvis or calyx.

Fig. 25-85 Left vertebral artery injection. **A,** Basilar tip aneurysm *(arrow)*. **B,** Left vertebral artery injection postembolization with the use of Guglielmi detachable coils (GDCs).

When the needle tip has entered the desired target, a guidewire is passed through the needle into the renal pelvis and is then maneuvered into the proximal ureter for additional support. The needle is then removed, the tract is dilated, and the drainage catheter is passed over the guidewire and into the renal pelvis. The pigtail end of the catheter must be placed well within the renal pelvis and not outside the kidney itself or in the proximal ureter (Figs. 25-86 and 25-87). The catheter's position is maintained by attaching it to a fixation disk or other device that is then sutured or taped to the body wall. A dressing is applied over the entry site. Either the fixation device or the dressing must prevent the catheter from becoming kinked, which would prevent the drainage of urine through the catheter. Periodic antegrade nephrograms may be performed by injecting the drainage catheter to evaluate anatomy and catheter function.

Nephrostomy tubes may be placed for temporary or permanent external drainage of urine. Nephrostomy tubes that are left in place for a long period of time need to be exchanged periodically for new ones. A guidewire is inserted through the existing catheter, and the catheter is removed, leaving the guidewire in place. A new nephrostomy tube is then passed over the guidewire and positioned in the renal pelvis. Nephrostomy tubes can be permanently removed by simply pulling them out. The tract from the body wall to the renal pelvis usually closes in a day or so without complication.

Fig. 25-86 Left nephrostogram through Coop Loop drainage tube. Note the high-grade stenosis of the distal ureter causing hydronephrosis.

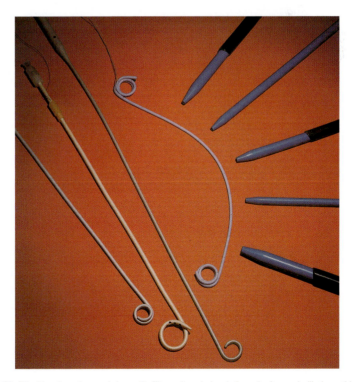

Fig. 25-87 Nephrostomy tubes *(left)*, ureteral stent *(center)*, and dilators *(right)*.

(Courtesy Cook, Inc., Bloomington, Ind.)

Angioplasty of stenoses in the ureteral system, renal cyst puncture with drainage, and percutaneous antegrade ureteral stent placement are additional procedures. A ureteral stent is a double-ended pigtail catheter that is passed into the ureter and remains inside the body, with one end placed into the renal pelvis and the other into the bladder (Fig. 25-88). This catheter is used when a constriction of the ureter or ureterovesicular junction is blocking the drainage of urine from the renal pelvis. The multiple side holes at both pigtail ends allow urine to drain into one end of the stent and exit the other end.

The stent provides an internal passageway for urine across the area of blockage. A nephrostomy tube is initially placed to provide access to the renal pelvis and to allow a tract to form in the body. At a later time, a guidewire is passed through the nephrostomy tube and down the ureter into the bladder. The nephrostomy tube is removed, and the stent is inserted over the guidewire using a pusher. The nephrostomy tube is replaced to provide external drainage until it is known that the stent is providing internal drainage. The stent can usually be removed through the urethra by a cystoscopic procedure.

Inferior Vena Cava Filter Placement

The idea of interrupting the pathway of an embolus is not a new one. Surgical interruption of the common femoral vein was first described in 1784, and surgical interruption of the inferior vena cava was described in 1868. These procedures and the partial surgical interruption procedures that evolved from them had a high rate of complications, not only due to the surgical process but also due to inadequate venous drainage from the lower limbs. Catheterization technology led to the development of detachable balloons for occluding the inferior vena cava, but that procedure also resulted in complications because of inadequate venous flow from the lower limbs.

Nephrostomy tube

Proximal pigtail in renal pelvis

Stent catheter in ureter

Distal pigtail in bladder

Fig. 25-88 Image of left ureteral stent and left nephrostomy after catheter placement.

Right popliteal vein

Thrombus

Thrombus

Fig. 25-89 Lower limb venogram.

Pulmonary angiography primarily evaluates embolic disease of the lungs. However, computed tomography angiography has been shown to be just as accurate as pulmonary angiography. A pulmonary embolus is a blood clot, which forms as a thrombus and usually develops in the deep veins of the leg (Fig. 25-89). When such a thrombus becomes dislodged and migrates, it is called an *embolus*. An embolus originating in the leg may migrate through the inferior vena cava and right side of the heart and finally lodge in the pulmonary arteries. A filter can be percutaneously placed in the inferior vena cava to trap such an embolus.

Lower limb vein thrombosis is not necessarily an indication for inferior vena cava filter placement. Normally, blood-thinning medications are administered to treat deep vein thrombosis. When anticoagulant therapy is contraindicated because of bleeding or the risk of hemorrhage, filter placement may be indicated. Filter placement itself has associated risks, including thrombosis of the vein through which the filter is introduced and thrombosis of the vena cava. However, these risks normally are not life threatening. It is important to note that inferior vena cava filter placement is not a treatment for deep vein thrombosis of the leg but a therapy intended to reduce the chance of pulmonary embolism.

The first true filter designed to trap emboli while maintaining vena cava patency was introduced in 1967 by Mobin-Uddin. It consisted of six metal struts joined at one end to form a conical shape that was covered by a perforated plastic canopy. The plastic canopy proved to be too occlusive, which is the reason that the Mobin-Uddin filter is no longer in use. Because of this filter's striking resemblance to an open umbrella, vena cava filters of all types were for many years referred to as "umbrella filters."

Inferior vena cava filters are available in a variety of shapes. All of these filters are initially compacted inside an introducer catheter delivery system and assume their functional shape as they are released (Fig. 25-90). The introducers are passed through sheaths ranging in size from 6 to 15 Fr.

Most filters are designed as a conical shape to trap clots in the central lumen. They are also designed to be placed in vena cavae ranging up to 20 to 30 mm in diameter. Each filter has its own mechanism of clot trapping. Fig. 25-90 demonstrates the most currently available permanent inferior vena cava filters. These filters would be employed as a temporary means to prevent new pulmonary embolus. While patients are in an acute high-risk state, these temporary filters may help prevent pulmonary embolus. Regardless of whether the filter is permanent or temporary, the purpose is to prevent and trap new onset of pulmonary embolus. These do treat preexisting clots, however.

Fig. 25-90 Vena cava filters: *I,* Kimray-Greenfield; *II,* Titanium Greenfield; *III,* Simon Nitinol; *IV,* Gianturco-Roehm Bird's Nest; *V,* Vena Tech. **A,** Photographic image. **B,** Radiographic image.

Fig. 25-91 Inferior vena cavogram. Note reflux into the renal veins *(large arrows)* and hepatic veins *(small arrows)*.

Fig. 25-92 Post-placement image showing Greenfield filter in place *(arrow)*.

Several filters are designed for temporary placement. They have hooks on the top and the bottom that allow them to be grasped by a catheter snare device and be removed percutaneously. Another temporary filter remains attached to its introducer catheter, which is used to retrieve it. Some temporary filters must be removed within approximately 10 days or they become permanently attached to the vena cava endothelium. Various filter designs are in use in countries other than the United States. Inferior vena cava filter development continues, and new designs will certainly become available.

The filters are percutaneously inserted through a femoral, jugular, or antecubital vein, usually for placement in the inferior vena cava just inferior to the renal veins. Placement inferior to the renal veins is important to prevent renal vein thrombosis, which can occur if the vena cava is occluded superior to the level of the renal veins by a large thrombus in a filter. An inferior vena cavogram is performed using the Seldinger technique, usually from the femoral vein approach. The inferior vena cavogram defines the anatomy, including the level of the renal veins, determines the diameter of the vena cava, and rules out the presence of a thrombus (Fig. 25-91). Filter insertion from the jugular or antecubital approach may be indicated if a thrombus is present in the inferior vena cava.

The diameter of the vena cava may influence the choice of filter because each filter has a maximum diameter. The filter insertion site is dilated to accommodate the filter introducer. The filter remains sheathed until it reaches the desired level and is released from its introducer by the angiographer. The introducing system is then removed, and external compression is applied to the venotomy site until hemostasis is achieved. A post-placement image is obtained to document the location of the filter (Fig. 25-92).

Transjugular Intrahepatic Portosystemic Shunt

The *portal circulation* consists of blood from the digestive organs, which drains into the liver. The portal system consists of the splenic vein, the superior mesenteric vein, and the inferior mesenteric vein. The blood passes through the liver tissue and is returned to the inferior vena cava via the hepatic veins. Disease processes can increase the resistance of blood flow through the liver, elevating the portal circulation's blood pressure—a condition known as *portal hypertension.* It may cause the blood to flow through collateral veins. Venous *varices* are the result and can be life-threatening if they bleed. The creation of a portosystemic shunt can decrease portal hypertension and the associated variceal bleeding by allowing the portal venous circulation to bypass its normal course through the liver. The percutaneous intervention for creating an artificial low-pressure pathway between the portal and hepatic veins is called a *transjugular intrahepatic portosystemic shunt* (TIPS).

Portography and hepatic venography are usually performed before a TIPS procedure to delineate anatomy and confirm *patency* of these vessels. Ultrasonography may be used for this purpose. Transcatheter blood pressure measurements may also confirm the existence of a pressure gradient between the portal and hepatic veins.

The most common approach for a TIPS procedure is from a right internal jugular venous puncture site to the middle or right hepatic vein. A hepatic venogram may be obtained using contrast material and/or CO_2. A special long needle is passed into the hepatic vein and advanced through the liver tissue into the portal vein. The needle is exchanged for an angioplasty balloon catheter, and the tract through the liver tissue is dilated. An angiographic catheter may be passed through the tract and advanced into the splenic vein for a splenoportal venogram. An intravascular stent is positioned across the tract to maintain its patency (Fig. 25-93). The tract and stent may be further enlarged with an angioplasty balloon catheter until the desired reduction in pressure gradient between the portal and hepatic veins is achieved. The sheath is then removed from the internal jugular vein, and external pressure is applied until hemostasis at the venotomy occurs.

Other Procedures

When an angiogram demonstrates thrombosis, the procedure may be continued for thrombolytic therapy. Blood clot–dissolving medications can be infused through an angiographic catheter positioned against the thrombus. Special infusion catheters that have side holes may be manipulated directly into the clot. Periodic repeat *angiograms* evaluate the progress of *lysis* (dissolution). The catheter may have to be advanced under fluoroscopic control to keep it against or in the clot as lysis progresses.

Catheters can also be used to percutaneously remove foreign bodies, such as catheter fragments or broken guidewires, from the vasculature. A variety of snares can be used for this purpose. A snare catheter introduced using the Seldinger technique is manipulated under fluoroscopic control to grasp the foreign body. Then the snare and foreign body are withdrawn as a unit.

Fig. 25-93 Intravascular stent placement in a TIPS procedure.

Lymphography is a general term applied to radiologic examinations of the lymph vessels and nodes after they have been opacified by an injected oil-based contrast medium (Figs. 25-94 and 25-95). The study of the lymph vessels, which may be called *lymphangiography*, is carried out within the first hour after injection of the contrast material. The study of the lymph nodes, which may be called *lymphadenography*, is performed 24 hours after injection of the contrast medium. The lymph vessels empty the contrast agent within a few hours. The nodes normally retain the contrast substance for 3 to 4 weeks. Abnormal nodes may retain the medium for several months, so delayed lymphadenograms may be made, as indicated, without further injection.

Lymphography is seldom performed in current practice because of the superior imaging capabilities of newer modalities such as MRI and CT. At present its primary purpose is to assess the clinical extent of lymphomas or for staging of radiation treatment. Lymphography may also be indicated in patients who demonstrate clinical evidence of obstruction or other impairment of the lymphatic system. A more detailed description of lymphography is provided in previous editions of this text.

Injections for lymphography are limited to easily accessible sites such as those of the hands and feet (Table 25-2). (Lymphatics of the feet are most commonly used.) For opacification of the lymphatic vessels and nodes, the vessels must be isolated and cannulated. Ordinarily the peripheral lymphatic vessels cannot be easily identified because of their small size and lack of color. For identification of the lymphatic vessels on the dorsum of the feet and hands, a blue dye that is selectively absorbed by the lymphatics is injected subcutaneously into the first and second interdigital web spaces about 15 minutes before the examination. (After patent blue violet is injected, the patient's urine and skin are tinted blue. This condition disappears within a few hours.)

A longitudinal incision is made on the dorsum of each hand or foot to locate the dye-filled lymphatic vessels. A 27- or 30-gauge needle is used to cannulate the isolated vessels. Iodinated oily contrast media is then slowly injected into the

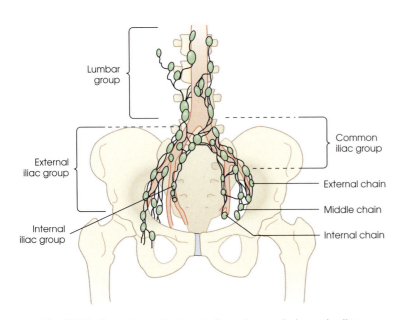

Fig. 25-94 Iliopelvic-aortic lymphatic system: anterior projection.

Fig. 25-95 AP projection of iliopelvic-abdominoaortic lymph nodes.

vessels over a 30-minute period. (As in any procedure involving the injection of foreign materials, untoward reactions must be anticipated. The patient must be observed closely, and appropriate medications and resuscitation equipment must be nearby.) Confirmation that the injection is intralymphatic is usually obtained fluoroscopically. After the injection, the needles are removed and the wounds sutured.

Injection of the feet provides visualization of the lymphatic structures of the lower limb (Fig. 25-96), groin, iliopelvic-abdominoaortic region, and thoracic duct. Injection of the lymphatics of the hands provides visualization of the upper limb and the axillary, infraclavicular, and supraclavicular regions.

IMAGING

For demonstration of the lymph vessels, radiographs are made within the first hour after the contrast agent is injected. A second series of radiographs is made 24 hours later to demonstrate the lymph nodes. The exposure factors employed for lymphographic studies are the same as those used for bone studies of the respective region. Table 25-2 summarizes the most common radiographic projections and the associated anatomic structures visualized.

Interventional radiologic procedures performed in the biliary system include biliary drainage and biliary stone removal (see Chapter 16).

TABLE 25-2

Projections and anatomy demonstrated with lymphography

Injection site	Projections	Anatomy demonstrated
Feet	AP abdomen	Iliopelvic and paraaortic lymph nodes
	RPO and LPO abdomen	
	AP thorax	Thoracic duct
	Left lateral thorax	
	Bilateral AP tibias	Lower limb lymphatic vessels
	Bilateral AP femora	Inguinal lymph nodes
	AP pelvis	
Hands	AP and lateral arm (centered at elbow)	Upper limb lymphatic vessels and nodes
	AP and 45-degree AP oblique shoulder	Axillary lymph nodes

AP, Anteroposterior; *LPO*, left posterior oblique; *RPO*, right posterior oblique.

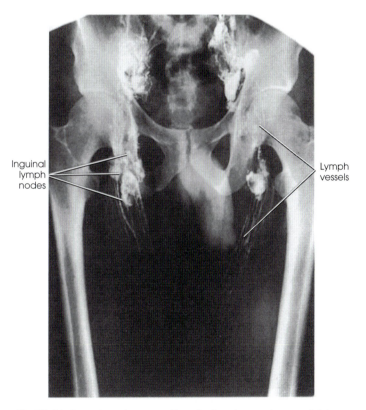

Fig. 25-96 Lymphangiogram of inguinal region and upper thighs.

Interventional Radiology: Present and Future

Interventional procedures bring therapeutic capabilities into the hands of the interventional radiologist. Procedures are done for diagnosis and treatment of multiple lesions. The treatment procedures can be performed at the same time as the diagnostic procedure. New equipment is continually becoming available to improve techniques and broaden the scope of percutaneous intervention. Although use of the catheter for angiographic diagnosis may wane, its ability to provide therapy percutaneously ensures a future for angiography. These procedures are highly technical and a team approach is most important. The cardiovascular and interventional technologist plays an active role on this interventional team[1] (Fig. 25-97). Along with the interventional technologist, the other members of the team would be the nurse, support personnel, and the interventionalist. Although these procedures are performed in an angiographic suite, this subspecialty of radiology can be considered less invasive surgery. The field can also be called *surgical angiography* and *surgical neuroangiography*. This field of interventional radiology has a bright future as more sophisticated equipment is developed.

[1]Scanlon PJ et al: ACC/AHA guidelines for coronary angiography: a report of the American College of Cardiology/American Heart Association Task Force on Practice Guidelines (Committee on Coronary Angiography), *J Am Coll Cardiol* 33:1758, 1999.

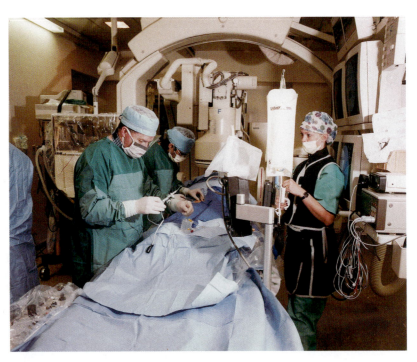

Fig. 25-97 The CIT plays an active role on the interventional team by assisting the interventionalist (*left*) or by circulating within the angiosuite (*right*).

Cardiac catheterization is a comprehensive term used to describe a minor surgical procedure involving the introduction of specialized catheters into the heart and surrounding vasculature for the purpose of diagnostic evaluation and therapy (intervention) associated with a variety of cardiovascular-related disorders in both children and adults. Therefore cardiac catheterization is classified as either a diagnostic procedure or an interventional procedure. The primary purpose of diagnostic procedures is to collect data necessary to evaluate the patient's condition. Cardiac interventional procedures involve the application of therapeutic measures through catheter-based systems or other mechanical means to treat disorders of the vascular and conduction systems within the heart.

Historical Development

As early as 1844, experimental placement of catheters into the hearts of animals led to the successful catheterization of both the right and left ventricles of a horse by Claude Bernard, a French physiologist. The first human cardiac catheterization was reported in 1929 by Forssman, a 25-year-old surgical resident who placed a catheter into his own heart and then walked to the radiology department where a chest radiograph was produced to document his medical achievement.

Catheterization of the heart soon became a valuable tool used primarily for diagnostic purposes. Through the 1940s, the basic catheterization study remained relatively uncomplicated and easy for physicians to perform; however, the risk to the patient was significant.

In the years that followed, catheterization methods and techniques increased in number and complexity and were refined. The refinements included the development of the Seldinger technique (see Fig. 25-15) and the introduction of transseptal left heart catheterization. Selective coronary *angiography* was first reported by Sones in 1959, when he inadvertently injected contrast medium into the right coronary artery of a patient who was undergoing routine aortography. In 1962, Ricketts and Abrams described the first percutaneous method for selective coronary angiography. This method was further perfected in the late 1960s with the introduction of preformed catheters designed to engage the ostium of both the right and left coronary arteries.

The 1960s and 1970s brought tremendous advances in radiologic and cardiovascular medicine and technology. Radiographic imaging and recording equipment, physiologic monitoring equipment, and cardiovascular pharmaceuticals and supplies became increasingly reliable. Since the 1970s, major efforts have been made to increase the dependability, applicability, and diversity of cardiac catheterization interventional techniques. The use of computers in the catheterization laboratory has facilitated the development of this rapidly growing subspecialty of the cardiovascular medical and surgical sciences. These advances and trends have enabled cardiac catheterization to evolve from a simple diagnostic investigation to its current state as a sophisticated diagnostic study and interventional procedure.

In the early 1990s, cardiac catheterization became the second most frequently performed inpatient operative procedure in the United States. More notably, it has become the most frequently performed procedure in patients older than age 65. Currently, more than 1.5 million cardiac catheterizations are performed. Based on predictions of an increased growth in patients older than 45 years, it is estimated that nearly 3 million cardiac catheterization procedures will be performed annually in the United States by the year 2010.

Principles of Cardiac Catheterization

General indications, contraindications, and risks are associated with diagnostic and interventional cardiac catheterizations. The physician must consider these factors when attempting to determine the appropriateness of any type of catheterization.

GENERAL INDICATIONS

Cardiac catheterization is performed to identify the anatomic and physiologic condition of the heart. The data gathered during catheterization provide the physician with information to develop management strategies for patients who have cardiovascular disorders. *Coronary angiography* is currently the most definitive procedure for visualizing the coronary anatomy. The anatomic information gained from this procedure may include the presence and extent of obstructive coronary artery disease, thrombus formation, coronary artery collateral flow, coronary anomalies, aneurysms, and spasm. Coronary artery size can also be determined.

Coronary artery disease is the most common disorder necessitating catheterization of the adult heart. This disease is caused primarily by the accumulation of fatty intracoronary *atheromatous* plaque, which leads to *stenosis* and *occlusion* of the coronary arteries. Coronary artery disease is symptomatically characterized by chest pain (angina pectoris) or a heart attack (myocardial infarction [MI]). Treatment of coronary artery disease includes both medical and surgical intervention.

Diagnostic cardiac catheterization of the adult patient with coronary artery disease is conducted to assess the appropriateness and feasibility of various therapeutic options. For example, cardiac catheterization is performed before open-heart surgery to provide *hemodynamic* and *angiographic* data to document the presence and severity of disease. In selected circumstances, postoperative catheterization is performed to assess the results of surgery. An interventional procedure (e.g., PTCA, intracoronary stent, or atherectomy) may be indicated for the relief of arteriosclerotic coronary artery stenosis.

Diagnostic studies of the adult heart also aid in evaluating the patient who has confusing or obscure symptoms (e.g., chest pain of undetermined cause). These studies are also used to assess diseases of the heart not requiring surgical intervention, such as certain cardiomyopathies.

TABLE 25-3

Indications for cardiac catheterization

Indications	Procedures
1. Suspected or known coronary artery disease	
a. New-onset angina	LV, COR
b. Unstable angina	LV, COR
c. Evaluation before a major surgical procedure	LV, COR
d. Silent ischemia	LV, COR, ERGO
e. Positive ETT	LV, COR, ERGO
f. Atypical chest pain or coronary artery spasm	LV, COR, ERGO
2. Myocardial infarction	
a. Unstable angina postinfarction	LV, COR
b. Failed thrombolysis	LV, COR, RH
c. Shock	LV, COR, RH
d. Mechanical complications (ventricular septal defect, rupture of wall or papillary muscle)	LV, COR, RH
3. Sudden cardiovascular death	LV, COR, R + L
4. Valvular heart disease	LV, COR, R + L, AO
5. Congenital heart disease (before anticipated corrective surgery)	LV, COR, R + L, AO
6. Aortic dissection	AO, COR
7. Pericardial constriction or tamponade	LV, COR, R + L
8. Cardiomyopathy	LV, COR, R + L, BX
9. Initial and follow-up assessment for heart transplant	LV, COR, R + L, BX

From Kern MJ: *The cardiac catheterization handbook*, ed 3, St Louis, 2003, Mosby.
AO, Aortography; *BX,* endomyocardial biopsy; *COR,* coronary angiography; *ERGO,* ergonovine provocation of coronary spasm; *ETT,* exercise tolerance test; *LV,* left ventriculography; *R + L,* right and left heart hemodynamics; *RH,* right heart oxygen saturations and hemodynamics (e.g., placement of Swan-Ganz catheter).

In children, diagnostic heart catheterization is employed in the evaluation of congenital and valvular disease, disorders of the cardiac conduction system, and selected cardiomyopathies. Interventional techniques are also performed in children, primarily to alleviate the symptoms associated with certain congenital heart defects.

The indications for cardiac catheterization as established by a special task force to the American College of Cardiology and the American Heart Association (ACC/AHA) are summarized in Table 25-3. The commonly performed procedures based on diagnosis are also presented. Furthermore, the ACC/AHA[1] has classified the indications and appropriateness for coronary angiography by placing the previously discussed disease categories into three classifications:

Class 1—Conditions for which there is general agreement that coronary angiography is justified.

[1]Scanlon PJ et al: ACC/AHA guidelines for coronary angiography: a report of the American College of Cardiology/American Heart Association Task Force on Practice Guidelines (Committee on Coronary Angiography), *J Am Coll Cardiol* 33:1758,1999.

Class 2—Conditions for which coronary angiography is frequently performed, but for which a divergence of opinion exists with respect to its justification in terms of value and appropriateness.

Class 3—Conditions for which coronary angiography ordinarily is not justified.

Other procedures that may be performed concurrently with coronary angiography are listed in Table 25-4. Discussion of some of these procedures occurs later in the text.

TABLE 25-4

Procedures that may accompany coronary angiography

Procedures	Comment
1. Central venous access (femoral, internal jugular, subclavian)	Used as IV access for emergency medications or fluids, temporary pacemaker (pacemaker not mandatory for coronary angiography)
2. Hemodynamic assessment	
a. Left heart pressures (aorta, left ventricle)	Routine for all studies
b. Right and left heart combined pressures	Not routine for coronary artery disease; mandatory for valvular heart disease; routine for CHF, right ventricular dysfunction, pericardial diseases, cardiomyopathy, intracardiac shunts, congenital abnormalities
3. Left ventricular angiography	Routine for all studies; may be excluded with high-risk patients, left main coronary or aortic stenosis, severe CHF
4. Internal mammary selective angiography	Not routine unless used as coronary bypass conduit
5. Pharmacologic studies	
a. Ergonovine	Routine for coronary vasospasm
b. IC/IV/sublingual nitroglycerin	Optionally routine for all studies
6. Aortography	Routine for aortic insufficiency, aortic dissection, aortic aneurysm, with or without aortic stenosis; routine to locate bypass grafts not visualized by selective angiography
7. Digital subtraction angiography	Not routine for coronary angiography; excellent for peripheral vascular disease
8. Cardiac pacing and electrophysiologic studies	Arrhythmia evaluation
9. Interventional and special techniques	Intracoronary flow-pressure for lesion assessment Coronary angioplasty (PTCA) Myocardial biopsy Transseptal or direct left ventricular puncture Balloon catheter valvuloplasty Conduction tract catheter ablation
10. Arterial closure devices	Available for patients with conditions prone to puncture site bleeding

From Kern MJ: *The cardiac catheterization handbook,* ed 3, St Louis, 2003, Mosby.
IV, Intravenous; *CHF,* congestive heart failure; *PTCA,* percutaneous transluminal coronary angioplasty.

CONTRAINDICATIONS, COMPLICATIONS, AND ASSOCIATED RISKS

Cardiac catheterization has associated inherent risk factors. However, many physicians agree that the only absolute contraindications to this procedure are the refusal of the procedure by a mentally competent person and the lack of adequate equipment or catheterization facilities.

Contraindications for cardiac catheterization are relatively few when the appropriateness of the procedure is based on the benefit-risk ratio. Relative contraindications according to the guidelines of the ACC/AHA[1] include the following:

- Active gastrointestinal bleeding
- Acute or chronic renal failure
- Recent stroke
- Fever from infection or the presence of an active infection
- Severe electrolyte imbalance
- Severe anemia
- Short life expectancy because of other illness
- Digitalis intoxication
- Patient refusal of therapeutic treatment such as PTCA or bypass surgery

[1]Scanlon PJ et al: ACC/AHA guidelines for coronary angiography: a report of the American College of Cardiology/American Heart Association Task Force on Practice Guidelines (Committee on Coronary Angiography), *J Am Coll Cardiol* 33:1758,1999.

- Severe uncontrolled hypertension
- Coagulopathy and bleeding disorders
- Acute pulmonary edema
- Uncontrolled ventricular arrhythmias
- Aortic valve endocarditis
- Previous anaphylactic reaction to contrast media

Some of these conditions may be temporary, or they may be treated and reversed before cardiac catheterization is attempted. Cardiac catheterization may proceed if any of the above conditions exist in a patient who is deemed to be unstable from a suspected cardiac cause.

As with any invasive procedure, complications can be expected during cardiac catheterization. The Society for Cardiac Angiography and Interventions (SCA&I) reviewed the catheterizations in more than 300,000 patients from three different time periods and found the major complication rate for the entire group was less than 2%. Those complications are listed in Table 25-5. The risks associated with cardiac catheterization have decreased since the early days of the procedure. However, as the severity of the patient's disease increases, so do the risks associated with the procedure. The risks of cardiac catheterization vary according to the type of procedure and the status of the patient undergoing the procedure. Significantly influencing the outcome of the procedure

is the stability of the patient's condition before the procedure. For example, patients presenting with left main coronary stenosis have a greater than twofold higher risk of complications from coronary angiography than those who have no left main coronary stenosis. The SCA&I database identified the main predictors of major complications following cardiac catheterization and determined that the following increased the risk of complications[1]:

- Moribund patient (patient with poor response to life-threatening condition)
- Cardiogenic shock
- Acute MI (within 24 hours)
- Renal insufficiency
- Cardiomyopathy

Risk variables of less significance include the anatomy to be studied, type of catheter and approach used, history of drug allergy, presence of basic cardiovascular disease or noncardiac disease such as asthma or diabetes, hemodynamic status, and age or other patient characteristics.

Therefore the benefits expected to be derived from cardiac catheterization must be weighed against the associated risks of the procedure when determining whether to perform the procedure.

[1]Laskey W, Boyle J, Johnson LW: Multivariable model for prediction of risk of significant complication during diagnostic cardiac catheterization: the Registry Committee of the Society for Cardiac Angiography and Interventions, *Cathet Cardiovasc Diagn* 30:185, 1993.

TABLE 25-5

Comparison of major complications for diagnostic catheterization

	1979-1998 (N = 53,581 pts) Percent	1984-1987 (N = 222,553 pts) Percent	1984-1987 (N = 59,792 pts) Percent
Death	0.14	0.10	0.11
Myocardial infarction	0.07	0.06	0.05
Cerebrovascular accident (neurologic)	0.07	0.07	0.07
Arrhythmia	0.56	0.47	0.38
Vascular	0.57	0.46	0.43
Hemorrhage	—	0.07	—
Contrast	—	0.23	0.37
Hemodynamic	—	—	0.26
Perforation	—	—	0.03
Other	0.4	0.28	0.28
TOTAL	1.77	1.74	1.70

From Noto TJ et al: Cardiac catheterization 1990: a report to the Registry of the Society for Cardiac Angiography and Interventions (SCA&I), *Cathet Cardiovasc Diagn* 24:75, 1991. *pts,* Patients.

Specialized Equipment

Cardiac catheterization has developed into a highly complex, sophisticated procedure requiring specialized equipment and supplies. Unlike earlier radiographic examinations of the intracardiac structures, modern cardiac catheterization requires more than a simple fluoroscope and a recording modality such as that used in overhead radiography.

Equipment and supplies required for cardiac catheterization can be categorized in three groups: (1) angiographic supplies and equipment, (2) imaging, and (3) ancillary equipment and supplies. The following are examples of equipment typically contained in each group.

ANGIOGRAPHIC SUPPLIES AND EQUIPMENT

Cardiovascular equipment consists of those supplies and equipment needed to perform the procedure. In addition to the equipment mentioned previously for angiographic procedures, there are variations in catheter design to accommodate the coronary arteries. The guidewires used also have several variations in length, stiffness, and coatings depending on the tortuosity of the aorta and iliacs leading to the heart. Because of the complexity and types of procedures performed in a cardiac catheterization laboratory, only a few of the main component items are discussed.

Catheters

The catheters used for left heart cardiac catheterization are similar to those angiographic catheters previously described, except that cardiac catheters are preformed for the cardiac vasculature (Fig. 25-98). Specialized catheters are used for right heart catheterization procedures. Unlike angiographic catheters whose main purpose is as a conduit for contrast media, right heart catheters are typically flow-directed catheters that use an inflated balloon on the tip of the catheter to ease passage through the various chambers of the heart. Moreover, various types of flow-directed catheters are capable of performing more tasks than the standard angiographic catheter. Depending on the type of procedure to be performed, the physician will decide which catheter to use.

Therefore the catheter (or catheters) placed in a patient's vasculature can function as a fluid-filled column for hemodynamic data or as a conduit for contrast media, thrombolytic agents, and mechanical devices. Blood samples can be drawn directly from selected cardiac chambers for the purpose of oximetry or other laboratory analysis. To perform these and other tasks, three or four valves (*stopcocks*) are combined to form a *manifold*, which is attached to the proximal end of the catheter (Fig. 25-99). Using a manifold allows such functions as drawing blood samples, administering medications, and recording blood pressures without disconnecting from the catheter.

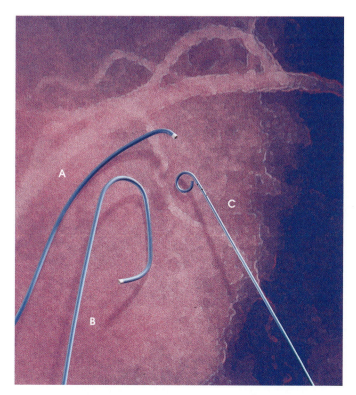

Fig. 25-98 Catheters used during cardiac catheterization. **A,** Judkins right. **B,** Judkins left. **C,** Pigtail.

(Courtesy Cordis Corp., Miami, Fla.)

Fig. 25-99 Disposable three-valve Compensator Morse manifold, with a Selector catheter **(A),** rotating adapter **(B),** pressure transducer **(C),** and angiographic control syringe **(D).**

(Courtesy SCHNEIDER/NAMIC, Glens Falls, NY.)

Contrast media

Injection of contrast media is essential for angiographic visualization of the cardiac anatomy. Several iodinated radiographic contrast media are approved for intravascular, intracardiac, and intracoronary use in both adults and children. However, many of these high-osmolar ionic contrast media have been noted to cause hemodynamic and electrophysiologic effects during administration. Transient (temporary) electrocardiographic (ECG) changes during and immediately after the injection of contrast medium are common.

Less viscous (low-osmolar), nonionic contrast agents that were developed in the 1980s have been found to exhibit the same radiopacity as their counterparts. Because of their properties, nonionic contrast media and ionic low-osmolar contrast media have gained acceptance and are now used in many cardiac catheterization laboratories. Nonionic contrast media have some definite advantages over ionic high-osmolar contrast media. For example, they are associated with a reduced incidence of cardiovascular reactions and side effects as a result of their lower osmotic pressure. Unfortunately, the newer contrast media are considerably more expensive. Due to their cost, most catheterization laboratories now restrict the use of the low-osmolality agents for those patients who are considered to be at a higher risk for contrast agent reactions.

Pressure injector

The pressure injector for the administration of radiographic contrast medium (Fig. 25-100) as previously discussed in Injection Techniques is also used during cardiac catheterization. In the catheterization laboratory, the pressure injector is used to inject a large amount (25 to 50 mL) of contrast material into either the right or left ventricle (the main pumping chambers of the heart), the aortic root, or the pulmonary vessels. Because the coronary arteries are of small caliber and of low flow rate, administration of contrast medium into these structures generally does not require a high-pressure injector. Instead, most physicians opt for manual injection using an angiographic control syringe (see Fig. 25-99). At some facilities, power injectors with a 4-Fr catheter system are used so that the least amount of contrast media is used and the possibility of introducing air into a coronary artery is reduced.

IMAGING

Image chain

The imaging equipment found in the cardiac catheterization laboratory is essentially the same as that found in the vascular angiography suite. The catheterization laboratory requires a system capable of producing fluoroscopic images with the greatest amount of recorded detail available. Maximum resolution from the optical system is crucial due to the small size of the cardiac anatomy, which must be imaged while in motion.

Angiographic x-ray tubes must be capable of producing ionizing radiation for the long periods of time necessary for fluoroscopy and therefore must be designed

Fig. 25-100 The Angiomat (ILLUMENA) high-pressure injector for radiographic contrast medium.

(Courtesy Liebel-Flarsheim, a product of Mallinckrodt, Inc., Cincinnati, Ohio.)

to withstand greater heat loading. Ideally angiographic tubes should have a heat load capacity of 1.5 million heat units or greater. For most cardiac imaging, multifocal-spot, high-speed rotating fluoroscopic tubes are desirable. Extremely short exposure times are required to accommodate the rapid-exposure sequencing of the various recording systems.

A high-resolution imaging and recording system requires several pieces of equipment, including an image intensifier tube. This tube should produce the maximum recorded detail necessary for cardiac catheterization. The image intensifier used in the cardiac catheterization laboratory generally comes with three different field of view modes (5 in, 7 in, 9 in) to allow for enhanced visualization of small anatomic structures. A video camera is optically coupled to the output phosphor of the image intensifier, and its signal is fed to television monitors placed so that the fluoroscopic images can be easily viewed during the procedure.

The imaging used for cardiac studies is typically 15 to 30 frames per second compared with 2 to 6 frames per second for peripheral imaging. The motion of the heart beating requires this increased frame rate to properly visualize these small arteries well.

Digital angiography imaging equipment

Digital angiography has gained universal acceptance in the catheterization laboratory. Digital imaging now produces resolution comparable with that of the 35-mm cineangiographic film image. The resolution possible with early digital equipment was a drawback to the use of digital imaging in the catheterization laboratory. Larger matrix size, the obvious solution to this problem, allowed for acceptable resolution but also created another problem: how to acquire and store large volumes of digital information.

In the late 1970s and early 1980s, the high-speed parallel transfer disk was introduced to solve the acquisition and short-term storage problem. This new disk acquired and stored an entire coronary angiogram and made real-time digital playback during the procedure possible. However, permanent storage of the digital images remained a problem. Floppy disk and computer tape storage were not adequate solutions because they required significant amounts of time and supplies.

Recently, long-term storage of large amounts of digital images has benefited from advances in computer technology. Larger hard drives, digital tape storage, optical disks, compact discs, and digital video disks (DVDs) are a few of the new storage media. These storage devices provide a high-speed, large-capacity method of storage, capable of acquiring large amounts of data (terabytes) with very high resolution. However, the long-term stability of these media has not been tested, and the need to routinely update the images recorded on them have been raised.

A problem incumbent with digital imaging is the incompatibility of the storage media from one system to the other. As more laboratories are becoming equipped with digital systems, the tendency has been to configure digital systems that can be easily updated and interfaced to image networks. A committee composed of industry representatives was established to set standards for digital imaging. The *Digital Communications Committee* (DICOM) has set guidelines for a universal exchange standard in digital imaging. The committee determined that the compact disc recordable (CD-R) would be the preferred transfer medium for single-patient study transfer between institutions. The CD-R, which is the same size as the compact disc read-only memory (CD-ROM), is a one-time recording medium capable of storing 650 megabytes (MB) of information. Because the CD-R can store such a large amount of information, it is quickly becoming the equivalent of a cineangiography film. Applications involving DVD are still evolving. Eventually it will be possible to store up to 14 GB of information on one DVD. Following the introduction of the computer in medicine, the practice and development of radiologic procedures rapidly expanded. Specifically in procedures discussed in this chapter, the computer assisted in major advancements.

One disadvantage of the CD-R is the need to purchase the equipment to download and play back the images. Until recently, all catheterization laboratories had a cineangiographic projector to view 35-mm film angiograms. Now, most laboratories are completely digital. The speculation that digital imaging systems will someday replace cineangiography film as the standard for cardiac catheterization imaging is now a reality. Problems regarding ways to transport and view digital images easily have been addressed by the DICOM standard. To conform to this standard, equipment manufacturers continue to produce digital products that can be accessed by any other manufacturer's product line.

Fig. 25-101 Computer-based physiologic monitor used to monitor patient ECG and hemodynamic pressures during cardiac catheterization.

(Courtesy Quinton Instrument Co., Bothell, Wash.)

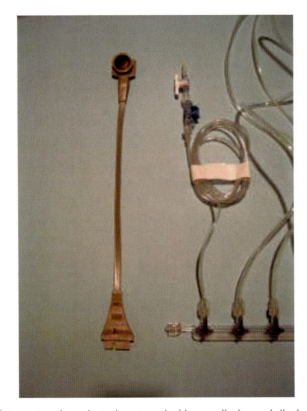

Fig. 25-102 The pressure transducer is connected to a catheter such that a patient's pressure is transmitted along the catheter and converted to an electrical signal that is displayed on a hemodynamic monitor. A manifold used in cardiac studies is on the right.

ANCILLARY EQUIPMENT AND SUPPLIES
Physiologic equipment

The physiologic monitor is essential to cardiac catheterization procedures. It is used to monitor and record vital patient functions, including electrical activity (ECG)* within the heart and blood pressure (hemodynamic) within the various intracardiac chambers (Fig. 25-101). The patient's ECG and hemodynamic pressures are continuously displayed throughout the various types of procedures. (Selective samplings of ECG and hemodynamic pressures are recorded for permanent documentation.)

For the collection of hemodynamic data during catheterization, the physiologic recorder (receiving information in electrical form) must be connected to the catheter (carrying information as physical fluid pressure). Devices called *pressure transducers* are interfaced between the manifold and the physiologic recorder to convert fluid (blood) pressure into an electrical signal (Fig. 25-102).

For a standard cardiac catheterization procedure, four channels of the physiologic recorder are usually prepared: two for ECG recordings and two for pressure recordings. However, a physiologic recorder can have as many as 32 *channels*. A channel, or module, is an electrical component of the physiologic recorder that is capable of measuring an individual parameter such as a specific type of ECG or intravascular pressure. The number of channels required for a particular catheterization increases as the amount of detailed information required increases. Increasingly these monitoring systems are produced with detailed procedural databases for the collection and maintenance of patient clinical data as well as the concurrent generation of a procedural report at the time of catheterization.

---

*Interpretation of ECG is beyond the scope of this chapter.

In addition to the basic coronary angiogram and left and right heart studies, there are many effective tools used to diagnose and treat coronary artery disease (Table 25-6).

Other equipment

Because of the nature of the patient's condition, the inherent risks of cardiac catheterization, and the types of procedures performed, each catheterization room should have the following equipment available:

- A fully equipped emergency cart. The cart typically contains emergency medications, cardiopulmonary resuscitation equipment, intubation equipment, and other related supplies.

- Oxygen and suction.
- Whole blood oximeters used to determine the oxygen saturation of the blood samples obtained during adult and pediatric catheterizations (Fig. 25-103).
- Defibrillator, used to treat life-threatening arrhythmias. Ideally, the defibrillator would also have external pacemaking capabilities.
- Temporary pacemaker to treat potential asystole or symptomatic bradycardia.
- Pulse oximeter to noninvasively monitor and assess level of oxygenation during sedation.
- Noninvasive blood pressure cuff.
- Equipment to perform cardiac output studies.
- Intraaortic balloon pump console and catheters to treat cardiogenic shock.
- ACT (activated clotting time) machine to measure levels of heparinization during interventional procedures.

Fig. 25-103 Oximeter used to measure oxygen saturation in blood.

TABLE 25-6

Tools for diagnosis and treatment of coronary artery disease

Equipment	Use	Diagnostic or Therapeutic
Pressure wire	Measures blood flow across lesion to determine severity of stenosis	Diagnostic
IVUS	Internal vessel visualization of stenosis, plaque, stent position	Diagnostic
Rotablator	Rotational atherectomy of intraluminal plaque/calcium	Therapeutic
Rhelytic thrombectomy device	High-velocity saline spray for thrombectomy	Therapeutic
The Crosser	Study device to cross CTOs	Therapeutic

CTOs, Chronic total occlusions; IVUS, intravascular ultrasound.

Patient Positioning for Cardiac Catheterization

Procedures such as selective coronary arteriography and certain pediatric catheterizations require imaging equipment to be positioned to reduce the superimposition created by the cardiac vasculature. Moving the patient during the catheterization is not desirable, particularly when catheters have been carefully positioned to demonstrate specific anatomic structures or to record certain data.

In most catheterization laboratories, the image intensifier and fluoroscopic tube are mechanically suspended in a C-arm configuration to allow for equipment rotation around the patient and to provide cranial or caudal angulation. In this configuration, the image intensifier is above the plane of the table, and the fluoroscopic tube is beneath the table. During catheterization procedures, the patient is placed on the examination table in a supine position. For optimal images, the imaging equipment should be rotated around the patient. In some interventional procedures, biplane C-arms are advantageous because they allow simultaneous imaging of cardiac structures in two different planes (Fig. 25-104).

Adult and pediatric coronary anatomy has both normal and pathologic variations. Therefore projections for each type of catheterization procedure cannot be specified. Instead, each patient's anatomy must be fluoroscopically evaluated to ascertain the optimum degree of rotation and cranial or caudal angulation necessary to visualize each structure of interest.

Fig. 25-104 A, Biplane radiology equipment used in the cardiac catheterization laboratory. **B,** Modern single-plane digital catheterization with "smart handle" technology.

(Courtesy Toshiba America Medical Systems.)

Catheterization Methods and Techniques

Different cardiac catheterizations require various combinations of methods and techniques to allow for precise data acquisition and the application of therapeutic interventions. Some methods and techniques common to most cardiac catheterizations are discussed in the following sections.

PRECATHETERIZATION CARE

Before the catheterization is performed, the procedure is explained and informed consent is obtained. Testing before catheterization normally includes the following:

- Patient history
- Physical examination
- Chest x-ray examination
- Blood work
- ECG
- Echocardiogram
- Exercise stress test
- Nuclear medicine cardiac perfusion studies

Various medications are frequently administered for sedation and control of nausea. Patients brought to the catheterization laboratory typically are not allowed anything to eat or drink for 4 to 6 hours before the procedure. During all catheterizations, a protocol (or detailed record) of the procedure is maintained. The record includes hemodynamic data, fluoroscopy time, medications administered, supplies used, and other pertinent information.

CATHETER INTRODUCTION

After the patient has been transported to the catheterization laboratory, ECG, noninvasive blood pressure monitoring, and, in some institutions, *pulse oximetry* are initiated. The appropriate site for catheter introduction must be prepared using aseptic technique to minimize the risk of subsequent infection. The area of the body to be entered is shaved, and an antiseptic solution is applied. Numerous sites can be used for catheter introduction. The specific sites vary according to the age and body habitus of the patient, the preference of the physician, and the procedure attempted. The most frequent site used for catheterization is the femoral area. However, the radial, brachial,

axillary, jugular (neck), and subclavian (chest) areas may also be chosen.

For catheterization of the femoral artery or vein, the percutaneous approach is employed (see the Seldinger technique, which is described and illustrated in Fig. 25-15). Once vascular access is obtained, an introducer sheath is placed over the guidewire and advanced into the vessel. This creates a controlled access into which catheters may be introduced with very little blood loss. The catheter is placed over the guidewire and advanced toward the heart. The guidewire may be removed or temporarily left in place to facilitate further placement of the catheter. When the catheter is in the proper position, the guidewire is removed, the catheter is connected to the manifold, and the coronary angiogram may begin.

If the percutaneous approach cannot be used, a cut-down technique is employed. This technique requires that a small incision be made in the skin to allow for direct visualization of the artery or vein that the physician wants to catheterize. The skin is aseptically prepared and infiltrated with local anesthetic, and the vessel or vessels are bluntly dissected and exposed. After an opening is created in the desired vessel (arteriotomy or venotomy), the catheter is introduced and advanced toward the heart. Cut-down procedures are frequently performed in the right antecubital fossa to access the basilic vein or brachial artery.

DATA COLLECTION

The acquisition of certain data is essential, regardless of the type of catheterization performed. Physiologic data typically collected include hemodynamic parameters, ECG, and oximetry readings.

Hemodynamic parameters include blood pressure and cardiac output. The monitoring and recording of both intracardiac (within the heart) and extracardiac (outside the heart) vascular pressures require the use of the physiologic-transducer system described previously in this chapter. Cardiac output, an important indicator of the overall ability of the heart to pump blood, can be measured in the catheterization laboratory. Several methods are used to obtain estimates of cardiac output. The ECG is continuously monitored during catheterization and can be simultaneously recorded with intracardiac or extracardiac pressures (Fig. 25-105). Blood samples are obtained from the various chambers of the heart to determine oxygen saturation levels and the presence of any intracardiac shunts.

Fig. 25-105 Simulated electrocardiogram *(top)* and aortic pressure *(bottom)*.

(Courtesy Quinton Instrument Co., Bothell, Wash.)

Catheterization Studies and Procedures

The primary purpose of the diagnostic cardiac catheterization is data collection, whereas the primary purpose of the interventional procedure is therapy. The following sections briefly describe some of the more commonly performed diagnostic and interventional heart catheterizations.

BASIC DIAGNOSTIC STUDIES OF THE VASCULAR SYSTEM

Adults

Catheterization of the left side of the heart is a widely performed, basic diagnostic cardiac study. The catheter may be introduced through the radial, brachial, or femoral artery and advanced over a guidewire to the ascending aorta. Once in the ascending aorta, the guidewire is removed and the catheter aspirated and flushed to prevent migration of any air bubbles. Aortic root angiography may be performed to document the competence of the aortic valve. A normal aortic valve prevents backward flow of contrast media into the left ventricle during injection, whereas an insufficient valve does not (Fig. 25-106). Arterial oximetry and blood pressure measurements within the aorta are taken using the manifold system. Once this has been accomplished, the catheter is passed through the aortic valve into the left ventricle.

Once again, arterial oximetry is performed, and blood pressure measurements are taken in the left ventricle. Angiography of the left ventricle is performed in nearly all catheterization studies of the left side of the heart (Fig. 25-107). Left ventriculography provides information about valvular competence, interventricular septal integrity, and the efficiency of the pumping action of the left ventricle (ejection fraction). Mitral regurgitation is another example of valvular incompetence and angiographically it is seen as the backward flow of contrast media from the left ventricle into the left atrium or pulmonary veins (Fig. 25-108). The *ejection fraction* (EF) of the left ventricle is determined angiographically by superimposing images of the left ventricle at end *diastole* and at end *systole* and expressed as a percentage. Computer *planimetry* software, which is now available on most digital systems, then calculates how well the ventricle functions (Fig. 25-109). Following left ventriculography, the presence of aortic valve stenosis is determined as the blood pressure measurements are repeated while the catheter is withdrawn across the aortic valve. Normal flow of blood through the aortic valve allows the systolic pressure in the left ventricle to match the systolic pressure in the aorta. When the systolic blood pressure in the left ventricle is greater than the systolic blood pressure in the aorta, aortic stenosis is present (Fig. 25-110).

Following a catheter exchange, selective angiography of the right coronary artery and left coronary artery is performed, with different projections used for each coronary artery to prevent superimposition with overlapping structures. Coronary angiography allows the extent of intracoronary stenosis to be evaluated (Figs. 25-111 and 25-112).

Fig. 25-106 Left ventriculogram demonstrating aortic insufficiency with contrast flowing back into the left ventricle *(white arrowheads)*.

Fig. 25-107 Normal left ventriculogram during diastole.

Fig. 25-108 Left ventriculogram demonstrating mitral valve regurgitation.

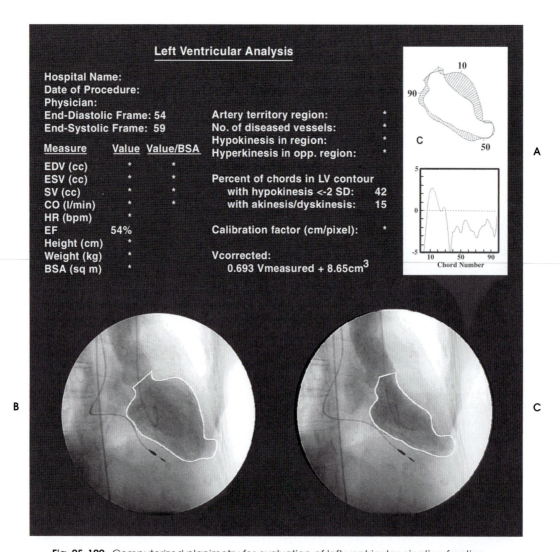

Left Ventricular Analysis

Hospital Name:
Date of Procedure:
Physician:
End-Diastolic Frame: 54
End-Systolic Frame: 59

Measure	Value	Value/BSA
EDV (cc)	*	*
ESV (cc)	*	*
SV (cc)	*	*
CO (l/min)	*	*
HR (bpm)	*	
EF	54%	
Height (cm)	*	
Weight (kg)	*	
BSA (sq m)	*	

Artery territory region: *
No. of diseased vessels: *
Hypokinesis in region: *
Hyperkinesis in opp. region: *

Percent of chords in LV contour
  with hypokinesis <-2 SD: 42
  with akinesis/dyskinesis: 15

Calibration factor (cm/pixel): *

Vcorrected:
  0.693 Vmeasured + 8.65cm^3

Fig. 25-109 Computerized planimetry for evaluation of left ventricular ejection fraction. **A,** Diastolic phase of the heart's contraction. **B,** Systolic phase of the heart's contraction. **C,** Digital representation of when the diastolic and systolic phases of the heart's contraction are superimposed.

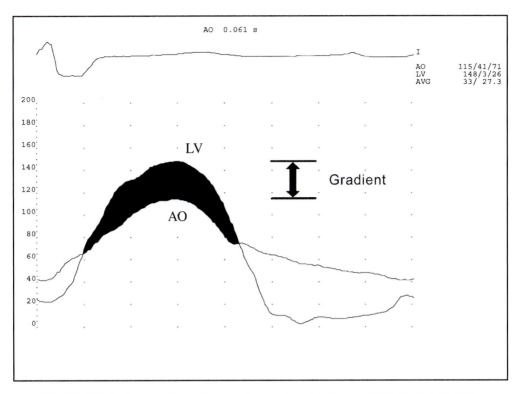

AO	115/41/71
LV	148/3/26
AVG	33/ 27.3

AO 0.061 s

Fig. 25-110 Aortic stenosis results when the aortic valve does not fully open during systole, resulting in an increase in left ventricular pressure.

Fig. 25-111 Normal right coronary artery.

Fig. 25-112 Normal left coronary artery.

Because of the complexity of the anatomy involved, the variations in patient body habitus, and the presence of anomalies, a comprehensive guide for angiographic projections is difficult to establish. Projections commonly used during coronary angiography are included in Table 25-7. The physician determines the projections that best demonstrate the artery of interest. Coronary arteriograms are obtained in nearly all catheterizations of the left side of the heart.

Catheterization of the right side of the heart is another commonly performed procedure. During right heart catheterization, a catheter is inserted into a vein in the groin, antecubital fossa, internal jugular, or subclavian and advanced to the vena cava, into the right atrium, across the tricuspid valve, to the right ventricle, and through the pulmonary valve to the pulmonary artery, until it is wedged distally in the pulmonary artery. Pressure measurements and oximetry are performed in each of the heart chambers as the catheter is advanced. The pressure measurements are used to determine the presence of such disorders as valvular heart disease, congestive heart failure, pulmonary hypertension and certain cardiomyopathies. The oximetry data are used to determine the presence of an intracardiac shunt. Cineangiography is performed as appropriate.

Exercise hemodynamics are often required in the evaluation of valvular heart disease when symptoms of fatigue and dyspnea are present. In such cases, simultaneous catheterization and pressure measurements of the right and left heart are performed at rest and during peak exercise. Exercise often consists of pedaling a stationary bicycle, exercise-type device—an ergometer—that is placed on top of the examination table. During simultaneous catheterization, a catheter is placed in a vein (femoral or basilic) and an artery (femoral or brachial).

Children

A primary indication for diagnostic catheterization studies in children is the evaluation and documentation of specific anatomy, hemodynamic data, and selected aspects of cardiac function associated with congenital heart defects. Methods and techniques used for catheterization of the pediatric heart vary depending on age, heart size, type and extent of defect, and other coincident pathophysiologic conditions.

Pediatric cardiac catheters are often introduced percutaneously into the femoral vein and, in older children, sometimes into the femoral artery. In very young patients, it may be possible to pass a catheter from the right atrium to the left atrium (thereby allowing access to the left side of the heart) through either a patent foramen ovale or a preexisting atrial septal defect. If the atrial septum is intact, temporary access to the left atrium may be obtained using a transseptal catheter system. With the transseptal catheter system, a long introducer and needle are used to puncture the right atrial septum of the heart to gain access to the left atrium if access cannot be attained as previously described.

TABLE 25-7
Common angiographic angles for specific coronary arteries

Coronary artery	Vessel segment	Projections
Left coronary artery	Left main	PA or RAO 5-15 degrees
	Left anterior descending	LAO 30-40 degrees, cranial 20-40 degrees
		RAO 5-15 degrees, cranial 15-45 degrees
		RAO 20-40 degrees, caudal 15-30 degrees
		RAO 30-50 degrees
		Lateral
	Circumflex	RAO 20-40 degrees, caudal 15-30 degrees
		LAO 40-55 degrees, caudal 15-30 degrees
		LAO 40-60 degrees
Right coronary artery	Middle right	LAO 20-40 degrees
		RAO 20-40 degrees
	Posterior descending	LAO 5-30 degrees, cranial 15-30 degrees

LAO, Left anterior oblique; *PA,* posteroanterior; *RAO,* right anterior oblique.

ADVANCED DIAGNOSTIC STUDIES OF THE VASCULAR SYSTEM: ADULTS AND CHILDREN

An example of an advanced diagnostic study of the vascular system is endomyocardial biopsy, which is performed to provide a tissue sample for direct pathologic evaluation of cardiac muscle. A special biopsy catheter with a bioptome tip (Fig. 25-113) is advanced under fluoroscopic control from either the jugular or femoral vein to the right ventricle (Fig. 25-114). After the bioptome is advanced into the ventricle, the jaws of the device are opened and the catheter is advanced to the ventricular septum. After the bioptome is in contact with the septum, its jaws are closed and a gentle tugging motion is applied to retrieve the tissue sample. Several biopsy specimens are acquired in this manner. The specimens are immediately fixed in either glutaraldehyde or buffered formalin before being sent for pathologic evaluation. Endomyocardial biopsy is frequently used to monitor cardiac transplantation patients for early signs of tissue rejection and to differentiate between various types of cardiomyopathies.

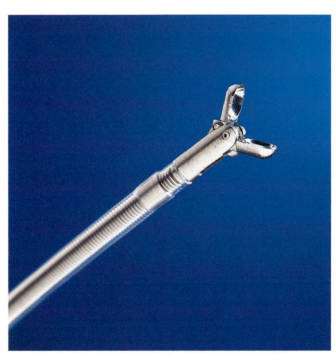

A   B

Fig. 25-113 A, Standard biopsy catheters. **B,** Bioptome catheter tip used for myocardial biopsy. The jaws on the tip close and take a "bite" from the inside of the heart muscle.

(Courtesy Cordis Corp., Miami, Fla.)

Fig. 25-114 The bioptome tip in the right ventricular apex points toward the ventricular septum.

ADVANCED DIAGNOSTIC STUDIES OF THE CONDUCTION SYSTEM: ADULTS AND CHILDREN

Electrophysiology studies involve the collection of sophisticated data to facilitate detailed mapping of the electrical conduction system within the heart. The procedures involve the placement of numerous multipolar catheters within the heart (Fig. 25-115). Electrophysiology studies are used to analyze the conduction system, induce and evaluate arrhythmias, and determine the effects of therapeutic measures in treating arrhythmias.

Electrode catheters are introduced into the femoral vein, internal jugular vein, or subclavian vein. Because several catheters are used, multiple access sites are needed. It is not uncommon to have three introducer sheaths placed within the same vein. The catheters consist of several insulated wires, each of which is attached to an electrode on the catheter tip that serves as an interface with the intracardiac surface. The arrangements of the electrodes on the catheter allow its dual function of recording the electrical signals of the heart (intracardiac electrograms) and pacing the heart. The pacemaker function is performed to introduce premature electrical impulses to determine possible arrhythmias. After characterization of the precise defect occurs, an appropriate course of therapy can be undertaken.

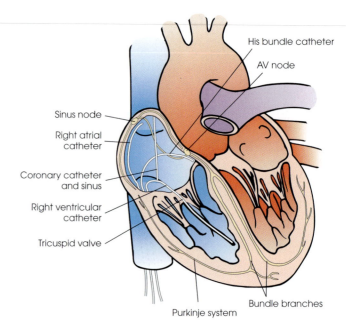

Fig. 25-115 Catheter positions for routine electrophysiologic study. Multipolar catheters are positioned in the high right atrium near the sinus node, in the area of the atrioventricular apex, and in the coronary sinus.

INTERVENTIONAL PROCEDURES OF THE VASCULAR SYSTEM
Adults

Interventional cardiac catheterization techniques requiring special-purpose catheters have expanded significantly since the late 1970s. PTCA is a technique that employs balloon dilation of a coronary artery stenosis to increase blood flow to the heart muscle. Gruentzig performed the first successful PTCA in 1977.

During PTCA, a specially designed guiding catheter is placed into the orifice of the stenotic coronary artery as determined by coronary angiography (Fig. 25-116). A steerable guidewire is inserted into the balloon catheter and advanced within the guiding catheter (Fig. 25-117). The guidewire is advanced across the stenotic area; it serves as a support platform so that the balloon catheter can be advanced and centered across the steno-

sis. Controlled and precise inflation of the balloon fractures and compresses the fatty deposits into the muscular wall of the artery. This compression, in conjunction with the stretching of the external vessel diameter, is necessary for successful angioplasty. The balloon is deflated to allow rapid reperfusion of blood to the heart muscle. The inflation procedure, followed by arteriography, may be repeated several times until a satisfactory degree

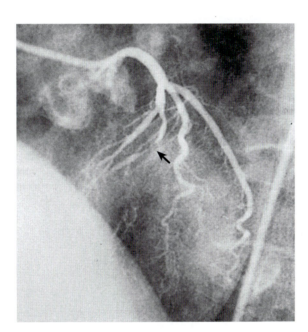

Fig. 25-116 Stenotic coronary artery before PTCA. The arrow indicates the stenotic area, estimated at 95%, with minimum blood flow distal to the lesion.

Fig. 25-117 Catheter system for PTCA. The three sections of the system are the outer guiding catheter *(right)*, central balloon catheter *(middle)*, and internal steerable guidewire *(left)*.

(Courtesy Cordis Corp., Miami, Fla.)

Fig. 25-118 Coronary arteriogram after PTCA in the same patient as in Fig. 25-116. The blood flow is estimated to be 100%.

of patency is observed (Fig. 25-118). The limiting factor of PTCA is restenosis, which occurs in approximately 30% to 50% of the patients who undergo the procedure.

Another interventional procedure being performed most frequently on adult patients with coronary artery stenosis is the placement of an expandable intracoronary stent. The procedure is similar to PTCA and is performed in the same manner, except that a metallic stent is mounted on the PTCA balloon (Fig. 25-119). For optimum stent deployment, the stent is centered across the entire length of the stenosis. Deployment of the stent is achieved with the inflation and deflation of the PTCA balloon. After the stent is deployed, the angioplasty balloon is removed and a high-pressure balloon is advanced within the stent. Inflation of the high-pressure balloon is performed to embed the metallic struts of the stent in the walls of the blood vessel. Restenosis rates are lower in patients receiving intracoronary stents than in those who undergo conventional angioplasty.

A

B

Fig. 25-119 Balloon expandable intracoronary stent: **A,** before stent balloon inflation; **B,** after stent balloon inflation.

Atherectomy devices have also been used in the treatment of coronary artery disease. Unlike PTCA balloons, atherectomy devices remove the fatty deposit or thrombus material from within the artery (Fig. 25-120). The directional coronary atherectomy (DCA) procedure uses a specially designed cutting device to shave the plaque out of the lumen of the artery. As the cutting blade is advanced, the excised atheroma is pushed forward into the distal nose-cone collection chamber.

Another type of atherectomy device called a Rotablator has been indicated in the use of atherosclerotic coronary artery disease. Commonly referred to as PTCRA (percutaneous transluminal coronary rotational atherectomy), it can be used in conjunction with PTCA and/or stenting. The tip of the catheter (1.25 to 2.5 mm in diameter) resembles a football and is embedded with microscopic diamond particles on the front half and is rotated on a special torque guidewire between 160,000 and 200,000 rpm (Fig. 25-121 and 25-122).

Fig. 25-120 Coronary atherectomy device used during directional coronary atherectomy. The balloon on the inferior aspect of the cutting device is inflated inside the coronary artery; plaque is forced into the opening, then shaved off and collected in the tip.

(Courtesy Guidant Vascular Intervention, Santa Clara, Calif.)

Fig. 25-121 Rotational atherectomy catheter with advancer unit. Insert shows "football"-shaped burr.

Fig. 25-122 Cart that is used with Rotablator with the nitrogen tank to run the burr in blue on the side, with the power unit on top and boxes with equipment below.

Standard angioplasty catheter positioning techniques are used to position a guidewire distal to the targeted lesion. A rotational atherectomy burr size is selected and advanced over the special torque guidewire just proximal to the lesion. At this point, the burr is activated and the plaque is pulverized and reduced to the size of a blood cell. The pulverized plaque is removed by the reticuloendothelial system. After an adequate amount of plaque is cleared, standard PTCA and/or stenting techniques are employed to maintain artery patency (Fig. 25-123). PTCRA has proven to be a benefit in the treatment of in-stent restenosis when compared with PTCA alone.

While coronary angiography remains the "gold standard" for the diagnosis of coronary artery disease, *intravascular ultrasound* (IVUS) offers further diagnostic and interventional information that cannot be appreciated by angiography alone. IVUS allows a full 360-degree circumference visualization of the vessel wall, permits information regarding vascular pathology and longitudinal and volumetric measurements, and facilitates guidance of catheter-based interventions. The intervention-associated potential of IVUS is the ability to optimize the type and size of device (i.e., PTCA/stent vs. Rotablator, atherectomy) being used and to determine proper apposition of the stent after deployment against the artery wall.

PTCA and/or stent interventions by far remain the bulk of the coronary interventions being performed today. Of major concern are dissection at the proximal and distal ends of the stent and complete apposition of the stent against the vessel wall (Fig. 25-124). A large observational study following angiography-guided stent deployment revealed an average residual plaque area of 51%, comparing minimum stent diameter with the normal artery. Additional balloon inflations resulted in a final average residual stenosis of 34%, even though the final angiographic percentage stenosis was negative (−0.7%).[1]

[1]Colombo A, Hall P, Nakamura S, et al: Intracoronary stenting without anticoagulation accomplished with intravascular ultrasound guidance, *Circulation* 91:1676, 1995.

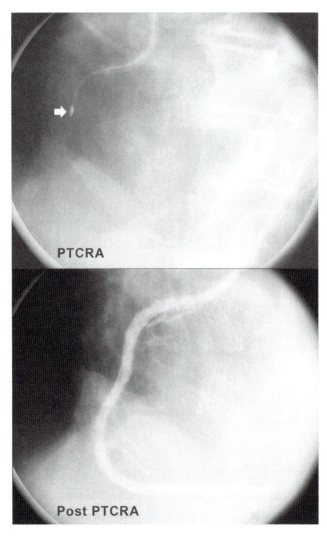

Fig. 25-123 PTCRA. Arrow points to burr of catheter. Post PTCRA shows a widely patent right coronary artery.

Fig. 25-124 IVUS images shown on the right correlated with angiography images on the left. Arrows in **B** show the echogenicity of the stent struts during IVUS.

Components consist of the ultrasound unit, recording device (usually stored on the hard drive and available for recording onto a VCR, CD-ROM, or floppy disk), printer, transducer, pullback device, and catheter (Fig. 25-125). The intravascular catheters being used today use 20- to 40-MHz silicon piezoelectric crystals and range in size from 5 Fr on the proximal end of the catheter to 2.9 Fr at the distal end (Fig. 25-126). During the procedure, the IVUS catheter is advanced over the guidewire that was previously placed within the artery being imaged. The IVUS catheter is advanced distal to the targeted lesion, at which time the transducer and recording device are turned on. Slowly, the catheter is withdrawn using the pullback device to maintain a consistent withdrawal of the catheter and to help ascertain the length of the targeted lesion. A recording device such as a VCR is used to store the acquired dynamic images and the cardiologist's audio dictation during IVUS acquisition. Documentation of IVUS catheter position can be obtained with angiography. This allows the cardiologist to later review, take measurements, and print images from the videotape.

At present, IVUS remains an integral part of coronary interventions being performed. With advances in stent designs, brachytherapy, local drug delivery, and future technologies, IVUS will remain a vital source for information in improving the outcomes of percutaneous coronary interventions. Equipment under investigation combines an imaging transducer with an interventional device, permitting guidance during the interventional procedure. The clinical use of IVUS imaging and other improved computerized image enhancements should allow for more precise data collection and more tailored methods of determining the interventional method to use in treating coronary artery disease.

Because of the risks associated with mechanical interventions of the vascular system, open-heart surgical facilities must be immediately available. Coronary occlusion, for example, is a major complication requiring emergency surgery in patients undergoing catheter-based mechanical interventions.

Interventional pharmacologic procedures in adults consist of the therapeutic administration of medications during cardiac catheterization. An example is the intracoronary infusion of urokinase, which is a thrombolytic agent used in the early hours of an acute MI in an effort to modify its course. Estimates indicate that thrombotic coronary artery occlusion is present in 75% to 85% of patients with acute MI. If reperfusion of the ischemic myocardium is effective, scarring is reduced. Reperfusion in the early stages of MI offers greater potential for heart muscle salvage.

Fig. 25-125 Intravascular ultrasound unit. Shown here are the keyboard, monitor, VCR, and printer.

Fig. 25-126 Intravascular ultrasound catheter and transducer.

Children

A number of congenital cardiac defects in children are amenable to interventional procedures performed in the catheterization laboratory. As with PTCA procedures, cardiovascular surgical support services must be readily available.

When successful, certain pediatric interventional procedures negate the need for surgical correction of defects. However, some procedures are performed for palliative purposes to allow the child to grow to a size and weight at which subsequent open-heart surgery is feasible.

One such technique, *balloon septostomy,* may be used to enlarge a patent foramen ovale or preexisting *atrial septal defect.* Enlargement of the opening enhances the mixing of right and left atrial blood, resulting in an improved level of systemic arterial oxygenation. Transposition of the great arteries is a condition for which atrial septostomy is performed.

Balloon septostomy requires a catheter similar to the type used in PTCA. The balloon is passed through the atrial septal opening into the left atrium, inflated with contrast medium, and then snapped back through the septal orifice. This causes the septum to tear. Often the technique must be repeated until the septal opening is sufficiently enlarged to allow the desired level of blood mixing as documented by oximetry, intracardiac pressures, and angiography.

If the atrial septum does not contain a preexisting opening, an artificial defect can be created. A transseptal system approach is employed, and a special catheter containing an internal folding knife-like blade is advanced into the left atrium (Fig. 25-127). After the catheter is inside the left atrium, the blade is advanced out of its protective outer housing and pulled back to the right atrium, creating an incision in the septal wall. This technique may be repeated. A balloon septostomy is then performed to widen the new opening, and the condition of the patient is monitored by oximetry, blood pressures, and angiography.

A patent ductus arteriosus is sometimes evident in the newborn. In utero the pulmonary artery shunts its blood flow into the aorta through the ductus arteriosus, which normally closes after birth. Patent ductus arteriosus occurs when this channel fails to close spontaneously. In some instances, closure can be induced with medication. If this measure is unsuccessful and the residual shunt is deemed significant, surgical closure (ligation) of the vessel is appropriate.

For some patients, occlusion of a patent ductus arteriosus can be accomplished in the catheterization laboratory. A catheter containing an occlusion device, such as an umbrella, is advanced to the ductus. After the position of the lesion is confirmed by angiography, the occluder is released. Subsequent clotting and fibrous infiltration permanently stop the flow and subsequent mixing of blood.

Fig. 25-127 Blade on catheter tip used to incise septal walls in pediatric interventional procedures.

INTERVENTIONAL PROCEDURES OF THE CONDUCTION SYSTEM: ADULTS AND CHILDREN

Permanent implantation of an antiarrhythmic device is a manipulative procedure that is being performed with greater frequency in cardiac catheterization laboratories, rather than in operating rooms (Fig. 25-128). Antiarrhythmic devices include pacemakers for patients with bradyarrhythmias and/or disease of the electrical conduction system of the heart and implantable cardioverter defibrillators (ICDs) for patients with lethal ventricular tachyarrhythmias originating from the bottom of the heart.

Pacemaker implantation can be successfully performed under local anesthesia in selected adult and pediatric patients. ICD implantation requires conscious sedation or general anesthesia because of the type of testing required at the time of implantation. Insertion of either a pacemaker or an ICD involves puncturing the subclavian or cephalic vein and introducing leads (electrically insulated wires with distal electrodes). The leads are manipulated so that their tips are in direct contact with the right ventricular or right atrial endocardium, or both. The leads are then tested for stimulation and sensing properties to ascertain proper functioning before they

A

B

Fig. 25-128 A, Single-chamber and dual-chamber pacemakers. **B,** Implantable cardioverter defibrillator.

(Courtesy Guidant Corp., Cardiac Pacemakers, Inc., St Paul, Minn.)

are attached to the pulse generator. During ICD implantation, defibrillation threshold testing is performed to determine the amount of energy required to defibrillate a patient from ventricular tachycardia or fibrillation. After testing is completed, the proximal end of the lead(s) is then attached to a battery pack (pacemaker or ICD) and implanted in a subcutaneous or subpectoral pocket created in the thorax (Fig. 25-129). Current pacemakers have longevity of 5 to 10 years, and ICDs have longevity of 6 to 8 years.

Another interventional procedure being performed to treat disorders of the conduction system in the cardiac catheterization laboratory is radiofrequency (RF) ablation. Several different arrhythmias previously treated with ICD implantation or drug therapy can now be treated with RF ablation. The procedure is normally performed at the time of the diagnostic electrophysiology study if an underlying mechanism or arrhythmogenic focus is identified.

RF ablation is achieved by delivering a low-voltage, high-frequency alternating current directly to the endocardial tissue through a specially designed ablation catheter. The current desiccates the underlying abnormal myocardial conduction tissue and creates a small, discrete burn lesion. Localized RF lesions create areas of tissue necrosis and scar, subsequently destroying the arrhythmogenic focus. Several RF lesions may be necessary to eliminate the abnormal conduction circuit.

Follow-up electrophysiologic testing is performed to document the resolution of the arrhythmia. RF ablation of the atrioventricular (AV) node and pacemaker insertion are quickly becoming the preferred treatment for chronic atrial fibrillation with rapid, irregular responses. The AV junction is destroyed intentionally; consequently the rapid, irregular electrical impulses from the atrium are not conducted into the ventricle. A pacemaker is then implanted, and a more consistent, regular heart rate is achieved.

Postcatheterization Care

When the catheterization procedure is completed, all catheters are removed. If a cut-down approach was used, the arteriotomy or venotomy is repaired as appropriate. If a percutaneous approach was used, pressure is placed on the puncture site until the bleeding is controlled. Wound sites are cleaned and dressed to minimize the risk of infection. Elastic dressings are often used to encourage hemostasis.

Postcatheterization medications are prescribed by the physician. The puncture site must be observed for hemorrhage or hematoma, and the status of the distal pulse is recorded on the protocol record before the patient leaves the catheterization laboratory. Vital signs should be monitored regularly for at least 24 hours after the catheterization. The ingestion of fluids should be encouraged, and pain medication may be indicated.

Cardiac catheterization may also be performed on an outpatient or same-day treatment basis. The patient is monitored for 4 to 8 hours in a recovery area and then allowed to go home. Instructions for home-care recovery procedures are usually given to the patient or a family member before the patient leaves the recovery area.

Fig. 25-129 Chest radiograph of a patient with a permanent pacemaker implanted. Note the pacemaker location in the superior and anterior chest wall, with the distal leads located in both the right ventricle and right atrium of the heart.

Cardiac Catheterization Trends

VASCULAR BRACHYTHERAPY

Vascular brachytherapy, also termed *vascular radiotherapy*, is a technique wherein radiation is delivered to an area of a previously stented artery using endovascular techniques. Current radiation sources under consideration are gamma- and beta-emitting sources. Brachytherapy has fallen out of favor after only a few years of regular use. Patients have not responded well to this treatment for in-stent restenosis, coming back still symptomatic, which requires another procedure typically involving a drug-eluting stent placed inside the narrowed area.

The renarrowing *(restenosis)* of the coronary artery in the months following a successful PTCA and/or stenting remains the major limitation to percutaneous coronary revascularization. Studies have shown that following percutaneous coronary revascularization, a complex process whereby remodeling of the angioplasty and/or stented portion of the artery takes place. One such remodeling process is the growth of a new lining of cells over the revascularized site. When this new lining of cells occurs rapidly, the term *neointimal hyperplasia* is used. Neointimal hyperplasia is the result of smooth muscle hyperplasia and matrix proliferation secondary to the revascularization process. Neointimal hyperplasia remains the biggest factor in restenosis after intervention.

An alternative approach to delivered vascular brachytherapy involves the use of stents impregnated with beta isotopes. The isotope slowly decays over a period of 6 months. Studies have shown that in-stent restenosis is minimized with radioactive stents. However, stenoses along the edges of the stent have occurred. Further investigation regarding the type of isotope, radiation dosage, and the effects of radiation on the arterial wall and surrounding tissues are being studied.

DRUG-ELUTING STENT

As previously discussed, restenosis of the coronary artery after revascularization is the major factor in failed long-term outcomes. Drug-coated or drug-eluting stents are now routinely used for the treatment of coronary artery disease. The goal is to reduce or inhibit restenosis that occurs after a revascularization procedure. Two such products on the market have drugs that are chemically bound or coated on a stent; over time, the drug is released in small amounts to inhibit restenosis. The various drugs reduce restenosis by limiting the proliferation of smooth muscle cells and/or reducing the rate at which this occurs. The prevention of restenosis after revascularization remains to be proven. Short-term data have been quite positive. Long-term clinical data from large randomized trials are being investigated.

MAGNETIC RESONANCE IMAGING

Techniques and methods for cardiac catheterization continue to be developed and refined. Angiographic imaging and recording devices are becoming even more sophisticated and therefore yielding ever-greater resolution and detail. MRI (see Chapter 33) of the cardiovascular system is now a well-recognized investigational technique. Magnetic resonance coronary arteriography is now able to reliably assess anomalous coronary artery anatomy and to identify the presence of calcification in the coronary arteries and bypass grafts.

ELECTRON BEAM COMPUTED TOMOGRAPHY

Recently, an area receiving much recognition in the study of coronary artery disease is the use of electron beam tomography (EBT) imaging. Many manufacturers are working on similar imaging equipment by using ultrafast CT scanning coupled with software reconstruction algorithms to accomplish the goal of noninvasive coronary angiography (see Chapter 31). EBT can detect heart disease at its earliest and most treatable stages by measuring the amount of coronary calcium. The coronary calcium score provides a good indication of the amount of artery blockage.

The patient lies on a table similar to that for a conventional CT scan. The significant difference between a conventional CT scanner and EBT is the exposure time. Exposure time for the EBT is approximately 100 milliseconds. This typically results in about 30 to 40 scans and the ability to scan the entire heart in a single breath hold.

Another technique using the EBT involves the injection of contrast media intravenously. The term *electron beam angiography* (EBA) is a simple and noninvasive technique that uses an IV venous injection of contrast media. EBA is effective for visualization of the heart, great vessels, carotid arteries, and peripheral vasculature. EBA demonstrates the coronary arteries with a high degree of accuracy when compared with conventional angiography.

Many experts believe that the greatest area for growth in the field of cardiac catheterization is in interventional procedures. Despite the use of such techniques as PTCA, intracoronary stenting, and atherectomy in coronary artery disease, restenosis continues to be prevalent and of major concern. The majority of the research in interventional procedures is geared toward finding a technique to prevent or greatly limit restenosis after an intervention. Procedures classified as experimental or investigational in the late 1980s are now being performed regularly. Existing and new interventional procedures should continue to provide patients with viable, relatively low-risk, financially reasonable alternatives to open-heart surgery. Current trends indicate that the number and variety of outpatient cardiac catheterizations will continue to increase. The equipment used and procedures performed in the cardiac catheterization laboratories of the future are likely to be significantly different from those associated with existing facilities and techniques employed today. However, despite changes in cardiovascular technology and medical techniques, cardiac catheterization laboratories will continue to provide essential patient care services necessary for the diagnosis and treatment of a vast number of cardiovascular-related diseases.

Definition of Terms

afferent lymph vessel Vessel carrying lymph toward a lymph vessel.

anastomose Join.

aneurysm Sac formed by local enlargement of a weakened artery wall.

angina pectoris Severe form of chest pain and constriction near the heart; usually caused by a decrease in the blood supply to cardiac tissue; most often associated with stenosis of a coronary artery as a result of atherosclerotic accumulations or spasm. The pain generally lasts for a few minutes and is more likely to occur after stress, exercise, or other activity resulting in increased heart rate.

angiography Radiographic demonstration of blood vessels after the introduction of a contrast medium.

anomaly Variation from the normal pattern.

aortic dissection Tear in the inner lining of the aortic wall that allows blood to enter and track along the muscular coat.

aortography Radiographic examination of the aorta.

arrhythmia Variation from normal heart rhythm.

arrhythmogenic Producing an arrhythmia.

arteriography Radiologic examination of arteries after the injection of a radiopaque contrast medium.

arteriole Very small arterial vessel.

arteriosclerotic Indicative of a general pathologic condition characterized by thickening and hardening of arterial walls, leading to general loss of elasticity.

arteriotomy Surgical opening of an artery.

arteriovenous malformation Abnormal anastomosis or communication between an artery and a vein.

artery Large blood vessel carrying blood away from the heart.

atherectomy Excision of atherosclerotic plaque.

atheromatous Characteristic of degenerative change in the inner lining of arteries caused by the deposition of fatty tissue and subsequent thickening of arterial walls that occurs in atherosclerosis.

atherosclerosis Condition in which fibrous and fatty deposits on the luminal wall of an artery may cause obstruction of the vessel.

atrium One of the two upper chambers of the heart.

bifurcation Place where a structure divides into two branches.

biplane Two x-ray exposure planes 90 degrees from one another, usually frontal and lateral.

blood vascular system Vascular system comprised of arteries, capillaries, and veins, which convey blood.

bradyarrhythmia Irregular heart rhythm in conjunction with bradycardia.

bradycardia Any heart rhythm with an average heart rate of less than 60 beats per minute.

capillary Tiny blood vessel through which blood and tissue cells exchange substances.

cardiac output Amount of blood pumped from the heart per given unit of time; can be calculated by multiplying stroke volume (amount of blood in milliliters ejected from the left ventricle during each heartbeat) by heart rate (number of heartbeats per minute). A normal, resting adult with a stroke volume of 70 mL and a heart rate of 72 beats per minute has a cardiac output of approximately 5 L per minute.

cardiomyopathies Relatively serious group of heart diseases typically characterized by enlargement of the myocardial layer of the left ventricle and resulting in decreased cardiac output; hypertrophic cardiomyopathy is a condition often studied in the catheterization laboratory.

cardiovascular and interventional technologist Technologists specializing in angiographic and interventional procedures.

cerebral angiography Imaging of vascular system of the brain.

cineangiography High-speed, 35-mm motion picture film recording of a fluoroscopic image of structures containing radiographic contrast medium.

cinefluorography Same as cineradiography; the production of a motion picture record of successive images on a fluoroscopic screen.

claudication Cramping of the leg muscles after physical exertion because of chronically inadequate blood supply.

coagulopathy Any disorder that affects the blood-clotting mechanism.

collateral Secondary or accessory.

diastole Relaxed phase of the atria or ventricles of the heart during which blood enters the chambers; in the cardiac cycle at which the heart is not contracting (at rest).

directional coronary atherectomy (DCA) Excision of atheroma through a percutaneous transcatheter approach using a rotating cutting device supported by a balloon positioned on the back of the catheter.

dyspnea Labored breathing.

efferent lymph vessel Vessel carrying lymph away from a node.

ejection fraction Measurements of ventricular contractility expressed as the percentage of blood pumped out of the left ventricle during contraction; can be estimated by evaluating the left ventriculogram; normal range is between 57% and 73%, with an average of 65%. A low ejection fraction indicates failure of the left ventricle to pump effectively.

embolus Foreign material, often thrombus, that detaches and moves freely in the bloodstream.

endocardium Interior lining of heart chambers.

ergometer Device used to imitate the muscular, metabolic, and respiratory effects of exercise.

epicardium Exterior layer of heart wall.

extravasation Escape of fluid from a vessel into the surrounding tissue.

fibrillation Involuntary, chaotic muscular contractions resulting from spontaneous activation of single muscle cells or muscle fibers.

French size A measurement of catheter sizes; 1 French = 0.33 mm.

guidewire Tightly wound metallic wire over which angiographic catheters are placed.

hematoma Collection of extravasated blood in an organ or a tissue space.

hemodynamics Study of factors involved in circulation of blood. Hemodynamic data typically collected during heart catheterization are cardiac output and intracardiac pressures.

hemostasis Stopping of blood flow in a hemorrhage.

hydronephrosis Distention of the pelvis and calices of the kidney with urine; caused by ureteral obstruction.

iatrogenic Caused by a therapeutic or diagnostic procedure.

innominate or brachiocephalic artery The first major artery of the aortic arch supplying the cerebral circulation.

in-stent restenosis Renarrowing of an artery inside a previously placed stent.

intervention Therapeutic modality—mechanical or pharmacologic—used to modify the course of a disease process.

interventional Improving a condition; therapeutic.

interventricular septal integrity Continuity of the membranous partition that separates the right and left ventricles of the heart.

intracoronary stent Metallic device placed within a coronary artery across a region of stenosis.

introducer sheath Plastic tubing placed within the vasculature through which other catheters may be passed.

ischemic Indicative of a local decrease of blood supply to myocardial tissue associated with temporary obstruction of a coronary vessel, typically as a result of thrombus (blood clot).

lesion Injury or other damaging change to an organ or tissue.

lymph Body fluid circulated by the lymphatic vessels and filtered by the lymph nodes.

lymph vessels See *afferent* and/or *efferent lymph vessel.*

lymphadenography Radiographic study of the lymph nodes.

lymphangiography Radiographic study of the lymph vessels.

lymphography Radiographic evaluation of the lymphatic channels and lymph nodes.

mandrel Inner metallic core of a spiral wound guidewire.

meninges Three membranes that envelop the brain and spinal cord.

misregistration Occurs when the two images used to form a subtraction image are slightly displaced from one another.

myocardial infarction (MI) Acute ischemic episode resulting in myocardial damage and pain; commonly referred to as a heart attack.

myocardium Muscular heart wall.

neointimal hyperplasia Hyperproliferation of smooth muscle cells and extracellular matrix secondary to revascularization.

nephrectomy Surgical removal of the kidney.

nephrostomy Surgical opening into the kidney's collecting system.

nephrotoxic Chemically damaging to the kidney cells.

nonocclusive Not completely closed or shut; allowing blood flow.

occlusion Obstruction or closure of a vessel, such as a coronary vessel, as a result of foreign material, thrombus, or spasm.

oximetry Measurement of oxygen saturation in blood.

oxygen saturation Amount of oxygen bound to hemoglobin in blood, expressed as a percentage.

patency State of being open or unobstructed.

patent foramen ovale Opening between the right atrium and left atrium that normally exists in fetal life to allow for the essential mixing of blood. The opening normally closes shortly after birth.

percutaneous Introduced through the skin.

percutaneous nephrolithotomy Uroradiologic procedure performed to extract stones from within the kidney or proximal ureter.

percutaneous transluminal angioplasty (PTA) Surgical correction of a vessel from within the vessel using catheter technology.

percutaneous transluminal coronary angioplasty (PTCA) Manipulative interventional procedure involving the placement and inflation of a balloon catheter in the lumen of a stenosed coronary artery for the purpose of compressing and fracturing the diseased material, thereby allowing subsequent increased distal blood flow to the myocardium.

percutaneous transluminal coronary rotational atherectomy (PTCRA) Manipulative interventional procedure involving a device called a Rotablator to remove atherosclerotic plaque from within the coronary artery using a high-speed rotational burr.

percutaneously Performed through the skin.

pericardium Fibrous sac that surrounds the heart.

planimetry Mechanical tracing to determine the volume of a structure.

pledget Small piece of material used as a dressing or plug.

portal circulation System of vessels carrying blood from the organs of digestion to the liver.

postprocessing Image processing operations performed when reviewing an imaging sequence.

pulmonary circulation System of vessels carrying blood from the heart to the lungs and back to the heart.

pulse Regular expansion and contraction of an artery that is produced by the ejection of blood from the heart.

pulse oximetry Measurement of oxygen saturation in the blood via an optic sensor placed on an extremity.

reperfusion Reestablishment of blood flow to the heart muscle through a previously occluded artery.

restenosis Narrowing or constriction of a vessel, orifice, or other type of passageway after interventional correction of primary condition.

rotational burr atherectomy Ablation of atheroma through a percutaneous transcatheter approach using a high-speed rotational burr.

serial imaging Acquisition of images in rapid succession.

stenosis Narrowing or constriction of a vessel, an orifice, or another type of passageway.

stent Wire mesh or plastic conduit placed to maintain flow.

systemic circulation System of vessels carrying blood from the heart out to the body (except the lungs) and back to the heart.

systole Contraction phase of the atria or ventricles of the heart during which blood is ejected from the chambers; point in the cardiac cycle at which the heart is contracting (at work).

tachyarrhythmia Irregular heart rhythm in conjunction with tachycardia.

tachycardia Any heart rhythm having an average heart rate in excess of 100 beats per minute.

targeted lesion Area of narrowing within an artery where a revascularization procedure is planned.

thrombogenesis Formation of a blood clot.

thrombolytic Capable of causing the breakup of a thrombus.

thrombosis Formation or existence of a blood clot.

thrombus Blood clot obstructing a blood vessel or cavity of the heart.

transducer Device used to convert one form of energy into another. Transducers used in cardiac catheterization convert fluid (blood) pressure into an electrical signal displayed on a physiologic monitor.

transposition of the great arteries Congenital heart defect requiring interventional therapy. In this defect the aorta arises from the right side of the heart and the pulmonary artery arises from the left side of the heart.

umbrella Prosthetic interventional device consisting of two opposing polyurethane disks connected by a central loop mounted on a spring-loaded assembly to provide opposing tension.

uroradiology Radiologic and interventional study of the urinary tract.

valvular competence Ability of the valve to prevent backward flow while not inhibiting forward flow.

varices Irregularly swollen veins.

vasoconstriction Temporary closure of a blood vessel using drug therapy.

vein Vessel that carries blood from the capillaries to the heart.

venography Radiologic study of veins after the injection of radiopaque contrast medium.

venotomy Surgical opening of a vein.

ventricle One of two larger pumping chambers of the heart.

venule Any of the small blood vessels that collect blood from the capillaries and join to become veins.

Selected bibliography

Abrams HL: *Abrams angiography: vascular and interventional radiology*, ed 3, Boston, 1983, Little, Brown.

Ahn SS, Concepcion B: Current status of atherectomy for peripheral arterial occlusive disease, *World J Surg* 20:635, 1996.

Athanasoulis CA et al: *Interventional radiology*, Philadelphia, 1982, Saunders.

Berenstein A, Lasjaunias P: *Surgical neuroangiography*, vol 1-5, Berlin, 1992, Springer-Verlag.

Brooks B: The treatment of traumatic arteriovenous fistula, *South Med J* 23:100, 1930.

Brooks B: Discussion. In Nolan L, Taylor AS: Pulsating exophthalmos, *Trans South Surg Assoc* 43:176, 1931.

Burke TH, Shetty PC, Sanders WP: Cardiovascular and interventional technologists: their growing role in the interventional suite, *J Vasc Interv Radiol* 8:720, 1997.

Caldwell DM, Stokes KR, Yakes WF: Embolotherapy: agents, clinical applications, and techniques, *Radiographics* 14:623, 1994.

Castaneda-Zuniga WR, Tadavarthy SM: *Interventional radiology*, vol 1-2, ed 2, Baltimore, 1988, Williams & Wilkins.

Colombo A et al: Intracoronary stenting without anticoagulation accomplished with intravascular ultrasound guidance, *Circulation* 91:1676, 1995.

Comerota AJ: *Thrombolytic therapy for peripheral vascular disease*, Philadelphia, 1995, JB Lippincott.

Conners B, Wojak J: *Interventional neuroradiology strategies and practical techniques*, Philadelphia, 1999, Saunders.

Cope C, Burke DR, Meranze S: *Atlas of interventional radiology*, Philadelphia, 1990, JB Lippincott.

Dorffner R et al: Treatment of abdominal aortic aneurysms with transfemoral placement of stent-grafts: complications and secondary radiologic intervention, *Radiology* 204:79, 1997.

Dyet JF: Endovascular stents in the arterial system—current status, *Clin Radiol* 52:83, 1997.

Eustace S et al: Magnetic resonance angiography in transjugular intrahepatic portosystemic stenting: comparison with contrast hepatic and portal venography, *Eur J Radiol* 19:43, 1994.

Ferrucci JT et al: *Interventional radiology of the abdomen*, ed 2, Baltimore, 1985, Williams & Wilkins.

Fillmore DJ et al: Transjugular intrahepatic portosystemic shunt: midterm clinical and angiographic follow-up, *J Vasc Interv Radiol* 7:255, 1996.

Fogoros RN: *Electrophysiological testing*, ed 3, Malden, Mass, 1999, Blackwell Science.

Freed M, Grines C: *Manual of interventional cardiology*, Birmingham, Ala, 1992, Physicians Press.

Furman S, Hayes DL, Holmes DR: *A practice of cardiac pacing*, Mt. Kisco, NY, 1993, Futura Publishing.

Grossman W: *Cardiac catheterization and angiography*, ed 3, Philadelphia, 1986, Lea & Febiger.

Guglielmi G et al: Electrothrombosis of saccular aneurysms via endovascular approach. Part I: electrochemical basis, technique, and experimental results, *J Neurosurg* 75:1, 1991.

Guglielmi G et al: Electrothrombosis of saccular aneurysms via endovascular approach. Part II: preliminary clinical experience, *J Neurosurg* 75:8, 1991.

Hayes DL, Lloyd MA, Friedman PA: *Cardiac pacing and defibrillation: a clinical approach*, Armonk, NY, 2000, Futura Publishing.

Johnson LW et al: Coronary arteriography 1984-1987: a report of the Registry of the Society for Cardiac Angiography and Interventions. Part 1: results and complications, *Cathet Cardiovasc Diagn* 17:5, 1989.

Johnsrude IS et al: *A practical approach to angiography*, ed 2, Boston, 1987, Little, Brown.

Kadir S: *Diagnostic angiography*, Philadelphia, 1986, Saunders.

Kadir S: *Atlas of normal variant angiographic anatomy*, Philadelphia, 1991, Saunders.

Kadir S: *Current practice of interventional radiology*, Philadelphia, 1991, BC Decker.

Kandarpa K: Technical determinants of success in catheter-directed thrombolysis for peripheral arterial occlusions, *J Vasc Interv Radiol* 6(6 pt 2 suppl):55S, 1995.

Kandarpa K: *Handbook of cardiovascular and interventional radiologic procedures*, ed 2, Boston, 1996, Little, Brown.

Kern MJ: *The cardiac catheterization handbook*, St Louis, 1999, Mosby.

Kerns SR, Hawkins IF Jr, Sabatelli FW: Current status of carbon dioxide angiography, *Radiol Clin North Am* 33:15, 1995.

Laine C et al: Combined cardiac catheterization for uncomplicated ischemic heart disease in a Medicare population, *Am J Med* 105:373, 1998.

Laskey W, Boyle J, Johnson LW: Multivariable model for prediction of risk of significant complication during diagnostic cardiac catheterization: the Registry of the Committee of the Society for Cardiac Angiographers and Interventions, *Cathet Cardiovasc Diagn* 30:190, 1993.

Laudicina P, Wean D: *Applied angiography for radiographers*, Philadelphia, 1994, Saunders.

LeRoux PD, Winn HR: Current management of aneurysms, *Neurosurg Clin N Am* 9:421, 1998.

Morris P: *Practical neuroangiography*, Baltimore, 1997, Williams & Wilkins.

Moses HW: *Practical guide to cardiac pacing*, Boston, 1995, Little, Brown.

Nelson PK, Kricheff II: Cerebral angiography, *Neuroimaging Clin North Am* 6:1, 1996.

Newton TH, Potts DG: *Radiology of the skull and brain—angiography*, vol 2, book 1, St Louis, 1974, Mosby.

Norris TG: Principles of cardiac catheterization, *Radiol Technol* 72:109, 2000.

Noto JT Jr et al: Cardiac catheterization 1990: a report of the Registry of the Society for Cardiac Angiography and Interventions (SCA&I), *Cathet Cardiovasc Diagn* 24:75, 1991.

Orrison WW: *Neuroimaging*, vol 1, Philadelphia, 2000, Saunders.

Osborn AG: *Introduction of cerebral angiography*, 1980, Harper & Row.

Osborn AG: *Diagnostic neuroradiology*, St Louis, 1994, Mosby.

Pepine CJ, Hill JA, Lambert CR: *Diagnostic and therapeutic cardiac catheterization*, Baltimore, 1998, Williams & Wilkins.

Peterson KL, Nicod P: *Cardiac catheterization: methods, diagnosis, and therapy*, Philadelphia, 1997, Saunders.

Pieters PC, Miller WJ, DeMeo JH: Evaluation of the portal venous system: complementary roles of invasive and noninvasive imaging strategies, *Radiographics* 17: 879, 1997.

Rees CR et al: Use of carbon dioxide as a contrast medium for transjugular intrahepatic portosystemic shunt procedures, *J Vasc Interv Radiol* 5:383, 1994.

Reuter SR et al: *Gastrointestinal angiography*, ed 3, Philadelphia, 1986, Saunders.

Ring EJ, McLean GK: *Interventional radiology: principles and techniques*, Boston, 1981, Little, Brown.

Rogers CG Jr, Paolini RM, O'Leary JP: Intrahepatic vascular shunting for portal hypertension: early experience with the transjugular intrahepatic porto-systemic shunt, *Am Surg* 60:114, 1994.

Scanlon PJ et al: ACC/AHA guidelines for coronary angiography: a report of the American College of Cardiology/American Heart Association Task Force on Practice Guidelines (Committee on Coronary Angiography), *J Am Coll Cardiol* 33:1756, 1999.

Seldinger SI: Percutaneous selective angiography of the aorta: preliminary report, *Acta Radiol (Stockh)* 45:15, 1956.

Snopek AM: *Fundamentals of special radiographic procedures*, ed 3, Philadelphia, 1992, Saunders.

Strandness DE, VanBreda A: *Vascular diseases surgical and interventional therapy*, vols 1-2, New York, 1994, Churchill Livingstone.

Tortorici MR, Apfel PJ: *Advanced radiographic and angiographic procedures with an introduction to specialized imaging*, Philadelphia, 1995, FA Davis.

Uflacker R, Wholey M: *Interventional radiology*, New York, 1991, McGraw-Hill.

Warner JJ, Harrison JK, Sketch MH: Recognizing complications of cardiac catheterization, *Emerg Med* 32:12, 2000.

Vinuela F, Duckwiler G, Mawad M: Guglielmi detachable coil embolization of acute intracranial aneurysm: perioperative anatomical and clinical outcome in 403 patients, *J Neurosurg* 86:475, 1997.

Vinuela F, Halbach VV, Dion JE: *Interventional neuroradiology endovascular therapy of central nervous system*, New York, 1992, Raven Press.

Von Sonnenberg E, Mueller PR: *Practical interventional radiology*, Philadelphia, 1989, Saunders.

Wojtowycz M: *Handbooks of interventional radiology*, Chicago, 1990, Mosby.

Wojtowycz M: *Handbook of interventional radiology and angiography*, ed 2, St Louis, 1995, Mosby.

26

SECTIONAL ANATOMY
FOR RADIOGRAPHERS

TERRI BRUCKNER

MRI through midsagittal plane.

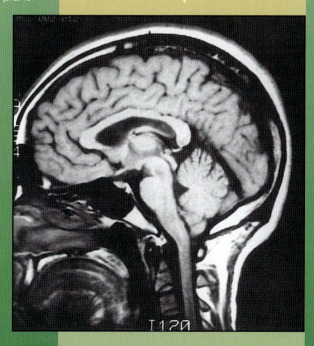

Overview

Imaging modalities, such as computed tomography (CT), magnetic resonance imaging (MRI), or sonography, require the technologist to look at anatomy in the resultant images in a totally different way than they are used to with general radiographs. These technologies create cross-sectional imaging planes, in effect visualizing a slice through the body. Cross-sectional images have the advantage of visualizing anatomic structures without the sometimes confusing superimposition of other anatomic parts. Images are generated in various planes, which makes it critical for the technologists working with these modalities to have a clear and complete understanding of general anatomic principles. Without a clear understanding of general anatomy, it is difficult to feel confident in the identification of normal and abnormal structures in cross-section. The purpose of this chapter is to provide the radiographer who possesses a background in general anatomy with an orientation to sectional anatomy and to correlate that anatomy with structures demonstrated on images from the various computer-generated imaging modalities.

In general, three major imaging planes exist: axial, coronal, and sagittal. Axial planes (sometimes referred to as *transverse planes*) transect the body from anterior to posterior and from side to side. In effect, this type of horizontal plane divides the body into superior and inferior portions. Most images generated by CT are examples of axial or transverse planes. When looking at an axial image, it is helpful to imagine standing at the patient's feet and looking up toward the head. With this orientation, the patient's right side is to the viewer's left and vice versa. The anterior aspect of the patient is usually at the top of the image. The coronal plane divides the body into anterior and posterior portions. Coronal planes pass from superior to inferior and from side to side. Images viewed in the coronal plane are similar to radiographs

in that the patient's right side is on the technologist's left (one can imagine facing the patient while viewing this type of image). Sagittal planes divide the body into right and left portions. These planes pass from superior to inferior and from anterior to posterior. Magnetic resonance (MR) images frequently use the coronal and sagittal planes to present the desired anatomy. CT images may be obtained in the coronal or sagittal planes, or the information from axial images may be reformatted by the computer to obtain images in these planes. Any plane that does not fit the previous descriptions is referred to as an *oblique plane*. Sonograms and MR images of some structures, such as the heart, are generated using oblique planes.

CT uses x-rays to generate images, so the various shades on the images correspond to the gray scale that radiographers are accustomed to seeing. Bones and other dense materials are white, whereas air and lower-density materials are closer to black. Fat, muscle, and organs are represented with various shades of gray. Hounsfield units or CT numbers represent the scale of white to black that is used in CT imaging. Lower numbers represent anatomic structures that are more easily penetrated by the x-ray and therefore appear closer to black on the image. Higher numbers are related to more radiopaque structures and are lighter gray or white on the image. Like routine radiographs, blood vessels and organs of the digestive system are not easily distinguishable from other structures. To be able to more accurately identify these structures, patients are frequently given radiopaque contrast media. Intravascular contrast will highlight vessels, making them appear radiopaque and therefore whiter on the image. To visualize the gastrointestinal system, patients may be given contrast by mouth or via the rectum. For a full description of CT fundamentals, the reader is referred to Chapter 31.

MRI uses magnetic fields and radiofrequencies to generate images. Anatomic structures are represented on the image

with regard to the signal generated from their protons. Structures that produce a strong signal are generally lighter gray or white on the image, and those that do not generate a strong signal tend to be darker on the image. The signal generated by these structures depends on many things including the strength of the magnetic fields and the characteristics of the radiofrequencies used. Contrast media may also be used when performing MRI to change the signal intensity of particular anatomic structures. Gadolinium, air, or fluid may be used as contrast agents depending on the organ of interest and the imaging sequences employed. MRI is discussed in depth in Chapter 33.

The cadaver sections depicted in this chapter are representative of major organ structures for each of the body regions, and they are *depicted from the inferior surface to correspond to the images*. Keep in mind that all relational terms are used in relation to the body in anatomic position (when a structure is described as being to the right of something, this refers to the *patient's* right, not the *viewer's* right). The major anatomic structures normally seen when using current imaging modalities are labeled. For each region of the body, a cadaver section is presented and representative images are included to provide an orientation to anatomic structures normally seen using the available imaging modalities. The cadaver sections and diagnostic images do not match exactly; therefore some structures are seen on only one of the illustrations for each body region. Major anatomic structures in each region of the body are reviewed in the following sections to assist identification of the images provided. Systematic review of the bones, vessels, major organs, and muscles begin each section. Selected images are presented in axial, sagittal, and coronal planes to demonstrate these structures. In practice, images should be examined collectively because the size, shape, and placement of these structures varies from slice to slice. "Following" a structure is frequently the ideal way to identify it.

Cranial Region

Fig. 26-1 is a cadaver image that can be used to distinguish bone, muscle, and other soft tissue structures. Referring to this image should be helpful in identifying the sometimes confusing shadows on the images. The head can be thought of systematically as being composed of the skull, the central nervous system structures, various sensory organs, the cranial blood supply, and the associated cranial and facial muscles. The bones of the skull are categorized as the 8 cranial bones and the 14 facial bones. The cranial bones include the frontal, occipital, and two parietal bones that surround and protect the external surface of the brain. The other four cranial bones include the ethmoid, sphenoid, and two temporal bones. The frontal bone forms the anterior surface of the skull, with a vertical portion that corresponds to the forehead and a horizontal portion that forms the roof of the orbits. Between the inner and outer layers of the vertical portion of the frontal bone, just superior to the level of the eyes, are the paired frontal paranasal sinuses. The vertex (most superior portion) of the skull is formed by the paired parietal bones. These roughly square-shaped bones articulate with the frontal bone at the coronal suture, with the temporal bones at the squamosal sutures, with the occipital bone at the lambdoidal suture, and with each other at the sagittal suture.

The posterior aspect of the skull is formed by the occipital bone, which is composed of a squamous (vertical) portion and a basilar portion. The foramen magnum is a large opening within the squamous portion that allows passage of the spinal cord into the brain. The external occipital protuberance is a large prominence on the posterior surface of this bone. Roughly corresponding in position to this landmark is the internal occipital protuberance. The ethmoid bone is found within the cranium and forms the medial walls of the orbits and part of the lateral walls of the nasal cavity. The ethmoid bone is divided into a horizontal portion called the *cribriform plane* and vertical portions called the *perpendicular plate* and *two labyrinths* or *lateral masses.*

The cribriform plate lies between the orbital plates of the frontal bone and supports the olfactory bulbs (cranial nerve I). The cribriform plate is perforated by many small foramina, which transmit nerves from the nose to this cranial nerve.

Projecting superiorly from the cribriform plate is a small ridge of bone called the *crista galli,* which serves as the anterior attachment for the falx cerebri. Projecting inferiorly from the center of the cribriform plate is the perpendicular plate. This thin strip of bone forms the superior part of the bony nasal septum. Extending inferiorly from the lateral edges of the cribriform plate are the labyrinths or lateral masses. These are perforated by multiple air spaces, which are collectively called the *ethmoidal paranasal sinuses.* From the medial surface of each labyrinth, two scroll-shaped ridges of bone project into the nasal cavity. These are the superior and middle nasal conchae.

In the center of the base of the skull is the sphenoid bone. This bone is sometimes referred to as the *anchor bone of the cranium* because it articulates with all of the cranial bones. Thinking of this bone as being composed of a body, two sets of wings, and a pterygoid portion is helpful. The body is the central portion of the bone and contains the easily identifiable landmark known as the *sella turcica.* The sella turcica forms a cup-shaped depression that surrounds and protects the pituitary gland. The anterior surface of the

Fig. 26-1 A, Line drawing of the gross anatomic section. **B,** Cadaver image of skull.

sella is called the *tuberculum sellae*, and the posterior portion is the *dorsum sellae*. Two posterior clinoid processes project from the superior edge of the dorsum sellae and are attachments for dura mater partitions. Within the body of the sphenoid and inferior to the sella turcica are the paired sphenoidal paranasal sinuses. The lesser wings of the sphenoid are triangular ridges of bone found posterior to the orbital plates of the frontal bone. Directly inferior to the medial edge of each lesser wing is the optic canal, which transmits the optic nerve (cranial nerve II). The larger, greater wings support the temporal lobes of the cerebrum and extend from the body to the external surface of the skull. The pterygoid processes project inferiorly from the body of the sphenoid and form the posterior walls of the nasal cavity.

The temporal bones form part of the lateral walls of the cranium and extend internally to meet the sphenoid and the basilar portion of the occipital bone. Parts of the temporal bone include the squamous, tympanic, mastoid, and petrous portions. The squamous portion is the thin, fan-shaped external part of the bone superior to the external ear. It articulates with the parietal and several other cranial bones. Its articulation with the parietal bone is called the *squamous suture*. The tympanic portion is the area of the bone surrounding the external ear canal. The zygomatic process arches anteriorly from just superior to the external ear canal. Just inferior to the origin of the zygomatic process is the mandibular fossa, in which the condyle of the mandible is found. On the inferior surface of the tympanic portion of the bone is the styloid process, which serves as an attachment for muscles. Posterior to the ear is the mastoid portion, which is perforated by many small, air-filled cavities. The mastoid portion extends inferiorly to form the cone-shaped mastoid process. The petrous portion of the bone lies within the cranium, normally forming an angle of approximately 45 degrees to the median sagittal plane. This dense ridge of bone surrounds and protects the organs of hearing and balance, the facial and vestibulocochlear nerves, and the internal carotid artery.

Fourteen bones surround and protect the organs associated with the face. Each of these bones is paired with the exception of the vomer and the mandible. The lacrimal bones are about the size of a fingernail and are found in the medial wall of the orbit between the maxilla and the labyrinth of the ethmoid bones. The nasal bones form the bridge of the nose and articulate superiorly with the frontal bone, laterally with the maxilla, and with each other in the midline. The zygomatic bones form the inferolateral walls of the orbits. Each of these bones articulate superiorly with the frontal bone, medially with the maxilla, and laterally with the zygomatic process of the temporal bone. The maxilla originates as two separate bones, which ultimately fuse along the midsagittal plane. This large bone forms the inferior surface of each orbit, the lateral walls of the nasal cavity, and the anterior portion of the roof of the mouth. On either side of the nasal cavity, large air-filled maxillary paranasal sinuses are embedded within the bone. The upper teeth are rooted within the alveolar process at the antero-inferior surface of the bone. The maxilla articulates with the nasal bones, the lacrimal bones, the frontal bone, the zygomatic bones, and the palatine bones. The inferior nasal conchae are scroll-shaped facial bones found in the nasal cavity, just inferior to the middle nasal conchae of the ethmoid bone. The posterior portion of the hard palate is formed by the L-shaped palatine bones. The vertical portions of the palatines extend superiorly along the posterior nasal cavity to form a small part of the posterior orbit.

The vomer is an unpaired facial bone that articulates with the inferior surface of the perpendicular plate of the ethmoid. It forms the inferior portion of the bony nasal septum. The mandible, which is also an unpaired facial bone, is formed by a body and two rami. The body comprises the anterior portion of the bone and presents an alveolar ridge in which the lower teeth are embedded. The rami extend superiorly from the body and end in anterior and posterior bony processes. The anterior process at the superior end of the ramus is the coronoid process, where muscles of mastication attach. The posterior process is the condyloid process, which rests in the mandibular fossa of the temporal bone. This articulation, the temporomandibular joint (TMJ), is the only movable articulation associated with the skull. (Refer to Chapter 20 for review of skull anatomy.)

The brain is surrounded by three layers of protective membranes called the *meninges.* From internal to external they are the pia mater, arachnoid, and dura mater. The pia mater adheres directly to the brain and is composed of a fine network of capillaries and supporting tissue. The arachnoid is a delicate membrane that resembles a cobweb. The subarachnoid space lies between the arachnoid and pia mater. Cerebrospinal fluid (CSF) circulates in this space. The arachnoid does not closely adhere to cerebral structures. As it bridges the gap between various parts of the brain, enlarged regions or cisterns are formed in the subarachnoid space. Some of the more crucial cisterns include the cisterna magna, pontine, interpeduncular, and superior (also known as the *ambient* or *quadrigeminal cistern*). The cisterna magna is the largest of these and is found just inside the foramen magnum, between the cerebellum and the medulla oblongata. This cistern receives CSF from the fourth ventricle. The pontine cistern lies anterior to the pons and contains the basilar artery. The interpeduncular cistern is anterior to the midbrain. The infundibulum (stalk) of the pituitary and the vessels of the circle of Willis are seen here. The cistern found posterior to the midbrain is the superior cistern. It surrounds the pineal gland and the great cerebral vein. The most external of the meninges is the double-layered dura mater. The outer layer of dura is attached to the inner surface of the cranial bones. The inner layer can be seen between cerebral structures and in large fissures. Dural sinuses are venous drainage channels formed where the inner dural layers separate from the outer layer. One of the largest dural flaps, the falx cerebri, is found in the longitudinal fissure between the cerebral hemispheres. It extends from the crista galli of the ethmoid to the occipital bone. The tentorium cerebelli extends between the cerebrum and the cerebellum. It attaches to the sella turcica and the internal surface of the occipital bones.

The structures of the central nervous system within the skull include the cerebrum, brainstem, and cerebellum. The cerebrum is the largest of these structures and is divided by the longitudinal fissure into two hemispheres. The hemispheres are connected to each other via a white matter tract called the *corpus callosum.* This arch-shaped structure is divided into the anterior genu, central body, and posterior splenium. Each cerebral hemisphere is divided into lobes that are named for the most adjacent cranial bone: frontal, parietal, temporal, and occipital. An additional lobe called the insula is buried deep to the temporal lobe. The cerebrum is thrown into numerous folds called *gyri,* which are separated by small fissures called *sulci.* The outer surface of the cerebrum consists of a thin layer of gray matter. The central portion of this part of the brain is mainly white matter (formed by myelinated nerve fibers). These fibers, referred to as the *corona radiata,* connect the gray matter of the cortex to deeper gray matter nuclei deep within each hemisphere. The buried gray matter centers are called *basal nuclei* or *basal ganglia* and include the claustrum, putamen, globus pallidus, and caudate nucleus. White matter tracts, or capsules, are found between these gray matter structures. Other gray matter structures found within the central cerebrum include the thalamus and hypothalamus. These form the walls of the third ventricle. Many of these gray and white matter structures are seen on the cadaver section in Fig. 26-1.

The brainstem is formed by the midbrain, pons, and medulla oblongata. It lies between the cerebrum and cerebellum and serves as a relay for nerve impulses between the spinal cord and these two structures. The midbrain is the most superior of the three. White matter tracts called the cerebral peduncles extend from the anterior midbrain to the cerebrum. Toward the posterior aspect of the midbrain are the corpora quadrigemina, which are formed by two superior and two inferior colliculi that lie just inferior to the splenium of the corpus callosum. The cerebral aqueduct drains CSF from the third ventricle to the fourth ventricle and passes through the posterior portion of the midbrain. The central portion of the brainstem is formed by the pons. It communicates with the medulla, the midbrain, and via white matter cerebellar peduncles to the cerebellum. The most inferior of the brainstem structures is the medulla oblongata, which is continuous with the spinal cord as it passes through the foramen magnum.

The cerebellum lies in the posteroinferior region of the cranium. Although smaller in size, it is similar in composition to the cerebrum. A midline fissure divides the cerebellum into hemispheres that are connected by a midline vermis. It

is also thrown into numerous small folds, here called folia, which are separated by numerous small fissures. The outer surface of the cerebellum is composed of gray matter, with white matter comprising most of the central portion of this part of the brain. Gray matter nuclei can be found here also, although they are difficult to distinguish on images and are not discussed in this chapter.

Four large cavities called *ventricles* are found in the brain. The ventricles' major function is to produce CSF. This is accomplished as blood is filtered through capillary networks called *choroid plexuses* in each of the ventricles. The largest of these chambers are the lateral ventricles, one of which is found in each cerebral hemisphere. The lateral ventricles are divided into body and anterior, posterior, and inferior horns. CSF from these chambers passes into the midline third ventricle through the interventricular foramina. The third ventricle is found between the cerebral hemispheres inferior to the lateral ventricles. The cerebral aqueduct drains CSF from here to the fourth ventricle. This ventricle is found between the cerebellum and the brainstem. Its walls are formed by white matter tracts called *cerebellar peduncles,* which connect the brainstem and cerebellum. A central aperture and two lateral apertures allow CSF to pass from the fourth ventricle into the subarachnoid space.

The brain is a highly metabolic organ, and in order to function well it needs a rich blood supply. Four major arteries supply the brain and its related structures: the two internal carotid arteries and the two vertebral arteries. The internal carotid arteries supply the anterior structures of the brain. After passing superiorly through the neck, these arteries enter the skull by way of the carotid canals in the petrous portion of the temporal bones. After exiting the petrous portion, the internal carotid arteries pass along the lateral aspect of the sella turcica, ultimately dividing into the anterior and middle cerebral arteries. The posterior communicating artery arises from the internal carotid just before this bifurcation. The anterior cerebral arteries pass anteriorly and superiorly to the longitudinal fissure, where they curl around the external aspect of the corpus callosum and supply the anterior portion of the brain. The middle cerebral arteries pass laterally to the lateral fis-

sures, where their branches supply the middle portion of the brain. The posterior communicating arteries pass posteriorly to join with the branches from the vertebrobasilar arterial system. The vertebral arteries traverse the neck in the transverse foramina of the cervical spine and enter the posterior skull by way of the foramen magnum. These arteries pass superiorly along the anterior aspect of the medulla and, at the base of the pons, join to form the basilar artery. At the superior aspect of the pons, the basilar artery splits to form the posterior cerebral arteries. A unique arterial anastomosis exists in the brain to protect it from sudden loss of blood supply. This vascular connection is called the *circle of Willis.* The blood supply to the anterior brain is connected to the blood supply for the posterior brain as the posterior communicating arteries extend from the internal carotid arteries to the posterior cerebral arteries. This communication lies in the interpeduncular cistern, just anterior to the midbrain.

Venous drainage in the cranium is accomplished by two systems: cerebral veins and dural venous sinuses. The dural sinuses are created by gaps formed between the inner and outer layers of the dura mater. These gaps are found in the areas where the dura invaginates between the various structures of the brain. The superior sagittal sinus is found in the superior border of the falx cerebri, and the inferior sagittal sinus is found in its inferior margin. The channel formed where the falx cerebri meets the tentorium cerebelli is the straight sinus. This sinus is a continuation of the inferior sagittal sinus as it joins with the great cerebral vein. The transverse or lateral sinuses are found along the lateral aspect of the tentorium cerebelli as it meets the occipital bone. At the level of the petrous portions of the temporal bones, the transverse sinuses curl medially and inferiorly and become known as the *sigmoid sinuses.* As the sigmoid sinuses pass out of the cranium via the jugular foramina, these vessels change names again and become the internal jugular veins. One of the major veins within the skull is the great cerebral vein. This large venous structure is found in the superior cistern and there it joins the inferior sagittal sinus to form the straight sinus.

Many muscles are associated with the face, only a few of which are referred to

Fig. 26-2 CT localizer (scout) image of skull.

in the following sections. The temporalis muscle is found on the external surface of the squamous portion of the temporal bone. Its inferior attachment is to the coronoid process of the mandible. On the external surface of the mandibular rami are the masseter muscles, and on the internal surface of the rami are the pterygoid muscles. These muscles are all associated with moving the mandible and with swallowing.

The CT localizer, or scout, image (Fig. 26-2) provides a lateral image of the cranium. CT imaging for the cranium may be performed with the gantry parallel to or angled 15 to 20 degrees to the orbitomeatal line (OML). MRI of the cranium generally results in images that are parallel to the orbitomeatal or infraorbitomeatal plane. More details on patient positioning for CT are provided in Chapter 31, and information on patient positioning for MRI is provided in Chapter 33. Because the imaging planes may be different for the CT and MRI images, some variation exists in the anatomic structures visualized on corresponding illustrations in this section. Seven identifying lines represent the approximate levels for each of the labeled images for this region.

The cranial CT image seen in Fig. 26-3 represents a CT slice obtained through the frontal and parietal bones, and Fig. 26-4 is a corresponding MR image. The *cortex*, or outer layer of gray matter, can be differentiated from the deeper *white matter.*

Fig. 26-3 A, Line drawing of CT section. **B,** CT image representing the anatomic structures located at level A in Fig. 26-2.

Fig. 26-4 MR image corresponding to level A in Fig. 26-2.

The numerous *gyri*, or *convolutions*, and *sulci* are demonstrated and are surrounded by the darker-appearing CSF in the subarachnoid space. The *cerebral hemispheres* are separated by the *longitudinal cerebral fissure*. Invaginated in this fissure is a fold of *dura mater*, the *falx cerebri*. The *superior sagittal sinus*, which passes through the superior margin of the falx, follows the contour of the superior skull margin. In cross section, the anterior and posterior aspects of this sinus can normally be seen in the midline deep to the bony plates when the patient has been given intravenous contrast and appear as triangular-shaped expansions near the bones easily seen on the MR image. Two of the five *cerebral lobes* are seen (frontal and parietal). The *corona radiata* is the central tract of white matter in the cerebrum and is somewhat darker than the cortex on the CT image. This section passes through the most superior portion of the *corpus callosum*, which separates the anterior and posterior portions of the falx cerebri.

Fig. 26-5 is an axial CT slice through the superior portions of the lateral ventricles; Fig. 26-6 is the corresponding MR image. Visualized bony structures on the CT scan include the *frontal bone* and the two *parietal bones*. The falx cerebri is seen within the *longitudinal fissure*. The *frontal lobes* and *parietal lobes* of the cerebrum are demonstrated. In the center of each image, the *lateral ventricles* are

easily seen due to the dark appearance of the CSF circulating within each. The posterior portions of the ventricles also have the contrast-filled capillary network of the *choroid plexuses* visualized. A thin membrane called the *septum pellucidum* can be seen separating the ventricles. The corpus callosum is an arch-shaped structure; therefore in cross section at this level only the anterior *genu* and the posterior *splenium* can be seen. The *caudate nuclei* lie along the lateral surfaces of the ventricles and tend to follow their curves. Several contrast-filled vascular structures are visible. The *anterior cerebral arteries* lie within the longitudinal fissure just anterior to the genu of the corpus callosum. A few branches of the *middle cerebral arteries* are seen near the lateral aspect of the skull on the CT scan. The anterior and posterior portions of the superior sagittal sinus are seen in the periphery of the falx cerebri. The *inferior sagittal sinus* lies in the internal edges of the falx. The thin strips of muscle seen on the external surface of the frontal bone correspond to the superior edges of the *temporalis muscles*.

The axial sections through the midportion of the cerebrum demonstrate many of the central structures of the cerebral hemispheres (Fig. 26-7 is a CT image, and Fig. 26-8 is the corresponding MR image). The *frontal sinuses* are seen on the CT image between the inner and outer cortical layers of the frontal bone. On the

lateral surface of the skull, images at this level pass through the greater wing of the *sphenoid* and the squamous portion of the *temporal bones*. The posterior portion of the skull is composed of the top edge of the *occipital bone* at this level. The falx cerebri is shown within the longitudinal fissure, with the superior sagittal sinus best demonstrated in the posterior margin. In the CT image the genu of the corpus callosum is found between the anterior

Fig. 26-6 MR image corresponding to level B in Fig. 26-2.

A — Anterior cerebral arteries, Genu of corpus callosum, Lateral ventricles, Choroid plexus, Splenium of corpus callosum, Falx cerebri in longitudinal fissure, Superior sagittal sinus, Frontal bone, Frontal lobe, Caudate nucleus, Septum pellucidum, Inferior sagittal sinus, Parietal lobe, Parietal bone — B

Fig. 26-5 A, Line drawing of CT section. **B,** CT image representing the structures located at level B in Fig. 26-2.

horns of the lateral ventricles; however, this slice is just inferior to the level of the splenium. The MR image demonstrates both the genu and the splenium. At this level the *frontal, temporal,* and *occipital lobes* are visualized along with the *insula* (fifth lobe or island of Reil), which is deep to the temporal lobe at the lateral fissure.

The anterior and posterior horns of the lateral ventricles are seen on both the CT and MR images. Within each posterior horn is a portion of the choroid plexus, which appears bright due to the presence of contrast media in the capillaries. The heads of the caudate nuclei lie along the external surfaces of the anterior horns of each lateral ventricles. Several areas of gray matter can be discerned on the CT image deep within the white matter of the cerebrum and comprise the basal nuclei. The major components of the basal nuclei seen at this level are (from lateral to medial) the *claustrum, lentiform nucleus* (composed of the putamen and globus pallidus), and the *caudate nucleus.* The lentiform nucleus is separated from the caudate nucleus and thalamus by a tract of white matter known as the *internal capsule.* These sections pass through the superior portion of the midline *third ventricle.* The *thalamus,* which serves as a central relay station for sensory impulses to the cerebral cortex, forms its lateral walls. On the CT image, a thin strip of thalamic tissue, the *massa intermedia,* can be seen connecting the two halves of the thalamus across the third ventricle. The large white region at the posterior border of the third ventricle is contrast in the choroid plexus (only on the CT image). Another contrast-enhanced vessel, the great cerebral vein, is found just posterior

Frontal sinuses
Frontal lobe
Genu of corpus callosum
Head of caudate nucleus
Anterior horn of lateral ventricle
Internal capsule
Sphenoid bone
Insula
Middle cerebral artery
Temporalis muscle
Temporal bone
Lateral fissure
Lentiform nucleus
Temporal lobe
Thalamus
Third ventricle
Choroid plexus
Great cerebral vein
Parietal bone
Superior cistern
Posterior horn of lateral ventricle
Occipital lobe
Falx cerebri
Superior sagittal sinus
Occipital bone

A

B

Fig. 26-7 A, Line drawing of CT section. **B,** CT image representing the anatomic structures located at level C in Fig. 26-2.

Fig. 26-8 MR image representing the anatomic structures located at level C in Fig. 26-2.

to the third ventricle on the CT image and posterior to the splenium of the corpus callosum on the MR image. It passes through the upper portion of the *superior cistern*. The pineal gland is also found in this cistern but is not clearly visualized in either image. This is an important radiographic landmark because of its tendency to calcify in adults. Branches of the middle cerebral artery are again visible within the lateral fissures, and the anterior cerebral

arteries can be seen in the anterior portion of the longitudinal fissure. The temporalis muscles are seen on the external surfaces on either side of the cranium.

The CT scan in Fig. 26-9 and the MR image in Fig. 26-10 pass through the superior portions of the orbits. In this CT image the frontal sinuses are again demonstrated. The orbital plates of the frontal bone are visualized here. The dark circles in the center of the orbital plates represent

the curved portion of this section of the bone where fat and the *superior rectus muscles* within the orbits curve upward. The *crista galli* of the ethmoid bone appears posterior to the frontal sinuses. The wings of the sphenoid bone are seen projecting medially into the cranium. The ridge of bone on the internal surface of the occipital bone is the upper portion of the *internal occipital protuberance*. The frontal, temporal, and occipital lobes of

Fig. 26-9 A, Line drawing of CT section. **B,** CT image representing the anatomic structures located at level D in Fig. 26-2.

Fig. 26-10 MR image corresponding to level D in Fig. 26-2.

the cerebrum, as well as the insula, are demonstrated on both images. These scans pass through the level of the midbrain. The *cerebral peduncles* form the anterior portions of the midbrain, and the *corpora quadrigemina* forms the posterior portion. In each image the small black circle anterior to the colliculi is the CSF-filled *cerebral aqueduct.* Posterior to the midbrain is the *cerebellum,* which is surrounded by the *tentorium cerebelli.* The dark region anterior to the midbrain is the *interpeduncular cistern,* and the one posterior to the midbrain is the superior cistern. On the MR image, within the interpeduncular cistern, the *optic tracts, hypothalamus,* inferior portion of the third ventricle, and the *mammillary bodies* can be seen. At this level several important vascular structures can be seen. The anterior and middle cerebral arteries are located at the anterior

edge of the interpeduncular cistern. One of the *posterior cerebral arteries* is visualized at the posterior edge of this cistern on the CT image; both can be seen on the MR image circling posteriorly around the cerebral peduncles of the midbrain. These vessels are part of the circle of Willis (although it is not seen in its entirety in either image). The posterior portion of the superior sagittal sinus is located near the internal occipital protuberance; the *straight sinus* can be seen in the edge of the tentorium cerebelli, just posterior to the cerebellum.

The CT and MR images seen in Figs. 26-11 and 26-12 were obtained through the center of the orbits and the tops of the ears. The *nasal bones* are visible in the anterior skull. Between the eyes the *ethmoidal sinuses* are seen, as well as the *cribriform plate* of the ethmoid bone. Several parts

of the sphenoid bone are visible on the CT scan. The greater wings are seen at the posterior wall of the orbit. The *sphenoidal sinuses* lie posterior to the ethmoidal sinuses. The *sella turcica* and *dorsum sellae* are seen surrounding the *pituitary gland.* The temporal bone constitutes most of the lateral portions of the skull, and the right *petrous ridge* can be seen on the CT image extending toward the median sagittal plane. The black air spaces near the lateral aspect of the petrous bone correspond to *mastoid air cells,* and those farther medial are associated with the internal structures of the ear. The internal occipital protuberance is seen in the posterior skull. Both *globes* are visible within the orbits. Rectus muscles lie along the medial and lateral walls of each. The *optic nerves* are seen in the centers of the posterior orbits passing from the eyes

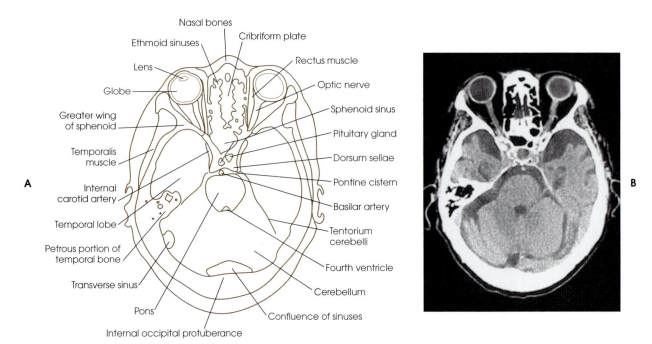

Fig. 26-11 A, Line drawing of CT section. **B,** CT image corresponding to level E in Fig. 26-2.

toward the brain via the optic canal. The bright area (on the CT image) in the right globe is the *lens* of the eye. The temporal lobes are found lateral to the sella turcica, resting in the middle cranial fossa. The *pons* lies posterior to the sella, and the cerebellum is seen filling the posterior cranial fossa. The edges of the tentorium cerebelli can faintly be seen between the temporal lobes and the cerebellum. The dark region anterior to the pons corresponds to the CSF-filled *pontine cistern* in which the contrast-filled *basilar artery* is easily visualized. At this level the *internal carotid arteries* lie lateral to the body of the sphenoid bone in an almost horizontal orientation. The dark region between the pons and the cerebellum is the superior region of the *fourth ventricle*. The *confluence of sinuses* can be seen just anterior to the internal occipital protuberance on the

CT image. The confluence is the region where the superior sagittal sinus and the straight sinus meet the transverse sinuses. The *transverse sinuses* are seen on the MR image at this level, and a portion of the right transverse sinus is also seen near the petrous ridge on the CT image. On the external surface of the skull, the temporalis muscles lie along the temporal bones. The *auricle*, or cartilaginous portion of each ear, lies external to the temporal bone.

The sectional images through the lower cranium demonstrate the inferior portions of the cerebrum, brainstem, cerebellum, and associated major skeletal structures (Fig. 26-13 is a CT image, Fig. 26-14 is an MR image). The maxilla, *maxillary sinuses*, and nasal bones are seen in the anterior skull (note the mass within the right maxillary sinus on the MR image).

The *zygomatic bones* form the lateral walls of the orbits, and the *maxillae* form the medial walls. The middle nasal conchae and the inferior ethmoidal sinuses are found within the nasal cavity (the MR image lies inferior to the ethmoidal sinuses). The *perpendicular plate* and *vomer* form the bony nasal septum seen in the center of the nasal cavity. Posterior to the nasal cavity, the sphenoidal sinuses are seen between the lower aspects of the greater wings. The right *zygomatic arch* is seen in its entirety; however, just the anterior portion is seen on the left in the CT scan. Both petrous ridges extend toward the midline; these are seen as dark areas on the MR image due to the lack of signal from this dense region of bone. Extending into the right petrous ridge is the *external auditory canal*. Just anterior to the canal is the *condyle of the mandible* resting in

Fig. 26-12 MR image corresponding to level E in Fig. 26-2.

the mandibular fossa. Mastoid air cells lie posterior to the external acoustic meatus. In the center of the skull the greater wings of the sphenoid, petrous ridges, and basilar portion of the occipital bone meet. The lowest parts of the globes are seen on the CT image within the orbits, surrounded by the radiolucent orbital fat. The most inferior folds of the temporal lobes are found in the middle cranial fossa resting on the greater wings of the sphenoid. The *medulla oblongata* lies posterior to the basilar portion of the occipital bone. The cerebellum is seen within the posterior fossa. The small, dark space between the medulla and the cerebellum is the lower extent of the fourth ventricle. CSF in the *cisterna magna* circulates around the anterior and lateral reaches of the medulla. At the level of this image the internal carotid arteries are found within the carotid canal of the temporal bone and thus are not visible on the CT scan; however, both are clearly visible as bright circles on the MR image. The *internal jugular veins* can also be seen on the MR scan just posterior to the internal carotid arteries. The two *vertebral arteries* lie anterior to the medulla. The MR image shows the junction of these two vessels, and the

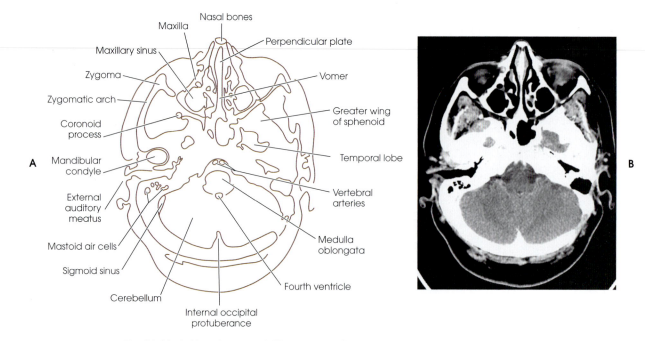

Fig. 26-13 **A,** Line drawing of CT section. **B,** CT image representing the anatomic structures located at level F in Fig. 26-2.

Fig. 26-14 MR image representing the anatomic structures located at level F in Fig. 26-2.

CT scan was obtained just inferior to the level where these vessels join to become the basilar artery. The transverse venous sinuses have passed anteriorly to the level of the petrous ridges. At this point they will change position and change names to become the *sigmoid sinuses*.

Fig. 26-15 is a CT scan, and Fig. 26-16 is an MR image through the lower part of the skull. The large, air-filled maxillary sinuses lie on either side of the nose. Within the nasal cavity, the *inferior nasal conchae* and the vomer are seen. Posterior to the nasal cavity, the medial and lateral

plates of the *pterygoid processes* lie at the back of the maxillary sinuses on the CT, and the nasopharynx is seen on the MR image. Portions of the zygomatic arches are seen extending posteriorly from the sides of the sinuses on the CT. The *condyles* and *coronoid processes* of the mandibular rami are deep to the zygomatic arches on the CT. These two processes are separated from each other by the mandibular notch. The MR image is slightly more inferior and demonstrates the rami of the mandible. The left *styloid process* of the temporal bone is seen medial to the left

mandibular condyle. The CT scan passes through the lowest regions of the petrous ridges and the mastoid processes; the MR image passes through the mastoid processes and the top of the vertebral column. The lowest reaches of the occipital bone are visible at the back of the skull, along with the foramen magnum on the CT. The *cerebellar tonsils* and the junction of the *spinal cord* and the medulla oblongata are seen at the foramen magnum, and the most inferior parts of the cerebellum can be seen through the occipital bone. The MR image demonstrates the spinal cord because the

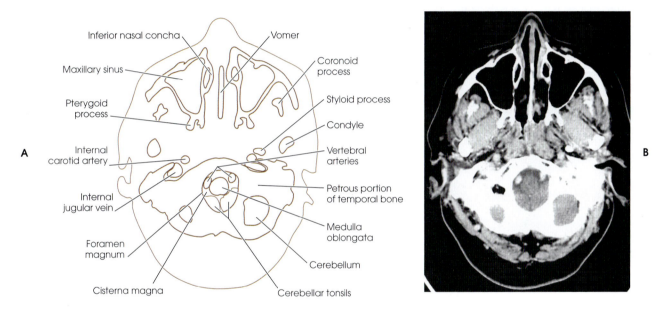

Fig. 26-15 **A,** Line drawing of CT section. **B,** CT image corresponding to level G in Fig. 26-2.

Fig. 26-16 MR image corresponding to level G in Fig. 26-2.

structures in this image lie inferior to the foramen magnum. The contrast-filled internal carotid arteries lie anterior and lateral to the foramen magnum and spinal cord. As the sigmoid venous sinuses pass through the jugular foramina, they become the internal jugular veins. These veins are visible in the images posterior to the internal carotid arteries. The contrast-filled vertebral arteries are seen along the anterolateral aspects of the medulla and spinal cord. Muscular structures on the external surface of the mandible are the *masseters*, and those on the internal surface are the *pterygoids*.

Finding images in sagittal, coronal, and oblique planes is increasingly common. CT scanners have the capability to generate images in the axial and coronal planes and to reconstruct the information in alternate planes. MRI, on the other hand, is capable of direct axial, sagittal, oblique, and coronal imaging. Representative images have been selected in the sagittal and coronal planes to help interpret the anatomy demonstrated.

Fig. 26-17 is a midsagittal MR image of the cranium. The relationship between the cerebral hemisphere, cerebellum, and brainstem is demonstrated. In this image the frontal, parietal, and occipital lobes of the cerebrum are seen and correspond to the cranial bones. The corpus callosum is a white matter tract that connects the hemispheres and is found at the inferior aspect of the frontal and parietal lobes. CSF appears dark on this T1-weighted image, making it relatively easy to trace the ventricular system. The anterior horn of the lateral ventricle is inferior to the genu of the corpus callosum. The third ventricle lies in the midline, between the two lateral ventricles. The lateral ventricles produce a great deal of CSF, which is transported to the third ventricle by way of the *intraventricular foramina (of Monro)*. The third ventricle is not optimally visualized in this image. What is actually seen is the thalamus, which forms the lateral wall of the third ventricle. CSF drains from the third ventricle via the *cerebral aqueduct (of Sylvius)*, which can be found within the midbrain (between the *corpora quadrigemina* and the *cerebral peduncles*). The *fourth ventricle* is also a midline structure and is situated between the pons and cerebellum. The large air-filled sphenoidal sinus is located anterior to the pons. Superior to this, the pituitary gland rests within hypophyseal fossa formed by the sella turcica. Directly superior to the pituitary gland is the optic chiasm.

A

B

Fig. 26-17 A, Line drawing of MR section. **B,** MR image through midsagittal plane.

Several vascular structures are well demonstrated in Fig. 26-17. The basilar artery appears between the clivus and pons. Portions of the superior sagittal sinus can be seen between the cerebrum and the cranial bones. Between the cerebrum and cerebellum, the *straight sinus* (one of the dural venous sinuses) is noted within the tentorium cerebelli. This vessel is formed by the junction of the inferior sagittal sinus and the great cerebral vein (of Galen).

A CT localizer, or scout, image (Fig. 26-18) is included as a reference for the next three coronal images. Fig. 26-19 is a coronal MR image through the anterior horns of the lateral ventricles and the pharyngeal structures. The anterior portions of the cerebral hemispheres are joined by the corpus callosum, which is immediately superior to the lateral ventricles. The membrane between the anterior horns of the lateral ventricles is the *septum pellucidum.* On the lateral aspect of each cerebral hemisphere is the *lateral fissure,* which divides the frontal lobe from the temporal lobe. The insula lies deep to this fissure.

Structures of the basal nuclei can again be identified. The caudate nucleus is lateral to the anterior horns. Inferolateral to the caudate nuclei are the internal capsules, white matter tracts that connect the cortex to deeper gray matter

structures. The anterior portion of the third ventricle is found in the midline inferior to the lateral ventricles. Inferior to the third ventricle are the optic chiasm and hypophysis cerebri. The *superior* and *inferior sagittal sinuses* occupy the margins of the falx cerebri in the longitudinal fissure between the hemispheres of the cerebrum. The internal carotid arteries occupy the *cavernous sinus* along

with several cranial nerves and are found lateral to the pituitary gland and sella turcica. Branches of the middle cerebral arteries occupy the lateral fissures of the cerebrum. Several air-filled structures are seen on this image; they are (from superior to inferior) the sphenoidal sinus and the *nasopharynx.* This image also demonstrates the external carotid arteries within the parotid salivary glands.

Fig. 26-18 CT localizer (scout) image of the skull.

Fig. 26-19 A, Line drawing of MR section. **B,** Coronal MR image corresponding to level A in Fig. 26-18.

A

B

Fig. 26-20 **A,** Line drawing of MR section. **B,** Coronal MR image corresponding to level B in Fig. 26-18.

Fig. 26-20 is a coronal MR image through the bodies of the lateral ventricles, the brainstem, and the bodies of the cervical vertebrae. The third ventricle is well demonstrated and bordered laterally by the thalamus. The cartilaginous structures of the *external ear* surround the *external acoustic meatus* and *canal.* The dark region (low signal return) medial to the external acoustic canal corresponds to the *petrous portion of the temporal bone.* The first two cervical vertebrae are detailed in this section with the *dens* of the *axis* (C2) seen between the lateral masses of the *atlas* (C1). The large, whitish masses inferior to the external acoustic canals are the *parotid glands.*

Fig. 26-21 shows a coronal MR image through the lateral ventricles and cerebellum. The splenium of the corpus callosum is found between the lateral ventricles. Inferior to the splenium is the superior cistern. Portions of the cerebellum are visualized superior and inferior to the middle cerebellar peduncles. The large, dark area near the center of the cerebellum is the fourth ventricle. The dark line between the cerebellum and cerebrum represents the tentorium cerebelli. The large, dark areas (signal void) lateral to the cerebellum correspond to the bony mastoid portions of the temporal bone.

A

B

Fig. 26-21 **A,** Line drawing of MR section. **B,** Coronal MR image corresponding to level C in Fig. 26-18.

Thoracic Region

The thorax extends from the thoracic inlet to the diaphragm. The inlet is an imaginary plane through the first thoracic vertebra and the top of the manubrium. Sectional images of the thorax are obtained to include all structures between these boundaries. Two cadaver images are included to assist in identifying some of the structures of the thorax. Fig. 26-22 is a cadaver image that corresponds to a level just superior to the sternoclavicular joints. Fig. 26-23 lies near the level of the sixth thoracic vertebra and demonstrates the chambers of the heart and other surrounding structures.

The bones of the thorax include the thoracic vertebrae, ribs, sternum, clavicles, and scapulae. Each of the 12 thoracic vertebra is subdivided into a body and a vertebral arch. The opening formed between these divisions is the vertebral foramen, through which the spinal cord travels. Two pedicles, two laminae, two transverse processes, and one spinous process constitute the arch. The pedicles are more anterior and unite with the body of the vertebra; the laminae form the posterior part of the arch and unite to give rise to the spinous process. Transverse processes arise from the lateral arch where pedicles and laminae meet. Two superior articular processes arise from the superior arch, and two inferior articular processes arise from the inferior arch. Superior and inferior articular processes from adjacent vertebrae articulate to form zygapophyseal joints. Intervertebral foramina are formed by notches between succeeding arches. These foramina transmit spinal nerves. Articular disks are found between the vertebral bodies. These disks are composed of a dense cartilaginous outer rim called the *annulus fibrosus* and a gelatinous central core called the *nucleus pulposus.* Twelve pairs of ribs curl around the lateral thorax to protect the lungs and heart. The head of each rib is posterior and articulates with the body of a thoracic vertebra. These joints are called *costovertebral joints.* Tubercles of the ribs are lateral to the heads and articulate with transverse processes of the vertebrae, forming costotransverse joints. Anteriorly, the first 10 pairs of ribs articulate with the sternum either directly or indirectly via costal cartilage. The sternum lies in the midline

Fig. 26-22 A, Line drawing of gross anatomic section. **B,** Cadaver image of the superior thorax.

of the anterior chest wall. From superior to inferior the parts are the manubrium, body, and xiphoid process. An indentation at the superior edge of the sternum, the jugular or sternal notch, lies at the level of the interspace between the second and third thoracic vertebrae. The manubrium joins the body of the sternum at the sternal angle, which corresponds to the interspace between the fourth and fifth thoracic vertebrae. The xiphoid process lies at approximately the level of the tenth thoracic vertebra. Familiarity with these vertebral levels can be helpful in orienting oneself when looking at thoracic sectional images.

The clavicles are slender, S-shaped bones that extend across the upper anterior thorax. The medial end of each clavicle articulates with the superolateral edge of the manubrium to form sternoclavicular (SC) joints. Acromioclavicular (AC) joints are formed where the lateral extremity of the clavicle articulates with the acromion process of the scapula. The scapulae are triangular bones in the superior posterior thorax. Thinking of the scapula as having two surfaces (anterior and posterior), three borders (superior, medial, lateral), and three angles (superior, lateral, inferior) is helpful. The posterior surface is divided into a superior fossa and an inferior fossa by the scapular spine. This bony ridge extends laterally and

superiorly to end as the acromion process. The coracoid process projects from the superior anterior surface near the glenoid. The lateral angle is formed by the glenoid cavity, which articulates with the humeral head. Many of these bony structures are identifiable on Fig. 26-22.

Major components of the respiratory system are seen in the thorax. The trachea originates at the level of the sixth cervical vertebra (near the bottom of the thyroid cartilage). The trachea is formed by incomplete cartilage rings, which are open along its posterior surface. The trachea passes into the thorax and bifurcates into the right and left main bronchi near the level of the sternal angle (T4/5). The carina is the last cartilage ring of the trachea. The main bronchi pass through the hila of the lungs and branch to secondary bronchi, one for each lobe. The lungs are triangular organs enclosed in the thoracic cavity by the double-walled pleural membrane. The portion of the lung that lies superior to the clavicle is the apex; the part that rests on the diaphragm is the base. The most inferior and posterior reaches of the base is a region called the *costophrenic angle*. The bronchi and vascular structures enter and exit the center of the medial aspect of the lung at the hilum. Each lung is divided into superior and inferior lobes by an oblique fissure. The upper lobe of the right lung is further

divided by a horizontal fissure to form a middle lobe that lies lateral to the heart. The portion of the left lung that corresponds in position to the right middle lobe is called the *lingula*.

The area between the lungs is the mediastinum. Within this cavity are the heart, trachea and bronchi, esophagus, major blood vessels, nerves, and lymphatic structures. The heart lies obliquely oriented in the lower mediastinum, surrounded by a double-walled fibrous sac called the *pericardium*. It rests on the diaphragm between the sternum and the thoracic spine. The superior surface is the base, and the inferior portion is the apex. The heart is divided into four chambers: two atria and two ventricles. The atria receive blood, and the ventricles pump blood away from the heart. The right atrium forms the right border of the heart and receives blood from the superior vena cava, inferior vena cava, and the coronary sinus (the venous drainage channel for the heart muscle). Blood passes from here through the tricuspid (right atrioventricular) valve into the right ventricle. This chamber forms most of the anterior surface of the heart. As this ventricle contracts, blood passes through the infundibulum (pulmonary outflow tract), through the pulmonary semilunar valve, and into the main pulmonary artery toward the lungs. The left atrium forms the posterior border of the heart

A

B

Fig. 26-23 A, Line drawing of gross anatomic section **B,** Cadaver image of the central thorax.

and receives blood from four pulmonary veins. Blood passes through the mitral (bicuspid or left atrioventricular) valve into the left ventricle. The most muscular of the chambers, the left ventricle forms the left side and most inferior portion of the heart. Blood is pumped out through the aortic semilunar valve and into the aorta as this ventricle contracts. A muscular wall, the interventricular septum, can be seen between the ventricles. Chambers of the heart are seen in Fig. 26-23.

One portion of the digestive system is typically found in the thorax. The esophagus originates at the level of the sixth cervical vertebra as the posterior continuation of the pharynx. It continues into the thorax, at first posterior to the trachea, then posterior to the left atrium and ventricle of the heart. At the lower thorax, the esophagus pierces the diaphragm to continue into the abdomen.

The vascular system in the upper thorax can be confusing. In order to identify these structures, one must clearly understand the vascular anatomy. Tracing the paths of vessels through the scan can help alleviate some of the confusion. This discussion follows the path of circulation through the vessels. The discussion of arterial structures starts at the heart and follows the vessels toward the periphery. Veins are discussed from their peripheral origins and followed as they travel toward the heart.

The aorta originates from the left ventricle of the heart. Just distal to the aortic semilunar valve are the origins of the right and left coronary arteries, which supply the heart muscle. The aorta ascends along the posterior sternum, arches posterior and toward the left behind the sternal angle, and then turns inferiorly to become the descending aorta. The descending aorta passes down the posterior thorax, resting against the left anterolateral sur-

faces of the vertebral bodies. The major vessels that supply the head and upper limbs arise from the aortic arch. From anterior to posterior, these are the brachiocephalic, left common carotid, and left subclavian arteries. The brachiocephalic artery passes superiorly and bifurcates into the right subclavian and right common carotid arteries posterior to the sternoclavicular joint. The right and left common carotid arteries ascend the neck along the lateral surface of the trachea. At approximately the level of the third cervical vertebra, each common carotid artery exhibits a dilatation called the *carotid sinus* just proximal to bifurcating into internal and external carotid arteries. The subclavian arteries pass laterally across the upper thorax, just deep to the clavicles. At the outer edges of the first ribs, the subclavian arteries become the axillary arteries.

Venous drainage from the head is mainly through the jugular veins. The internal jugular veins accompany the carotid arteries down through the neck, lateral to the trachea. The subclavian veins are continuations of the axillary veins draining the upper limbs. These veins pass toward the midline deep to the clavicles. At the sternoclavicular joints, the internal jugular veins and the subclavian veins unite to form the brachiocephalic veins. The right brachiocephalic vein passes vertically downward; the left passes obliquely down, posterior to the manubrium. These two vessels unite to form the superior vena cava (SVC). The SVC lies posterior to the right border of the sternum and enters the right atrium just below the level of the sternal angle. Venous drainage from the lower body is via the inferior vena cava (IVC). This vessel is found along the right anterior surface of the vertebral bodies and empties into the inferior aspect

of the right atrium. The azygos vein is a small vessel that passes up the posterior thorax along the right anterior aspect of the vertebral bodies. It arches anteriorly (near the level of the aortic arch) to drain into the SVC.

The pulmonary vascular system transports blood between the lungs and heart. The main pulmonary artery receives deoxygenated blood from the right ventricle. At the level of the sternal angle, this vessel gives rise to the right and left pulmonary arteries, which pass laterally toward the hila of the lungs. The bifurcation of the main pulmonary artery is just inferior to the aortic arch. Four pulmonary veins exit the hila, two from each lung, and pass medially to enter the superolateral aspect of the left atrium.

Many muscles can be seen in the thorax, especially in the shoulder region. The pectoralis major is a large, fan-shaped muscle superficially located along the anterior chest wall. The pectoralis minor lies just deep to the pectoralis major. The trapezius is the most superficial of the posterior thoracic muscles. The rhomboid major and minor muscles are deep to the trapezius and lie between the medial scapular borders and the spinous processes of the upper thoracic spine. The serratus anterior muscles attach to the medial side of the anterior scapula and blanket the external surface of the rib cage. Several muscles are associated with the scapula; many of these also attach to the humerus. The subscapularis muscle lines the anterior surface. Supraspinatus and infraspinatus muscles lie in the supraspinous and infraspinous fossae, respectively. The teres major and minor also lie along the infraspinous fossa. Four of these muscles are collectively known as the rotator cuff: subscapularis, supraspinatus, infraspinatus, and teres minor.

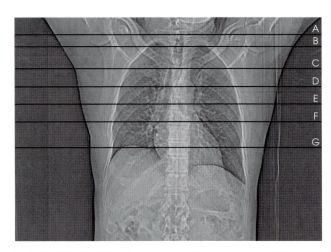

Fig. 26-24 CT localizer (scout) image of the thorax.

Fig. 26-25 A, Line drawing of CT section. **B,** CT image corresponding to level A in Fig. 26-24 through the first thoracic vertebra.

The CT localizer, or scout, image represents an anteroposterior (AP) projection of the thoracic region with identifying lines (Fig. 26-24). These lines demonstrate the approximate levels for each of the labeled images for this region. Most of the images for this region will be CT scans. When performing scans of the thorax, the patient's arms are extended above the head. This fact must be kept in mind when looking at upper thoracic scans because some anatomic structures will not correspond to the normal anatomic position. MR images are frequently degraded by motion artifact in the thorax, so only a few representative images are included.

Fig. 26-25 represents a CT image at the level of T1 and demonstrates the relationship between the vertebral column, esophagus, and trachea. The body and *vertebral arch* of the first thoracic vertebra can be identified, and the spinal cord is seen in the vertebral foramen. The *costotransverse joint* between the first rib and the transverse process of the first thoracic vertebra is seen on the left. The acromial extremity of the *clavicle* lies near the *acromion* on the left side, and the AC joint is seen on the right. Because the patient's arms are raised, this scan passes through the surgical neck of the humerus. The inferior portion of the *thyroid gland,* which extends from C6 to T1, is positioned lateral to the *trachea.* The soft tissue shadow immediately posterior to the trachea is the *esophagus.* The *vertebral arteries* are positioned lateral to the vertebral column, and the *common carotid arteries* are found lateral to the trachea. At this level the *internal jugular veins* are positioned to the lateral aspect of the carotid arteries. The contrast-filled axillary arteries can be seen in the medial aspect of the arms. The *sternocleidomastoid muscles* are found lateral to the thyroid gland. The *trapezius* is the most superficial muscle of the posterior thorax, with the levator scapulae muscles lying just anterior.

Fig. 26-26 is a CT image through the lower edge of T2. This scan passes through the *jugular notch* of the sternum and is just superior to the sternoclavicular joints. The costovertebral and costotransverse joints are seen between the ribs and the spine. On the right, the glenoid portion and the acromion process of the scapula are seen. The humerus is visible where it articulates with the glenoid cavity. On the left, the spine and the body of the scapula are seen. The *trachea* and esophagus are located anterior to the vertebral body. The major vessels of the superior thorax are visualized posterior to the clavicles. The right and left *brachiocephalic veins* are formed by the junction of the *subclavian veins* and the internal jugular veins. Because contrast media was injected for this scan, the axillary and most of the right subclavian vein are filled with contrast. Posterior to the right clavicle, the right subclavian vein and internal jugular vein have joined. Because the image is slightly more inferior on the left, the image plane passes through the left brachiocephalic vein (below the junction of these two vessels). The brachiocephalic veins will unite and form the *superior vena cava* at a more inferior level. The arterial branches to the head and upper limb are also visualized on this image. From the patient's right to left, they are the *right subclavian artery, right common carotid artery, left common carotid artery,* and *left subclavian artery.* The brachiocephalic artery gives rise to the right subclavian and right common carotid arteries and is inferior to this level. The *pectoralis major and minor* lie along the anterior thoracic wall. The trapezius is the most superficial of the posterior muscles and is seen between the scapula and the spine on each side. The *subscapularis muscle* lines the left anterior scapula, the *infraspinatus* and *teres minor* line the posterior portion of this bone, and the *supraspinatus* is seen between the body and the scapular spine.

Fig. 26-26 A, Line drawing of CT section. **B,** CT image corresponding to level B in Fig. 26-24 through the jugular notch.

Brachiocephalic veins

Pectoralis muscles
Sternoclavicular joint
Brahiocephalic artery

Rib
Manubrium

Subscapularis
muscle
Common
carotid artery

A

Lung

T3

Scapula

Infraspinatus and
teres muscles
Trachea
Subclavian
artery

Trapezius
muscle
Rhomboid
muscles

Esophagus

Fig. 26-27 A, Line drawing of CT section. **B,** CT image corresponding to level C in Fig. 26-24 just superior to the aortic arch.

Fig. 26-27 is a CT image through the level of T3. Bony structures depicted in this image include the *manubrium* and sternoclavicular joints anteriorly, the ribs laterally, and the scapulae and vertebra posteriorly. Both the spine and the body of the right scapula are visible at this level. Costovertebral and costotransverse joints are again noted along the right side of the vertebra. Several vascular structures, highlighted with contrast, are visible posterior to the manubrium. The right and left brachiocephalic veins are seen just posterior to the right sternoclavicular joint. This level is just superior to where the vessels join to form the superior vena cava. The brachiocephalic artery, left common carotid artery, and left subclavian artery curl around the left side of the trachea. This scan is just superior to the arch of the aorta and thus visualizes the origins of these three vessels. Posterior to the vessels are the trachea and esophagus. The upper lobes of each lung lie lateral to the mediastinal structures. The pectoralis major and minor lie external to the anterior ribs. Rotator cuff muscles (subscapularis, infraspinatus, teres minor) are demonstrated anterior and posterior to the scapulae. The trapezius and *rhomboid muscles* lie between the scapulae and the spinous process of the vertebra in this image.

Fig. 26-28 is a CT scan obtained through the lower edge of T4. At this level the brachiocephalic veins have joined to form the *superior vena cava*. The large contrast-filled structure in the left antero-lateral mediastinum is the *aortic arch*.

Fig. 26-29 represents a CT image at the level of T5 and demonstrates the great vessels superior to the heart. (The heart is normally positioned between T7 and T11, with the majority of the organ lying left of the midline.) The *ascending aorta* is found anteriorly in the midline; the *descending aorta* is related to the left anterolateral surface of the vertebral bodies. (This relationship between the descending aorta and vertebral column is continuous through the thorax and abdomen.) Note the normal difference in caliber between the ascending and descending aorta. The superior vena cava

Fig. 26-28 A, Line drawing of CT section. **B,** CT image corresponding to level D in Fig. 26-24 through the aortic arch.

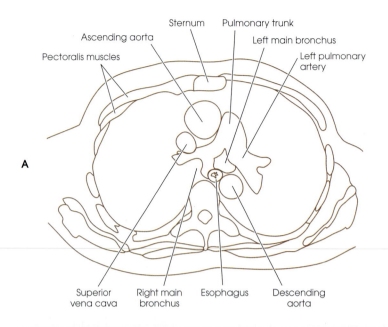

Ascending aorta   Sternum   Pulmonary trunk

Pectoralis muscles   Left main bronchus

Left pulmonary artery

A

Superior vena cava   Right main bronchus   Esophagus   Descending aorta

B

Fig. 26-29 **A,** Line drawing of CT section. **B,** CT image corresponding to level E in Fig. 26-24 through the pulmonary trunk.

is located to the right of the ascending aorta, and the pulmonary trunk and left and right pulmonary arteries are located to the left of the ascending aorta at this level. The *pulmonary trunk* originates from the right ventricle of the heart and divides into the right and left *pulmonary arteries,* which carry deoxygenated blood to the lungs. The left pulmonary artery is seen bifurcating into the two lobar branches at the hilum of the left lung. Near the T5 level the trachea divides into the left and right *primary bronchi.* The esophagus (in which a small amount of air is seen) is found just posterior to the left main bronchus. Fig. 26-30 is an MR image that corresponds in position to the previous CT image. Notice on this image that the main pulmonary artery and the left pulmonary artery are seen, although the right pulmonary artery is not visible. Muscular structures are easily differentiated. The spinal cord is seen within the vertebral canal, where it is surrounded by CSF.

Fig. 26-30 MR image corresponding to level E in Fig. 26-24.

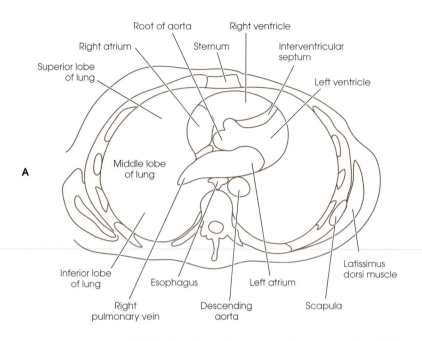

A

Root of aorta

Right ventricle

Right atrium

Sternum

Interventricular septum

Superior lobe of lung

Left ventricle

Middle lobe of lung

Inferior lobe of lung

Esophagus

Left atrium

Latissimus dorsi muscle

Right pulmonary vein

Descending aorta

Scapula

B

Fig. 26-31 A, Line drawing of CT section. **B,** CT image corresponding to level F in Fig. 26-24 through the base of the heart.

The CT image depicted in Fig. 26-31 demonstrates the *lungs* and the base of the *heart.* Generally when the heart is imaged in cross section, the *left atrium* is the most superior structure encountered and the *pulmonary veins* are seen emptying into it (one of the right pulmonary veins can be seen here). The *right atrium* is seen lying the farthest toward the right side of the body, anterior and somewhat inferior to the left atrium. The SVC may be seen at this level as it enters the right atrium. The *right ventricle* lies to the left of the right atrium and anterior to the more muscular *left ventricle.* Contrast-enhanced blood is seen here as blood exits the left ventricle to enter the root of the aorta. The *interventricular septum* can be seen between the ventricles.

The lungs are divided into superior and inferior lobes by the diagonally oriented *oblique fissure.* The *superior lobes* lie superior and anterior to the inferior lobes. The *superior lobe* of the right lung is further divided by the *horizontal fissure,* with the lower portion termed the *middle lobe.* The left lung has no horizontal fissure. The inferior and anterior portion of the left lung (corresponding to the right middle lobe) is termed the *lingula.* Although the fissures are not seen, the approximate locations of these lobes are identified here.

Muscular structures that can be seen at this level include the inferior insertions of the trapezius, the *latissimus dorsi,* and the *serratus anterior muscles.* The esophagus lies between the left atrium and the vertebral column at this level.

Fig. 26-32 lies at approximately T9 and demonstrates the lower sternum and ribs. The descending aorta normally lies along the left anterolateral surface of the vertebral column, and the *azygos vein* is normally on the right anterolateral surface. Because this scan is inferior to the right ventricle, the *inferior vena cava* is seen between the heart and the liver. The superior portion of the liver is bulging against the base of the right lung, and the most superior portion of the left hemidiaphragm is seen at the base of the left lung.

The right and left ventricles of the heart, as well as the interventricular septum, can be seen surrounded by pericardium. Major muscle structures visible are the serratus anterior, latissimus dorsi, and the deep back muscles.

Fig. 26-33 presents a sagittal MR image through the midline structures of the neck and upper thorax. The air-filled pharynx and trachea are easily identified. The cartilaginous flap within the laryngeal portion of the pharynx is the *epiglottis*. Spinal structures are clearly visible in this image, and the relationship between the *intervertebral disks* and *spinal cord* is demonstrated. The major blood vessels of the superior thorax are seen posterior to the *manubrium*. The most anterior of these vessels is the left brachiocephalic vein, which ultimately unites with the right brachiocephalic vein to form the superior vena cava. Posterior to the brachiocephalic vein is a portion of the aortic arch with the origin of the brachiocephalic artery. Inferior to the arch is the right pulmonary artery.

The coronal MR image in Fig. 26-34 is slightly posterior to the midcoronal plane and also demonstrates structures of the neck and superior thorax. The distal cervical and superior thoracic vertebrae are identifiable. On the patient's left side, the *humeral head, clavicle, acromion process,* and *acromioclavicular joint* are seen. The *tracheal bifurcation* is visualized on this image. The aortic arch and left pulmonary artery are found in close proximity to the left main bronchus. From the superior aspect of the arch extends the left subcla-

Fig. 26-32 A, Line drawing of CT section. **B,** CT image corresponding to level G in Fig. 26-24 through the right hemidiaphragm.

Pharynx
Tongue
Epiglottis

Trachea

Left brachiocephalic vein

Manubrium of sternum

C2 vertebra

Spinal cord

Intervertebral disk

Brachiocephalic artery

Aortic arch

Right pulmonary artery

Fig. 26-33 Midline sagittal MR image through neck and upper thorax.

Spinal cord
Sternocleidomastoid muscle

Right lung

Tracheal bifurcation

Heart

Left subclavian artery

Clavicle

Acromion

Humeral head

Arch of aorta
Pulmonary trunk

Fig. 26-34 MR image of neck and thorax through midcoronal plane.

vian artery. The heart and lungs are not ideally imaged in this scan because of motion artifacts.

Abdominopelvic Region

The abdominopelvic region includes the diaphragm and everything inferior to it. Fig. 26-35 is a cadaver image at the level of the second lumbar vertebra. Major abdominal organs and vascular structures can be identified in this image. In the abdomen, five lumbar vertebrae are visible. Although these vertebrae are slightly larger than those in the thorax, the anatomic components are roughly the same. In the pelvis the lower spine and hip bones (os coxae or innominate) form an attachment for the lower limbs and support for the trunk. The sacrum and coccyx comprise the lower spine. These are triangular bones with their broad bases oriented superiorly. Each os coxae lies obliquely situated in the pelvis, articulating with the sacrum (sacroiliac joint) posteriorly and with the opposite os coxae anteriorly (symphysis pubis). At birth, this bone consists of three components: the ilium, ischium, and pubis. Ultimately these three fuse at the acetabulum. The superior, wing-shaped portion of the os coxae is the ilium. The superior edge is the crest, which lies at the level of the lower fourth lumbar vertebra. The anterior superior and anterior inferior iliac spines lie along the anterior surface of the ilium. At the posterior ilium, posterior superior and posterior inferior iliac spines are found at the top and bottom of the sacral articular surface. Below the posterior inferior iliac spine, the greater sciatic notch curves sharply toward the front of the bone. The inferior and anterior os coxae are composed of the pubis. The pubic bone extends from the acetabulum toward the midline, then curves inferiorly. The pubic bones articulate with each other at the symphysis pubis. The posterior inferior os coxae is formed by the ischium. This portion extends inferiorly from the acetabulum, then curls forward to meet the lower part of the pubis. The obturator foramen is a circular opening formed by the junction of the pubis and ischium.

The abdominal cavity is lined by a double-walled membrane called the *peritoneum.* Some organs develop posterior to the peritoneum and are referred to as *retroperitoneal.* Others invaginate into the peritoneum and are referred to as *intraperitoneal.* Several large folds of the peritoneum are identifiable on sectional images because of the large amount of fat found within it. The greater omentum extends from the greater curvature of the stomach and the transverse colon to blanket the anterior surface of the abdominal organs, especially the digestive organs. The small intestines invaginate into the peritoneum as they develop, and a large flap of peritoneum—the mesentery—anchors this part of the digestive system to the posterior abdominal wall.

The spleen is an organ belonging to the lymphatic system. It lies inferior to the left hemidiaphragm and posterior to the fundus of the stomach. On the medial surface of the spleen, blood vessels enter and exit at the hilum.

The organs of the alimentary tract include the esophagus, stomach, small intestine, and large intestine. The esophagus lies anterior to the spine and passes through the diaphragm to enter the abdomen at about the level of T10. Once in the abdomen, it passes toward the left to enter the stomach. The opening into the stomach is the cardiac orifice, and the junction is the esophagogastric (EG) junction. The stomach is a somewhat J-shaped pouch in the left upper quadrant. The region above the level of the EG junction is the fundus, the central region is the body, and the distal part is the pyloric antrum. This last portion normally lies at about the level of the second lumbar vertebra. The medial and lateral borders are referred to as the *lesser and greater curvatures.* Internally the stomach is thrown into multiple folds termed *rugae.* Food passes from the distal stomach through the pyloric canal into the

Fig. 26-35 A, Line drawing of gross anatomic section. **B,** Cadaver section through the central abdomen at the level of L2.

small intestine. Passage through the canal is controlled by a muscle called the *pyloric sphincter.* The small intestine consists of the duodenum, jejunum, and ileum. The first portion or duodenum extends from the stomach, laterally to the liver where the remainder curls inferiorly and medially to form a C-shaped loop around the head of the pancreas. The duodenum is approximately 10 to 12 inches long, and at the ligament of Treitz it continues as the jejunum. The jejunum is approximately 8 feet long and mainly occupies the left upper abdomen. It continues as the ileum. This most distal part of the small bowel is about 10 feet long and occupies the right inferior abdominal cavity and the pelvis. The large intestine is about 6 feet long. It frames the periphery of the abdominal cavity and comprises the cecum; colon (ascending, transverse, descending, and sigmoid portions); rectum; and anus. The ileum empties into the saclike cecum in the right lower quadrant via the ileocecal valve. The vermiform appendix can frequently be seen projecting off the cecum. From the cecum the ascending portion of the colon passes superiorly. Just below the liver, this portion curves anteriorly and medially at the hepatic (right colic) flexure. From here the transverse portion passes across the anterior abdomen. This portion dips inferiorly into the abdomen to a variable degree depending on the body habitus of the patient. As the colon reaches the spleen, it turns posteriorly and inferiorly at the splenic (left colic) flexure to become the descending colon. This portion passes down the posterior aspect of the left side of the abdomen toward the pelvis, where it continues as the sigmoid colon. The sigmoid colon curls medially and posteriorly in the pelvis, and at the midsacrum it curves inferiorly as the rectum. The rectum lies anterior to and follows the curve of the sacrum to become the anal canal as the large intestine exits the pelvis.

Several accessory organs of the digestive system are located in the upper abdomen. The liver occupies most of the right upper quadrant. This triangular organ is divided anatomically into a large right lobe and a much smaller left lobe. The falciform ligament is located along the division between these lobes on the anterior surface, and the ligamentum venosum and ligamentum teres are found along the division on the posterior surface of the liver. On the posteroinferior surface of the right lobe are two smaller lobes: the caudate (superior) and the quadrate (inferior). These two lobes are separated by the porta hepatis (hilum) of the liver. The hepatic artery, portal vein, and hepatic bile ducts enter and exit the liver here. The gallbladder rests against the undersurface of the liver. This organ functions as a storage vessel for bile, which is produced in the liver. Bile drains from the liver through the right and left hepatic ducts. These ducts unite to form the common hepatic duct, which meets the cystic duct from the gallbladder. Distal to this junction, the continuation of this duct is known as the *common bile duct.* Bile passes through this duct to empty into the second part of the duodenum at the hepatopancreatic ampulla (ampulla of Vater). The pancreas, which functions as both an endocrine and exocrine gland, lies transversely across the abdomen near the level of the second lumbar vertebra. The divisions of this retroperitoneal organ, from right to left, are the head, neck, body, and tail. The head is the most inferior portion and is encircled by the duodenum. The tail is located near the hilum of the spleen. The pancreatic duct traverses the length of the organ and enters the second part of the duodenum at or near the common bile duct.

The urinary system includes the two kidneys and ureters, the bladder, and the urethra. The kidneys are retroperitoneal and lie between the twelfth thoracic and third lumbar vertebrae. The center or hilar region is normally near the interspace between L1 and L2. Suprarenal (adrenal) glands are perched on the upper surface of each kidney. The right adrenal gland can be seen between the liver and the right diaphragmatic crus, and the left lies between the left crus and the pancreatic tail and spleen. Each kidney is surrounded by a dense membrane, the renal fasciae, and a layer of fat, the perirenal fat. Urine is formed in the parenchyma of the kidney and collects in the calyceal system. The calyces unite to form the renal pelvis, which is continuous with the ureter. The ureters are musculomembranous tubes that extend down the posterior abdomen resting along the anterior surface of the psoas muscles. They are difficult to visualize unless filled with radiopaque contrast. In the pelvis the ureters empty into the posteroinferior region of the bladder. The bladder is a collapsible muscular sac, which serves as a reservoir for urine until it is expelled from the body. The bladder rests on or near the pelvic floor, posterior to the symphysis pubis and anterior to the rectum in males or the vagina in females. The urethra is the muscular passageway that originates from the apex (inferior surface) of the bladder and by which urine is expelled. The urethra is relatively short in females, passing through the floor of the pelvis. The urethra is much longer in males because it passes through the prostate gland and the membranous and cavernous portions of the penis.

The internal organs of the male reproductive system include the ductus deferens, seminal vesicles, and prostate. Internal and external reproductive structures are connected by the spermatic cord, which includes the ductus deferens, testicular vessels, nerves, and lymphatic structures. The spermatic cord is seen anterior and medial to the femoral artery and vein and anterior and lateral to the pubis. The ductus deferens enters the pelvis through the spermatic cord and then arches over the anterior and lateral aspect of the bladder. It passes down the posterior surface of the bladder and enters the superior prostate. The seminal vesicles are found on the posterior and inferior surface of the bladder near the insertion of the ureters. The prostate gland lies inferior to the bladder, between the symphysis pubis and the rectum. The prostatic portion of the urethra passes through the prostate.

The organs of the female reproductive system include the uterus, uterine (fallopian) tubes, ovaries, and vagina. The uterus, which normally lies superior and posterior to the urinary bladder, is divided into a fundus, body, isthmus, and cervix. The fundus is the upper, rounded portion of the organ, superior to the orifices of the uterine tubes. The central portion is the body, which narrows at its lower end to become the isthmus. The narrowed lower 2 cm of the uterus is the cervix, which is continuous with the vagina. The uterus is suspended in the pelvis by folds of peritoneum called the *broad ligaments.* The ovaries lie lateral to the body of the uterus within the broad ligament. They are normally found near the lateral pelvic wall, at or slightly below the level of the anterior superior iliac spine. Extending between the ovaries and uterus, in the superior rim of the broad ligament, are the uterine tubes. The medial ends open into the upper body of the uterus. The lateral end of each tube, the infundibulum, is expanded and terminates in multiple fingerlike projections called *fimbriae*. This end of the tube is superior to the ovary but not attached. The most inferior part of the internal female reproductive system is the vagina. This muscular tube lies between the rectum and the bladder and opens to the external body surface posterior to the urethral meatus.

Three vascular systems can be described in the abdomen: arterial, venous, and portal. The descending, or abdominal, aorta passes through the diaphragm at approximately the level of T11 and extends to the pelvis along the left anterolateral surface of the vertebral bodies. Just below the diaphragm, at approximately the level of the twelfth thoracic vertebra, the celiac artery originates from the anterior aorta. This fairly short vessel divides into the splenic, common hepatic, and left gastric arteries. The splenic artery passes toward the left to enter the hilum of the spleen. The common hepatic extends to the right to the porta hepatis. The superior mesenteric artery arises from the left anterior aorta near the first lumbar vertebra. The origin of this vessel is posterior to the neck of the pancreas. It extends anteriorly for a short distance and then turns inferiorly as it sends its branches to supply the small intestine and the proximal half of the large intestine. Near the level of the second lumbar vertebra, the renal arteries arise from the lateral surface of the aorta. The renal arteries pass laterally to enter the hila of the kidneys. The right renal artery is somewhat longer than the left because it must cross the spine to reach the right kidney. The inferior mesenteric artery arises from the abdominal aorta at L3 and supplies the distal half of the large bowel. At the fourth lumbar vertebra, the abdominal aorta bifurcates to form the right and left common iliac arteries. Each common iliac divides into internal and external iliac arteries near the top of the sacrum. Internal iliac arteries divide rapidly as branches are sent to various structures within the pelvis. The external iliac arteries pass anteriorly and inferiorly through the pelvis. These vessels pass deep to the inguinal ligaments and become the femoral arteries.

The femoral vein carries venous blood from the lower limbs toward the pelvis.

The femoral vein becomes the external iliac vein as it passes deep to the inguinal ligament. Within the pelvis it is joined by the internal iliac vein to form the common iliac vein. The two common iliac veins unite at the level of the fifth lumbar vertebra to form the inferior vena cava. The inferior vena cava passes up the right anterolateral surface of the vertebral bodies, pierces the diaphragm, and empties into the inferior surface of the right atrium. The major tributaries of the IVC are the renal veins and the hepatic veins. The renal veins enter the lateral IVC near L2; the three hepatic veins enter near the top of the liver.

The vessels that drain the spleen and digestive system form the portal venous system. The major tributaries of this system are the superior and inferior mesenteric veins and the splenic vein. The inferior mesenteric vein empties into the splenic vein, which meets the superior mesenteric vein just posterior to the head of the pancreas. The junction of these two vessels forms the portal vein. These vessels extend superiorly to enter the porta hepatis of the liver.

Fig. 26-36 is a CT localizer, or scout, image representing an AP projection of the abdominopelvic region. The figure has 11 identifying lines demonstrating the levels for each of the labeled images for this region.

Fig. 26-36 CT localizer (scout) image of abdominopelvic region.

Fig. 26-37 A, Line drawing of CT section. **B,** CT image corresponding to level A in Fig. 26-36.

Fig. 26-37 represents structures seen at the T9 level. The tip of the xiphoid process and lower ribs are seen. The image demonstrates the *right hemidiaphragm* surrounding the superior portion of the *liver* and the *left hemidiaphragm* encircling the pericardial fat surrounding the apex of the heart and the *fundus* of the stomach. A small amount of oral contrast can be seen in the dependent portion of the stomach in this image. The *esophagus,* posterior to the liver, has migrated toward the patient's left as it nears its entrance into the stomach. The lower lobes of each lung are seen external to the diaphragm. The *aorta* is in its normal position, anterior and slightly left of the vertebral body; the azygos vein lies to the right of the aorta. The IVC appears embedded within the liver. Three *hepatic veins* drain into the IVC at this level. Serratus anterior muscles are seen external to the lateral aspects of the ribs; latissimus dorsi muscles extend superficially across the posterior abdomen.

Fig. 26-38 is a CT image at the level of the tenth thoracic vertebra. The aorta and inferior vena cava are seen, as well as contrast-enhanced vessels within the liver. These represent branches of the hepatic and portal venous circulation. The right, left, and *caudate lobes* of the liver are visible. On the patient's left, the contrast-filled body of the stomach and the *spleen* can be identified. This is normally the level at which the esophagus enters the cardiac portion of the stomach (the approximate location is identified). The *greater omentum* (a large fold of peritoneum) lies along the greater curvature of the stomach. Fig. 26-38 shows the greater omentum anterior and lateral to the stomach. The inferior lobes of the lungs are seen posterior to the liver and the spleen. The *crura of the diaphragm* are the lower tendinous insertions of this muscle. They can be seen extending around the anterior aorta and the posterior liver and spleen. This scan demonstrates the latissimus dorsi and the lower reaches of the serratus anterior. The upper portions of the anterior abdominal muscles (rectus abdominis, external oblique) can also be seen.

Fig. 26-38 A, Line drawing of CT section. **B,** CT image corresponding to level B in Fig. 26-36.

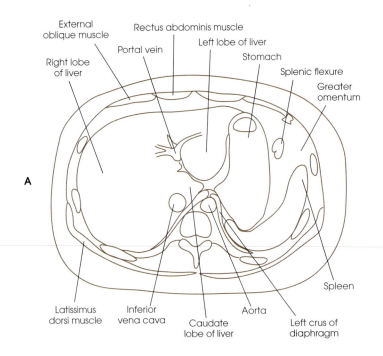

A

External
oblique muscle — Rectus abdominis muscle

Right lobe — Portal vein — Left lobe of liver
of liver — Stomach — Splenic flexure

Greater
omentum

Spleen

Latissimus — Inferior — Aorta
dorsi muscle — vena cava — Left crus of
Caudate — diaphragm
lobe of liver

B

Fig. 26-39 A, Line drawing of CT section. **B,** CT image corresponding to level C in Fig. 26-36.

The CT image at the level of T11 (Fig. 26-39) demonstrates the relationships among the liver, stomach, and spleen. The cardiac portion of the stomach is located at approximately the T10/11 level in the anterior aspect of the left upper quadrant, and the *pyloric portion* normally lies anterior to L2. This scan passes through the center or body of the stomach. An air-fluid level exists between the gas in the anterior stomach and the contrast in the posterior stomach. The spleen, located between the levels of T12 and L1, is in the posterolateral aspect of the left upper quadrant posterior to the fundus and body of the stomach. Contrast in the patient's colon is seen at the *splenic flexure,* seen here between the body of the stomach and the spleen. The liver is generally found between T11 and L3 and occupies the entire right upper quadrant. The right lobe of the liver has two small subdivisions, the caudate and *quadrate lobes,* which are bounded by the *gallbladder, ligamentum teres,* and IVC. The left lobe of the liver stretches across the midline and into the left upper quadrant. The *porta hepatis,* or hilum of the liver, is visible between the right and left lobes at this level. The inferior vena cava is found between the right and caudate lobes of the liver. In this image it is isodense with liver tissue and thus has been outlined for clarity. Large branches of the portal vein are seen at the porta hepatis.

Fig. 26-40 lies at the inferior edge of T11. The right, left, and caudate lobes of the liver are seen, as well as the porta hepatis. Anteriorly, the falciform ligament lies near the fissure between the right and left lobes (not seen on this image). The pyloric antrum of the stomach lies near the left lobe of the liver. This scan is inferior to the splenic flexure, so both *the transverse and descending portions of the colon* can be differentiated. The spleen lies along the left posterior abdominal wall. This scan lies near the hilum, and vascular structures are seen in this region. The tail of the pancreas normally lies near the spleen and can be seen here between the stomach and spleen. The *suprarenal glands* are normally located superior to the kidney. The right suprarenal gland is found at this level between the liver and the right diaphragmatic crus. The left suprarenal gland is medial to the pancreas and spleen. The abdominal aorta is positioned anterior and to the left of the vertebral column; the IVC is between the right and caudate lobes of the liver. The portal vein is seen within the porta hepatis along with branches of the hepatic artery. The splenic artery is normally tortuous and not seen in its entirety. At this level, the bright circles along the posterior pancreas most likely represent portions of the contrast-filled *splenic artery*.

A

B

Fig. 26-40 A, Line drawing of CT section. **B,** CT image corresponding to level D in Fig. 26-36.

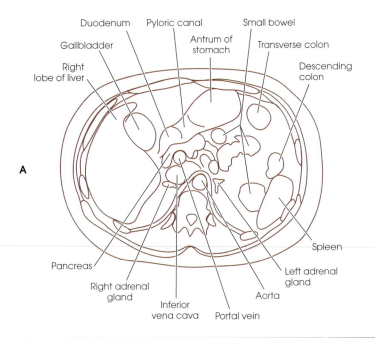

A

Duodenum · Pyloric canal · Small bowel
Gallbladder · Antrum of stomach · Transverse colon
Right lobe of liver · Descending colon

Spleen

Pancreas
Right adrenal gland · Inferior vena cava · Portal vein · Aorta · Left adrenal gland

B

Fig. 26-41 A, Line drawing of CT section. **B,** CT image corresponding to level E in Fig. 26-36.

The CT scan in Fig. 26-41 passes through the upper portion of T12. The difference in density between the liver tissue and the bile-filled *gallbladder* makes these organs easy to differentiate. The antrum of the stomach, pyloric canal, and bulb (first portion) of the *duodenum* are seen in the anterior abdomen. The neck of the pancreas is posterior to the pyloric canal of the stomach in this image. The transverse and descending colon lie in the anterior left abdomen. The spleen is posterior to the descending colon. Loops of *jejunum*, the second part of the small bowel, are posterior to the antrum of the stomach. The left adrenal gland is lateral to the aorta and left diaphragmatic crus. The right adrenal gland is posterior to the IVC. The three branches of the *celiac trunk* (hepatic, splenic, left gastric arteries) supply the liver, spleen, pancreas, and stomach with oxygen-rich blood. In this image the celiac trunk is seen as it divides into the *common hepatic artery* and the splenic artery. The left gastric artery is not seen. The splenic artery runs a tortuous course and normally cannot be visualized in its entirety in axial sections. Here, branches of the splenic artery and vein lie in close proximity and are difficult to differentiate. The IVC can be seen in its normal position anterior and to the right of the vertebral column. The main portion of the portal vein is just posterior to the duodenal bulb.

The muscles of the abdomen are located between the lower rib cage and the iliac crests. This group of muscles includes the *external oblique, internal oblique,* and *transverse abdominal muscles.* The two *rectus abdominis muscles* are located on the anterior aspect of the abdomen on either side of the midline and extend from the *pubic symphysis* to the xiphoid process.

The CT image in Fig. 26-42 is through the level of the first lumbar vertebra. The lower right lobe of the liver lies along the right side of the abdomen. The hepatic (right colic) flexure lies just medial to the liver. The duodenum forms a C-shaped loop around the head of the pancreas. In this scan, the head of the pancreas is seen between the duodenum (second portion) and the superior mesenteric vein. On the left side of the abdomen, loops of small bowel and the transverse and descending colon are seen. Folds of *mesentery* can be seen connecting some of the small bowel loops. The most inferior edge of the spleen lies along the left posterior abdomen. The upper poles of the kidneys appear on either side of the vertebral body. At this level the *superior mesenteric artery* is seen as it originates from the anterior aorta. The *left renal vein* can also be seen as it empties into the lateral aspect of the IVC.

A

B

Fig. 26-42 A, Line drawing of CT section. **B,** CT image corresponding to level F in Fig. 26-36.

Transverse colon   Small bowel

Ascending colon   Descending colon

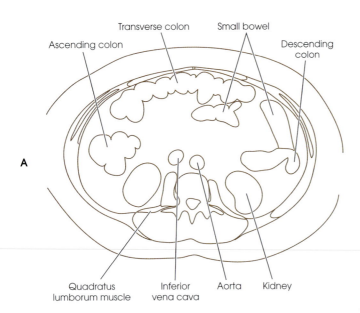

A

Quadratus lumborum muscle   Inferior vena cava   Aorta   Kidney

B

Fig. 26-43 **A,** Line drawing of CT section. **B,** CT image corresponding to level G in Fig. 26-36.

Fig. 26-43 is a CT scan through the third lumbar vertebra. The ascending colon is found on the right side of the abdomen. In this image most of the transverse colon can be seen across the anterior abdomen. The descending colon lies along the posterior left abdomen. Loops of small bowel are found in the central portion of the abdomen. Ileal loops are filled with contrast that has refluxed through the ileocecal valve from the colon. This level is just below the hila of the kidneys, and some of the central collecting system can be observed. The IVC and contrast-filled aorta lie anterior to the vertebral body. The rectus abdominis muscles lie on either side of the midline in the anterior abdomen. The three layers of the lateral abdominal muscles (external oblique, internal oblique, transverse abdominis) are separated by fat and can plainly be seen in this scan. The *psoas muscles* originate from the body of T12 and the transverse processes of the lumbar vertebrae and descend the abdomen lateral to the vertebral bodies. The *quadratus lumborum muscles* are located posterolateral to the psoas muscles through the abdomen. These muscles can be seen on either side of the vertebra. The *spinal cord* normally terminates at the level of L1. Inferior to L1 the *spinal nerves,* known as *cauda equina,* are seen within the spinal canal.

The CT scan in Fig. 26-44 lies near the interspace between the fourth and fifth lumbar vertebrae. The superior edge of the right *iliac crest* is visible in this image. The inferior portion of the cecum and the descending colon lie in the posterior abdomen on the right and left sides, respectively. Loops of small bowel are seen more anteriorly in the abdomen. The ureters normally lie just anterior to the psoas muscles. Due to peristalsis, no contrast is seen in the ureters on this image. At this level the aorta has bifurcated to form the right and left *common iliac vessels.* The common iliac veins are fairly close to each other, indicating this scan is just inferior to their junction (which forms the IVC).

A

B

Fig. 26-44 A, Line drawing of CT section. **B,** CT image corresponding to level H in Fig. 26-36.

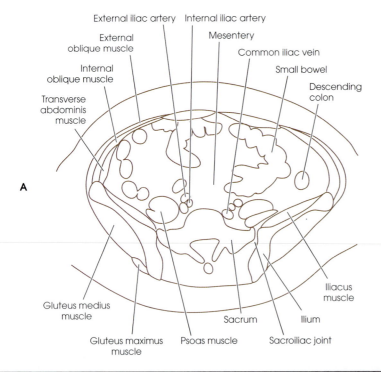

A

External iliac artery Internal iliac artery

External
oblique muscle

Mesentery

Common iliac vein

Internal
oblique muscle

Small bowel

Transverse
abdominis
muscle

Descending
colon

Iliacus
muscle

Gluteus medius
muscle

Sacrum   Ilium

Gluteus maximus
muscle   Psoas muscle   Sacroiliac joint

B

Fig. 26-45 **A,** Line drawing of CT section. **B,** CT image corresponding to level I in Fig. 26-36.

The CT image seen in Fig. 26-45 is of a female patient and was obtained at the upper sacral level. It demonstrates the *wings* of the *ilia,* the right *anterior superior iliac spine* (ASIS), and the *sacroiliac joints.* The descending colon is seen at the left lateral aspect of the pelvis, and multiple loops of *small intestine* are found throughout this level in the images. Three muscles lie posterior to the wings of the ilia: the gluteus minimus, gluteus medius, and gluteus maximus. The gluteus medius normally extends the farthest superiorly and is the first muscle visible as scans progress down through the pelvis. At the posterolateral aspect of the right ilium, two of the three *gluteal muscles* are visible—the gluteus medius and a small amount of the gluteus maximus—while on the left, only the gluteus medius is visible. The *iliacus muscle* is seen lining the internal aspect of the iliac wings near the psoas muscles. The two rectus abdominis muscles are found in the anterior abdomen on both sides of the midline. The external oblique, internal oblique, and transverse abdominis are seen extending anteriorly from the ilium on each side. The abdominal aorta bifurcates at L4 into the *common iliac arteries.* Each common iliac artery divides at the level of the ASIS into *internal* and *external iliac arteries.* The *internal iliac arteries* tend to be located in the posterior pelvis and branch to feed the pelvic structures. The *external iliac vessels* are found progressively anterior in succeeding inferior sections to become the femoral vessels at the superior aspect of the thigh. The internal and external iliac veins unite inferior to the ASIS to form the common iliac veins, and the IVC is formed anterior to L5 by the junction of the common iliac veins. This scan demonstrates the internal and external iliac arteries. At this level the internal and external iliac veins have joined to form the common iliac veins. The common iliac veins are positioned at the anterior aspects of the sacrum with the internal and external iliac arteries anterior and medial to the veins in these images.

Fig. 26-46 is a CT image obtained just superior to the level of the *acetabulum*. In this image the inferior sacrum is visible and the junction of the *ilium, ischium,* and *pubis* lies near the upper part of the acetabulum. Loops of ileum, filled with contrast, are seen in the anterior right pelvis. The haustral folds of the *sigmoid colon* are found in the center of the pelvis as this part of the large intestine curls toward the sacrum. A portion of the rectum is seen just anterior to the sacrum in this image. The fundus of the *uterus* lies medial to the right acetabulum and posterior to the ileal folds. The ureters are filled with contrast in this image and are easily identifiable in the posterior and lateral regions of the pelvic cavity. The external iliac arteries and veins run a diagonal course through the pelvis, lying near the sacrum in the upper part of the pelvis and passing anteriorly as they pass down through the pelvis toward the lower extremities. In this scan the external iliac vessels are seen just medial to the anterior edges of the acetabula. Multiple muscular structures are found at this level. The rectus abdominis muscles lie on either side of the midline in the anterior abdomen. The gluteal muscles (maximus, medius, and minimus) lie along the external surface of the posterior pelvis. Other muscles of the lower limbs are found just anterior to the acetabula. The large *sciatic nerve* can be plainly seen on the left between the gluteus maximus and medius muscles.

Fig. 26-46 A, Line drawing of CT section. **B,** CT image of the female pelvis corresponding to level J in Fig. 26-36.

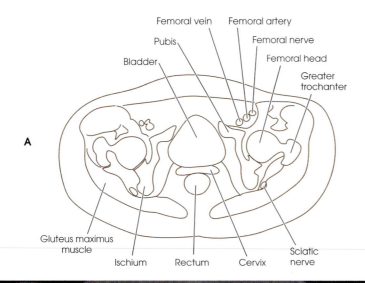

A

Femoral vein   Femoral artery

Pubis   Femoral nerve

Bladder   Femoral head

                                    Greater
                                    trochanter

Gluteus maximus
muscle

Ischium   Rectum   Cervix   Sciatic
                                    nerve

B

The CT scan in Fig. 26-47 is of a female patient and is at a level just superior to the pubic symphysis. The pubic bones, *ischia, acetabula, femoral heads,* and *greater trochanters* are visualized. The relationship between the *rectum, cervix,* and wall of the *bladder* is demonstrated from posterior to anterior in the pelvic region. The ureters entered the bladder just superior to this scan and so are no longer visible. The external iliac vessels are now referred to as the *femoral vessels,* with the name change occurring at the inguinal ligament, which is found between the pubic symphysis and the ASIS. The *iliopsoas muscles* (formed by the junction of the psoas and iliacus muscles) are found anterior to the femoral heads; the *obturator internus muscle,* with its characteristic right-angle bend, is found medial to the acetabulum.

Fig. 26-47 A, Line drawing of CT section. **B,** CT image of the female pelvis corresponding to level K in Fig. 26-36.

Fig. 26-48 is a CT scan through the lower pelvis of a male patient. This scan is at a slightly more inferior level than the previous scan. The symphysis pubis is seen here, as well as the acetabula, the *ischial spines,* and the *femoral heads* and *greater trochanters. The tip of the coccyx* is visible in the posterior pelvis. In the male pelvis the prostate gland lies inferior to the bladder and is traversed by the *urethra.* In this image the prostate gland, seminal vesicles, and rectum occupy the pelvic cavity from anterior to posterior. The bright spot within the prostate gland is the contrast-filled urethra. The *spermatic cords* transmit the ductus deferens and vascular structures between the pelvis and the testicular structures and are found on either side of the midline just anterior to the symphysis pubis.

Fig. 26-48 A, Line drawing of CT section. **B,** CT image of the male pelvis corresponding to level K in Fig. 26-36.

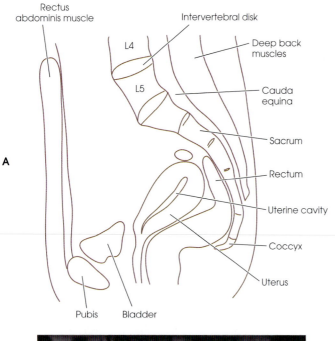

Rectus
abdominis muscle

Intervertebral disk

L4

Deep back
muscles

L5

Cauda
equina

A

Sacrum

Rectum

Uterine cavity

Coccyx

Uterus

Pubis   Bladder

B

Fig. 26-49 is a sagittal MR image of the female pelvis near the midline. The fourth and fifth lumbar vertebrae, the sacrum, and the coccyx are visualized. The cauda equina is seen descending the spinal canal. The areas of signal void anterior to the sacrum represent the rectum. The musculature and cavity of the uterus are visible anterior to the rectum. In the anterior pelvis, the bladder is seen posterior and superior to the symphysis pubis. Multiple loops of small bowel fill the upper anterior region of the pelvis but are somewhat blurry due to peristaltic motion. The rectus abdominis muscle extends superiorly from the pubis in the anterior abdominal wall. Fig. 26-50 is a sagittal MR image of a male patient. Note the prostate gland lying inferior to the bladder. A portion of the urethra can be seen passing through the prostate in this image.

Fig. 26-49 A, Line drawing of MR section. **B,** MR image of the female abdominopelvic region at the midsagittal plane.

A coronal MR image through the femoral heads and greater trochanters is presented in Fig. 26-51. The femoral heads are demonstrated within the *acetabula.* The crests of the ilia are visualized with their associated musculature. The internal surface of the iliac bone is lined by the iliac muscle. In this image the psoas muscles are seen joining the iliac muscles to form the iliopsoas muscles. (Iliopsoas muscles are visualized on more anterior sections of the pelvis.) *Gluteus medius* and *minimus* muscles are found external to the iliac bones. The bladder and prostate are seen within the pelvic cavity. Superior to the bladder is a portion of the *sigmoid colon.* The right ductus deferens is found lateral to the neck of the bladder. Between the rami of the pubic bones are the corpus spongiosum and corpora cavernosa. The *scrotum* is seen inferior to the *penis* and between the *gracilis muscles* of the thighs.

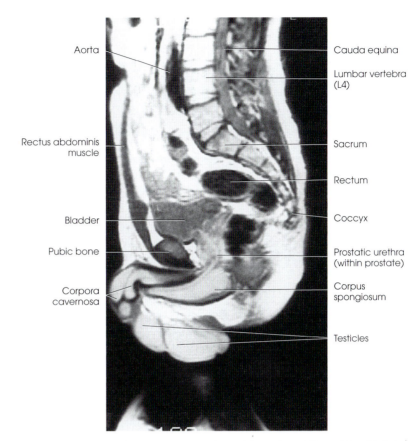

Fig. 26-50 MR image of the male abdominopelvic region at the midsagittal plane.

Fig. 26-51 MR image of the abdominopelvic region at the midcoronal plane.

Selected bibliography

Applegate E: *The sectional anatomy learning system,* ed 2, Philadelphia, 2001, Saunders.

Bo WJ et al: *Basic atlas of sectional anatomy,* ed 3, Philadelphia, 1998, Saunders.

Cahill DR et al: *Atlas of human cross-sectional anatomy,* ed 3, New York, 1995, Wiley-Liss.

Carter BL et al: *Cross-sectional anatomy: computed tomography and ultrasound correlation,* Englewood Cliffs, NJ, 1977, Appleton-Century-Crofts.

Dean D, Herbener TE: *Cross-sectional human anatomy,* Philadelphia, 2000, Lippincott Williams & Wilkins.

El-Khoury GY, Bergman RA, Montgomery WJ: *Sectional anatomy by MRI,* ed 2, New York, 1995, Churchill Livingstone.

Ellis H et al: *Human cross-sectional anatomy: atlas of body sections and CT images,* ed 2, Oxford, 1999, Butterworth-Heinemann.

Farkas ML: *Cross-sectional anatomy for computed tomography: a self-study guide,* New York, 1988, Springer.

Hagen-Ansert S: *The anatomy workbook,* Philadelphia, 1986, Lippincott.

Keiffer S, Heitzman E: *An atlas of cross-sectional anatomy,* Hagerstown, Md, 1979, Harper Collins.

Kelley LL, Petersen CM: *Sectional anatomy for imaging professionals,* St Louis, 1997, Mosby.

Koritke J, Sick H: *Atlas of sectional human anatomy,* Germany, 1988, Urban & Schwarzenberg.

Lazo DL: *Fundamentals of sectional anatomy: an imaging approach,* Clifton Park, NY, 2005, Thompson Delmar Learning.

Ledley RS, Huang HK, Mazziotta JC: *Cross-sectional anatomy: an atlas for computerized tomography,* Baltimore, 1977, Williams & Wilkins.

Madden ME: *Introduction to sectional anatomy,* Philadelphia, 2001, Lippincott Williams & Wilkins.

Moller TB, Reif E: *Pocket atlas of cross-sectional anatomy: computed tomography and magnetic resonance imaging: head, neck, spine and joints,* New York, 1994, Thieme Medical.

National Institutes of Health: *The visible human project* (website): http://www.nlm. nih.gov/research/visible/visible_human. html. Accessed June 12, 2006.

Novelline R, Squire L: *Living anatomy: a working atlas using computed tomography, magnetic resonance and angiography images,* St Louis, 1986, Mosby.

Poritsky R: *Cross-sectional anatomy to color and study,* Philadelphia, 1996, Hanley & Belfus.

Robert D: *Acland's cross-sectional navigator,* Philadelphia, 2005, Lippincott Williams & Wilkins.

Spitzer VM, Whitlock AG: *Atlas of the visible human male,* Sudsbury, Mass, 1997, Jones and Bartlett.

27

PEDIATRIC IMAGING

ALBERT AZIZA
ELLEN CHARKOT

In planning corrective surgery, orthopedic surgeons generally observe the bending images as if looking at the patient's back. The structures to be demonstrated include the uppermost non–wedge-shaped vertebrae and the iliac crests.

Principles of Pediatric Imaging

Understanding that *children are not just small adults* and appreciating that they need to be approached on their level are essential ingredients for successful encounters with children in the imaging department. Radiographers often lack confidence in two main areas of pediatric radiography—pediatric communication skills and immobilization techniques. The basic steps of pediatric radiography can be explained, but they must also be practiced.

Although pediatric imaging and adult radiography have many similarities, including basic positioning and image quality assessment, some significant differences remain. The way to *approach* the child tops the list of differences. It may help novice pediatric radiographers to think about children of various ages whom they know and to imagine how they would explain a particular radiographic examination to those children. This strategy, along with the descriptions that follow, will prove quite effective. Working successfully with children requires an open mind, patience, creativity, the willingness to learn, and the ability to look at the world through the eyes of a child.

Atmosphere

The environment in which patients are treated and recover plays a significant role in the recovery process. Research studies have compared the recovery course of patients whose hospital rooms looked out over parks with the recovery course of those whose view was a brick wall. The patients who faced the park had a much shorter hospital stay than the other patients, and they required considerably fewer pain killers. With these differences in mind, the patient care center at the Hospital for Sick Children (Toronto) was designed and built as an atrium (Fig. 27-1). Each patient room receives natural light, either by facing outside or overlooking the atrium, which receives natural light from the glass roof. Although it is easy to see how children can be amused by Miss Piggy and the barnyard animals that fly across the atrium, the environment does not have to be this elaborate to be appreciated by children. Small measures can be taken at relatively little cost to make a child's hospital stay more comfortable.

Fig. 27-1 Atrium of the Hospital for Sick Children (Toronto), which provides inpatient care and directly related support services.

WAITING ROOM

Parents of pediatric patients often arrive at the reception desk feeling anxious. They may be worried about what is involved in a procedure because they have not had the specifics explained to them or because they *did not hear* all that was explained to them. They also may be worried about the amount of time the care of their child will take, not to mention the outcome.

Feelings of anxiousness and tension are often transferred from parent to child—the child senses a parent's tension through the parent's tone of voice or actions. A well-equipped waiting room (this does not have to be expensive) can reduce this tension. Children are attracted to and amused by the toys, leaving the parents free to check in or register and ask pertinent questions.

Gender-neutral toys or activities such as a small table and chairs with crayons and coloring pages are most appropriate. (Children should be supervised to prevent them from putting the crayons in their mouths.) Books or magazines for older children are also good investments. The child life department of the hospital can provide advice and recommendations (Fig. 27-2).

IMAGING ROOM

Time can pass quickly for lengthy procedures if age-appropriate music or videos are available. A child who is absorbed in a video often requires little or no immobilization (other than the usual safety precautions designed to prevent the child from rolling off the table). Charitable and fundraising organizations are often happy to donate televisions, VCRs, DVD players, and computer games for this purpose.

Experience has shown that children are less likely to become upset or agitated if they are brought into a room that has been prepared before they enter. This preparation should include placement of the image receptor (IR), approximate centering of the tube to the IR, and placement of all immobilization tools likely to be needed at one end of the table.

Young children are often afraid of the dark. They dislike having the lights turned out but are often comfortable with low levels of illumination. Dimming the lights enough to see the collimator light before the child enters can prevent the need to explain why the lights have to be dimmed. Busy radiographers often turn the lights down without explanation, causing unnecessary anxiety.

After the procedure is complete, the radiographer or other imaging professional should take a moment to emphasize, *even overemphasize,* how helpful the child was and to explain where the child should wait or what the child should do next, *ensuring that the parent is comprehending the instructions.*

Fig. 27-2 Children in waiting area enjoying *normal activity* before being radiographed.

Approach

APPROACHING THE PARENT

No discussion of dealing with children is complete without mentioning ways to approach the parent(s). Although children are sometimes brought for medical care by someone other than the parents, in this discussion, the caregiver is referred to as the *parent*.

In many cases, radiographers find that they are dealing with two patients—the child and the parent. They may wonder to whom they should primarily speak. The answer, however, is easy:

- If the child is capable of understanding, direct the explanation to the child but use age-appropriate language (discussed later). The parents will listen and consequently understand what is expected. Communicating in this way puts the parents more at ease and increases their confidence in the radiographer's skills. They appreciate the fact that their child has been made the focus of attention.
- If the child is too young to comprehend, direct the explanation to the parent, explaining in simple sentences what is going to happen and what is expected of the parent. The importance and value of simple sentences cannot be emphasized enough. People in stress-filled situations do not think as clearly as they normally do, and many parents in this setting are under stress. Successful communication involves the use of short sentences repeated once or twice in a soothing tone.

Dealing with the agitated parent

When approaching the agitated parent, the radiographer should observe the following guidelines:

- Remain calm and speak in an even tone, remembering that fear and frustration may be the cause of the agitation.
- Use phrases such as "My name is. . . . I can identify with how you must be feeling and can appreciate your concern," followed by "Let me explain to you what is happening."
- If possible, escort the parent to a nearby room to continue the explanation and listen to their concerns without interruption. This can avoid an unwanted scene in the waiting room.

Parent participation

The degree of parent participation depends on several factors:

1. The general philosophy of the department
2. The wishes of the parent and patient
3. The laws of the province or state regarding radiation protection

The advantages of parental participation can be great for everyone concerned—patients, parents, radiographers, and departmental administrators. Experience has shown that both parents should have the basic procedure explained to them. However, it is advisable that only *one* parent be present in the imaging room. The presence of both parents often causes the room to become crowded; moreover, it is distracting and can actually lengthen the procedure. Many provincial or state laws permit only one additional person in the room, and this serves nicely as a rationale when the radiographer explains the policy to parents. Posting signs to this effect in strategic locations also can be helpful.

Some parents insist on participating and many pediatric radiographers advocate parent participation for the following reasons:

1. The parent can watch the child if the attention of the radiographer or radiologist is directed to the equipment or the fluoroscopic monitor.
2. The radiographer may need to leave the room.
3. The parent can assist with immobilization if needed (where permitted).
4. The parent who witnesses an entire procedure has little room for doubt about professional conduct.

This last point illustrates a benefit to parents as well as to medical personnel. The parent's presence ensures that no action, explanation, or question is misinterpreted by the child or adolescent. At the same time, the parent can take comfort in seeing that the child is being cared for in a professional manner. Although parental participation is perhaps less controversial now than it was in the past, radiographers can put the situation in perspective by imagining themselves in the position of parents and asking whether they would want to be present. With increasing public knowledge and the ever-present threat of litigation, parents are participating in more procedures.

Informed parents, whether physically present in the imaging room or not, can usually help to explain the procedure to the child. Most hospitals and commercial organizations have prepared pamphlets describing procedures and answering many commonly asked questions.

In some situations, parental presence is not advised. For example, some children are further agitated by their parents' presence, or some parents may find certain procedures too disturbing, such as those performed in the interventional suites.

Whenever parents are in the room during a radiographic exposure, they should be protected from scatter radiation. Parents should also be given lead gloves if their hands will be near the primary radiation beam.

APPROACHING THE CHILD

Naturally, good communication is essential to obtaining maximum cooperation. Thus children should be spoken to at their level in words that they can understand. Fortunately, this is not as difficult as learning a new language, and it can be made even easier if the radiographer keeps a few strategies in mind:

- Greet the patient and parent in the waiting area with a smile.
- Bend down to talk to the child at the child's eye level.
- Take a moment to *introduce yourself and ensure that you are meeting with the correct patient;* then state briefly what you are going to do.
- Suggest, rather than ask, the child to come and *help* you with some pictures. This *firm, yet gentle* approach avoids creating the idea that the child has a choice. After all, the patient may be tempted to be emphatic and say *"no."*
- Use sincere *praise.* This is a powerful motivator, no matter what the age of the patient. Praise for young children (3 to 7 years old) should be immediate. Children have short attention spans and often expect to receive rewards immediately. The reward should be linked directly to the task that has been well done. Use phrases such as "You sat very still for me, thank you" or "You took a nice, big breath in for that picture, and I am going to ask you to do it again for the next one."
- When the outcome will be the same, *give children an option:* "Would you like Mom to help lift you up on the table, or may I help you?" or "We have two pictures to do. Which would you like first—the one with you sitting down or the one with you lying down?"

- Employ distraction techniques. As radiographers develop confidence in basic radiography skills and adapting these skills for children, they find themselves able to engage in *chatter* and *distraction techniques,* thus making the experience as pleasant as possible for the child. Ask the child about brothers, sisters, pets, school, or friends—the topics are limitless. As homework, watch a few popular children's cartoons. Communication is improved when the radiographer can build rapport with a child, and learning a few more distraction techniques is helpful.
- Answer all questions truthfully—regardless of their nature. Maintaining honesty is crucial in all communications with children. Confidence and credibility built by the previous strategies can be lost if the truth is withheld. The secret is to not volunteer information too early or dwell on unpleasantness.

The child's age should greatly influence the approach. Children are unique individuals with unique social styles, of course, but the following guidelines may still prove helpful.

Infants

The basic needs of infants to the age of 6 months are warmth, security, and, of course, nourishment. They do not make an appreciable distinction among caregivers. They are often calmed by the use of a pacifier or soother. As they get older, they become attached to familiar objects, which they should be allowed to keep with them. Because infants are easily startled, care should be taken to minimize loud stimuli.

Children 6 months to 2 years old

Children between 6 months and 2 years of age are particularly fearful of pain, separation from their parents, and limitation of their freedom of movement. This helps explain why they are very disturbed by immobilization. Unfortunately, children in this age group usually require the most assertive immobilization techniques. Experience has shown that it is less disturbing to children to be well immobilized than to have a number of adults in lead aprons trying to hold them in the correct positions.

Although radiographers should be knowledgeable in the art of immobilization for children in this age group (particularly 2-year-olds), one of the most valuable forms of immobilization is natural sleep. The challenge, of course, is to complete the entire radiographic sequence without waking the child. This can be done by carefully transferring the child to the table and taking care to maintain warmth, comfort, and safety.

Parental participation is especially valuable with this age group, as it is with children between the ages of 2 and 4 years. Radiographers can easily pick up tips for communicating with children by taking cues from parents as they explain procedures to their children. Parents are also helpful because they can act as "baby-sitters" during the procedure.

NOTE: Chest radiography must be performed while children are awake. Because respirations are generally shallow during sleep, it is not possible to obtain an adequate degree of inspiration.

Children 2 to 4 years old

Preschoolers can test the power of the radiographer's imagination. They are extremely curious—their favorite question is "Why?" They enjoy fantasy and may readily cooperate if the situation is treated like a game or distraction techniques are used. The following strategies can be useful:

- Give explanations at the child's eye level by bending down or by sitting the child on the radiographic or scanner table.
- Take a moment to show the child how the collimator light works and let the child turn it on (Fig. 27-3)—for a child, this is as much fun as pressing the buttons in an elevator.
- Use the camera analogy to describe the x-ray tube, taking care to explain that the tube may move sideways but will never come down and touch the child.
- Avoid any unnecessary equipment manipulation.
- Encourage the child gently as the child attempts to cooperate—then praise the cooperation.

Children between 2 and 4 years of age can be verbally and physically aggressive. A child who is having a tantrum will not respond to games and distraction techniques. Making the procedure as short as possible through the use of practiced and kind, yet effective, immobilization techniques is the best approach. Young patients generally calm down quickly when they are back in their parents' arms or resume the activity they were involved in before the examination.

The 5-year-old

The 5-year-old has typically reached a time that is rich in new experiences. Reactions can differ widely, depending on how at ease the child feels with a given environment. Children in this age group generally want to perform tasks correctly, and they enjoy mimicking adults. When a 5-year-old feels confident, that child will act like a 6-, 7-, or 8-year-old; however, when afraid or worried, that same child may cling to parents and become reticent and uncooperative. Constant reassurance and simple explanations help in such moments.

School-age children 6 to 8 years old

For the radiographer who is not accustomed to working with children, the perfect group to start with is the 6- to 8-year-olds. These children are generally accommodating and eager to please. They are modest and embarrass easily, so their privacy should be protected. These children are the easiest age group with which to communicate; they appreciate being talked through the procedure, which gives them less time to worry about their surroundings or the procedure itself. Anatomic landmarks are easy to locate for positioning, and body habitus evens out nicely—the "big belly" of the toddler disappears. From an imaging standpoint, the bones are maturing, with the increased calcium content enhancing subject contrast (Fig. 27-4).

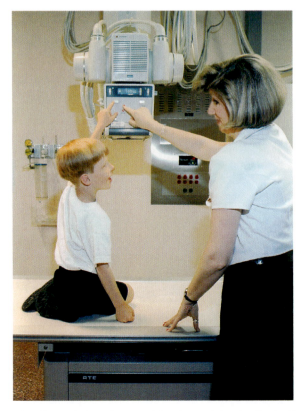

Fig. 27-3 The radiographer should make an introduction to the child and show the child how the collimator light is used. The child can be allowed to turn on the light.

Fig. 27-4 Child properly positioned and shielded for a lateral elbow radiograph.

Adolescents

Image is important to preteens and adolescents. Although they are better able to understand the need for hospitalization, they are upset by interference in their social and school activities. They are particularly concerned that as a result of the injury they may not be able to return to their preinjury state. These patients require, and often demand, clear explanations. Health care workers should not be surprised by the frankness of their questions and should be prepared for some discussion.[1]

Adolescents want to be treated as adults, and the radiographer must exercise judgment in assessing the patient's degree of maturity. The radiographer should become familiar with the local statutes regarding consent in order to understand when children are deemed to be responsible for themselves.[2]

Sensitive issues, such as the possibility of pregnancy in the postpubescent girl, must be approached discreetly. Honest responses are more likely to be elicited if the girl is alone with the radiographer (i.e., the parent is not present), and the following guidelines are observed:

- Preface the questioning by stating that information of a sensitive nature needs to be obtained for radiation safety.
- Ask the 10-, 11-, 12-, or 13-year-old girl if she has started menstruating. If the response is affirmative, continue by saying that a slightly more sensitive question needs to be asked. Then ask if there is any possibility of pregnancy.
- Simply but tactfully ask girls 14 years and older if there is any chance of pregnancy. Judging from the patient's expression and response, decide how to continue.
- Differing levels of maturity call for different explanations. If necessary, apologize for the need to ask sensitive questions and assure the patient that the same questions are asked of all girls of this age.
- Follow the questioning with an explanation that it is unsafe for unborn babies to receive radiation.
- If possible, have the questioning performed by a female.

[1]Wilmot DM, Sharko GA: *Pediatric imaging for the technologist,* New York, 1987, Springer-Verlag.
[2]Torres LS: *Basic medical techniques and patient care in imaging technology,* ed 5, Philadelphia, 1997, Lippincott-Raven.

APPROACHING PATIENTS WITH SPECIAL NEEDS
Children with physical and mental disabilities

The radiographer should consider age when approaching children with physical and mental disabilities. Children older than 8 years of age with disabilities strive to achieve as much autonomy and independence as possible. They are sensitive to the fact that they are less independent than their peers. The radiographer should observe the following guidelines:

- Direct communication toward the child first. All children appreciate being given the opportunity to listen and respond. Like any patients, these children also want to be talked to rather than talked about.
- If this approach proves ineffective, turn to the parents. As a general rule, the parents of these patients are present and can be very helpful. In strange environments, younger children may trust only one person—the parent. In that case, the medical team can gain cooperation from the child by communicating through the parent. Parents often know the best way to lift and transfer the child from the wheelchair or stretcher to the table. Children with physical disabilities often have a fear of falling and may want only a parent's assistance.
- After introducing yourself, briefly explain the procedure to the child.
- Place the wheelchair or stretcher parallel to the imaging table, taking care to explain that you have locked the wheelchair or stretcher and will be getting help for the transfer. These children often know the way they should be lifted—*ask them.* They can tell you which areas to support and which actions they prefer to do themselves.

Finally, children with spastic contractions are often frustrated by muscle movements that are counterproductive to the intended action. Gentle massage should be used to help relax the muscle, and a compression band should be applied to maintain the position.

Communicating with a child who has a mental disability can be difficult, depending on the severity of the disability. Some patients react to verbal stimuli. Loud or abrupt phrases can startle and consequently agitate them.

Patient Care: Psychologic Considerations

Although pediatric patients have many of the same psychologic characteristics as adults, some factors are worthy of mention to better prepare the radiographer for interactions with children and their parents.

EMERGENCY PATIENT

When an accident happens, emotions run high, thought processes are clouded, and the ability to rationalize is often lost. For the parents of the child who has been injured, another powerful factor is often involved—guilt. As parents try to absorb information about the child's condition, they also ask themselves how they could have let the accident happen. Dealing with these questions often prevents parents from hearing or understanding all that is being explained. In addition, fearing that permanent damage has been done, the child can feel extremely traumatized by a relatively minor injury. The radiographer should observe the following guidelines in dealing with emergency patients and their parents:

- Greet the patient and parents, and then describe the procedure using short, simple, and often-repeated sentences.
- Remember that when patients and parents speak with a tone of urgency and frustration, this usually stems from fear. Maintaining a calm perspective in these situations can ensure a smooth examination.
- Increase the level of confidence the parents and child have in your abilities with frequent reassurance presented in a calming tone. (The *reassurance* referred to here is reassurance that the radiographer knows how to approach the situation, not reassurance that all will be well with respect to the injury.)
- In emergency examinations, as with any other examination, ensure that only one caregiver is giving the child instructions and explanations. (Caregivers include parents, nurses, doctors, and radiographers, all of whom may be present.) Much greater success is achieved when only one person speaks to the child.
- After completing the procedure, ensure that you have the parents' attention. Speaking slowly, give clear instructions about where to wait and what to expect.

OUTPATIENT

Generally speaking, outpatients and their parents are easier to approach than inpatients. For the radiographer who has had little experience with children, these are among the best patients with whom to begin. Outpatient visits are frequently a form of progress report, and patients are usually ambulatory and relatively healthy. For the most part, parents are calm because they are not dealing with the emotions of an emergency situation or perhaps the tension or fear that the parents of inpatients can experience. However, they can become agitated if kept waiting too long, which unfortunately happens often in the outpatient clinical setting.

INPATIENT

A child must usually be very sick to be admitted to a hospital. Children often become acutely ill in a much shorter period than adults. However, they generally heal quicker than adults, which decreases the length of the hospital stay. The stresses the child experiences involve fear and separation from parents, family, and friends. It also is a stressful time for the parents who, while worrying about their child's health, must often juggle time for work and for taking care of other family members. By understanding that these responsibilities weigh heavily on parents' minds and by remembering to provide reassurance and simple explanations, the radiographer can make the child's visit to the imaging department easier.

Patient Care: Physical Considerations

GENERAL MEASURES

Depending on the level of care being provided, children may arrive in the imaging department with chest tubes, intravenous (IV) infusions (including central venous lines), colostomies, ileostomies, or urine collection systems. Usually these children are inpatients, but in many instances outpatients (particularly in interventional cases) arrive in the department with various tubes in situ (e.g., gastrostomy or gastrojejunostomy tube placements). The radiographer must be aware of the purpose and significance of these medical adjuncts and know the ways to care for the patient with them (see Figs. 27-46 and 27-47).

The competent and caring radiographer takes note of the following:
1. What are the specific instructions regarding the care and management of the child during the child's stay in the department?
2. Will a nurse or another health care professional accompany the child?
3. Will physical limitations influence the way the examination is performed?

Many inpatients are on a 24-hour urine and stool collection routine. Therefore medical personnel who change diapers on these patients should save the old diaper for the ward/floor personnel to weigh or assess.

Hospital policy and the availability of nursing staff within the imaging department determine the amount of involvement the radiographer has with the management of IV lines. The radiographer must be able to assess the integrity of the line and must know the measures to take in the event of problems.[1]

ISOLATION PROTOCOLS AND STANDARD BLOOD AND BODY FLUID PRECAUTIONS

Prevention of the spread of contagious disease is of primary importance in a health care facility for children. Microorganisms are most commonly spread from one person to another by human hands. *Careful handwashing* is the single most important precaution, but unfortunately, it is often the most neglected. In addition, all

---

[1]Torres LS: *Basic medical techniques and patient care in imaging technology,* ed 5, Philadelphia, 1997, Lippincott-Raven.

equipment that comes in contact with the radiographer and patient during isolation cases must be washed with an appropriate cleanser.

The premise of standard blood and body fluid precautions is that *all blood and body fluids* are to be considered *infected.* The Centers for Disease Control and Prevention recommend that health care workers practice blood and body fluid precautions when caring for all patients. These precautions are designed to protect both patients and medical personnel from the diseases spread by infected blood and body fluids. All blood and body fluids, including secretions and excretions, must be treated as if they contain infective microorganisms. Working under this assumption, personnel can protect themselves not only from patients in whom a known infective organism is present but also from the unknown. The management of patients in isolation varies according to the type of organism or preexisting condition, the procedure itself (some can alternatively be performed with a mobile unit), and hospital/departmental policies. Decisions regarding when to bring an infectious patient to the department also often depend on the condition of other patients who may be in the vicinity. For example, patients with *multiresistant organisms* should not be close to immunocompromised patients.

The radiographer should follow all precautions outlined by the physician and nursing unit responsible for the child. Respiratory, enteric, or wound precautions for handling a patient are usually instituted to protect staff members and other patients. Isolation procedures are instituted to protect a patient from infection. Protective isolation is used, for example, with burn victims and patients with immunologic disorders. The protective clothing worn by staff members may be the same in either situation, but the method of discarding the clothing will be different.[1]

---

[1]Torres LS: *Basic medical techniques and patient care in imaging technology,* ed 5, Philadelphia, 1997, Lippincott-Raven.

Patient Care: Special Concerns

As with most pediatric examinations, a team approach produces the best results. Cooperation among all caregivers and the child provides for a smooth examination. A few special situations that deserve individual mention are discussed in the following sections.

PREMATURE INFANT

One of the greatest dangers facing the premature and sometimes the full-term neonate is *hypothermia* (below normal body temperature). *Thermoregulation,* the balance of heat losses and gains, is crucial to the care and survival of the premature infant. The sources of heat loss—evaporation, convection, conduction, and radiation—are greater in the preterm infant. Premature babies have a greater surface area in comparison with body mass. Furthermore, they are not capable of storing the fat needed for warmth, and they have increased metabolic rates.

So that hypothermia does not occur, premature infants should be examined within the infant warmer or isolette whenever possible. Therefore general radiography must be performed with a portable or mobile unit. (See Chapter 29 for a discussion on mobile radiography.) The radiographer should take great care to prevent the infant's skin from coming in contact with IRs. Covering the IR with one or two layers of a cloth diaper (or equivalent) works well; however, the material should be free of creases because these produce significant artifacts on neonatal radiographs.

When the premature infant is brought to the imaging department for gastrointestinal (GI) procedures or various types of scans, the radiographer should observe the following guidelines:

- Elevate the temperature in the room 20 to 30 minutes before the arrival of the child. The ambient temperature of the imaging room is usually cool compared with the temperature of the neonatal nursery.
- When raising the temperature is impossible, prepare the infant for the procedure while the infant is still in the isolette and remove the infant for as brief a period as possible.
- Use heating pads and radiant heaters to help maintain the infant's body temperature; however, these adjuncts are often of limited usefulness because of necessary obstructions such as the image intensifier. If heaters are used, position them at least 3 feet from the infant.
- Place large bags of IV solutions, prewarmed by soaking in a sink of warm water, beside the infant to serve as small hot water bottles.
- Monitor the infant's temperature throughout the procedure, and keep the isolette plugged in to maintain the appropriate temperature.

Because of the risk of infection to infants in the neonatal intensive care unit (NICU), most units insist on adherence to isolation protocols such as gowning and hand washing.

NOTE: *Neonatal* refers to newborn. Although premature babies comprise the highest percentage of patients in NICUs, all of the infants in these units are not necessarily premature. Full-term babies experiencing distress are also cared for in NICUs.

The radiographer must take care when positioning an infant from the NICU. Many of these infants can tolerate only minimal handling without their heart rates becoming irregular.

MYELOMENINGOCELE

A *myelomeningocele* is a *congenital* defect characterized by a cystic protrusion of the meninges and the spinal cord tissue and fluid. It occurs as a result of spina bifida, a cleft in the neural arches of a vertebra. It can be recognized by fetal ultrasonography at the seventeenth or eighteenth week of gestation. Myelomeningoceles may cause varying degrees of paralysis and hydrocephalus. The higher the location of the myelomeningocele, the worse the neurologic symptoms.

Patients with myelomeningoceles are cared for in the prone position. Therefore, whenever possible, radiographic examinations on these patients should be performed using the prone position until the defect has been surgically repaired and the wound healed. The primary imaging modalities used in the investigation and follow-up care of myelomeningoceles include ultrasonography, computed tomography (CT), and magnetic resonance imaging (MRI) (Fig. 27-5).

Fig. 27-5 Five-year-old with severe herniation of cerebellar structures into cervical spine. Note medullary kink and extreme angled kyphosis at site of myelomeningocele.

OMPHALOCELE AND GASTROSCHISIS

An *omphalocele* is a congenital defect that resembles an enormous umbilical hernia. Omphaloceles are covered in a thin, translucent, membranous sac of peritoneum, and their contents include bowel and perhaps liver. *Gastroschisis* is a similar condition in which a portion of bowel herniates through a defect near the naval. The difference is that in gastroschisis the bowel is not included within a sac.

In both omphalocele and gastroschisis, the herniated abdominal contents must be kept warm and moist. This is especially important with gastroschisis. A responsible physician or nurse should be present when patients with these conditions are examined radiographically because such patients become rapidly hypothermic.

EPIGLOTTITIS

Epiglottitis is one of the most dangerous causes of acute upper airway obstruction in children and must be treated as an EMERGENCY. Its peak incidence occurs in children between the ages of 3 and 6 years. Epiglottitis is usually caused by *Haemophilus influenzae,* and the symptoms include acute respiratory obstruction, high temperature, and *dysphasia* (inability to swallow or difficulty in swallowing). When epiglottitis is clinically suspected, the radiographer observes the following steps:

- **Insist** that the patient be accompanied by and transported **into** the radiographic room with the responsible physician. The patient must be supported in the upright position with an emergency physician monitoring the airway at all times.
- **Do not proceed with the necessary lateral radiograph of the nasopharynx or soft tissues of the neck without the presence of the physician.**
- Perform the single upright lateral image without moving the patient's head or neck (Fig. 27-6).
- Take extreme care to ensure the child does not panic, cry, or become agitated.

OSTEOGENESIS IMPERFECTA

Osteogenesis imperfecta, a disease characterized by brittle bones, is often referred to by its abbreviation, OI. Because the approach and management need to be altered significantly in the imaging department to accommodate patients with OI, radiographers should be aware of this commonly used abbreviation. Children with OI are prone to spontaneous fractures or fractures that occur with minimal trauma. Although OI can vary in severity, patients with this disease need to be handled with extreme care by an experienced radiographer (Fig. 27-7).

Children with OI are almost always accompanied by a key caregiver—usually a parent. Experience has shown that these patients are best handled with a team approach in an unhurried atmosphere. The team is comprised of the patient, parent (caregiver), and radiographer, with the radiographer observing the following guidelines:

- Constantly reassure the parent and patient that every part of the procedure will be explained before it is attempted.

Fig. 27-6 There is diffuse swelling of the epiglottis, aryepiglottic folds, and the retropharyngeal soft tissues. These findings are consistent with epiglottitis.

A   B

Fig. 27-7 Left forearm AP **(A)** and lateral **(B)** projections show healing fractures of radius and ulna with abundant remodeling bony callus.

- For the best results, explain the desired position to the parent in simple terms. For example, "the knee needs to point to the side" for a lateral image. Then allow the parent to do the positioning.
- Ask the older child for advice on the way the child should be moved or lifted.
- If possible, take the radiographs with the child in the bed or on the stretcher. This is often possible, given the patient's small physical stature.

Practical tip: It is wise to evaluate the technical factors by checking the first radiograph before proceeding with the rest of the series. (Generally speaking, the technical factors can be halved.) The radiographer should remember that an introduction and a few moments of explanation and reassurance that the radiograph will be done using a team approach can ensure a smooth examination in most OI patients.

SUSPECTED CHILD ABUSE

Although no *universal* agreement exists on the definition of child abuse, the radiographer should have an appreciation of the all-encompassing nature of this problem. *Child abuse* has been described as "the involvement of physical injury, sexual abuse or deprivation of nutrition, care or affection in circumstances, which indicate that injury or deprivation may not be accidental or may have occurred through neglect."[1] Although diagnostic imaging staff members are usually involved only in cases in which physical abuse is a possibility, they should realize that sexual abuse and nutritional neglect are also prevalent.

It is mandatory in all provinces and states in North America for health care professionals to *report suspected cases* of abuse or neglect. The radiographer, while

[1]Robinson MJ: *Practical pediatrics,* ed 2, New York, 1990, Churchill Livingstone.

preparing or positioning the patient, may be the first person to suspect abuse or neglect (Fig. 27-8). The first course of action for the radiographer should be to consult a radiologist (when available) or the attending physician. After this consultation, the radiographer may no longer have cause for suspicion because some naturally occurring skin markings mimic bruising. *If the radiographer's doubts persist, the suspicions must be reported to the proper authority, regardless of the physician's opinion.* Recognizing the complexity of child abuse issues, many health care facilities have developed a multidisciplinary team of health care workers to respond to these issues. Radiographers working in hospitals have access to this team of physicians, social workers, and psychologists for the purposes of reporting their concerns; others are advised to work through their local Children's Aid Society or appropriate organization.

Fig. 27-8 Seven-year-old with loop marks representative of forceful blows by a looped belt.

Plain image radiography, often the initial imaging tool, can reveal characteristic radiologic patterns of skeletal injury. Clear evidence of posterior rib fractures, corner fractures, and "bucket-handle" fractures of limbs are considered *classic indicators* of physical abuse (Fig. 27-9). All imaging modalities can and do play a role in the investigation of suspected child abuse. After plain radiography, nuclear medicine is often the next investigative tool of choice (Fig. 27-10). CT with three-dimensional (3D) reconstruction has contributed to differentiating cases of actual abuse from accidental trauma (Fig. 27-11). The presence of numerous fracture sites at varied or multiple stages of healing can also indicate long-term or ongoing abuse. These cases are often viewed by nonradiologic staff members (e.g., lawyers), as well as imaging professionals. Therefore evidence of injury must be readily apparent, especially because pediatric fractures at an early age can remodel totally over a period of time, thus providing no clear evidence of earlier fractures.

A   B   C

Fig. 27-9 Radiographs demonstrating physical abuse. Left and right corner fractures (*arrows,* **A** and **B**) and bucket-handle fractures (*arrow,* **C**) are considered classic indicators of physical abuse in children. The bucket-handle appearance is subtle and demonstrated only if the "ring" is seen on profile (*arrow*).

Fig. 27-10 Delayed image of bone scintigraphy (nuclear medicine) demonstrating focal increased uptake in the posterior lower six ribs bilaterally in a linear fashion indicative of child abuse.

Fig. 27-11 CT axial noncontrast image of the brain demonstrating a hyperdense crescent-shaped collection in the subdural space consistent with acute hemorrhage (*arrows*). There is also evidence of old resolving subdural hematomas (*arrowheads*). This is characteristic of child abuse.

The radiographer's role is to provide physicians with diagnostic radiographs that *demonstrate bone and soft tissue equally well.* Referring physicians depend on the expertise of the diagnostic imaging service for the detection of physical abuse, and radiologists are able to estimate the date of the injury based on the degree of callous formation or the amount of healing.

The radiographer observes the following guidelines when dealing with a case of possible child abuse:

- Give careful attention to exposure factors and the recorded detail demonstrated for limb radiography. Imaging systems yielding high detail are recommended for cases of suspected child abuse because the associated skeletal injuries are often very subtle (Fig. 27-12).
- Performing a *babygram*—a 35 × 43 cm (14 × 17 inch) IR of the entire baby—should be avoided because the resultant images are of reduced diagnostic quality. Distortion because of improper centering, scatter, and underexposure *or overexposure* of the radiograph all play a part in the degradation of the image. Babygrams are no longer considered an acceptable imaging protocol for the investigation of child abuse. Instead, *skeletal surveys* with *multiple images of individual areas* should be performed using appropriate centering points, collimation, and technical factors. The following guidelines were developed based on routines performed at the Hospital for Sick Children in Toronto:

AP Skull
Lateral Skull
AP Complete Spine
Lateral Complete Spine
AP Both Humeri
AP Both Radii and Ulnae
PA Both Hands and Wrists
AP Pelvis
AP Both Femora
AP Both Tibiae and Fibulae
AP Both Feet
AP Chest for Ribs
Lateral Chest for Ribs

All images must be performed separately with exposure factors adjusted to maximize recorded detail. Visualization of joints is an essential component of the study. Chest x-rays are done primarily for visualizing ribs and therefore can be done with the patient lying on the table using lower kVp (kilovolt [peak]) and Bucky grid.

- Although it may be difficult to do, give the parents of these children the same courtesy as any other parent. Remember that the parent who is present may not be responsible for the injuries. Deal with the parent in a nonjudgmental manner aimed at not jeopardizing further relations between the parent and health care providers.

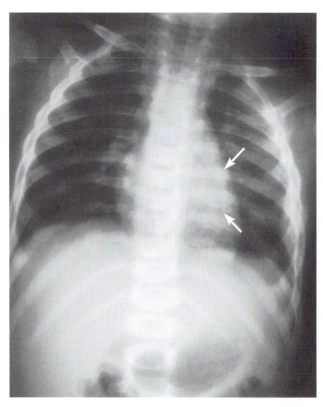

Fig. 27-12 Chest radiograph showing different stages of healing posterior rib fractures (arrows).

SUMMARY OF PATHOLOGY: PEDIATRIC IMAGING

Condition	Definition
Congenital Club Foot	Abnormal twisting of the foot, usually inward and downward
Congenital Hip Dysplasia	Malformation of the acetabulum, causing displacement of the femoral head
Cystic Fibrosis	Disorder associated with widespread dysfunction of exocrine glands, abnormal secretion of sweat and saliva, and accumulation of thick mucus in the lungs
Fracture	Disruption in the continuity of bone
Greenstick	Incomplete fracture of a bone
Torus or Buckle	Impacted fracture with bulging of the periosteum
Hirschsprung's or Congenital Aganglionic Megacolon	Absence of parasympathetic ganglia, usually in the distal colon, resulting in the absence of peristalsis
Hyaline Membrane Disease or Respiratory Distress Syndrome	Underaeration of the lungs due to a lack of surfactant
Intussusception	Prolapse of a portion of the bowel into the lumen of an adjacent portion
Legg-Calvé-Perthes Disease	Flattening of the femoral head due to vascular interruption
Osgood-Schlatter Disease	Incomplete separation or avulsion of the tibial tuberosity
Osteomalacia or Rickets	Softening of the bones due to a vitamin D deficiency
Pyloric Stenosis	Narrowing of the pyloric canal, causing obstruction
Scheuermann's Disease or Adolescent Kyphosis	Kyphosis with onset in adolescence
Slipped Epiphysis	Proximal portion of femur dislocated from distal portion at the proximal epiphysis
Tumor	New tissue growth where cell proliferation is uncontrolled
Ewing's Sarcoma	Malignant tumor of bone arising in medullary tissue
Osteochondroma	Benign bone tumor projection with a cartilaginous cap
Osteosarcoma	Malignant, primary tumor of bone with bone or cartilage formation
Wilms' Tumor	Most common childhood abdominal neoplasm affecting the kidney

Patient care: special concerns

Protection of the Child

PROTECTION FROM INJURY

The diagnostic imaging department is responsible for ensuring that children neither injure themselves nor are injured during their stay in the department. Emphasis on quality assurance and risk management dictates that many hospitals (and, consequently, radiology departments) perform routine safety inspections to take a proactive stance in minimizing the potential for harm. These inspections are often performed by a two-person team that includes: (1) the supervising or charge radiographer and (2) a frontline worker, whose input is vital because the worker uses the equipment on a daily basis. The following guidelines are observed:

- To *avoid the possibility of injury*, supervise children while they are in the department or being transported to and from the department. Some departments clearly delineate in their policy and procedure manuals what safety precautions are to be carried out while patients are in the imaging room. Such policies relate to the use of Velcro or compression bands designed to prevent patients from rolling off the imaging table (Fig. 27-13). See also Fig. 27-19.

- Regularly inspect all immobilization tools to ensure that they are maintained in working order. Experienced radiographers should instruct all novice pediatric radiographers in proper immobilization techniques, and novice radiographers' practices should be observed by senior or supervising radiographers.

- In the event of an injury, however minor, file a report documenting the specifics of the incident and the actions taken. Some departments require that reports be filed even in the event that there was *potential* for an injury to occur.

PROTECTION FROM UNNECESSARY RADIATION

The conscientious radiographer can do much to protect children from exposure to unnecessary radiation. Radiographers should remember that bone marrow, active in the formation of blood cells, is distributed throughout the pediatric skeleton and that tissue damage is associated with ionizing radiation. Radiographers should observe the following steps:

- Direct efforts toward proper centering and selection of exposure factors, precise collimation, and appropriate use of filters (where required), which all contribute to safe practice.

- Use strategic placement of gonadal and breast shielding and employ effective immobilization techniques to reduce the need for repeat examinations.

- Instead of the AP projection, use the PA projection of the thorax and skull to reduce the amount of radiation reaching the breast tissue and lens of the eye, respectively.

- During radiography of the upper limbs, protect the upper torsos of all children.

- Employ diagonal placement of small gonadal aprons along the thorax and abdomen to protect the sternum and gonads of infants and toddlers during supine radiography.

- Have older children wear child-size full lead aprons or adult aprons. (See Common Pediatric Examinations, Limb Radiography, later in this chapter.)

Radiographers in supervisory and management positions have additional responsibilities. In addition to ensuring that the previously described practices are followed, supervising radiographers should take into account the clinical needs of the radiologist and follow the ALARA (As Low As Reasonably Achievable) principle of radiation exposure when developing technique charts or programming exposure consoles. Pediatric imaging poses conflicting demands on imaging protocols. High kVp is desired to keep the

Fig. 27-13 Three tools frequently used in pediatric immobilization: *(left to right)* a Velcro band, often called a Bucky or body band; a strip of reusable Velcro; and a "bookend."

milliampere-seconds (mAs) low (thereby reducing the absorbed dose), but low mAs values can present *quantum mottle* problems in the radiographic examination of small body parts, specifically pediatric limbs and neonatal chests. For acceptable diagnostic quality, relatively high resolution is needed. Practically speaking, these needs are often met by the development of a multispeed film-screen combination or *computed radiography* (CR) system. Slow-speed systems are used to demonstrate small parts (limbs and neonatal chests), and faster speeds are used for procedures involving the spine, abdomen, and GI tract. The least confusing approach is to purchase one type of film and *screens of varying speeds,* when a film-screen system is used. The IRs are then color coded along their outer edges, and the user can be directed to a corresponding color-coded chart to select the appropriate combination.

Used judiciously by experienced and knowledgeable personnel, CR can reduce the radiation dose. This technique significantly shortens the time needed to perform the procedure and optimizes or tailors the images to suit individual patient requirements. As a result of increased familiarity with the power of window-level adjustments in CT (see Chapter 31) and MRI (see Chapter 33), radiologists have developed a deeper appreciation and acceptance of the digital format. Automatic, laser-printed spot images in GI barium studies are a common general application of *image intensifier–based digital radiography.* Pulsed fluoroscopy with "last image hold" also reduces patient dose and length of examination. Furthermore, the ability to transmit the digital image directly to a laser printer to produce hard copies or to PACS (picture archive and communication system) saves valuable radiographer time. This savings often allows the radiographer to spend more time with the patient or to assist the next child sooner.

A *cautionary note:* The fact that digitally acquired images can be "postprocessed," thereby correcting some exposure errors, does not negate an important truth—images of proper density are achieved by proper positioning. The anatomy to be demonstrated must be in proper alignment with the photocell or ionization chamber.

Immobilization: Principles and Tools

Perhaps the two most successful tools for pediatric radiography are *effective immobilization* and *good communication skills.* Respected pediatric radiographers approach patients and parents with kindness and take care to maintain patient comfort throughout the procedure.

Naturally, a willingness to cooperate on the child's part allows for more *passive,* less aggressive immobilization techniques. *Reassurance, praise,* and conversational *distraction* are the three ingredients of successful communication. Reassurance is perhaps second only to sleep as the best passive immobilization technique. A sleeping child who is moved gently, kept comfortable and warm, and not startled by sudden or loud noises often remains asleep throughout the procedure. However, as previously noted, all chest images must be taken while the child is awake because the rate of respiration is too shallow during sleep to provide full inspiration images.

Despite effective communication, it is often necessary to restrain children during radiography. If immobilization is not handled appropriately, difficulties can arise for the radiographer, patient, and parent. Immobilization should never become a traumatic, torturous event for the child, and no immobilization technique should cause harm to the child. Experienced radiographers should teach novice pediatric radiographers how to *carefully* restrain a child. A radiographer's lack of experience, coupled with the parent's and child's fear, can often lead to frustration on *everyone's* part. With practice, the radiographer can keep patients both comfortable and immobilized with a minimum of frustration.

The radiographer can prevent a great deal of frustration by using the communication strategies described at the beginning of this chapter and applying some *practiced* immobilization techniques. It is important to remember that the parent (presuming one is present) can do only one job. For example, a parent who assists with the radiographic examination of her 2-year-old's forearm can help only by holding the humerus and the hand; the radiographer or some other staff member must immobilize the other arm and both legs.

Aside from the regular sponges and sandbags, three tools frequently used in pediatric immobilization deserve mention. They are the Velcro compression band (sometimes referred to as a Bucky or body band), a strip of reusable Velcro, and a "bookend" (see Fig. 27-13). These devices are effective for the immobilization of children, although their applications are not limited to pediatric radiography.

Other tools, such as the Pigg-o-stat (Modern Way Immobilizers, Clifton, Tenn.) and the octagonal infant immobilization cradle, are described in the following sections.

Common Pediatric Examinations

CHEST RADIOGRAPHY

The most common radiographic procedure performed in hospitals and clinics is of the chest. Radiologists agree that for most diagnostic chest radiographs in pediatric patients, upright images yield a great deal more information than supine radiographs. It is, however, important to know the way to achieve diagnostic quality in both positions. Regardless of body position, accurate diagnosis depends on high-quality images made with short exposure times to reduce motion. *Expiratory images can lead to erroneous radiologic interpretations.* Therefore images acquired *on maximal inspiration* are crucially important for accurate diagnosis. Well-positioned, nonrotated radiographs are also essential for proper diagnosis because even minor degrees of rotation can significantly distort the normal anatomy.

Upright radiograph on the newborn to 3-year-old

The many challenges of obtaining upright images include preventing motion and rotation, freeing the lung fields of superimposition of humeri and scapulae, and obtaining a good inspiratory radiograph. Various methods of immobilization are used to achieve these images, often with somewhat mixed results. Fortunately these challenges are easily met with the use of a pediatric positioner and immobilization tool called the *Pigg-o-stat* (Fig. 27-14). Although the Pigg-o-stat is primarily used for chest radiography, other applications include upright abdominal images and radiography of the thoracic and lumbar spine.

The Pigg-o-stat is composed of a large support base on wheels, a small adjustable seat, and Plexiglas supports called *sleeves*. These sleeves come in two sizes. The seat, sleeves, and "turntable" base rotate as a unit to facilitate quick positioning from PA to lateral projections. Although some physicians do not favor use of the Pigg-o-stat (for aesthetic reasons and because of the possibility of sleeve artifacts), the device has been shown to be one of the safest and most versatile restraining methods available for chest and upright abdominal radiography.

Communication with parents

The Pigg-o-stat requires explanation for parents unfamiliar with its use. The radiographer should offer an explanation similar to this: "Doctors prefer chest x-rays to be performed with the child in the upright position. To help your child remain still, we have the child sit on this little seat. These plastic supports fit snugly around the child's sides and keep the arms raised. The device looks funny, and your child will probably cry, but this is usually an expression of frustration about being confined. The crying actually helps to obtain a good x-ray image because at the end of a cry, your child will take a big gasp of air. At that moment the exposure will be taken."

A complete explanation is worthwhile and essential. The parent can be shown how to help place the child on the seat by guiding in the feet. Then the parent can assist by holding the arms above the child's head.

Radiographers should realize that positioning a child in a Pigg-o-stat is a *two-person job.* Radiographers can safely take children out of the Pigg-o-stat without assistance, but an extra pair of hands is needed in the initial positioning. The properly instructed parent is generally willing and able to assist.

Fig. 27-14 Position for PA chest radiograph. The Pigg-o-stat (Modern Way Immobilizers, Clifton, Tenn) is a pediatric positioner and immobilization tool. The IR is held in the metal extension stand.

Method

The following steps are observed:

- Have the patient undress completely from the waist up, so that after the patient is positioned, the ribs are visible on inspiration.
- Choose the appropriate sleeve size. Sleeves should fit snugly, which often requires Velcro strips or adhesive tape wrapped around the base of the sleeves (see Fig. 27-14).
- Adjust the seat height to approximately the correct level. The seat is at the correct height if, when the patient is sitting up straight, the face fits in the contours or cutout portions of the sleeves.

This one-step positioning, in which the child is sitting straight on the seat with the arms raised evenly above the head, ensures motionless and nonrotated images (Fig. 27-15). The orientation of the room (i.e., where the chest stand or IR holder is located relative to the control panel) and the image requested determine how well the radiographer can see the child's thorax to ensure that the exposure is made during inspiration. The radiographer can detect inspiration by doing the following (listed in decreasing order of reliability):

1. Waiting for the end of a cry—the child will take a big gasp of air
2. Watching the abdomen—the child's abdomen will extend on inspiration
3. Watching the chest wall—the ribs will be outlined on inspiration
4. Watching the rise and fall of the sternum

Centering and collimation

The central ray for both PA and lateral projections is directed to the level of T6-T7, but the collimated field should extend from and include the mastoid tips to just above the iliac crests. Inclusion of the mastoid tips demonstrates the upper airway; narrowed or stenotic airways are a common source of respiratory problems in pediatric patients. By collimating just above the crests of the ilia, the radiographer can include the inferior costal margins. A significant number of children arrive in the imaging department with long lung fields resulting from hyperinflation. Noted examples include patients with cardiac disorders and asthma.

Fig. 27-15 PA **(A)** and lateral **(B)** chest images of a 10-day-old patient with a pathologic cardiac condition. The Pigg-o-stat provides motionless, nonrotated radiographs of good inspiration. Note the presence of sternal wires *(arrows)*, cardiac pacing wires *(arrowheads)*, and a central venous line *(dashed line)*. The nasogastric tube is seen well.

A   B

Fig. 27-16 A, PA chest radiographs should be performed on the 3- to 18-year-old with the child sitting. **B,** The parent, if present, can assist with immobilization for the lateral image by holding the child's head between the child's arms. Metal extension stands *(arrows on **A** and **B**)* are commercially available from companies that market diagnostic imaging accessories.

Upright radiograph on the 3- to 18-year-old

Upright radiographs on 3- to 18-year-olds are easily obtained by observing the following steps:

- Help the child sit on a large wooden box, a wide-based trolley with brakes, or a stool, with the IR supported using a metal extension stand. Young children of this age are curious and have short attention spans. By having them sit, the radiographer can prevent them from wiggling from the waist down.
- For the PA radiograph, have the child hold onto the side supports of the extension stand, with the chin on top of or next to the IR. This prevents upper body movement.
- When positioning for the lateral radiograph, have the parent (if presence is permitted) assist by raising the child's arms above the head and holding the head between the arms (Fig. 27-16). PA and lateral chest images of a 6-year-old patient are shown in Fig. 27-17.

A   B

Fig. 27-17 PA **(A)** and lateral **(B)** radiographs of a seated 6-year-old boy. Large wooden boxes have the advantage of being sturdier than stools or trolleys, which often have wheels.

Supine radiograph

Infants needing supine and cross-table lateral radiographs can be immobilized using Velcro straps around the knees and Velcro band across the legs (Fig. 27-18). The patient is raised on a sponge with the arms held up, and a cross-table lateral is performed. This is particularly useful for patients with chest tubes, delicately positioned gastrostomy tubes, or soft tissue swellings or protrusions that may be compromised by the sleeves of the Pigg-o-stat.

Evaluating the image

As in adult chest radiography, the use of kVp is also desirable in pediatric chest work; however, this is relative. In adult work, high kVp generally ranges between 110 and 130, but for pediatric PA projections, kVp ranges between 80 and 90. Practically speaking, the use of a higher kVp is impossible because the corresponding mAs are too low to produce a diagnostic image. Relatively high kVp helps to provide images with long-scale contrast.

The criteria used to evaluate recorded detail include the resolution of peripheral lung markings. Evaluating any image for adequate density involves assessing the most and least dense areas of the demonstrated anatomy. In the PA chest image, the ideal technical factor is a selection that permits visualization of the intervertebral disk spaces through the heart (the most dense area) while still demonstrating the peripheral lung markings (the least dense area). Rotation should be assessed by evaluating the position of midline structures. Posterior and anterior midline structures (i.e., sternum, airway, and vertebral bodies) should be superimposed. The anatomic structures to be demonstrated include the airway (trachea) to the costophrenic angles. Similar to chest radiography in adults, the visualization of 9 to 10 posterior ribs is a reliable indicator of a radiograph taken with good inspiration (Table 27-1).

Fig. 27-18 The patient is raised on a sponge with arms held up by the head, and the legs are immobilized using Velcro straps. The IR is in place for the horizontal lateral beam (cross-table lateral).

TABLE 27-1

Quick reference guide for radiograph assessment

	Density			Contrast			
	Most dense	Least dense	Recorded detail	Long scale >3 shades	Short scale >3 shades	Anatomy	Rotation check
PA Chest	Midline; intervertebral disk spaces, heart	Peripheral lung markings	Peripheral lung markings	Airway, heart, apices, bases, mediastinum, lung markings behind diaphragm and heart		Airway to bases	Airway position, SC joints, lung field measurement, cardiac silhouette
PA Chest	Heart	Retrocardiac space	Peripheral lung markings	Airway, heart, apices, bases		Airway to bases, spinous process to sternum	Superimposition of ribs, spinous processes on profile
Abdomen	Lumbar spine	Peripheral edges, soft tissue above the iliac crests	Organ silhouettes	Diaphragm, liver, kidney, spine, gas shadows		Right and left hemidiaphragm, pubic symphysis, right and left skin edges	
Limbs	Bone	Soft tissue	Bony trabecular patterns		Bone, muscle, soft tissue	Joints above and below injury, all soft tissue	AP and lateral images must not resemble obliques
Hips	Hip joints	Iliac crests	Bony trabecular patterns		Bone, soft tissue	Iliac crests, lesser trochanter	Symmetric iliac crests
Lateral Lumbar Spine	L5-S1	Spinous processes	Bony trabecular patterns		Bone	T12 to coccyx, spinous processes to vertebral bodies	Alignment of posterior surfaces of vertebral bodies

Evaluating the radiograph to determine its diagnostic quality is a practiced skill. This chart, designed as a quick reference guide, outlines the five important technical criteria and the related anatomic indicators used in critiquing radiographs.
SC, Sternoclavicular; *AP,* anteroposterior.

HIP RADIOGRAPHY

The hip and pelvis are commonly examined radiographically in both the pediatric and adult population. However, the clinical rationale for ordering these examinations varies tremendously. The informed radiographer who understands these differences can be of great assistance. With a basic comprehension of some of the common pediatric pathologies and disease processes, the radiographer is better able to appreciate the skills required of the radiologist to make an accurate diagnosis.

General principles

Both hips are examined, using the same projection for comparison. Hip examinations on children are most often ordered to assess for Legg-Calvé-Perthes disease (aseptic avascular necrosis of the femoral head of unknown etiology) and congenital dislocation of the hip and to diagnose nonspecific hip pain. Because these conditions require evaluation of the symmetry of the acetabula, joint spaces, and soft tissue, symmetric positioning is crucial.

Despite the importance of radiation protection, little written literature is available to guide radiographers on the placement of gonadal shields and when to use shielding. The radiographer should observe the following guidelines:

- *Always* use gonadal shielding on males. However, take care to prevent potential lesions of the pubic symphysis from being obscured.
- In females, use gonadal protection on all radiographs *except* the first AP projection of the *initial* examination of the hips and pelvis.
- After sacral abnormality or sacral involvement has been ruled out, use shielding on subsequent images in females.
- Before proceeding, check the girl's records or seek clarification from the parents regarding whether this is the child's first examination.
- Because the female reproductive organs are located in the mid-pelvis with their exact position varying, ensure that the shield covers the sacrum and part or all of the sacroiliac joints, making sure it does not cover the hip joints or pubic symphysis.

NOTE: Many children have been taught that no one should touch their "private parts." Radiographers need to be sensitive and use discretion when explaining and carrying out the procedure.

- *Never touch the pubic symphysis in a child,* regardless of whether you are positioning the patient or placing the gonadal shield.

- The superior border of the pubic symphysis is always at the level of the greater trochanters. Use the trochanters as a guide for both positioning and shield placement. The CR should be located midline at a point midway between the anterior superior iliac spine (ASIS) and the symphysis.
- In males, keep the gonadal shield from touching the scrotum by laying a 15-degree sponge or a cloth over the top of the femora. The top of the shield can be placed level with the trochanters and the bottom half of the shield can rest on top of the sponge or cloth (Fig. 27-19, *A*).
- In females, place the top, widest part of the shield in the midline, level with the ASIS.

Initial images

The preliminary examination of the hips and pelvis on children includes a well-collimated AP projection (see Fig. 27-19, *B*) and a projection in what is commonly referred to as the "frog leg" position. This position is more correctly described as a coronal image of the pelvis with the thighs in abduction and external rotation, or the frog (Lauenstein) lateral projection (see Chapter 7).

A   B

Fig. 27-19 A, The male gonadal shield should cover the scrotum without obscuring the pubic symphysis. The greater trochanters indicate the upper border of the pubic symphysis; the top of the shield should be placed approximately ½ inch below this level. The gonadal shield rests on a 15-degree sponge, which prevents the radiographer's hands from coming close to or touching the scrotal area. **B,** A 3½-year-old normal pelvis; note the shielding.

Preparation and communication

All images of the abdomen and pelvic girdle should be performed with the diaper completely removed. This is *essential* for radiography of the hips and pelvis. Diapers, especially wet diapers, produce significant artifacts on radiographs, often rendering them undiagnostic. The radiographer or imaging department staff member should place all necessary sponges, gonadal shielding, Velcro strips, and Velcro restraining bands on the table before beginning the examination.

Positioning and immobilization

As described previously, *symmetric positioning* is of great importance. However, as in many examinations, the hip positions that are the most uncomfortable for the patient are often the most crucial.

When a child suffers from hip pain or dislocation, symmetric positioning is difficult to achieve because the patient often tries to compensate for the discomfort by rotating the pelvis. The radiographer should observe the following steps when positioning the patient:

- As with hip examinations on any patient, check that the ASISs are equidistant from the table.
- After carefully observing and communicating with the patient to discover the location of pain, the radiographer can use sponges to compensate for rotation. Sponges should routinely be used to support the thighs in the frog leg position. This can help prevent motion artifacts.
- Do not accept poorly positioned images. Expend considerable effort in attempting to achieve optimal positioning. This effort may include giving instructions, or repeating instructions to the novice pediatric radiographer.

Because *immobilization techniques* should vary according to the aggressiveness of the patient, the radiographer can follow these additional guidelines:

- Make every effort to use explanation and reassurance as part of the immobilization method. The child may require only a Velcro band placed across the legs as a safety precaution (see Fig. 27-19, *A*).
- For the active (or potentially active) child, wrap a Velcro strip around the knees and place large sandbags over the arms (Fig. 27-20). The Velcro strip around the knees keeps the child from wiggling one leg out from under the Velcro band. After getting one leg out, the child may get the other out and possibly roll off the table.

Fig. 27-20 Immobilization of the active child: sandbags over the arms, Velcro strips around the knees, and a Velcro band beside the patient's feet to be secured over the legs, as in Fig. 27-18.

- If the child has enough strength to free the arms from the sandbags, ask a parent to stand on the opposite side of the table from the radiographer and hold the child's humeri. The parent's thumbs should be placed directly over the child's shoulders (Fig. 27-21). This method of immobilization is used extensively. It works well for supine abdominal images, intravenous urograms (IVUs), intravenous pyelograms (IVPs), overhead GI procedures, and spinal radiography.

Evaluating the images

Rotation or symmetry can be evaluated by ensuring that midline structures are, in fact, in the midline and that the ilia appear symmetric. Depending on the degree of skeletal maturation, visualization of the trochanters can indicate the position of the legs when the radiograph was taken. Symmetry in the skin folds is also an important evaluation criterion for the diagnostician. The anatomy to be demonstrated includes the crests of the ilia to the upper quarter of the femora. The density should be such that the bony trabecular pattern is visible in the hip joints, the thickest and most dense area within the region. The visualization of the bony trabecular pattern is used as an indicator that sufficient recorded detail has been demonstrated. This, of course, should not be at the expense of demonstrating the soft tissues—the muscles and skin folds (see Table 27-1).

Fig. 27-21 If the child is strong enough or aggressive enough to remove the sandbags, the parent can hold the child's humeri by placing the thumbs directly over the child's shoulders.

SKULL RADIOGRAPHY

Along with radiography of the limbs, skull radiography presents some of the greatest challenges to the radiographer. Indeed, cranial radiography is usually one of the last areas that students become comfortable with during their clinical education. The reasons are twofold: (1) anatomically speaking, the skull is complex, and (2) the frequency of skull examinations has steadily decreased with the increased availability of CT (see Chapter 31) and MRI (see Chapter 33). Pediatric patients such as the 3-year-old in Fig. 27-22 are an even greater challenge.

The problems associated with cranial radiography in children can be lessened by *preparing the room* before the patient and parent enter (Fig. 27-23) and avoiding *two common pitfalls:* (1) ineffective immobilization and (2) forgetting (or not taking the time) to check the first radiograph of a skull series. The first image should be treated as a *scout radiograph,* an image that permits assessment of the exposure factors and allows the radiographer to tailor the remaining images to suit the peculiarities of the individual patient. The clinical rationale for performing skull radiography differs tremendously between pediatric and adult patients. Children who arrive in the imaging department for skull examinations may have congenital abnormalities that significantly alter the bone density. Their age and consequent degree of skeletal maturation also affect bone density. These factors need to be considered as the technical factors are selected. Therefore the viewing of the initial image is very important.

Immobilization

Unless the child is asleep, all patients 3 years old and younger should be immobilized using the "bunny" technique illustrated in Fig. 27-24. A well-wrapped child remains that way through five to seven images. Mastering this technique is clearly one of the secrets to successful immobilization. A few words of explanation to the parent regarding the need to wrap the child, along with some instructions for ways the parent can help, are also very beneficial. Experience has shown that although children initially do not like being wrapped up using this technique, after their initial frustration and perhaps the use of a pacifier, they often settle down and occasionally fall asleep. If beneficial, the pacifier can be left in the patient's mouth for every image except the reverse AP projection. The parent must be cautioned not to unwrap the child until all radiographs have been checked for diagnostic quality.

Fig. 27-22 This little girl's face indicates a challenge for skull radiography.

Fig. 27-23 The well-prepared radiographer can make a potentially difficult skull examination go smoothly. Note the gonadal shield, Velcro band, and head clamps in place. A standard hospital sheet has been unfolded and placed on the table to prepare for immobilization using the "bunny" technique.

Fig. 27-24 The "bunny" method used to immobilize the patient for cranial radiography. **A** to **D** focus on immobilization of the shoulders, **E** to **G** concentrate on the humeri, and **H** to **K** illustrate the way the sheet is folded and wrapped to immobilize the legs. **A,** Begin with a standard hospital sheet folded in half lengthwise. Make a 6-inch fold at the top, and lay the child down about 2 feet from the end of the sheet. **B,** Wrap the end of the sheet over the left shoulder, and pass the sheet under the child. **C,** This step makes use of the 6-inch fold. Reach under, undo the fold, and wrap it over the right shoulder. (Steps **B** and **C** are crucial to the success of this immobilization technique because they prevent the child from wiggling the shoulders free.) **D,** After wrapping the right shoulder, pass the end of the sheet under the child. Pull it through to keep the right arm snug against the body. **E,** Begin wrapping, keeping the sheet snug over the upper body to immobilize the humeri. **F,** Lift the lower body and pass the sheet underneath, keeping the child's head on the table. Repeat steps **E** and **F** if material permits. **G,** Make sure the material is evenly wrapped around the upper body. (Extra rolls around the shoulder and neck area produce artifacts on 30-degree fronto-occipital and submentovertical radiographs.) **H,** Make a diagonal fold with the remaining material (approximately 2 feet). **I,** Roll the material together. **J,** Snugly wrap this over the child's femora. (The tendency to misjudge the location of the femora and thus wrap too snugly around the lower legs should be avoided.) **K,** Tuck the end of the rolled material in front. (If not enough material remains to tuck in, use a Velcro strip or tape to secure it.)

(From The Michener Institute for Applied Health Sciences, Toronto.)

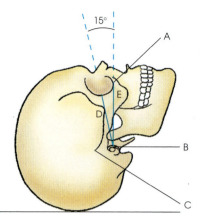

Fig. 27-25 Established tube angles and positions modified to suit the pediatric patient: *A*, infraorbital margin; *B*, EAM; *C*, petrous ridge; *D*, OML; *E*, IOML. Note that in the young child the OML and IOML are 15 degrees apart (in contrast to older children and adults, where the difference can be 15 to 20 degrees). For simplicity, these diagrams adopt a convention of 15 degrees.

(Courtesy K. Edgell, Cook, Inc., Toronto.)

Fig. 27-26 PA projection with OML (*A*) perpendicular to the table. In the older child, teenager, and adult, a 15- to 20-degree caudal angulation results in the petrous ridges being projected in the lower third of the orbits. In infants and young children, a 10- to 15-degree caudal angulation achieves the same result.

Fig. 27-27 AP projection with the OML perpendicular to the table. This projection requires a 15-degree cephalad angulation to project the petrous ridges in the lower third of the orbits.

Fig. 27-28 The IOML (*A*) is positioned perpendicular to the table with the patient in a *comfortable* position—one that the head and neck naturally assume as the patient lies down. (A comfortable patient is more likely to remain still.) With the patient positioned this way, the tube does not have to be angled cephalad to project the petrous ridges in the lower third of the orbits (represented by *dotted line, C*). With the necessary head clamps positioned, the IOML remains perpendicular to the film. With the IOML perpendicular to the IR, the forehead and chin are parallel to the IR (*dotted line, B*).

Positioning

The skull grows rapidly in the first 2½ years of life, approaching the 75th percentile of adult size by that age. The radiographer must understand the way this growth and the rate at which the cranium grows relative to the facial bones alter the position of the various radiographic landmarks and angles.

Practical tip: The established cranial angulations (see Chapter 20) can be adapted to suit young children by decreasing the angulation of the central ray by 5 degrees. The line diagrams in Figs. 27-25 to 27-28 put this in perspective. The PA projection is used as the basis for these diagrams because this image projects the petrous ridges in the lower third of the orbits, which is a common baseline radiograph for many departments.

Head clamps should be used on all children, even sleeping children. Although motion may not be a factor, the sleeping child's head needs some support to maintain the required positions. (The lateral image may be an exception if the child has fallen asleep on the back with the head turned to the side.) Many radiographers believe that the use of head clamps further agitates some children.

As with any form of immobilization, acceptance of the method depends greatly on the way it is introduced to the patient and parent. If the room is prepared before the patient enters, the head clamps should already be in position. Attention need not be drawn to the head clamps until they are about to be used, and they can then be referred to as "earmuffs" (Fig. 27-29). This avoids the unnecessary anxiety that may otherwise be experienced. The degree to which the clamps are tightened depends on the situation. Some children need them only as a reminder to keep still, whereas others need to have them adjusted more tightly. Although various kinds of head clamps are available, clamps with a suction-cup base are particularly effective and versatile. (The problem some users experience with the suction cups not sticking to the table is often eliminated by lightly wetting the rubber cups.)

Fig. 27-29 AP projection with head clamps in place.

TABLE 27-2

Protocols for neurologic and trauma/injury radiographic routines

Neurologic routine	Trauma/injury routine
PA or AP projection (see Fig. 27-29)	PA or AP projection (see Fig. 27-29)
AP axial projection (Towne method)	AP axial projection (Towne method)
Lateral with vertical beam (see Fig. 27-30)	Lateral with horizontal beam (see Fig. 27-31)
Submentovertical projection (see Fig. 27-32)	

The important differences between neurologic and trauma/injury routines are the inclusion of a submentovertical projection in the neurologic routine and the need for the lateral image to be performed using a horizontal beam in the trauma/injury routine. This lateral image with a horizontal beam is often referred to as a *cross-table lateral* and is performed to assess possible air-fluid levels that may occur as a result of the injury.

Fig. 27-30 When other methods prove unsuccessful, effective immobilization for a lateral skull radiograph with a vertical beam can be achieved with the use of a second Velcro band—*and some additional explanation* to the parent. Some radiographers question the technique because it covers the child's eyes. Turning the child's head and placing the Velcro band should be the last step (apart from a quick collimation check) before the exposure is made. Anxiousness can be alleviated if the parent bends down facing the child and talks to the child for the few seconds the radiographer needs to make the exposure.

Routines and protocols

Physicians order skull radiographs to assess neurologic problems and evaluate the extent of trauma or injury. For these reasons, many departments develop two routines: neurologic and trauma (Table 27-2; Figs. 27-30 to 27-32; see also Fig. 27-29).

A

B

Fig. 27-31 A, Effective immobilization for lateral skull images with a horizontal beam can be achieved using the infant head and neck immobilizer. **B,** The resultant image reveals a well-positioned, nonrotated lateral skull image, including the upper cervical spine.

Fig. 27-32 Positioning for a submentovertical projection. Note the use of tape over the forehead to help maintain extension. (The tape is flipped over so that the nonsticky surface is in contact with the child's forehead.)

LIMB RADIOGRAPHY

Limb radiography, which accounts for a high percentage of pediatric general radiographic procedures in most clinics and hospitals, requires some explanation. The child's age and demeanor determine the method of immobilization to be employed. The immobilization methods are described here according to age group. In planning the approach, the radiographer should consider the chronologic age and psychologic outlook of the patient. For example, a very active 3-year-old may be better managed using the approach for newborns to 2-year-olds.

Immobilization
Newborn to 2-year-old

Limb radiography on the newborn to 2-year-old is probably the most challenging; however, it is made easier when the patient is wrapped in a towel. (A pillowcase will suffice if a towel is not available.) This wrapping technique, a modification of the "bunny" method described previously, keeps the baby warm and allows the radiographer (and the parent, if assisting) to concentrate on immobilizing the injured arm. Fig. 27-33 demonstrates the method by which a piece of Plexiglas and "bookends" can be used to immobilize the hand.

Lower limbs on patients in this age group pose the greatest challenge in all pediatric limb work. In general, both arms should be wrapped in the towel and a Velcro band should be placed across the abdomen. A large sandbag is then placed over the unaffected leg (Fig. 27-34).

A

B

Fig. 27-33 A, With a simple modification of the "bunny" technique using a towel (or pillowcase), the child can be immobilized for upper limb radiography. Plexiglas *(dashed lines)* and "bookends" *(B)* can be used to immobilize the hands of children 2 years old and younger. Note that after the child is wrapped, a Velcro band is used for safety and a small apron is placed diagonally over the body to protect the sternum and gonads. The IR is placed on a lead mat, which prevents the image receptor from sliding on the table. **B,** Nine-month-old normal right hand.

Fig. 27-34 A, The challenges of immobilizing lower limbs are greater than those of immobilizing upper limbs. After wrapping both of the patient's arms in a towel and placing a Velcro band over the abdomen, the radiographer can place a large sandbag over the unaffected leg. With careful collimation and proper instruction, the parent can hold the limb as demonstrated. Normal 21-month-old AP **(B)** and lateral **(C)** tibia and fibula.

Preschoolers

The upper limbs of preschoolers are best examined radiographically with the child sitting on the parent's lap as shown in Fig. 27-35. If the parent is unable to participate, these children can be immobilized as described previously.

With parental participation, radiography of the lower limbs can be accomplished with the child sitting or lying on the table. Preventing the patient from falling from the table is always a primary concern with preschoolers. The parent must be instructed to remain by the child's side if the child is seated on the table. If the examination is performed with the child lying on the table, a Velcro band should be placed over the child.

School-age children

School-age children can generally be managed in the same way as adult patients for both upper and lower limb examinations.

Radiation protection

The upper body should be protected in all examinations of the upper limbs because of the close proximity of the thymus, sternum, and breast tissue to the scatter of the primary beam. Child-sized lead aprons with cartoon characters are both popular and practical (Fig. 27-36).

Management of fractures

As with adult patients who arrive in the imaging department with obvious fractures, the child with an obvious fracture *must* have the limb properly splinted by qualified personnel before the radiographer commences the examination. The splint protects both the patient and the radiographer, because the radiographer could cause further injury by manipulating an unsplinted limb.

Patients with fractures often arrive in the imaging department on a stretcher. The radiographer skilled at adapting routines can often obtain the necessary radiographs without moving the patient onto the table.

Ways to manage patients with osteogenesis imperfecta were discussed previously in Patient Care: Special Concerns.

Fig. 27-35 Preschoolers are best managed sitting on a parent's lap. A lead mat is used to keep the IR from sliding. Note use of Plexiglas to immobilize fingers. (The parent's hands are shown without lead gloves and not draped in lead for illustration purposes only.)

Fig. 27-36 The teddy bear on this full-length apron *(left)* makes it appropriate for young children.

Evaluating the image

One of the most striking differences between adult and pediatric patients is the radiographic appearance of the limb. Radiographers develop an appreciation for these differences, which are caused by the presence of epiphyseal lines, as they gain experience in evaluating pediatric images. In departments in which the patient mixture includes children and adults, preliminary limb work may require the *contralateral* side to be examined for comparison purposes. To the uneducated eye, a normally developing epiphysis may mimic a fracture. For this reason and because fractures can occur through the epiphyseal plate, physicians must learn to recognize epiphyseal lines and their appearance at various stages of ossification. Fractures that occur through the epiphysis are called *growth plate fractures.* Fig. 27-37 illustrates five types of epiphyseal fractures, referred to as *Salter-Harris type fractures,* the most widely used form of classification.

Because the growth plates are composed of cartilaginous tissue, the *density* of the radiographic image must be such that soft tissue is demonstrated in addition to bone (see Table 27-1). As previously described for radiography of the hip, the visualization of the bony trabecular pattern is used as an indicator that sufficient *recorded detail* has been demonstrated. Because of the smallness of pediatric limbs, an imaging system that provides better resolving power is usually required. As a general rule, the speed of the imaging system used for limb radiography should be half that used for spines and abdomens.

| A | B | C | D | E |

Fig. 27-37 Salter-Harris fractures. The black lines represent the fracture lines. **A,** A type 1 fracture occurs directly through the growth plate. **B,** A type 2 fracture extends through the growth plate and into the metaphyses. **C,** A type 3 fracture line extends through the growth plate and into the epiphyses. **D,** A type 4 fracture line extends through the metaphyses, across or sometimes along the growth plate, and through the epiphyses. **E,** A type 5 fracture involves a crushing of all or part of the growth plate. Fractures that occur through the epiphyses are significant injuries because they can affect growth if not recognized and treated properly. Proper radiographic technique is required for the demonstration of both soft tissue and bone. This is especially important with type 1 fractures, in which the growth plate is separated as a result of a lateral blow, and type 5 fractures, in which the growth plate has sustained a compression injury. Types 1 and 5 fractures do not occur through the bone.

ABDOMINAL RADIOGRAPHY

Abdominal radiography on children is requested for different reasons than it is on adults. Consequently, the initial procedure or protocol differs significantly. In addition to the supine and upright images, the assessment for acute abdomen conditions or the abdominal series in adult radiography usually includes radiographs obtained in the left lateral decubitus position. Often the series is not considered complete without a PA projection of the chest. To keep radiation exposure to a minimum, the pediatric abdominal series need only include two images: the supine abdomen and an image to demonstrate air-fluid levels. The upright image is preferred over the lateral decubitus in patients younger than 2 or 3 years of age because, from an immobilization and patient-comfort perspective, it is much easier to perform. The upright image can be obtained with a slight modification of the Pigg-o-stat, whereas the lateral decubitus position requires significant modification of the Pigg-o-stat. As mentioned for hip radiography, the diaper should be completely removed for all abdomen and pelvic imaging to avoid artifacts.

Positioning and immobilization

Young children can be immobilized for supine abdomen imaging with the same methods described for radiography of the hips and pelvis (see Fig. 27-20), methods that provide basic immobilization of a patient for supine table radiography. All males should be shielded using methods described for radiography of the hips and pelvis. The CR should be located midway at the level of L2. The radiographer should observe the following guidelines for upright abdominal imaging:

- Effectively immobilize newborns and children as old as 3 years for the upright image using the Pigg-o-stat.
- Raise the seat of the Pigg-o-stat to avoid projecting artifacts from the bases of the sleeves over the lower abdomen (Fig. 27-38).
- For the best results in the older child, have the child sit on a large box, trolley, or stool and spread the legs apart to prevent superimposition of the upper femora over the pelvis.

Fig. 27-38 The Pigg-o-stat, modified with the seat raised to suit upright abdominal radiography. The sleeves and seat are cleaned, and the seat is covered with a cloth diaper or thick tissue before the patient is positioned. (Note the gonad shield placed anterior.)

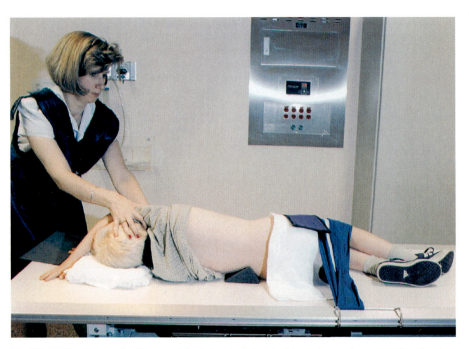

Fig. 27-39 The immobilization used for lateral abdominal imaging is also very effective for lateral thoracic and lumbosacral spine images. A 45-degree sponge and sandbag are used anteriorly.

Lateral images of the abdomen are occasionally required in children, generally to localize something in the AP plane. Immobilization for lateral images is quite challenging; this difficulty, along with the fact that patient immobilization is the same as for lateral spine images, makes it worthy of mention here. Properly instructed, the parent can be helpful with this radiograph. The radiographer should observe the following steps:

- Remember that the *parent can do only one job*.
- Ask the parent to stand on the opposite side of the table and hold the child's head and arms.
- Immobilize the rest of the child's body using available immobilization tools. These tools include large 45-degree sponges, sandbags (large and small), a "bookend," and a Velcro band.
- Accomplish immobilization by rolling the child on the side and placing a small sponge or sandbag between the knees.
- Snugly wrap the Velcro band over the hips; to prevent backward arching, place the "bookend" against the child's back with the 45-degree sponge and sandbag positioned anteriorly (Fig. 27-39).

Practical tip: It is common for pediatric clinicians to request "two projections of the abdomen." The accompanying clinical information should support this request; if it does not, the radiographer should seek *clarification before proceeding*. Depending on the clinical reason for the radiographs, the two images may need to be supine and lateral. Abdominal images requested for infants in the NICU illustrate this point well. The neonatal patient with *necrotizing enterocolitis* requires supine and left lateral decubitus radiographs to rule out air-fluid levels indicative of bowel obstruction. However, the patient with an umbilical catheter needs supine and lateral images to verify the location and position of the catheter.

GASTROINTESTINAL AND GENITOURINARY PROCEDURES

In the interest of limiting radiation exposure to the GI and genitourinary systems, examinations are tailored to the individual patient. After a brief introduction, the radiographer should explain the procedure and check that the patient has undergone proper bowel preparation. The radiographer can then proceed with preparation (e.g., enema tip insertion) and immobilization of the patient.

Most procedures are performed by the radiologist. Exceptions include IVUs and, in some hospitals, voiding cystourethrograms (VCUGs). Notwithstanding, the radiographer has an integral role in the success of all examinations. Optimal hardcopy images require a thorough understanding of the equipment, its capabilities, and its limitations. Good patient care and organizational skills can also make the examination proceed more smoothly.

Immobilization for gastrointestinal procedures

As with other immobilization techniques, various beliefs exist regarding immobilization methods for the fluoroscopic portion of GI procedures; two methods are described. (The child may be immobilized for the "overhead" images as per the method outlined for the supine abdomen examination.)

Modified "bunny" method

The child's torso and legs are wrapped in a small blanket or towel and secured with a Velcro strip or tape. The arms are left free, raised above the head, and held by the parent (if present) (Fig. 27-40). The radiologist can then operate the carriage with one hand, holding the child's legs with the other to rotate the patient, thus obtaining the necessary coating of barium. This technique, thought by many to be more comfortable for the child, is often preferred by radiologists because small blankets are more readily available than the octagonal infant immobilization device. Success with this technique depends on someone (often a parent) assisting.

Conventional fluoroscopic suites, in contrast to remote suites, are often preferred for GI examinations on children younger than 5 years old. Infants and preschoolers often require hands-on assistance to achieve desired positions and ensure their safety. In addition, the scattered dose is easier to minimize in conventional suites (see Radiation Protection for Gastrointestinal Procedures).

Fig. 27-40 Another modification of the "bunny" technique. The arms are left free and are raised above the head to prevent superimposition over the esophagus. In this example, tape is used to secure the blanket; however, Velcro strips are easier to use if a parent is not available to assist. (Note lead under patient when tube is under the table.)

Octagonal infant immobilization method

The octagonal infant immobilization method, although effective, is less comfortable and appears more traumatic. However, with some creativity on the part of staff members, much of the child's fear can be averted by playing the "rocket ship game." The 3-year-old in Fig. 27-41 was told he would be dressed in a space suit (the hospital gown) and would go for a ride in the rocket ship.

By virtue of its construction, the octagonal immobilizer provides immobilization of the child in a variety of positions. As with the Pigg-o-stat, initial positioning of the child is a two-person process. The additional person does not have to be another radiographer; a well-instructed parent can assist. Because this technique immobilizes the head and arms, it is the method of choice when a parent is unable to provide assistance.

Radiation protection for gastrointestinal procedures

It is good practice to cover most of the tabletop of conventional fluoroscopic units with large mats of lead rubber (the equivalent of 0.5 mm of lead is recommended) (see Fig. 27-41). Effective protection for operators and patients can be achieved by positioning the mats so that only the areas being examined are exposed.

Voiding cystourethrogram for genitourinary procedures

A primary purpose of the VCUG is to assess vesicoureteral reflux (reflux from the bladder to the ureters). In addition, VCUG in males can identify and evaluate urethral strictures. Radiation protection for the fluoroscopic portion should be the same as outlined previously for GI examinations. The VCUG assesses bladder function and demonstrates ureteral and urethral anatomy.

Method

The patient is catheterized, a procedure that often requires two people—one to perform the catheterization and one to immobilize the legs in a frog leg position. The catheter is connected via tubing to a 500-mL bottle of contrast medium hung about 3 feet above the table. Under fluoroscopic guidance, contrast medium is dripped into the bladder until the bladder is full. Images are then taken while the patient is voiding to demonstrate reflux. This is often easier said than done! Preschoolers who have just been "toilet trained" and older children are often embarrassed. Techniques such as running tap water or pouring warm water over the genital area often encourage children to void.

Positioning

The female patient remains in the supine position, but the male patient must be placed in an oblique position during voiding to prevent the urethra from being superimposed over the pubic symphysis. After placing the male in an oblique position, the radiographer should take care to ensure the urethra is not superimposed over the femur.

Intravenous urogram for genitourinary procedures

Most pathologic conditions identified on an IVU or IVP can also be diagnosed with ultrasonography, a noninvasive, radiation-free examination. These advantages, combined with increased confidence on the part of urologists about ultrasound images and corresponding reports, are responsible for the dramatic decline in requests for IVUs. However, when IVUs are requested, most radiologists make a conscious effort to keep the number of exposures to a minimum; indeed, many examinations are completed with one preliminary radiograph and a late-stage filling radiography (between 5 and 15 minutes). Radiologists find it helpful to review previous radiographs at the time of the study so that the imaging sequence can be tailored to the patient, thereby keeping the radiation dose as low as possible.

Fig. 27-41 The octagonal immobilizer (or, for this child, a "rocket ship") permits the child to be immobilized in a variety of positions. (Note lead under patient when tube is under the table.)

Examinations Unique to the Pediatric Patient

BONE AGE

Children can arrive at the imaging department with either retarded skeletal development or advanced skeletal maturation. In either situation, the degree of skeletal maturation is determined by the appearance, size, and differentiation of various ossification centers. The most commonly used assessment technique, developed by Gruelich and Pyle,[1] compares an AP radiograph of the left hand and wrist with standards developed in the 1930s and 1940s and later revised. Although these standards recognize the differing degrees of skeletal maturation between males and females by using separate standards for each gender, their applications are limited. Variations can also occur as a result of genetic diversity, nutritional status, and race.

Radiologists evaluate the differentiation and degree of fusion between the epiphyses and shafts of the bones of the hand and wrist by comparing the patient's radiograph with the standards printed in the atlas to determine the best match. The Gruelich and Pyle method is considered extremely useful for most ages. Little change occurs in the ossification centers of the hand and wrist in the first 1 to 2 years of life, whereas the ossification of the knee and foot occurs rapidly during this time. Therefore bone age protocols for children 1 and 2 years old often include an AP radiograph of the left knee. Some department protocols specify that a knee radiograph be included for all children younger than the age of 2 years. In dedicated pediatric centers, others have found it more practical to specify that if, on reviewing the radiograph, the radiographer notes an apparent lack of ossification in the metacarpal epiphyses, the necessary radiograph of the left knee should then be obtained.

[1]Gruelich WW, Pyle SI: *Radiographic atlas of skeletal development of the hand and wrist*, ed 2, Stanford, Calif, 1959, Stanford University Press.

RADIOGRAPHY FOR SUSPECTED FOREIGN BODIES
Aspirated foreign body

A significant number of pediatric patients examined in emergency departments have a history that leads the physician to suspect a foreign body has been aspirated into the bronchial tree. This is a common cause of respiratory distress in children between the ages of 6 months and 3 years. In many cases the foreign body is nonopaque or radiolucent.

The foreign body, if slightly opaque and lodged in the *trachea,* may be demonstrated with filtered, high-kVp radiography of the *soft tissues of the neck.* From a radiologist's perspective, these images must be performed with the child's neck adequately extended and the shoulders lowered as much as possible. From the radiographer's perspective, this can be difficult to accomplish on the 6-month-old to 3-year-old. This challenge, however, is made easier with the use of the mc Infant Head and Neck Immobilizer (Fig. 27-42).

Method

The radiographer observes the following guidelines:

- Have the child be undressed from the waist up. Then position the child with the head in the contoured/cut-out portion, the neck over the raised portion, and the chest on the sloped portion of the immobility device (see Fig. 27-42).
- Lower and immobilize the shoulders using the provided towelette; then immobilize the head and upper thorax using the foam-lined Velcro strips. The neck extension helps keep the trachea from appearing buckled, and the towelette and foam-lined Velcro shoulder straps keep the shoulders from being superimposed on the airway.

The mc Infant Head and Neck Immobilizer is specially designed for radiography of the soft tissue of the neck. However, if the device is not available, the radiographer can improvise with a 45-degree sponge and some Velcro strips.

Fig. 27-42 The mc Infant Head and Neck Immobilizer provides the necessary extension of the neck for radiography of the soft tissues of the neck. The shoulders are kept low with the use of a towelette.

Aspirated foreign bodies are *more commonly lodged in the bronchial tree,* more often in the right side than in the left. Air becomes trapped on the affected side because the lodged foreign body acts as a ball valve, permitting air to enter on inspiration but preventing it from being exhaled on expiration. The result is a relatively normal-appearing inspiratory PA chest image but an abnormal appearance on the expiratory radiograph. Consequently the *routine* or *protocol* for chest examinations in patients with suspected aspirated foreign bodies should be an *inspiratory PA projection,* an *expiratory PA projection,* and a *lateral projection.* If satisfactory inspiration and expiration images cannot be obtained, bilateral lateral decubitus images should be obtained. (The unaffected lung will show that the heart has migrated toward the dependent lung. The affected dependent lung will remain fully inflated, preventing any downward migration of the heart.)

Ingested foreign body

Children frequently put objects in their mouths. If swallowed, these objects can cause obstruction or respiratory distress. Coins are the most commonly ingested foreign body, and, being radiopaque, they are easily identified. When ingested foreign body is known or suspected, the first imaging examination should be radiographs of the neck and chest or radiographs of the nasopharynx, chest, and abdomen.

Practical tip: In small children (approximately 1 year of age), this examination can be performed using a 35- × 43-cm (14- × 17-inch) IR (Fig. 27-43). The radiographer needs to understand that the foreign body may be lodged anywhere between the nasopharynx and the anal canal. The presence of a foreign body cannot be ruled out if these areas are not well demonstrated. Esophageal studies are often required to demonstrate nonopaque foreign bodies.

Because of the anatomy of the esophagus and trachea, a coin identified in the coronal plane at the level of the thoracic inlet generally is lodged in the esophagus, whereas a coin found along the sagittal plane is generally lodged in the trachea.

Fig. 27-43 A radiograph of the nasopharynx, chest, and abdomen is used to rule out the presence of a foreign body. If the coin that this child ingested had not been visible, a separate radiograph of the nasopharynx would have been obtained. Note that the diagonal placement of the gonadal shield over the distal pubic symphysis prevents the lower rectum from being obscured by lead.

SCOLIOSIS

Scoliosis has been defined as "the presence of one or more lateral-rotatory curvatures of the spine."[1] *Lateral* means toward the side, and *rotary* refers to the fact that the vertebral column rotates around its axis. Scoliosis can be a congenital or an acquired (e.g., posttrauma) condition. When physicians suspect scoliosis, radiographers evaluate for it using a PA or an AP projection (preferably PA projection for a significant radiation exposure dose reduction; see Volume 1, Chapter 8, scoliosis projections for references) on a 3-foot-long IR of the entire spine. If the physician believes that the curve has progressed to the point that further intervention is needed, a full scoliosis series is requested. The full scoliosis series should consist of 3-foot PA and lateral projections of the spine and probably right- and left-bending images (Fig. 27-44; see also Figs. 8-130 and 8-131). A PA chest radiograph is included when the series is requested preoperatively. The purpose of the bending images is to assess or predict the degree of correction that can be obtained. The follow-up radiographic examination usually includes upright PA and lateral images.

[1]Silverman FN, Kuhn UP: *Caffey's pediatric x-ray diagnosis—an integrated approach*, St Louis, 1993, Mosby.

The radiographer should observe the following guidelines for obtaining the easiest and potentially most accurate method of accomplishing the bending images:
- Place the patient in the supine position on the radiographic table.
- Ask the patient to bend sideways as if reaching for the knees.
- Ensure that the ASISs remain equidistant to the table as the patient bends.
- Collimation and centering are crucial because the resultant image must include the first "normal" shaped (i.e., non–wedge-shaped) cervical or thoracic vertebra down to the crests of the ilia (see Fig. 27-44). (Experience has shown that curve progression usually stops coincident with the fusing of the epiphyses of the iliac crests.)
- The geometric measurements determine the degree of curvature. The selected method of treatment is determined in part by the measurement of the angles outlined.

Radiation protection

Because scoliosis images are obtained relatively frequently to assess the progression of the curves, effective methods of radiation protection must be used:
- Obtain the 3-foot AP projection using breast shields (the AP is used as it allows for more stability of the patient, especially after surgery) (see Fig. 8-133); alternatively, position the patient for the PA projection, with very careful placement of breast shields.
- Ensure that lead is draped over the patient's right breast tissue for the AP left-bending image, and vice versa.
- Protect gonads by placing a small lead apron at the level of the ASIS.

Fig. 27-44 In planning corrective surgery, orthopedic surgeons generally observe the bending images as if looking at the patient's back. The structures to be demonstrated include the uppermost non–wedge-shaped vertebrae and the iliac crests.

Overview of Advanced Modalities

It is beyond the scope of this chapter to discuss *all* the imaging advances that have had a recent impact on pediatric imaging. The following sections highlight some advances that have had a direct impact on previously established protocols or routines in general radiography.

MAGNETIC RESONANCE IMAGING

MRI is perhaps the most dramatic and widespread technologic advancement in imaging. MRI quickly gained acceptance in the evaluation of most organ systems in the adult population. Its acceptance has been slower in pediatrics. This is somewhat ironic, considering that some of the advantages of MRI (enhanced contrast resolution, multiplanar capabilities, and lack of ionizing radiation) are crucial considerations in pediatric imaging.

The explanation for the slower acceptance of pediatric MRI lies in the length of an MRI examination. For example, a spinal MRI procedure may take from 60 to 90 minutes. During this time, a child is required to remain still in an enclosed tunnel, hearing a loud and constant "hammering" noise that can be rather frightening. In a large proportion of the pediatric population, heavy sedation is often required to be able to complete an MRI examination. Conscious sedation is sometimes inadequate because the child can wake up during the scan. General anesthesia, with its risks and potential complications, is therefore needed. This being the case, MRI in young children may be a very serious and potentially risky procedure. Consequently, the MRI staff needs enhanced skills to care properly for these patients. It is preferable if the direct patient care team includes pediatric anesthetists and nurses. In addition, just as the successful radiologist of the twenty-first century will probably need to be proficient at MRI, the radiographer must be similarly proficient at providing high-quality diagnostic MRI studies.

MRI is documented as the method of choice for evaluating such pediatric spinal cord abnormalities as *tethered cords, lipomyelomeningoceles, neoplasms, myelination,* and *congenital anomalies.* MRI has also proved advantageous to cardiologists and cardiac surgeons. Diagnoses previously suggested on chest radiographs are now confirmed for the cardiologist. Cardiac surgeons are better able to plan corrective surgeries because MRI scans demonstrate the sites and full extent of collateral vessels necessary for grafting procedures.

As experience with pediatric limb radiography increases, the radiographer can appreciate the difficulties the physician has in diagnosing certain types of fractures of the epiphyseal plates (Salter-Harris fractures). MRI can demonstrate, through cartilaginous structures, fractures that would otherwise be missed because these areas appear lucent on the standard radiograph. Elbow surgery can be less complex for the orthopedic surgeon who can first rule out additional Salter-Harris fractures with multiplanar MRI scans. These multiplanar images include coronal, axial, and sagittal images.

MYELOGRAPHY

In imaging departments where MRI is available, the popularity of myelography has been steadily decreasing. This is especially true in the adult population, but a relatively significant number of myelograms are still performed in pediatric centers. Neonatal patients, for example, sometimes develop a weakness in their upper limbs after traumatic births. If the neonate has been removed too aggressively during vaginal delivery, the nerves of the brachial plexus can be injured. Small tears may resolve of their own accord. Alternatively, they may worsen and require surgical repair. The diagnostic procedure of choice in this instance is a CT myelogram (see Chapter 24). After introducing a contrast medium into the subarachnoid space using a spinal needle, the radiographer performs a spinal CT scan. This scan shows any abnormal collections of contrast material where the nerve roots have been pulled. A cervical CT scan with special reconstructions in the sagittal, coronal, and oblique planes helps visualize this condition best.

COMPUTED TOMOGRAPHY

CT has become a routine diagnostic tool—one that more and more general radiographers are using. Pediatric patients present unique challenges, even to the seasoned CT technologist.

In the pediatric population, CT is useful in diagnosing congenital anomalies, assessing metastases, and diagnosing bone sarcomas and sinus disease; it has virtually replaced radiographic scanography. Young children have difficulty following the instructions needed for a diagnostic scan. Suggestions regarding approach and atmosphere are presented at the beginning of this chapter. Some basic technical tips are given here. As in the care of any pediatric patient, the role of the CT technologist is important in the success of the examination. The technologist must gain the respect and confidence of the young patient and the caregiver, if present.

The CT scanner itself is an impressive piece of equipment, one that needs careful explanation to help allay the patient's fears. One of the most significant fears is claustrophobia. Techniques to reduce claustrophobia include the use of a television/VCR/DVD player and music for entertainment (Fig. 27-45). Parent participation is often encouraged for the same reasons outlined previously in the chapter.

The advent of faster scanners and the introduction of volumetric scanning have significantly reduced scan times, thereby lessening patient anxiety. For example, a neck, chest, abdomen, and pelvic scan can now be completed in a few seconds. However, patient preparation, the injection of IV contrast material, and the computer processing of images can bring the total time of this examination to 10 to 15 minutes.

For young children, 10 to 15 minutes can be a long time, sometimes long enough to warrant the use of conscious sedation. Nursing staff then become actively involved in monitoring the sedated patient. The CT technologist should be comfortable with the use of oxygen-delivery systems, suction apparatus, and basic emergency management techniques. Generally speaking, if a reaction occurs in a pediatric patient, the symptoms could worsen significantly faster than in an adult. This underscores the need for the technologist to be well versed in the signs and symptoms of a potential reaction and the appropriate emergency response measures.

Emphasis should also be placed on mechanisms of dose reduction in CT. Examples include reducing the field of view (FOV) to allow precise collimation for the body part being examined and performing scans using technical parameters based on age and following dose-conscious protocols.

Technical advances in CT are bringing even faster systems. In fact, most CT scanners produced today can acquire "real-time" images. In practice, this should reduce the number of patients requiring sedation, making the procedure faster, safer, and less costly. In addition to increasing scan speed, CT manufacturers have worked hard to include dose-minimizing software features and user-friendly protocol programming options. If optimized and used to their maximum potential, these features make routine CT examinations easier.

CT has largely replaced conventional radiographic examinations done to assess leg length discrepancy (LLD). *Spot scanography,* one of the relatively common conventional methods, is a technique in which three exposures of the lower limbs (centered over the hips, knees, and ankles in turn) are made on a single 35- × 43-cm (14- × 17-inch) IR (see Chapter 11). A radiopaque rule is included for the

purpose of calculating the discrepancy on the resulting image.

Studies have shown that CT digital radiography is an accurate technique for measuring LLD. It is reproducible, and positioning and centering errors are less likely to occur. More importantly, studies also report radiation dose to be less than that for conventional techniques, leading researchers to recommend that the CT scout image–type option be used particularly in young patients having serial examinations. Technical details beyond the scope of this atlas are provided in texts cited in the bibliography at the end of this chapter.

Fig. 27-45 Right coronal CT positioning is best tolerated when the patient is distracted by a television positioned behind the gantry.

THREE-DIMENSIONAL IMAGING

In the pediatric population, 3D images reconstructed from CT or MRI data have revolutionized surgical procedures. This new technique allows clinicians (predominantly neurosurgeons, but also orthopedic and plastic surgeons) to manipulate 3D images of their patients interactively on a computer screen, rotating the image in any angle. Using this information, they can develop strategies that may change the complete treatment, management, or operative approach. 3D images are extremely useful, if not vital, in "mapping" a course of treatment for many corrective procedures for congenital malformations. Examples include craniofacial syndromes, congenital hip dysplasia, and conditions requiring plastic correction. 3D imaging also plays a major role in the management of cervical spine trauma and rotary subluxation of the spine in children.

INTERVENTIONAL RADIOLOGY

Image-guided, minimally invasive interventions have dramatically changed the role of the radiology department in both teaching and nonteaching hospitals and clinics. In the past, the justifications and rationales for radiology departments were diagnostic ones. However, radiology departments with professionally instructed interventional staff can now offer hospitals therapeutic services in addition to diagnostic services. This heightened awareness has largely resulted from the nature and efficacy of the interventional procedures.

These therapeutic interventions often obviate the need for surgery. Therapeutic procedures performed in the pediatric imaging department provide an attractive alternative to surgery for the patient, parent, hospital administrator, and society. (A procedure performed in the imaging department is much less expensive than one performed in the operating room.) These procedures are minimally invasive compared with their surgical counterparts, thereby reducing recovery times. Shortened length of stay translates into economic savings for the parents of pediatric patients.

Although these interventional procedures are predominantly performed in suites previously referred to as *specials* or *angiographic suites,* many procedures, especially nonvascular procedures, are performed in digital radiography and fluoroscopy suites. These diverse locations of care and the postprocedural care involved with vascular-interventional cases provide expanded avenues for general-duty radiographers to come in contact with patients. Interventional radiology holds a privileged position in many imaging departments. Nevertheless, a detailed, descriptive explanation of this role is beyond the scope of this text. (Detailed discussions appear in texts cited in the bibliography at the end of this chapter.)

Interventional radiology presents an alternative to pediatric surgery for angioplasty (balloon dilation), stent placement, embolization, vascular access device insertion, and numerous other procedures. *Angioplasty* refers to the placement of a balloon-tipped catheter in the center of a narrowed vessel; the balloon is inflated and deflated several times to stretch or dilate the narrowed segment. *Embolization* refers to the occlusion of small feeder vessels with either tiny coils or specially formulated glue. This procedure is performed to cut off the blood supply to a tumor.

For simplicity, interventional radiology can be divided into vascular and nonvascular procedures. Vascular procedures are generally performed in angiographic suites. During these therapeutic interventions, angiography and ultrasonography are also performed for diagnostic and guidance purposes. Angiography can be arterial or venous; pediatric vasculature is well suited to both. IV injection is favored in infants because their relatively small blood volume and rapid circulation allow for good vascular images to be obtained after the injection of contrast material into a peripheral vein. In infants, hand injections are often preferred over power injections to help avoid extravasation. Intraarterial digital subtraction angiography (DSA) (see Chapter 25) has become a valuable tool for imaging professionals. DSA is performed using diluted contrast medium, which can reduce pain, and it provides a useful "road mapping" tool. Road mapping, a software tool available on newer angiographic equipment, uses the intraarterial injection to provide a fluoroscopic display of arterial anatomy—a very useful tool for imaging tortuous vessels.

Vascular-interventional procedures can be neurologic, cardiac, or systemic in nature. Nonvascular procedures often involve the digestive and urinary systems. Examples include the insertion of gastrostomy tubes to supplement the nutrition of pediatric patients and insertion of cecostomy tubes in chronically constipated patients with spina bifida. The following paragraphs focus on the vascular side of interventional radiology, more specifically the insertion of vascular access devices.

The reason for this is simple: given the number of chest radiographs ordered for pediatric patients, radiographers will far more frequently encounter patients with these devices.

Simply stated, vascular access devices are of three types: nontunneled, tunneled, and implanted. The selection of device is often determined by a combination of factors, including the purpose of the access and proposed indwelling time. Furthermore, the physician or patient may choose a particular device in the interests of compliance or after assessing underlying clinical considerations.

Nontunneled catheters are commonly referred to as *peripherally inserted central catheters*, or *PICC lines*. They are available with single or multiple lumens. The insertion point is usually the basilic or cephalic vein, at or above the antecubital space of the nondominant arm. Multiple lumens are desirable when a variety of different medications (including total parenteral nutrition) are to be administered (Fig. 27-46). These devices must be strongly anchored to the skin because children often pull on and displace the catheters, resulting in damage to the line and potential risk to themselves. To render the catheters more secure, pediatric clinicians often tailor their insertion and anchoring techniques to help prevent the catheter from being pulled out by the patient.

As with PICC lines, tunneled catheters can have multiple lumens. However, unlike PICC lines, they are not inserted into the peripheral circulation; rather, they are inserted via a subcutaneous tunnel into the subclavian or internal jugular veins. The tunneling acts as an anchoring mechanism for the catheter to facilitate long-term placement (Fig. 27-47). Tunneled catheters are used for the administration of chemotherapy, antibiotics, and fluids; they are also used for hemodialysis. (Technologists may see or hear these referred to as *Hickman lines*, a term that has been generalized to include tunneled catheters placed in subclavian or internal jugular veins.)

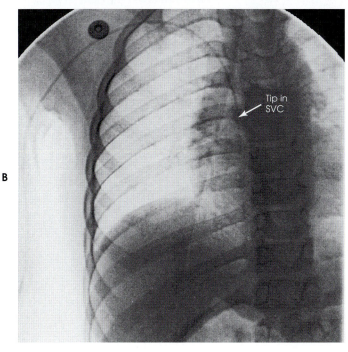

Tip in SVC

Fig. 27-46 **A,** Postinsertion image of a double-lumen PICC line in a 7-year-old boy (shown in the interventional suite). Conscious sedation was used for this procedure. **B,** Digital image of PICC line demonstrating the distal tip of the catheter positioned in the superior vena cava (*SVC*).

Fig. 27-47 External appearance of tunneled, double-lumen central venous access device. These catheters are used for long-term therapy. Their short track to the heart can increase the risk of infection, necessitating proper care for maintenance.

Implanted devices are often referred to as *ports*. These are titanium or polysulfone devices with silicone centers, and they are attached to catheters. The whole device is implanted subcutaneously with the distal end of the catheter tip further implanted, often into the superior vena cava or right atrium. A port is the device of choice for noncompliant children or adults who, for aesthetic purposes, would rather not have the limb of a catheter protruding from their chest (Fig. 27-48).

In summary, vascular access devices have dramatically changed the course of treatment for many patients in a positive way. Patients who would have previously been hospitalized for antibiotic therapy can now go home with the device in place and resume normal activity. This is good news. The increased prevalence of these devices means that patients with vascular access devices are in the community and visiting radiology departments everywhere. Therefore the need has grown for increased education for patients and those who come in contact with them. PICC lines have a smaller likelihood of introducing catheter-related infections; tunneled lines present a greater risk.

Radiographers must recognize vascular access devices and treat them with utmost care. They should report dislodged bandages and sites showing signs of infection (i.e., redness, exudate) *immediately.* Catheter-related infections compound recovery courses, sometimes in life-threatening ways. They cost hospitals many thousands of dollars each year.

Postprocedural care currently represents a significant and ongoing challenge for all personnel who treat, manage, and come in contact with patients who have vascular access devices. To date, this challenge has not been adequately addressed. *With whom does the responsibility of postprocedural care rest?* It is the responsibility of all these personnel.

NUCLEAR MEDICINE

If bladder function is the *only* concern for the physician who requests a VCUG, a nuclear medicine *direct radionuclide cystogram* (DRC) can be performed. The DRC emphasizes the assessment of bladder function. Radiographers should recognize that *nuclear medicine studies assess function rather than demonstrate anatomy.* The DRC permits observation of reflux during imaging over a longer period. In addition, it allows for accurate quantification of postvoiding residual volume. The radiation dose to the patient is less with this procedure than with the VCUG, making it an attractive option for the pediatric patient. (Technical details on nuclear medicine are presented in texts cited in the selected bibliography at the end of this chapter.)

Fig. 27-48 Digital image of port *(arrow).* Ports are vascular devices that must be accessed subcutaneously. They are preferred for active children and for aesthetic reasons.

Conclusion

Although no one can prevent a child from experiencing the fear engendered by a visit to the hospital, much can be done to allay that fear. Questions from children such as "Am I going to have a needle?" require a truthful response. However, the manner in which the response is delivered can make a tremendous difference. Children are impressionable and dependent on their caregivers, but they are also often the best teachers radiographers can have. Radiographers should watch and listen to these small patients, observe their body language and facial expressions, and note their questions and reactions for cues regarding ways to respond to them. The rewards—a child's smile and trust—are given more frequently than might be expected.

Acknowledgment

The authors wish to acknowledge the contributions of GE Medical Systems Canada, Mississauga, Ontario, and Cook (Canada), Inc., Stouffville, Ontario, which made the color illustration portion of this chapter possible.

Dedication

To the many children who have passed through the doors of the Hospital for Sick Children, and to those who will come in the future.

Selected bibliography

Aitken AGF et al: Leg length determination by CT digital radiography, *AJR* 144:613, 1985.

Dietrich RB: *The Raven MRI teaching file, pediatric MRI,* New York, 1991, Raven Press.

Duck S: Neonatal intravenous therapy, *J Intravenous Nurs* 20:366, 1997.

Godderidge C: *Pediatric imaging,* Philadelphia, 1995, Saunders.

Green RE, Oestman JW: *Computed digital radiography in clinical practice,* New York, 1992, Thieme.

Gruelich WW, Pyle SI: *Radiographic atlas of skeletal development of the hand and wrist,* ed 2, Stanford, Calif, 1959, Stanford University Press.

Harris VJ et al, editors: *Radiographic atlas of child abuse,* New York, 1996, Igaku-Shoin Medical.

Jones D, Gleason CA, Lipstein SU: *Hospital care of the recovering NICU infant,* Baltimore, 1991, Williams & Wilkins.

Kleinman PK: *Diagnostic imaging of child abuse,* Baltimore, 1987, Williams & Wilkins.

Maynar M et al: Vascular interventional procedures in the pediatric age group. In Casteneda-Zunigo WR, editor: *Interventional radiology,* Baltimore, 1992, Williams & Wilkins.

Milne DA et al: *Hospital for Sick Children diagnostic imaging—procedure manual,* Toronto, 1993, Hospital for Sick Children.

Reed ME: *Pediatric skeletal radiology,* Baltimore, 1992, Williams & Wilkins.

Robinson MJ: *Practical pediatrics,* ed 2, New York, 1990, Churchill Livingstone.

Silverman FN, Kuhn UP: *Caffey's pediatric x-ray diagnosis—an integrated imaging approach,* St Louis, 1993, Mosby.

Torres LS: *Basic medical techniques and patient care for radiologic technologists,* ed 5, Philadelphia, 1997, Lippincott.

Wilmot DM, Sharko GA: *Pediatric imaging for the technologist,* New York, 1987, Springer-Verlag.

28

GERIATRIC RADIOGRAPHY

SANDRA J. NAUMAN

Lateral chest radiograph on a
73-year-old with kyphosis and
compression fractures of T11
and T12.

Geriatrics is the branch of medicine dealing with the aged and the problems of the aging. The field of gerontology includes illness prevention and management, health maintenance, and promotion of quality of life for the aged. The ongoing increase in the numbers of elderly persons older than age 65 in the U.S. population is well known. An even more dramatic aging trend exists among those older than 85 years of age. The number of people aged 100 is approximately 100,000 and increasing. Every aspect of the health care delivery system is affected by this shift in the general population. The 1993 Pew Health Commission Report noted that "aging of the nation's society and the accompanying shift to chronic care that is occurring foretell major shifts in care needs in which allied health professionals are major providers of services." As members of the allied health professions, radiographers are an important component of the health care system. As the geriatric population increases, so does the number of medical imaging procedures performed on the elderly. Students and practitioners must be prepared to meet the challenges that this dramatic shift in patient population represents. An understanding of geriatrics will foster a positive interaction between the radiographer and the elderly patient.

A Special Population
DEMOGRAPHICS AND SOCIAL EFFECTS OF AGING

The acceleration of the "gray" American population began when those individuals born between 1946 and 1964 (known as the "baby boomers") began to turn age 50 in 1996. The number in the age 65 and older cohort is expected to reach 70.2 million by 2030 (Fig. 28-1). The U.S. experience regarding the increase in the elderly population is not unique; it is a global one. As of 1990, 28 countries had more than 2 million persons older than 65 and 12 additional countries had more than 5 million people. The entire elder population of the world has begun a predicted dramatic increase for the period from 1995 to 2030.

Research on a wide variety of topics ranging from family aspects of aging, economic resources, and the delivery of long-term care states that gender, race, ethnicity, and social class have consistently influenced the quality of the experience of aging. The experience of aging results from interaction of physical, mental, social, and cultural factors. Aging varies across cultures. Culturally, aging, as well as the treatment of the elderly, is often determined by the values of an ethnic group. Culture also may determine the way the older person views the process of aging, as well as the manner in which he or she adapts to growing older. A more heterogeneous elderly population than any generation that preceded it can be expected. This is a result of both increasing immigration from non-Caucasian countries and a lower fertility/reproductive rate among the Caucasian population. This group will contain a mix of cultural and ethnic backgrounds. The United States is a multicultural society in which a generalized view of aging in America would be difficult. *Health care professionals will need to know not only diseases and disorders common to a specific age group but those common to a particular ethnic group as well.* An appreciation of diverse backgrounds can help the health care professional provide a personal approach when dealing with and meeting the needs of elderly patients. Many universities are incorporating cultural diversity into their curriculum.

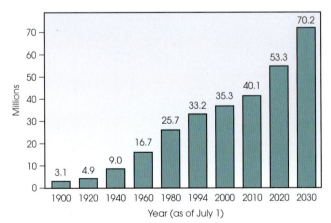

Fig. 28-1 Number of persons older than 65 years in millions; 1900 to 2030.

(Reprinted from U.S. Department of Commerce, Economics and Statistics Administration: *65+ in the United States,* Washington, DC, 1996, U.S. Bureau of the Census.)

The *economic status* of the elderly is varied and has an important influence on their health and well-being (Fig. 28-2). The majority of older people have an adequate income, but a substantial number of minority patients do not. Single elders are more likely to be below the poverty line. Economic hardships increase for single elders, especially women. Sixty percent of the population older than age 85 is women, making them twice as likely as men to be poor. By age 75, nearly two thirds of women are widows. Financial security is extremely important to an elderly person. Many elderly people are reluctant to spend money on what others may consider necessary for their well-being. A problem facing the American aging society is health care finances. Individuals in this situation will often base decisions regarding their care not on their needs but exclusively on the cost of those services. (An increase in health care and the aging population go hand in hand.) Heart disease, cancer, and stroke account for 7 of every 10 deaths among people older than 65. By the year 2025, an estimated two thirds of the U.S. health care budget will be devoted to services for the elderly.

Fig. 28-2 The economic status of the elderly is varied and an important influence on their health and well being.

Aging is a broad concept that includes physical changes in people's bodies over adult life, psychologic changes in their minds and mental capacities, social psychologic changes in what they think and believe, and social changes in how they are viewed, what they expect, and what is expected of them. Aging is a constantly evolving concept. Notions that biologic age is more critical than chronologic age when determining health status of the elderly are valid. Aging is an individual and extremely variable process. The functional capacity of major body organs varies with advancing age. As one grows older, environmental and lifestyle factors affect the age-related functional changes in the body organs. Advancements in medical technology have extended the average life expectancy in the United States by nearly 20 years over the past half-century, which has allowed senior citizens to be actively involved in every aspect of American society. People are healthier longer today because of advanced technology; the results of health promotion and secondary disease prevention; and lifestyle factors, such as diet, exercise, and smoking cessation, which have been effective in reducing the risk of disease (Fig. 28-3).

The majority of the elderly seen in the health care setting have been diagnosed with at least one chronic condition. Individuals who in the 1970s would not have survived a debilitating illness, such as cancer or a catastrophic health event like a heart attack, can now live for more extended periods of time, sometimes with a variety of concurrent debilitating conditions. Although age is the most consistent and strongest predictor of risk for cancer and for death from cancer, management of the elderly cancer patient becomes complex because other chronic conditions, such as osteoarthritis, diabetes, chronic obstructive pulmonary disease (COPD), and heart disease, must also be considered in their care. Box 28-1 lists the top 10 chronic conditions for people older than 65.

The attitudes of health care providers toward older adults affect their health care. Unfortunately, research indicates that health care professionals are significantly more negative in their attitudes toward older patients than younger ones. This attitude must change if the health care provider is to have a positive interaction with the elderly patient. These attitudes appear to be related to the pervasive stereotyping of the elderly, which serves to justify avoiding care and contact with them, as well as being reminders of our own mortality. *Ageism* is a term used to describe the stereotyping of and discrimination against elderly persons and is considered to be similar to that of racism and sexism. It emphasizes that frequently the elderly are perceived to be repulsive and that a distaste for the aging process itself exists. Ageism suggests that the majority of elderly are senile, miserable most of the time, and dependent rather than independent individuals. The media have also influenced ongoing stereotypical notions about the elderly. Commercials target the elderly as consumers of laxatives, wrinkle creams, and other products that promise to prolong their condition of being younger, more attractive, and desirable. Television sitcoms portray the elderly as stubborn and eccentric. Health care providers must learn to appreciate the positive aspects of aging so that they can assist the elderly in having a positive experience with their imaging procedure.

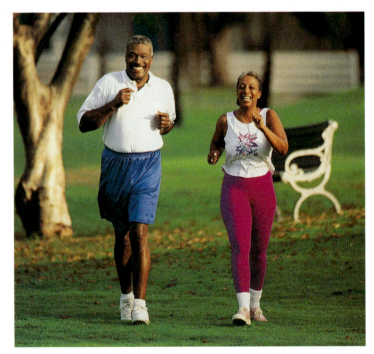

Fig. 28-3 Lifestyle factors, such as diet, exercise, and smoking cessation, reduce the risk of disease and increase life span.

BOX 28-1

Top 10 chronic conditions of people older than 65 years

Arthritis
Hypertension
Hearing impairment
Heart disease
Cataracts
Deformity or orthopedic impairment
Chronic sinusitis
Diabetes
Visual impairment
Varicose veins

A 1995 study by Rarey concluded that a large majority of the 835 radiographers surveyed in California were not well informed about gerontologic issues and were not prepared to meet the needs of their patients older than age 65.[1] Reuters Health reported from a Johns Hopkins study that medical students generally have poor knowledge and understanding of the elderly, and this translates to an inferior quality of care for older patients. More education in gerontology is necessary for radiographers and even physicians. Education will enable them to adapt imaging and therapeutic procedures to accommodate mental, emotional, and physiologic alterations associated with aging and to be sensitive to cultural, economic, and social influences in the provision of care for the elderly.

Physical, Cognitive, and Psychosocial Effects of Aging

The human body undergoes a multiplicity of physiologic changes second by second.

Little consideration is given regarding these changes unless they are brought on by sudden physical, psychologic, or cognitive events. Radiographers must remember that each elderly person they encounter is a unique individual with distinct characteristics. These individuals have experienced a life filled with memories and accomplishments.

Young or old, the definition of quality of life is an individual and personal one. Research has shown that health status is an excellent predictor of happiness. Greater social contact, health satisfaction, low vulnerable personality traits, and fewer stressful life events have been linked to successful aging. *Self-efficacy* can be defined as the level of control one has over one's future. Many elderly people feel they have no control over medical emergencies and fixed incomes. Many have fewer choices about their personal living arrangements. These environmental factors can lead to depression and decreased self-efficacy. An increase in illness will usually parallel a decrease in self-efficacy.

The elderly may experience changing roles from a life of independence to dependence. The family role of an adult caring for children and grandchildren may evolve into the children caring for their aging parents. It is also a time of loss. Losses may include the death of a spouse and friends, as well as loss of income due to retirement. The loss of health may be the reason for the health care visit. The overall loss of control may lead to isolation and depression in the elderly. Death and dying is also an imminent fact of life.

A positive attitude is an important aspect of aging. Many older people have the same negative stereotypes about aging that young people do.[1] For them, feeling "down" and depressed becomes a common consequence of aging. One of five people older than age 65 in a community will show signs of clinical depression. Yet health care professionals know that depression can affect both young and old. In general, research has shown the majority of elderly people rate their health status as good to excellent. How elderly persons perceive their health status depends largely on their successful adaptation to disabilities. Radiographers need to be sensitive to the fact that an elderly person may have had to deal with a number of losses, both social and physical, in a short period of time. More importantly, they must recognize symptoms resulting from these losses in order to communicate and interact effectively with this patient population.

Although as a health care provider the radiographer's contribution to a patient's quality of life may be minimal, it is not insignificant. The radiographer must remember that each elderly person is unique and deserves respect for his or her own opinions.

---

[1]Rowe JW, Kahn RL: *Successful aging,* New York, 1998, Dell.

---

[1]Rarey LK: Radiologic technologists' responses to elderly patients, *Radiol Tech* 69:566, 1996.

The aging process alone does not likely alter the essential core of the human being. Physical illness is not aging, and age-related changes in the body are often modest in magnitude. As one ages, the tendencies to prefer slower-paced activities, take longer to learn new tasks, become more forgetful, and lose portions of sensory processing skills increase slowly but perceptibly. Health care professionals need to be reminded that *aging and disease are not synonymous.* The more closely a function is tied to physical capabilities, the more likely it is to decline with age, whereas the closer a function depends on experience, the more likely it will increase with age. Box 28-2 lists the most common health complaints of the elderly.

Joint stiffness, weight gain, fatigue, and loss of bone mass can be slowed through proper nutritional interventions and low-impact exercise. The importance of exercise cannot be overstated. Exercise has been shown to increase aerobic capacity and mental speed. Exercise programs designed for the elderly should emphasize increased strength, flexibility, and endurance. One of the best predictors of good health in later years is the number and extent of healthy lifestyles that were established in earlier life.

The elderly person may show decreases in attention skills during complex tasks. Balance, coordination, strength, and reaction time all decrease with age. Falls associated with balance problems are common in the elderly population, resulting in a need to concentrate on walking. *Not overwhelming them with instructions is helpful.* Their hesitation to follow instructions may be a fear instilled from a previous fall. Sight, hearing, taste, and smell are all sensory modalities that decline with age. Older people have more difficulty with bright lights and tuning out background noise. Many elderly people become adept at lip reading to compensate for loss of hearing. For radiographers to assume that all elderly patients are hard of hearing is not unusual; they are not. Talking in a normal tone, while making volume adjustments only if necessary, is a good rule of thumb. Speaking slowly, directly, and distinctly when giving instructions allows older adults an opportunity to sort through directions and improves their ability to follow them with better accuracy (Fig. 28-4).

Cognitive impairment in the elderly can be caused by disease, aging, and disuse. *Dementia* is defined as progressive cognitive impairment that eventually interferes with daily functioning. It includes cognitive, psychologic, and functional deficits including memory impairment. With normal aging comes a slowing down and a gradual wearing out of bodily systems, but it does not include dementia. Yet the prevalence of dementia increases with age. Persistent disturbances in cognitive functioning, including memory and intellectual ability, accompany dementia. *Fears of cognitive loss, especially Alzheimer's disease, are widespread among older people.* Alzheimer's disease is the most common form of dementia. Therefore health care professionals are more likely to encounter people with this type. The majority of elderly people work at maintaining and keeping their mental functions by staying active through mental games and exercises and keeping engaged in regular conversation. When caring for patients with any degree of dementia, verbal conversation should be inclusive and respectful. One should never discuss these patients as though they are not in the room or are not active participants in the procedure.

BOX 28-2

Most common health complaints of the elderly

Weight gain
Fatigue
Loss of bone mass
Joint stiffness
Loneliness

Fig. 28-4 Speaking slowly, directly, and distinctly when giving instructions allows older adults an opportunity to sort through directions and improves their ability to follow them with better accuracy.

One of the first questions asked of any patient entering a health care facility for emergency service is, "Do you know where you are and what day it is?" The health care providers need to know just how alert the patient is. Although memory does decline with age, this is experienced mostly with short-term memory tasks. Long-term memory or subconscious memory tasks show little change over time and with increasing age. There can be a variety of reasons for confusion or disorientation. Medication, psychiatric disturbance, or retirement can confuse the patient. For some older people, retirement means creating a new set of routines and adjusting to them. The majority of elders like structure in their lives and have familiar routines for approaching each day.

Physiology of Aging

Health and well-being depend largely on the degree to which organ systems can successfully work together to maintain internal stability. With age, there is apparently a gradual impairment of these homeostatic mechanisms. Elderly people experience nonuniform, gradual, ongoing organ function failure in all systems. Many of the body organs gradually lose strength with advancing age. These changes place the elderly at risk for disease or dysfunction, especially in the presence of stress. At some point the likelihood of illness, disease, and death increases. Various physical diseases and disorders affect both the mental and physical health of people of all ages. They are more profound among elderly people because diseases and disorders among older people are more likely to be chronic in nature. *Although aging is inevitable, the aging experience is highly individual and is affected by heredity, lifestyle choices, physical health, and attitude.* A great portion of usual aging risks can be modified with positive shifts in lifestyle.

AGING OF THE ORGAN SYSTEMS
Integumentary system disorders
The integumentary system is one of the first apparent signs of aging. The most common skin diseases among the elderly are herpes zoster (shingles), malignant tumors, and decubitus ulcers. With age comes flattening of the skin membranes, making it vulnerable to abrasions and blisters. The number of melanocytes decreases, making ultraviolet light more dangerous, and the susceptibility to skin cancer increases. Wrinkling and thinning skin are noticeable among the elderly. This is attributable to decreases in collagen and elastin in the dermis. A gradual loss of functioning sweat glands and skin receptors occurs, which increases the threshold for pain stimuli, making the elderly person vulnerable to heat strokes. With age comes atrophy or thinning of the subcutaneous layer of skin in the face, back of the hands, and soles of the feet. Loss of this "fat pad" can cause many foot conditions in the elderly. The most striking age-related changes to the integumentary system are the graying, thinning, and loss of hair. With age, the number of hair follicles decreases and those follicles that remain grow at a slower rate with less concentration of melanin, causing the hair to become thin and white. A major problem with aging skin is chronic exposure to sunlight. The benefits of protecting one's skin with sunscreen and protective clothing cannot be overemphasized and will be more evident as one grows older. The three most common skin tumors in the elderly are basal cell carcinoma, malignant melanoma, and squamous cell carcinoma.

Nervous system disorders
The nervous system is the principle regulatory system of all other systems in the body. It is probably the least understood of all body systems. Central nervous system disorders are one of the most common causes of disability in the elderly, accounting for almost 50% of disability in those older than age 65. Loss of myelin in axons in some of the nervous system contributes to the decrease in nerve impulse velocity that is noted in aging. Like any other organ system, the nervous system is vulnerable to the effects of atherosclerosis with advancing age. When blood flow to the brain is blocked, brain tissue is damaged. Repeated episodes of cerebral infarction can eventually lead to multiinfarct dementia. Changes in the blood flow and oxygenation to the brain slow down the time to carry out motor and sensory tasks requiring speed, coordination, balance, and fine motor hand movements. This decrease in the function of motor control puts the elderly person at a higher risk for falls. Healthy changes in lifestyles can reduce the risk of disease. High blood pressure, for example, is a noted risk and can be decreased with medication, weight loss, proper nutritional diet, and exercise.

Sensory system disorders
All of the sensory systems undergo changes with age. Beginning around the age of 40, the ability to focus on near objects becomes increasingly difficult. The lens of the eye becomes less pliable; starts to yellow; and becomes cloudy, resulting in farsightedness (presbyopia). Distorted color perception and cataracts also begin. Changes in the retina affect the ability to adapt to changes in lighting, and there are decreased abilities to tolerate glare, making night vision more difficult for the elderly.

Hearing impairment is common in the elderly. The gradual progressive hearing loss of tone discrimination is called *presbycusis*. Men are affected more often than are women and the degree of loss is more severe for high-frequency sounds. Speech discrimination is problematic when in noisy surroundings, such as a room full of talking people.

There is a decline in sensitivity to taste and smell with age. The decline in taste is consistent with a decreased number of taste buds on the tongue, decreased saliva, and dry mouth that accompany the aging process. Hyposmia, the impairment of the ability to smell, accounts for much of the decreased appetite and irregular eating habits that are noted consistently in the elderly. Similar to taste, the degree of impairment varies with a particular odor, and the ability to identify odors in a mixture is gradually lost with age.

Musculoskeletal system disorders

Musculoskeletal dysfunction is the major cause of disability in the elderly. Osteoporosis, the reduction in bone mass and density, is one of the most significant age-related changes. Women are four times as likely as men to develop this disease. Risk factors for osteoporosis include estrogen depletion, calcium deficiency, physical inactivity, testosterone depletion, alcoholism, and cigarette smoking. The rate of new bone resorption surpasses the rate of new bone formation at approximately age 40. This accounts for a subsequent loss of 40% bone mass in women and 30% bone mass in men over the course of the life span. Osteoporosis is associated with an increased risk of fractures. Common fracture sites are the vertebral bodies, distal radius, femoral neck, ribs, and pubis. Changes in the shape of the vertebral bodies can indicate the degree and severity of osteoporosis. Advanced cases may demonstrate complete compression fractures of the vertebral bodies. Compression fractures can result in severe kyphosis of the thoracic spine (Fig. 28-5).

The incidence of degenerative joint disease, osteoarthritis, increases with age. Osteoarthritis is the chronic deterioration of the joint cartilage, and therefore the weight-bearing joints are the most commonly affected. Obesity is probably the most important single risk factor. Osteoarthritis of the joint cartilage causes pain, swelling, and a decrease in range of motion in the affected joint. Osteoarthritis is the second most common cause of disability in the United States, affecting more than 50 million Americans. At age 40, most adults have osteoarthritic changes visible on radiographic images of the cervical spine. The most progressive changes occur in weight-bearing joints and hands as age increases (Fig. 28-6).

Total joint replacement or arthroplasty procedures are common among elderly patients. Joint replacement may offer pain relief and improve joint mobility. Joint replacements can be performed on any joint including the hip, knee, ankle, foot, shoulder, elbow, wrist, and fingers. Hip and knee replacements are the most common, as well as the most effective (Fig. 28-7).

With age, women are more likely to store fat in their hips and thighs, whereas men store fat in their abdomen area. Without exercise, muscle mass declines, resulting in decreased strength and endurance, prolonged reaction time, and disturbed coordination. It cannot be overemphasized that regular physical training can improve muscle strength and endurance, along with cardiovascular fitness, even in the oldest population.

Cardiovascular system disorders

The cardiovascular system circulates the blood, which delivers oxygen and nutrients to all parts of the body and removes waste products. Therefore damage to this system can have negative implications for the entire body. Decreased blood flow to the digestive tract, liver, and kidneys affects the absorption, distribution, and elimination of substances, such as medications and alcohol.

Cardiovascular disease is the most common cause of death worldwide. The maximum heart rate during exercise decreases with age; thus the elderly become short

Fig. 28-5 Lateral chest radiograph on a 73-year-old with kyphosis and compression fractures of T11 and T12.

Fig. 28-6 Lateral knee radiograph showing severe arthritis.

of breath and tire quickly. Loss of arterial elasticity results in increased systolic blood pressure, increasing the risk for heart disease and stroke. Another prevalent problem is postural hypertension in which there is a fall in systemic blood pressure when rising from a supine to standing position. The predominant change that occurs in the blood vessels with age is atherosclerosis, a development of fatty plaques in the walls of the arteries. These fatty plaques within the artery wall can lead to ulcerations of the artery wall, subsequently making the artery prone to the formation of blood clots. The plaques also cause destruction of the artery wall, causing it to balloon, increasing the risk of an aneurysm. Complications can lead to an embolism, heart attack, or stroke.

Congestive heart failure (CHF) is due to an inability of the heart to propel blood at a sufficient rate and volume. This pathology is more common in elderly people, particularly in the age range of 75 to 85 years. People who are most at risk for developing CHF include those who have been diagnosed with coronary artery disease, heart attack, cardiomyopathy, untreated hypertension, and chronic kidney disease. Radiographically, the heart is enlarged and the hilar region of the lungs is congested with increased vascular markings. Exposure factors must be adjusted to visualize the heart borders despite the pulmonary edema.

Preventive health measures, such as control of high blood pressure, diet, exercise, and smoking cessation, decrease the risk of cardiovascular disease. These interventions are more effective if initiated early in life.

Gastrointestinal system disorders

Gastrointestinal disorders in the elderly can include malignancies, peptic ulcer disease, gastrointestinal bleeding, pancreatitis, difficulty swallowing, diverticulitis, gastric outlet obstruction, esophageal foreign bodies, constipation, and fecal incontinence. Mouth and teeth pain, side effects of medication, decreased saliva, and dry mouth can lead to nutritional deficiencies, malnutrition, and dehydration problems. The majority of gastrointestinal disorders are related to an age-related decrease in the rate of gastric acid production and secretions, as well as decreased motility of the smooth muscle in the large intestine. A decrease in acid production and secretion can lead to iron-deficiency anemia, peptic ulcers, and gastritis. Diverticulosis, a common problem in the elderly, develops when the large intestine herniates through the muscle wall (Fig. 28-8). Gallstone disease, hepatitis, and dehydration tend to be more common in the older population. Healthy lifestyle habits, such as smoking cessation, low alcohol intake, high fiber–low sugar diet, and regular exercise can decrease the risk of gastrointestinal problems. Gastrointestinal malignancies are second only to lung cancer as a cause of cancer mortality. The secret to survival for colon and rectal cancer lies in inexpensive early detection. Stool samples and rectal examinations are effective in detecting early cancer.

Fig. 28-7 AP proximal femur radiograph showing a "total hip" arthroplasty procedure.

Fig. 28-8 AP abdomen radiograph on an elderly patient demonstrating diverticulitis.

Immune system decline

Age takes its toll on the immune system. To be immune to an infection implies protection from that infection. The ability of one's body to remain free of infections requires the immune system to distinguish healthy cells from invading microorganisms or altered cancer cells. The age-related decline of the immune system functioning makes the elderly more vulnerable to diabetes mellitus, pneumonia, and nosocomial infections. The incidence of infectious disease rises in adulthood. Prevalent among the aged are influenza, pneumonia, tuberculosis, meningitis, and urinary tract infections. The three general categories of illness that preferentially afflict the elderly are infections, cancer, and autoimmune disease.[1]

[1]Chop WC, Robnett RH: *Gerontology for the health care professional,* Philadelphia, 1999, FA Davis.

Respiratory system disorders

Throughout the aging process the lungs lose some of their elastic recoil, trapping air in the alveoli. This decreases the rate of oxygen entering the bloodstream and the elimination of carbon dioxide. The muscles involved in breathing become a little more rigid, which can account for shortness of breath with physical stress. In the wall of the thorax the rib cage stiffens, causing kyphotic curvature of the thoracic spine. Respiratory diseases that increase in frequency with aging include emphysema, chronic bronchitis, pneumonia, and lung cancer.

Chronic obstructive pulmonary disease (COPD) refers to a variety of breathing disorders that cause a decreased ability of the lungs to perform their ventilation. Emphysema is the permanent destruction and distention of the alveoli. Cigarette smoking remains the most significant risk factor in the development of emphysema and is also the leading cause of chronic bronchitis. Chronic bronchitis is an inflammation of the mucous membrane of the bronchial tubes. These two conditions are considered irreversible. Chest radiographs may demonstrate hyperinflation of the lungs (Fig. 28-9).

Pneumonia is the most frequent type of lung infection and among the leading causes of death in the elderly. This population is also at an increased risk for aspiration pneumonia due to slower swallowing reflexes and other health conditions. Radiographically, pneumonia may appear as soft, patchy alveolar infiltrates or pulmonary densities (Fig. 28-10).

Lung cancer is the second most common cancer and the most common cause of cancer-related death in both men and women. In fact, more Americans die each year from lung cancer than from breast, prostate, and colorectal cancers combined.

There is a strong association between low lung function and the future development of coronary heart disease. Research has shown that the total amount of air inhaled in one's deepest breath and the fastest rate at which one can exhale are powerful predictors of how many more years one will live. Sedentary lifestyle is the greatest risk factor in lung function, and lifestyle habits are the critical factors over which one has control.

Fig. 28-9 PA chest radiograph demonstrating emphysema.

Fig. 28-10 PA chest radiograph with right middle lobe pneumonia and accompanying abscess.

Hematologic system disorders

A major hematologic concern in the elderly is the high prevalence of anemia. Individuals with anemia often have pale skin and shortness of breath, and they fatigue easily. As bone ages, the marrow of the bone has a harder time maintaining blood cell production than young bone marrow when the body is stressed. The high incidence of anemia in the elderly is believed to be not a result of aging per se but rather of the high frequency of other age-related illnesses that can cause anemia. Anemia is not a single disease but a syndrome that has several different causes. Insufficient dietary intake and inflammation or destruction of the gastrointestinal lining to absorb vitamin B_{12} causes a type of anemia that afflicts the elderly. Because of other physiologic stresses affecting marrow production, the elderly have an increased incidence of a variety of blood disorders.

Genitourinary system disorders

Familiar age-related genitourinary (GU) changes are those associated with incontinence. Changes in bladder capacity and muscle structure predispose the elderly to this problem. Urinary and bowel incontinence can also lead to social and hygiene concerns. Along with structural changes in the GU system, the number of nephrons in the kidneys decreases dramatically following the onset of adulthood. This decreased reserve capacity of the kidneys could cause what would otherwise be a regularly prescribed dose of medication to be an overdose in the elderly. The role of the kidneys to maintain the body's water balance and regulate the concentration according to the body's need diminishes with age. Acute and chronic renal failure can affect many elderly people in their later years.

Benign prostatic hyperplasia (BPH) affects up to 70% of men older than age 70. BPH is enlargement of the prostate gland, which can cause obstruction with the flow of urine. Surgical resection of the prostate may be necessary. Prostate cancer is primarily a disease of later life, and more than 80% of tumors are found in men older than 65 years of age. Prostate cancer is the most common cancer in males and the third most common cause of cancer deaths in men. Radiographic imaging of the male reproductive system comprises ureterograms, intravenous urography, and computed tomography. Ultrasound is commonly used to evaluate testicular masses as well as prostate nodules.

Endocrine system disorders

The endocrine system is another principle regulatory system of the body. Age-related changes in thyroid function result from inadequate responses of target cells to thyroid hormone. The most common age-related disease associated with the endocrine system is diabetes mellitus. Non–insulin-dependent diabetes mellitus increases in frequency with age and accounts for about 90% of all cases. Regular exercise and weight loss can significantly reduce the risk and delay the onset of non–insulin-dependent diabetes.

Aging is the one certainty in life. It starts at conception and continues throughout the life cycle. No two persons age in the same way. As stated earlier, aging is individualized and is affected by heredity, lifestyle choices, physical health, and attitude. Despite the changes that occur in the body systems observed with aging, the majority of older adults view themselves as healthy. They learn to adapt, adjust, and compensate for these disabilities. *Older people are stereotyped into two groups: diseased and normal.* The normal group is, in fact, at high risk of disease but is just not there yet. Although categorizing these older adults as normal, health professionals tend to underestimate their vulnerability. Modest increases in blood pressure, blood sugar, body weight, and low bone density are common among the normal elderly. These risk factors promote disease, and yet they can be modified. They may be age related in industrial societies, but they are not age determined or harmless. The power of lifestyle factors, such as diet, exercise, and smoking cessation reduces the risk of disease and improves the quality of life. Good health cannot be left to chance, and staying healthy depends to a large degree on lifestyle choices and attitude.

SUMMARY OF PATHOLOGY: GERIATRIC RADIOGRAPHY

Condition	Definition
Alzheimer's Disease	Progressive, irreversible mental disorder with loss of memory, deterioration of intellectual functions, speech and gait disturbances, and disorientation
Atherosclerosis	Condition in which fibrous and fatty deposits on the luminal wall of an artery may cause obstruction of the vessel
Benign Prostatic Hyperplasia	Enlargement of the prostate gland
Chronic Obstructive Pulmonary Disease	Chronic condition of persistent obstruction of bronchial airflow
Compression Fracture	Fracture that causes compaction of bone and a decrease in length or width
Congestive Heart Failure	Heart is unable to propel blood at a sufficient rate and volume
Contractures	Permanent contraction of a muscle due to spasm or paralysis
Dementia	Broad impairment of intellectual function that usually is progressive and interferes with normal social and occupational activities
Emphysema	Destructive and obstructive airway changes leading to an increased volume of air in the lungs
Geriatrics	Branch of medicine dealing with the aged and the problems of the aging
Gerontology	Branch of medicine dealing with illness prevention and management, health maintenance, and promotion of quality of life for the aged
Kyphosis	Abnormally increased convexity in the thoracic curvature
Osteoarthritis	Form of arthritis marked by progressive cartilage deterioration in synovial joints and vertebrae
Osteoporosis	Loss of bone density
Renal Failure	Failure of the kidney to perform its essential functions
Urinary Incontinence	Absence of voluntary control of urination

Patient Care of the Elderly

Box 28-3 lists some quick tips for working with the elderly. These tips are discussed in the following pages.

PATIENT AND FAMILY EDUCATION

Educating all patients, especially the elderly ones, about imaging procedures is crucial to obtain their confidence and compliance. More time with elderly patients may be necessary to accommodate their decreased ability to rapidly process information. The majority of elderly have been diagnosed with at least one chronic illness. They typically arrive at the clinical imaging environment with a natural anxiety because they are likely to have little knowledge of the procedure or the highly technical modalities employed for their procedures. Moreover, a fear concerning consequences resulting from the examination exacerbates their increased levels of anxiety. Taking time to educate patients and their families or significant caregivers in their support system about the procedures makes for a less stressful experience and improved patient compliance and satisfaction.

COMMUNICATION

Good communication and listening skills create a connection between the radiographer and his or her patient. Older people are unique and should be treated with dignity and respect. Each elderly person is a wealth of cultural and historical knowledge that in turn becomes a learning experience for the radiographer. If it is evident that the patient cannot hear or understand verbal directions, it is appropriate to speak lower and closer. Background noise can be disrupting to an older person and should be eliminated if possible when giving precise instructions. Giving instruction individually gives the elder person time to process a request. An empathetic, warm attitude and approach to the geriatric patient will result in a trusting and compliant patient.

TRANSPORTATION AND LIFTING

Balance and coordination of the elderly patient can be affected by normal aging changes. Their anxiety about falling can be diminished by assistance in and out of a wheelchair and to and from the examination table. Many elderly patients have decreased height perception resulting from some degree of vision impairment. Hesitation of the elderly person may be due to previous falls. Assisting an older patient when there is a need to step up or down throughout the procedure is more than a reassuring gesture. Preventing opportunities for falls is a necessity for the radiographer. The elderly patient will often experience vertigo and dizziness when going from a recumbent position to a sitting position. Giving the patient time to rest between positions will mitigate these disturbing, frightening, and uncomfortable sensations. The use of table handgrips and proper assistance from the radiographer creates a sense of security for the elderly patient. A sense of security will result in a compliant and trusting patient throughout the imaging procedure.

SKIN CARE

Acute age-related changes in the skin will cause it to become thin and fragile. The skin becomes more susceptible to bruising, tears, abrasions, and blisters. All health care professionals should use caution in turning and holding the elderly patient. Excessive pressure on the skin will cause it to break and tear. *Adhesive tape should be avoided because it can be irritating and can easily tear the skin of an older person.* The loss of fat pads makes it painful for the elderly patient to lie on a hard surface and can increase the possibility of developing ulcerations. Decubitus ulcers, or pressure sores, are commonly seen in bedridden people or those with decreased mobility. Bony areas such as the heels, ankles, elbow, and lateral hips are frequent sites for pressure sores. A decubitus ulcer can develop in 1 to 2 hours. Almost without exception, tables used for imaging procedures are hard surfaced and cannot be avoided. However, the use of a table pad can reduce the friction between the hard surface of the table and the patient's fragile skin. Sponges, blankets, and positioning aids will make the procedure much more bearable and comfortable for the elderly patient. Because skin plays a critical role in maintaining body temperature, the increasingly thinning process associated with aging skin renders the patient less able to retain normal body heat. Thus the regulation of body temperature of the elderly person varies from that of a younger person. To prevent hypothermia in rooms where the ambient air temperature is comfortable for the radiographer, it may be essential to provide blankets for the elderly patient.

> ## BOX 28-3
>
> Tips for working with the elderly patient
>
> Take time to educate the patient and his or her family
> Speak lower and closer
> Treat the patient with dignity and respect
> Give the patient time to rest between projections and procedures
> Avoid adhesive tape: elderly skin is thin and fragile
> Provide warm blankets in cold examination rooms
> Use table pads and hand rails
> Always access the patient's medical history before contrast media is administered

CONTRAST ADMINISTRATION

Because of age-related changes in kidney and liver functions, only the amount, not the type, of contrast media is varied when performing radiographic procedures on the elderly patient. The number of functioning nephrons in the kidneys steadily decreases from middle age throughout the life span. Compromised kidney function contributes to the elderly patient being more prone to electrolyte and fluid imbalance, which can create life-threatening consequences. They are also more susceptible to the effects of dehydration because of diabetes and decreased renal or adrenal function. The decision of type and amount of contrast media used for the geriatric patient usually follows some sort of routine protocol. Assessment for contrast agent administration accomplished by the imaging technologist must include age and history of liver, kidney, or thyroid disease; history of hypersensitivity reactions and previous reactions to medications or contrast agents; sensitivity to aspirin; over-the-counter and prescription drug history including acetaminophen (Tylenol); and history of diabetes and hypertension.[1] The imaging technologist must be selective in locating an appropriate vein for contrast administration on the elderly patient. They should consider the location and condition of the vein, decreased integrity of the skin, and duration of the therapy. Thin superficial veins, repeatedly used veins, and veins located in areas where the skin is bruised or scarred should be avoided. Assess the patient for any swallowing impairments, which could lead to difficulties with drinking liquid contrast agents. The patient should be instructed to drink slowly to avoid choking, and an upright position will help prevent aspiration.

---

[1]Norris T: *Special needs of geriatric patients,* American Society of Radiologic Technologists Homestudy Series, vol 4, no 5, 1999.

JOINT COMMISSION ON THE ACCREDITATION OF HEALTHCARE ORGANIZATIONS CRITERIA

The Joint Commission on the Accreditation of Healthcare Organizations (JCAHO) is the accrediting and standards-setting body for hospitals, clinics, and other health care organizations in the United States. Employees in institutions accredited by the JCAHO must demonstrate age-based communication competencies, which include the elderly. The standards were adopted as a means of demonstrating competence in meeting the physiologic and psychologic needs of patients in special populations. These populations include infants, children, adolescents, and the elderly.

Age-related competencies

Standard HR.5 of the Human Resources section of the JCAHO manual states: "When appropriate, the hospital considers special needs and behaviors of specific age groups in defining qualifications, duties, and responsibilities of staff members who do not have clinical privileges but who have regular clinical contact with patients (e.g., radiologic technologists and mental health technicians)." The intent of the standard is to ensure age-specific competency in technical and clinical matters but is not limited to equipment and technical performance. Age-specific competencies address the different needs people have at different ages. Examples of age-specific care for older adults may include the following: assessing visual or hearing impairments; assessing digestive and esophageal problems, such as reflux, bladder, and bowl problems; addressing grief concerns; providing warmth; and providing safety aids. Being able to apply age-specific care also includes the use of age-appropriate communication skills. Clear communication with the patient can be the key to providing age-specific care. Knowledge of age-related changes and disease processes assist all health care professionals, including those in the radiation sciences, in providing care that meets the needs of the elderly patient.

The Radiographer's Role

The role of the radiographer is no different than that of all other health professionals. The whole person must be treated, not just the manifested symptoms of an illness or injury. Medical imaging and therapeutic procedures reflect the impact of ongoing systemic aging in documentable and visual forms. Adapting procedures to accommodate disabilities and diseases of geriatric patients is a critical responsibility and a challenge based almost exclusively on the radiographer's knowledge, abilities, and skills. An understanding of the physiology and pathology of aging, in addition to an awareness of the social, psychologic, cognitive, and economic aspects of aging, are required to meet the needs of the elderly population. Conditions typically associated with elderly patients invariably require adaptations or modifications of routine imaging procedures. The radiographer must be able to differentiate between age-related changes and disease processes. Production of diagnostic images requiring professional decision making to compensate for physiologic changes, while maintaining the compliance, safety, and comfort of the patient, is the foundation of the contract between the elderly patient and the radiographer.

Radiographic Positioning for Geriatric Patients

The preceding discussions and understanding of the physical, cognitive, and psychosocial effects of aging can help radiographers adapt to the positioning challenges of the geriatric patient. In some cases routine examinations need to be modified to accommodate the limitations, safety, and comfort of the patient. Communicating clear instructions with the patient is important. The following discussion addresses positioning suggestions for various structures.

CHEST

The position of choice for the chest radiograph is the upright position; however, the elderly patient may not be able to stand without assistance for this examination. The traditional posteroanterior (PA) position is to have the "backs of hands on hips." This may be difficult for someone with impaired balance and flexibility. The radiographer can allow the patient to wrap his or her arms around the chest stand as a means of support and security. The patient may not be able to maintain his or her arms over the head for the lateral projection of the chest. Provide extra security and stability while moving the arms up and forward (Fig. 28-11).

When the patient cannot stand, the examination may be done seated in a wheelchair, but some issues will affect the radiographic quality. First, the radiologist needs to be aware that the radiograph is an anteroposterior (AP) instead of a PA projection, which may make comparison difficult. Hyperkyphosis can result in the lung apices being obscured, and the abdomen may obscure the lung bases. In a sitting position, respiration may be compromised, and the patient should be instructed on the importance of a deep inspiration.

Positioning of the image receptor for the kyphotic patient should be higher than normal because the shoulders and apices are in a higher position. Radiographic landmarks may change with age, and the centering may need to be lower if the patient is extremely kyphotic. When positioning the patient for the sitting lateral chest projection, the radiographer should place a large sponge behind the patient to lean him or her forward (Fig. 28-12).

SPINE

Radiographic spine examinations may be painful for the patient suffering from osteoporosis who is lying on the x-ray table. Positioning aids such as radiolucent sponges, sandbags, and a mattress may be used as long as the quality of the image is not compromised (Fig. 28-13). Performing upright radiographic examinations may also be appropriate if a patient can safely tolerate this position. The combination of cervical lordosis and thoracic kyphosis can make positioning and visualization of the cervical and thoracic spine difficult. Lateral cervical projections can be done with the patient standing, sitting, or lying supine. The AP projection in the sitting position may not visualize the upper cervical vertebrae because the chin may obscure this anatomy. In the supine position the head may not reach the table and result in magnification. The AP and open-mouth projections are difficult to do in a wheelchair.

Fig. 28-11 Radiographer positioning patient's arms around the chest stand for a PA chest radiograph. Having the patient hold on in this way provides stability.

Fig. 28-13 Positioning sponges and sandbags are commonly used as immobilization devices.

Fig. 28-12 Radiographer placing the image receptor (IR) behind a patient who is unable to stand. With careful positioning of the IR and x-ray tube, a quality image of the chest can be obtained.

Fig. 28-14 Recumbent lateral thoracic spine. Support placed under lower thoracic region; perpendicular central ray.

The thoracic and lumbar spines are sites for compression fractures. The use of positioning blocks may be necessary to help the patient remain in position. For the lateral projection, a lead blocker or shield behind the spine should be used to absorb as much scatter radiation as possible (Fig. 28-14).

PELVIS/HIP

Osteoarthritis, osteoporosis, and injuries as the result of falls contribute to hip pathologies. A common fracture in the elderly is the femoral neck. An AP projection of the pelvis should be done to examine the hip. If the indication is trauma, the radiographer should *not attempt to rotate the limbs*. The second view taken should be a cross-table lateral of the affected hip. If hip pain is the indication, assist the patient to internal rotation of the legs with the use of sandbags if necessary (Figs. 28-15 and 28-16).

Fig. 28-15 Legs inverted for an AP projection of the pelvis. Use of flexible sandbags to wrap around the feet can help the geriatric patient hold his or her legs in this position.

Fig. 28-16 Elderly patient with Alzheimer's disease was brought to the emergency department because he could not walk. Patient did not complain of pain. Note fracture of the right hip. Trauma radiograph was made with patient's pants on and zipper shown.

UPPER EXTREMITY

Positioning the geriatric patient for projections of the upper extremities can present its own challenges. Often the upper extremities have limited flexibility and mobility. A cerebrovascular accident or stroke may cause contractures of the affected limb. Contracted limbs cannot be forced into position, and cross-table views may need to be done. The inability of the patient to move his or her limb should not be interpreted as a lack of cooperation. Supination is often a problem in patients with contractures, fractures, and paralysis. The routine AP and lateral projections can be supported with the use of sponges, sandbags, and blocks to raise and support the extremity being imaged. The shoulder is also a site of decreased mobility, dislocation, and fractures. The therapist should assess how much movement the patient can do before attempting to move the arm. The use of finger sponges may also help with the contractures of the fingers (Fig. 28-17).

A

B

Fig. 28-17 Most projections of the upper limb can be obtained with the patient in a wheelchair and with some creativity. **A,** Patient being positioned for an AP hand radiograph. Note use of a 4-inch sponge to raise the image receptor (IR). **B,** Patient being positioned for a lateral wrist radiograph. A hospital food tray table provides a base for the IR and for ease of positioning.

LOWER EXTREMITY

The lower extremities may have limited flexibility and mobility. The ability to dorsiflex the ankle may be reduced as a result of neurologic disorders. Imaging on the x-ray table may need to be modified when a patient cannot turn on his or her side. Flexion of the knee may be impaired and require a cross-table lateral projection. If a tangential projection of the patella, such as the Settegast method, is necessary and the patient can turn on his or her side, place the image receptor superior to the knee and direct the central ray perpendicular through the patellofemoral joint. Projections of the feet and ankles may be obtained with the patient sitting in the wheelchair. The use of positioning sponges and sandbags support and maintain the position of the body part being imaged (Fig. 28-18).

TECHNICAL FACTORS

Exposure factors also need to be taken into consideration when imaging the geriatric patient. The loss of bone mass, as well as atrophy of tissues, often requires a lower kilovoltage (kVp) to maintain sufficient contrast. kVp is also a factor in chest radiographs when there may be a large heart and pleural fluid to penetrate. Patients with emphysema require a reduction in technical factors to prevent overexposure of the lung field. Patient assessment can help with the appropriate exposure adjustments.

Time may also be a major factor. Geriatric patients may have problems maintaining the positions necessary for the examinations. A short exposure time will help reduce any voluntary and involuntary motion and breathing. Ensure that the geriatric patient clearly hears and understands the breathing instructions.

A   B

Fig. 28-18 Projections of the lower limb, especially from the knee and lower, can be obtained with the patient in a wheelchair. **A,** AP projection of the ankle with the patient's leg and foot resting on a chair. **B,** Lateral projection of the ankle performed by using a chair as a rest and a sponge to raise the image receptor.

Conclusion

The imaging professional will continue to see a change in the health care delivery system with the dramatic shift in the population of persons older than age 65. This shift in the general population is resulting in an ongoing increase in the number of medical imaging procedures performed on elderly patients. Demographic and social effects of aging determine the way in which the elderly adapt to and view the process of aging. An individual's family size and perceptions of aging, economic resources, gender, race, ethnicity, social class, and the availability and delivery of health care will affect the quality of the aging experience. Biologic age will be much more critical than chronologic aging when determining the health status of the elderly. Healthier lifestyles and advancement in medical treatment will create a generation of successfully aging adults, which in turn should decrease the negative stereotyping of the elderly person. Attitudes of all health care professionals, whether positive or negative, will affect the care provided to the growing elderly population. Education about the mental and physiologic alterations associated with aging, along with the cultural, economic, and social influences accompanying aging, enables the radiographer to adapt imaging and therapeutic procedures to the elderly patient's disabilities resulting from age-related changes.

The human body undergoes a multiplicity of physiologic changes and failure in all organ systems. The aging experience is affected by heredity, lifestyle choices, physical health, and attitude, making it highly individualized. No individual's aging process is predictable and is never exactly the same as that of any other individual. Radiologic technologists must use their knowledge, abilities, and skills to adjust imaging procedures to accommodate for disabilities and diseases encountered with geriatric patients. Safety and comfort of the patient is essential in maintaining compliance throughout imaging procedures. Implementation of skills, such as communication, listening, sensitivity, and empathy, all lead to patient compliance. The JCAHO, recognizing the importance of age-based communication competencies for the elderly, requires documentation of achievement of these skills by the employees of accredited health care organizations. Knowledge of age-related changes and disease processes will enhance the radiographer's ability to provide diagnostic information and treatment when providing care that meets the needs of the increasing elderly patient population.

Selective bibliography

Aiken L: *Aging: an introduction to gerontology,* Thousand Oaks, Calif, 1995, Sage.

Byyny RL: *A clinical guide for the care of older women: primary and preventive care,* Philadelphia, 1996, Williams & Wilkins.

Chop WC, Robnett RH: *Gerontology for the health care professional,* Philadelphia, 1999, FA Davis.

Garfein AJ, Herzog AR: Robust aging among the young-old, old-old, and oldest-old, *J Gerontol Soc Sci* 50B(suppl):S77, 1995.

Health Professions in Service to the Nation, San Francisco, 1993, Pew Health Professions Commission.

Hollman FW: *U.S. population estimates by age, sex, race and Hispanic origin: 1989,* Washington, DC, 1990, U.S. Bureau of the Census, Current Population Reports Series, No. 1057.

Lindeman RH: Renal and urinary tract function. In Masoro EJ, editor: *Handbook of physiology-aging,* New York, 1995, Oxford University Press.

Maddox G, editor: *Encyclopedia of aging,* New York, 1987, Springer.

Mazess RB: On aging bone loss, *Clin Orthop* 165:239, 1982.

Norris T: *Special needs of geriatric patients,* American Society of Radiologic Technologists Homestudy Series, vol 4, no 5, 1999.

O'Malley TA, Blakeney BA: Physical health problems and treatment of the aged. In Satin DG, Blakeney TA, editors: *The clinical care of the aged person: an interdisciplinary perspective,* New York, 1994, Oxford University Press.

Rarey LK: Radiologic technologists' responses to elderly patients, *Radiol Technol* 69:566, 1996.

Rimer BK et al: Multistrategy health education program to increase mammography use among women ages 65 and older, *Public Health Rep* 107:369, 1992.

Sorensen LB: Rheumatology. In Cassel CK et al, editors: *Geriatric medicine,* ed 2, New York, 1990, Springer-Verlag.

Spencer G: *What are the demographic implications of an aging U.S. population from 1990 to 2030?* Washington, DC, 1993, American Association of Retired Persons and Resources for the Future.

Timiras PS: Aging of the nervous system: functional changes. In Timiras PS, editor: *Physiological basis of aging and geriatrics,* ed 2, Boca Raton, Fla, 1994, CRC Press.

U.S. Department of Commerce, Economics and Statistics Administration: *65+ in the United States,* Washington, DC, 1996, U.S. Bureau of the Census.

29

MOBILE RADIOGRAPHY

KARI J. WETTERLIN

Mobile AP chest and abdomen radiograph of a neonate. The exposure technique demonstrates the anatomy of the entire chest and abdomen. Note the gonad shield accurately positioned on this male infant *(arrow)*.

Principles of Mobile Radiography

Mobile radiography using transportable radiographic equipment allows imaging services to be brought to the patient. In contrast to the large stationary machines found in radiographic rooms, compact mobile radiography units can produce diagnostic images in virtually any location (Fig. 29-1). Mobile radiography is commonly performed in patient rooms, emergency departments, intensive care units, surgery and recovery rooms, as well as nursery and neonatal units. Some machines are designed for transport by automobile or van to nursing homes, extended care facilities, or other off-site locations requiring radiographic imaging services.

Mobile radiography was first used by the military for treating battlefield injuries during World War I. Small portable units were designed to be carried by soldiers and set up in field locations. Although mobile equipment is no longer "carried" to the patient, the term *portable* has persisted and is often used in reference to mobile procedures.

This chapter focuses on the most common projections performed with mobile radiography machines. The basic principles of mobile radiography are detailed, and helpful hints are provided for successful completion of the examinations. An understanding of common projections enables the radiographer to perform most mobile examinations ordered by the physician.

Mobile X-Ray Machines

Mobile x-ray machines are not as sophisticated as the larger stationary machines in the radiology department. Although mobile units are capable of producing images of most body parts, they vary in their exposure controls and power sources (or generators).

A typical mobile x-ray machine has controls for setting kilovolt (peak) (kVp) and milliampere-seconds (mAs). The mAs control automatically adjusts milliamperage (mA) and time to preset values. Maximum settings differ among manufacturers, but mAs typically range from 0.04 to 320 and kVp from 40 to 130. The total power of the unit varies between 15 and 25 kilowatts (kW), which is adequate for most mobile projections. By comparison, the power of a stationary radiography unit can reach 150 kW (150 kVp, 1000 mA) or more.

Some mobile x-ray machines have preset anatomic programs (APRs) similar to stationary units. The anatomic programs use exposure techniques with predetermined values based on the selected examination. The radiographer can adjust these settings as needed to compensate for differences in the size or condition of a patient. Automatic exposure control (AEC) may be available for some mobile machines. A paddle containing an ionization chamber is placed behind the image receptor (IR) and is used to determine the exposure time. However, with the increasing use of computed radiography (CR), AEC may not be as useful. The much wider dynamic range available with CR and the ability to manipulate the final image with computer software results in images of proper density without the use of automatic systems.

Mobile x-ray machines are classified into two categories—*battery operated* and *capacitor discharge*—depending on the power source.

Fig. 29-1 Radiographer driving a battery-operated mobile radiography machine to a patient's room.

BATTERY-OPERATED MOBILE UNITS

Battery-operated machines use two different sets of batteries. One set, consisting of as many as ten 12-volt lead acid batteries, controls the x-ray power output; the other set provides the power for the self-propelled driving ability. When the batteries are fully charged, these machines can be used for as many as 10 to 15 x-ray exposures and can be driven reasonable distances around the institution. Recharging after heavy use is necessary to ensure maximum consistency in radiation output. The driving mechanisms include forward and reverse speeds; because of the power drive, a strong "deadman" type of brake is standard. A deadman brake stops the machine instantly when the push-handle is released. The advantages of these machines are that they are cordless and provide constant kVp and mAs.

CAPACITOR-DISCHARGE MOBILE UNITS

Capacitor-discharge mobile machines contain a capacitor-discharge unit and do not operate on batteries. A capacitor is a device that stores electrical energy. The radiation is generated when an electrical discharge is sent across the x-ray tube electrodes from a bank of high-voltage capacitors. The capacitor must be charged briefly before each exposure, with the power coming from a standard 110-volt outlet. Larger capacitor-discharge machines may require a 220-volt outlet. These machines are not self-propelling, and they are typically much lighter as a result of not having batteries. Their lighter weight allows them to be driven manually.

In a capacitor-discharge system, the kVp drops constantly during the length of the exposure. For example, the kVp may start at 100 and then drop to 80 by the end of an exposure. This drop may result in inadequate penetration of thick body areas. Consequently, special attention must be given to creating a technique chart that uses higher kVp and lower mAs than would normally be used with a conventional generator. If the desired technique normally requires 90 kVp at 20 mAs on noncapacitor-discharge machines, using a technique of 100 kVp on a capacitor-discharge unit is preferred because the average kVp during the exposure is about 92. The advantages of capacitor-discharge machines are their smaller size and ease in movement. They also do not require long capacitor charging times before the exposure.

Technical Considerations

Mobile radiography presents the radiographer with challenges different from those experienced in performing examinations with stationary equipment in the radiology department. Although the positioning of the patient and placement of the central ray are essentially the same, three important technical matters must be clearly understood to perform optimum mobile examinations: the *grid*, the *anode heel effect*, and the *source–to–image-receptor distance* (SID). In addition, exposure technique charts must be available (see Fig. 29-4).

GRID

For optimum imaging, a *grid* must be level, centered to the central ray, and correctly used at the recommended focal distance, or radius. When a grid is placed on an unstable surface such as the mattress of a bed, the weight of the patient can cause the grid to tilt "off-level." If the grid tilts transversely while using a longitudinal grid, the central ray forms an angle across the long axis. Image density is lost as a result of grid "cutoff" (Fig. 29-2). If the grid tilts longitudinally, the central ray angles through the long axis. In this case, grid cutoff is avoided, but the image may be distorted or elongated.

A grid positioned under a patient can be difficult to center. If the central ray is directed to a point transversely off the midline of a grid more than 1 to 1½ inches (2.5 to 3.8 cm), a cutoff effect similar to that produced by an off-level grid results. The central ray can be centered longitudinally to any point along the midline of a grid without cutoff. Depending on the procedure, beam-restriction problems may occur. If this happens, a portion of the image is "collimated off," or patient exposure is excessive because of an oversized exposure field.

A   B

Fig. 29-2 Mobile radiograph of a proximal femur and hip, demonstrating comminuted fracture of the left acetabulum. **A,** Poor-quality radiograph resulted when the grid was transversely tilted far enough to produce significant grid cutoff. **B,** Excellent-quality repeat radiograph on the same patient, performed with the grid accurately positioned perpendicular to the central ray.

Fig. 29-3 Transverse and longitudinal grids mounted on rigid holder, many times referred to as "slip-on." Focal ranges are clearly identified for proper use.

TABLE 29-1

Cathode placement for mobile projections

Part	Projection	Cathode placement
Chest	AP	Diaphragm
	AP—decubitus	Down side of chest
Abdomen	AP	Diaphragm
	AP—decubitus	Down side of abdomen
Pelvis	AP	Upper pelvis
Femur	AP	Proximal femur
	Lateral	Proximal femur
Cervical spine	Lateral	Over lower vertebrae (40-inch (102-cm) SID only)
Chest and abdomen in neonate	All	No designation*

The cathode side of the beam has the greatest intensity.
AP, Anteroposterior; *SID,* source–to–image-receptor distance.
*Not necessary because of small field size of the collimator.

Grids used for mobile radiography are often of the focused type. However, some radiology departments continue to use the older, parallel-type grids. All focused grids have a recommended focal range, or radius, that varies with the grid ratio. Projections taken at distances greater or less than the recommended focal range can produce cutoff in which image density is reduced on lateral margins. Grids with a lower ratio have a greater focal range, but they are less efficient for cleaning up scatter radiation. The radiographer must be aware of the *exact* focal range for the grid used. Most focused grids used for mobile radiography have a ratio of 6:1 or 8:1 and a focal range of about 36 to 44 inches (91 to 112 cm). This focal range allows mobile examinations to be performed efficiently. Inverting a focused grid causes a pronounced cutoff effect similar to that produced by improper distance.

Today most grids are mounted on a protective frame, and the IR is easily inserted behind the grid (Fig. 29-3). A final concern regarding grids relates to the use of "tape-on" grids. If a grid is not mounted on an IR holder frame but instead is manually fastened to the surface of the IR with tape, care must be taken to ensure that the tube side of the grid faces the x-ray tube. The examinations described in this chapter present methods of ensuring proper grid and IR placement for projections that require a grid.

ANODE HEEL EFFECT

Another consideration in mobile radiography is the *anode heel effect.* The heel effect causes a decrease of image density under the anode side of the x-ray tube. The heel effect is more pronounced with the following:
- Short SID
- Larger field sizes
- Small anode angles

Short SIDs and large field sizes are common in mobile radiography. Furthermore, in mobile radiography, the radiographer has control of the anode-cathode axis of the x-ray tube relative to the body part. Therefore correct placement of the anode-cathode axis with regard to the anatomy is essential. When performing a mobile examination, the radiographer may not always be able to orient the anode-cathode axis of the tube to the desired position because of limited space and maneuverability in the room. For optimum mobile radiography, the anode and cathode sides of the x-ray tube should be clearly marked to indicate where the high-tension cables enter the x-ray tube, and the radiographer should use the heel effect maximally (Table 29-1).

SOURCE–TO–IMAGE-RECEPTOR DISTANCE

The SID should be maintained at 40 inches (102 cm) for most mobile examinations. A standardized distance for all patients and projections helps to ensure consistency in imaging. Longer SIDs—40 to 48 inches (102 to 122 cm)—require increased mAs to compensate for the additional distance. The mA limitations of a mobile unit necessitate longer exposure times when the SID exceeds 40 inches (102 cm). Despite the longer exposure time, a radiograph with motion artifacts may result if the SID is greater than 40 inches (102 cm). In addition, motion artifacts may occur in the radiographs of critically ill adult patients and infants or small children who require chest and abdominal examinations but may not be able to hold their breath.

RADIOGRAPHIC TECHNIQUE CHARTS

A radiographic technique chart should be available for use with every mobile machine. The chart should display, in an organized manner, the standardized technical factors for all the radiographic projections done with the machine (Fig. 29-4). A caliper should also be available; this device is used to measure the thickness of body parts to ensure that accurate and consistent exposure factors are used. Measuring the patient also allows the radiographer to determine the optimum kVp level for all exposures (Fig. 29-5).

MOBILE RADIOGRAPHIC TECHNIQUE CHART

AMX—4   40-inch SID   Lanex medium screens/TML   8:1 grid

Part	Projection	Position	cm—kVp	mAs	Grid
Chest	AP	Supine/upright	21—85	1.25	No
	AP	Lateral decubitus	21—85	6.25	Yes
Abdomen	AP	Supine	23—74	25	Yes
	AP	Lateral decubitus	23—74	32	Yes
Pelvis	AP	Supine	23—74	32	Yes
Femur (distal)	AP	Supine	15—70	10	Yes
	Lateral	Dorsal decubitus	15—70	10	Yes
C-spine	Lateral	Dorsal decubitus	10—62	20	Yes
NEONATAL					
Chest/abdomen	AP	Supine	7—64	0.8	No
	Lateral	Dorsal decubitus	10—72	1	No

Fig. 29-4 Sample radiographic technique chart showing the manual technical factors used for the 10 common mobile projections described in this chapter. The kVp and mAs factors are for the specific centimeter measurements indicated. Factors vary depending on the actual centimeter measurement. *AP,* Anteroposterior.

Fig. 29-5 Radiographer measuring the thickest portion of the femur to determine the exact technical factors needed for the examination.

Radiation Safety

Radiation protection for the radiographer, others in the immediate area, and the patient is of paramount importance when mobile examinations are performed. *Mobile radiography produces some of the highest occupational radiation exposures for radiographers.* The radiographer should wear a lead apron and stand as far away from the patient, x-ray tube, and useful beam as the room and the exposure cable allow. The recommended *minimal* distance is 6 feet (2 m). For a horizontal (cross-table) x-ray beam, or for an upright anteroposterior (AP) chest projection, the radiographer should stand at a right angle (90 degrees) to the primary beam and the object being radiographed. The least amount of scatter radiation occurs at this position (Fig. 29-6). However, shielding and distance have a greater effect on exposure reduction and therefore should always be considered first.

The single most effective means of radiation protection is *distance.* The radiographer should inform all persons in the immediate area that an x-ray exposure is about to occur so that they may leave to avoid exposure. Lead protection should be provided for any individuals who are unable to leave the room and for those who may have to hold a patient or IR.

The patient's gonads should be shielded with appropriate radiation protection devices for any of the following situations:

- X-ray examinations performed on children
- X-ray examinations performed on patients of reproductive age
- Any examination for which the patient requests protection
- Examinations in which the gonads lie in or near the useful beam
- Examinations in which shielding will not interfere with imaging of the anatomy that must be demonstrated (Fig. 29-7)

In addition, the source-to-skin distance (SSD) cannot be less than 12 inches (30 cm), in accordance with federal safety regulations.[1]

---

[1]National Council on Radiation Protection: *Report 102: Medical x-ray, electron beam and gamma ray protection for energies up to 50 MeV,* Bethesda, Md, 1989.

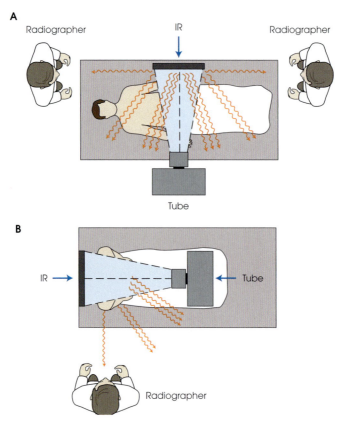

Fig. 29-6 Whenever possible, the radiographer should stand at least 6 feet (2 m) from the patient and useful beam. The lowest amount of scatter radiation occurs at a right angle (90 degrees) from the primary x-ray beam. **A,** Note radiographer standing at either the head or foot of the patient at a right angle to the x-ray beam for a dorsal decubitus position lateral projection of the abdomen. **B,** Radiographer standing at right angle to the x-ray beam for an AP projection of the chest. *IR,* Image receptor.

Mobile radiography

Isolation Considerations

Two types of patients are often cared for in isolation units: (1) patients who have infectious microorganisms that could be spread to health care workers and visitors and (2) patients who need protection from potentially lethal microorganisms that may be carried by health care workers and visitors. Optimally, a radiographer entering an isolation room should have a full knowledge of the patient's disease, the way it is transmitted, and the proper way to clean and disinfect equipment before and after use in the isolation unit. However, because of the confidentiality of patient records, the radiographer may not be able to obtain information about a patient's specific disease. Therefore all patients must be treated with universal precautions. If isolation is used to protect the patient from receiving microorganisms (reverse isolation), a different protocol may be required. Institutional policy regarding isolation procedures should be available and strictly followed.

When performing mobile procedures in an isolation unit, the radiographer should wear the required protective apparel for the specific situation—gown, cap, mask, shoe covers, and gloves. All of this apparel is not needed for every isolation patient. For example, all persons entering a strict isolation unit wear a mask, a gown, and gloves, but only gloves are worn for drainage secretion precautions. Radiographers should always wash their hands with warm, soapy water before putting on gloves. The x-ray machine is taken into the room and moved into position. The IR is placed into a clean, protective cover.

Pillowcases will not protect the IR or the patient if body fluids soak through them. A clean, impermeable cover should be used in situations in which body fluids may come into contact with the IR. For examinations of patients in strict isolation, two radiographers may be required to maintain a safe barrier (see Chapter 1).

After finishing the examination, the radiographer should remove and dispose of the mask, cap, gown, shoe covers, and the gloves according to institutional policies. All equipment that touched the patient or the patient's bed must be wiped with a disinfectant according to appropriate aseptic technique. The radiographer should wear new gloves, if necessary, while cleaning equipment. Handwashing is repeated before the radiographer leaves the room.

Fig. 29-7 Patient ready for a mobile chest examination. Note lead shield placed over the patient's pelvis. This shield does not interfere with the examination.

Performing Mobile Examinations

INITIAL PROCEDURES

The radiographer should plan for the trip out of the radiology department. Ensuring that all of the necessary devices (e.g., IR, grid, tape, caliper, markers, blocks) are transported with the mobile x-ray machine provides greater efficiency in performing examinations. Many mobile x-ray machines are equipped with a storage area for transporting IRs and supplies. If a battery-operated machine is used, the radiographer should check the machine to ensure that it is acceptably charged. An inadequately charged machine can interfere with performance and affect the quality of the radiograph.

Before entering the patient's room with the machine, the radiographer should follow several important steps (Box 29-1). The radiographer begins by checking that the correct patient is going to be examined. After confirming the identity of the patient, the radiographer enters, makes an introduction as a radiographer, and informs the patient about the x-ray examinations to be performed. While in the room, the radiographer observes any medical appliances, such as chest tube boxes, catheter bags, and IV poles, that may be positioned next to or hanging on the sides of the patient's bed. The radiographer should ask family members or visitors to step out of the room until the examination is finished. If necessary, the nursing staff should be alerted that assistance is required.

Communication and cooperation between the radiographer and nursing staff members are essential for proper patient care during mobile radiography. In addition, communication with the patient is *imperative,* even if the patient is or appears to be unconscious or unresponsive.

THE EXAMINATION

Chairs, stands, IV poles, wastebaskets, and other obstacles should be moved from the path of the mobile machine. Lighting should be adjusted if necessary. If the patient is to be examined in the supine position, the base of the mobile machine should be positioned toward the middle of the bed. If a seated patient position is used, the base of the machine should be toward the foot of the bed.

For lateral and decubitus radiographs, positioning the base of the mobile machine parallel to or directly perpendicular to the bed allows the greatest ease in positioning the x-ray tube. Room size can also influence the base position used.

At times, the radiographer may have difficulty accurately aligning the x-ray tube parallel to the IR while standing at the side of the bed. When positioning the tube above the patient, the radiographer may need to check the x-ray tube and IR alignment from the foot of the bed to ensure that the tube is not tilted.

For all projections, the primary x-ray beam must be collimated no larger than the size of the IR. When the central ray is correctly centered to the IR, the light field coincides with or fits within the borders of the IR.

A routine and consistent system for labeling and separating exposed and unexposed IRs should be developed and maintained. It is easy to "double expose" IRs during mobile radiography, particularly if many examinations are performed at one time. Most institutions require additional identification markers for mobile examinations. Typically the time of examination (especially for chest radiographs) and technical notes such as the position of the patient are indicated. A log may be maintained for each patient and kept in the patient's room. The log should contain the exposure factors used for the projections and other notes regarding the performance of the examination.

PATIENT CONSIDERATIONS

Patients requiring mobile radiography often are in extended care facilities or are immobile and among the most sick. They may be awake and lying in bed in traction because of a broken limb, or they may be critically ill and unconscious. A brief but total assessment of the patient must be conducted both before and during the examination. Some specific considerations to keep in mind are described in the following sections.

Assessment of the patient's condition

A thorough assessment of the patient's condition and room allows the radiographer to make necessary adaptations to ensure the best possible patient care and imaging outcome. The radiographer assesses the patient's level of alertness and respiration and then determines the extent to which the patient is able to cooperate and the limitations that may affect the procedure. Some patients may have varying degrees of drowsiness because of their medications or medical condition. Many mobile examinations are performed in patients' rooms immediately after surgery; these patients may be under the influence of various anesthetics.

BOX 29-1

Preliminary steps for the radiographer before mobile radiography is performed

- Announce your presence to the nursing staff, and ask for assistance if needed.
- Determine that the correct patient is in the room.
- Introduce yourself to the patient and family as a radiographer and explain the examination.
- Observe the medical equipment in the room, as well as other apparatus and IV poles with fluids. Move the equipment if necessary.
- Ask family members and visitors to leave.*

*A family member may need to be present for the examination of a small child.

Patient mobility

The radiographer must never move a patient or part of the patient's body without assessing the patient's ability to move or tolerate movement. At all times, *gentleness* and *caution* must prevail. If unsure, the radiographer should always check with the nursing staff or physician. For example, many patients who undergo total joint replacement may not be able to move the affected joint for a number of days or weeks. However, this may not be evident to the radiographer. Some patients may be able to indicate verbally their ability to move or their tolerance for movement. *The radiographer should never move a limb that has been operated on or is broken unless the nurse, the physician, or sometimes the patient grants permission.* Inappropriate movement of the patient by the radiographer during the examination may harm the patient.

Fractures

Patients can have a variety of fractures and fracture types, ranging from one simple fracture to multiple fractures of many bones. A patient lying awake in a traction bed with a simple femur fracture may be able to assist with a radiographic examination. However, another patient may be unconscious and have multiple broken ribs, spinal fractures, or a severe closed head injury.

Few patients with multiple fractures are able to move or tolerate movement. The radiographer must be cautious, resourceful, and work in accordance with the patient's condition and pain tolerance. If a patient's trunk or limb must be raised into position for a projection, the radiographer should have ample assistance so that the part can be raised safely without causing harm or intense pain.

Interfering devices

Patients who are in intensive care units or orthopedic beds because of fractures may be attached to a variety of devices, wires, and tubing. These objects may be in the direct path of the x-ray beam and consequently produce artifacts on the image. Experienced radiographers know which of these objects can be moved out of the x-ray beam. When devices such as fracture frames cannot be moved, it may be necessary to angle the central ray or adjust the IR to obtain the best radiograph possible. In many instances the objects have to be radiographed along with the body part (Fig. 29-8). The radiographer must exercise caution when handling any of these devices and should never remove traction devices without the assistance of a physician.

Positioning and asepsis

During positioning, the IR (with or without a grid) often is perceived by the patient as cold, hard, and uncomfortable. Therefore before the IR is put in place, the patient should be warned of possible discomfort and assured that the examination will be for as short a time as possible. The patient will appreciate the radiographer's concern and efficiency in completing the examination as quickly as possible.

If the surface of the IR touches bare skin, it can stick, making positioning adjustments difficult. *The skin of older patients may be thin and dry and can be torn by manipulation of the IR if care is not taken.* A cloth or paper cover over the IR can protect the patient's skin and alleviate some of the discomfort by making it feel less cold. The cover also helps to keep the IR clean. IRs that contact the patient directly should be wiped off with a disinfectant for asepsis and infection control.

The IR must be enclosed in an appropriate, impermeable barrier in any situation in which it may come in contact with blood, body fluids, and other potentially infectious material. A contaminated IR can be difficult and sometimes impossible to clean. Approved procedures for disposing of used barriers must be followed.

Fig. 29-8 A, Mobile radiograph of the chest. Note the variety of objects in the image that could not be removed for the exposure. **B,** Mobile radiograph of proximal femur and hip. Metal buckles could not be removed for the exposure.

AP PROJECTION*
Upright or supine

Image receptor: 35 × 43 cm lengthwise or crosswise, depending on body habitus; a non-grid or grid IR can be used, depending on patient size or institutional policy

Position of patient
Depending on the condition of the patient, elevate the head of the bed to a semierect or sitting position. The projection should be performed with the patient in the upright position or to the greatest angle tolerated by the patient whenever possible. Use the supine position for critically ill or injured patients.

_____

*The nonmobile projection is described in Chapter 10.

Position of part
Center the midsagittal plane to the IR.
- To include the entire chest, position the IR under the patient with the top about 2 inches (5 cm) above the *relaxed* shoulders. The exact distance depends on the size of the patient. When the patient is supine, the shoulders may move to a higher position relative to the lungs. Adjust accordingly.
- Be certain that the patient's shoulders are relaxed; then internally rotate the patient's arms to prevent scapular superimposition of the lung field, if not contraindicated.
- Ensure that the patient's upper torso is not rotated or leaning toward one side (Fig. 29-9).
- *Shield gonads.*
- *Respiration:* Inspiration, unless otherwise requested. If the patient is receiving respiratory assistance, carefully watch the patient's chest to determine the inspiratory phase for the exposure.

Central ray
- Perpendicular to the long axis of the sternum and the center of the IR. The central ray should enter about 3 inches (7.6 cm) below the jugular notch at the level of T7.

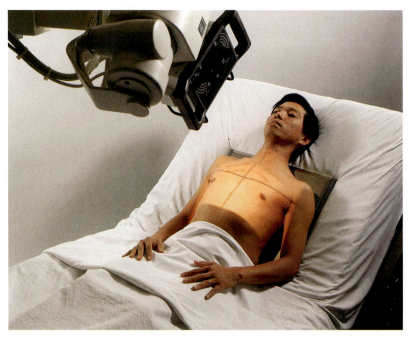

Fig. 29-9 Mobile AP chest: partially upright.

DIGITAL RADIOGRAPHY

A grid must be used for all mobile computed radiography chest examinations if the exposure technique is more than 90 kVp. (Review the manufacturer's protocol for the exact kVp levels for the unit that is used.) When a crosswise-positioned grid is used, the central ray must be perpendicular to the grid to prevent grid cutoff.

Structures shown

This projection demonstrates the anatomy of the thorax, including the heart, trachea, diaphragmatic domes, and most importantly the entire lung fields, including vascular markings (Fig. 29-10).

The following should be clearly demonstrated:

■ No motion; well-defined (not blurred) diaphragmatic domes and lung fields
■ Lung fields in their entirety, including costophrenic angles
■ Pleural markings
■ Ribs and thoracic intervertebral disk spaces faintly visible through heart shadow
■ No rotation, with medial portion of clavicles and lateral border of ribs equidistant from vertebral column

NOTE: To ensure the proper angle from the x-ray tube to the IR, the radiographer can double-check the shadow of the shoulders from the field light projected onto the IR. If the shadow of the shoulders is thrown far above the upper edge of the IR, the angle of the tube must be corrected.

Fig. 29-10 Mobile AP chest radiographs in critically ill patients. **A,** Patient with postoperative left thoracotomy and chest tube, infiltrate or atelectasis in the left base, segmental elevation of the right hemidiaphragm, and soft tissue emphysema on the left. **B,** Patient with small left pleural effusion and moderate right effusion, cardiomegaly, mild pulmonary vascular congestion, and calcification and torsion of the aorta.

AP OR PA PROJECTION*
Right or left lateral decubitus position

Image receptor: 35 × 43 cm lengthwise; a non-grid or grid IR can be used, depending on patient size

Position of patient
- Place the patient in the lateral recumbent position.
- Flex the patient's knees to provide stabilization, if possible.
- Place a firm support under the patient to elevate the body 2 to 3 inches (5 to 8 cm) and prevent the patient from sinking into the mattress.
- Raise both of the patient's arms up and away from the chest region, preferably above the head. An arm lying on the patient's side can imitate a region of free air.
- Ensure that the patient cannot roll off the bed.

*The nonmobile projection is described in Chapter 10.

Position of part
- Position the patient for the AP projection whenever possible. It is much easier to position an ill patient (particularly the arms) for an AP.
- Adjust the patient to ensure a lateral position. The coronal plane passing through the shoulders and hips should be vertical.
- Place the IR behind the patient and below the support so that the lower margin of the chest will be visualized.
- Adjust the grid so that it extends approximately 2 inches (5 cm) above the shoulders. The IR should be supported in position and not leaning against the patient to avoid distortion (Fig. 29-11).
- *Shield gonads.*
- *Respiration:* Inspiration unless otherwise requested.

Central ray
- Horizontal and perpendicular to the center of the IR, entering the patient at a level of 3 inches (7.6 cm) below the jugular notch

Fig. 29-11 Mobile AP chest: left lateral decubitus position. Note yellow block placed under the chest to elevate it. The block is necessary to ensure that the left side of the chest is included on the image.

Structures shown

This projection demonstrates the anatomy of the thorax, including the entire lung fields and any air or fluid levels that may be present (Fig. 29-12).

The following should be clearly demonstrated:

- No motion
- No rotation
- Affected side in its entirety (upper lung for free air and lower lung for fluid)
- Patient's arms out of region of interest
- Proper identification to indicate that decubitus position was used

NOTE: Fluid levels in the pleural cavity are best visualized with the affected side down, which also prevents mediastinal overlapping. Air levels are best visualized with the unaffected side down. The patient should be in position for at least 5 minutes before the exposure is made to allow air to rise and fluid levels to settle.

Fig. 29-12 Mobile AP chest radiographs performed in lateral decubitus positions in critically ill patients. **A,** Left lateral decubitus position. The patient has a large right pleural effusion *(arrow)* and no left effusion. Note that the complete left side of thorax is visualized because of elevation on a block. **B,** Right lateral decubitus position. The patient has right pleural effusion *(arrows)*, cardiomegaly, and mild pulmonary vascular congestion. Note that the complete right side of thorax is visualized because of elevation on a block.

♠ AP PROJECTION*

Image receptor: 35 × 43 cm lengthwise grid

Position of patient
- If necessary, adjust the patient's bed to achieve a horizontal bed position.
- Place the patient in a supine position.

*The nonmobile projection is described in Chapter 16.

Position of part
- Position the grid under the patient to demonstrate the abdominal anatomy from the pubic symphysis to the upper abdominal region.
- Keep the grid from tipping side to side by placing it in the center of the bed and stabilizing it with blankets or towels if necessary.
- Use the patient's draw sheet to roll the patient; this makes it easier to shift the patient from side to side during positioning of the IR, and it provides a barrier between the patient's skin and the grid.
- Center the midsagittal plane of the patient to the midline of the grid.

- Center the grid to the level of the iliac crests. If the emphasis is on the upper abdomen, center the grid 2 inches (5 cm) above the iliac crests or high enough to include the diaphragm.
- Adjust the patient's shoulders and pelvis to lie in the same plane (Fig. 29-13).
- Move the patient's arms out of the region of the abdomen.
- *Shield gonads.* Note that this may not be possible in a female patient.
- *Respiration:* Expiration.

Fig. 29-13 Mobile AP abdomen.

Central ray

- Perpendicular to the center of the grid along the midsagittal plane and at the level of the iliac crests or the tenth rib laterally

Structures shown

This projection demonstrates the following: the inferior margin of the liver; the spleen, kidneys, and psoas muscles; calcifications; and evidence of tumor masses. If the image includes the upper abdomen and diaphragm, the size and shape of the liver may be seen (Fig. 29-14).

EVALUATION CRITERIA

The following should be clearly demonstrated:

- No motion
- Outlines of the abdominal viscera
- Abdominal region, including pubic symphysis or diaphragm (both may be seen on some patients)
- Vertebral column in center of image
- Psoas muscles, lower margin of liver, and kidney margins
- No rotation
- Symmetric appearance of vertebral column and iliac wings

NOTE: Hypersthenic patients may require two separate projections using a crosswise grid. One grid is positioned for the upper abdomen and the other for the lower abdomen.

A

B

Fig. 29-14 Mobile AP abdomen radiographs. **A,** Abdomen without pathology. Note that the entire abdomen is seen in this patient. **B,** Patient with hepatomegaly encompassing the entire upper abdomen *(arrows).* Note that the diaphragm cannot be seen in this patient, who has a longer abdomen than the patient in **A.**

Mobile radiography

Fig. 29-15 Mobile AP abdomen radiograph: left lateral decubitus position. **A,** AP projection. **B,** PA projection. Note yellow blocks placed under the abdomen to level the abdomen and keep the patient from sinking into the mattress.

♠ AP OR PA PROJECTION*
Left lateral decubitus position

Image receptor: 35 × 43 cm lengthwise grid

Position of patient
- Place the patient in the left lateral recumbent position unless requested otherwise.
- Flex the patient's knees slightly to provide stabilization.
- If necessary, place a firm support under the patient to elevate the body and keep the patient from sinking into the mattress.
- Raise both of the patient's arms away from the abdominal region, if possible. The right arm lying on the side of the abdomen may imitate a region of free air.
- Ensure that the patient cannot fall out of bed.

Position of part
- Use the PA or AP projection, depending on the room layout.
- Adjust the patient to ensure a true lateral position. The coronal plane passing through the shoulders and hips should be vertical.
- Place the grid vertically in front of the patient for a PA projection and behind the patient for an AP projection. The grid should be supported in position and not leaned against the patient; this position prevents grid cutoff.
- Position the grid so that its center is 2 inches (5 cm) above the iliac crests to ensure that the diaphragm is included. The pubic symphysis and lower abdomen do not have to be visualized (Fig. 29-15).
- Before making the exposure, be certain that the patient has been in the lateral recumbent position for at least 5 minutes to allow air to rise and fluid levels to settle.
- *Shield gonads.*
- *Respiration:* Expiration.

---

*The nonmobile projection is described in Chapter 16.

Central ray
- Horizontal and perpendicular to the center of the grid, entering the patient along the midsagittal plane

Structures shown
Air or fluid levels within the abdominal cavity are demonstrated. These projections are especially helpful in assessing free air in the abdomen. The right border of the abdominal region must be visualized (Fig. 29-16).

The following should be clearly demonstrated:
- No motion
- Well-defined diaphragm and abdominal viscera
- Air or fluid levels, if present
- Right and left abdominal wall and flank structures
- No rotation
- Symmetric appearance of vertebral column and iliac wings

NOTE: Hypersthenic patients may require two projections with the 35- × 43-cm grid positioned crosswise to visualize the entire abdominal area. A patient with a long torso may require two projections with the grid lengthwise to visualize the entire abdominal region.

Fig. 29-16 Mobile AP abdomen radiograph: left lateral decubitus position. Free intraperitoneal air is seen on the upper or right side of the abdomen *(arrow)*. The radiograph is slightly underexposed to demonstrate the free air more easily.

♠ AP PROJECTION*

Image receptor: 35 × 43 cm grid crosswise

Position of patient
- Adjust the patient's bed horizontally so that the patient is in a supine patient position.
- Move the patient's arms out of the region of the pelvis.

---

*The nonmobile projection is described in Chapter 7.

Position of part
- Position the grid under the pelvis so that the center is midway between the anterior superior iliac spine (ASIS) and the pubic symphysis. This is about 2 inches (5 cm) inferior to the ASIS and 2 inches (5 cm) superior to the pubic symphysis.
- Center the midsagittal plane of the patient to the midline of the grid. The pelvis should not be rotated.
- Rotate the patient's legs medially approximately 15 degrees when not contraindicated (Fig. 29-17).
- *Shield gonads:* Note that this may not be possible in female patients.
- *Respiration*: Suspend.

Fig. 29-17 Mobile AP pelvis. Note that the grid is placed horizontal and perpendicular to the central ray.

Central ray

- Perpendicular to the midpoint of the grid, entering the midsagittal plane. The central ray should enter the patient 2 inches (5 cm) above the pubic symphysis and 2 inches (5 cm) below the ASIS.

Structures shown

This projection demonstrates the pelvis, including the following: both hip bones; the sacrum and coccyx; and the head, neck, trochanters, and proximal portion of the femurs (Fig. 29-18).

EVALUATION CRITERIA

The following should be clearly demonstrated:

- Entire pelvis, including proximal femurs and both hip bones
- No rotation
- Symmetric appearance of iliac wings and obturator foramina
- Both greater trochanters and ilia equidistant from edge of radiograph
- Femoral necks not foreshortened and greater trochanters in profile

NOTE: It is not uncommon for the weight of the patient to cause the bottom edge of the grid to tilt upward. The x-ray tube may need to be angled caudally to compensate and maintain proper grid alignment, thereby preventing grid cutoff. However, the exact angle needed is not always known or easy to determine. The radiographer may want to lower the foot of the bed slightly (Fowler's position), thereby shifting the patient's weight more evenly on the grid and allowing it to be flat. A rolled-up towel or blanket placed under the grid also may be useful to prevent lateral tilting. If the bed is equipped with an inflatable air mattress, the maximum inflate mode is recommended. Tilting the bottom edge of the grid downward is another possibility. Check the level of the grid carefully and compensate accordingly.

Fig. 29-18 Mobile AP pelvis radiograph. This patient has a comminuted fracture of the left acetabulum with medial displacement of the medial acetabular wall (*arrow*). Residual barium is seen in the colon, sigmoid, and rectum.

❄ AP PROJECTION*

Most mobile AP and lateral projections of the femur may be radiographs of the middle and distal femur taken while the patient is in traction. The femur cannot be moved, which presents a challenge to the radiographer.

Image receptor: 35 × 43 cm grid lengthwise

Position of patient

• The patient is in the supine position.

*The nonmobile projection is described in Chapter 6.

Position of part

• *Cautiously* place the grid lengthwise under the patient's femur, with the distal edge of the grid low enough to include the fracture site, pathologic region, and knee joint.
• Elevate the grid with towels, blankets, or blocks under each side, if necessary, to ensure proper grid alignment with the x-ray tube.
• Center the grid to the midline of the affected femur.
• Ensure that the grid is placed parallel to the plane of the femoral condyles (Fig. 29-19).
• *Shield gonads.*
• *Respiration:* Suspend.

Fig. 29-19 Mobile AP femur.

Femur

Central ray

- Perpendicular to the long axis of the femur and centered to the grid
- Be certain that the central ray and grid are aligned to prevent grid cutoff.

DIGITAL RADIOGRAPHY

The thickest portion of the femur (proximal area) must be carefully measured and an appropriate kVp must be selected to penetrate this area. The computer cannot form an image of the anatomy in this area if penetration does not occur. A light area of the entire proximal femur will result. Positioning the cathode over the proximal femur will improve CR image quality.

Structures shown

The distal two thirds of the femur, including the knee joint, are demonstrated (Fig. 29-20).

EVALUATION CRITERIA

The following should be clearly demonstrated:

- Majority of femur, including knee joint
- No knee rotation
- Adequate penetration of proximal portion of femur
- Any orthopedic appliance, such as plate and screw fixation

NOTE: If the entire length of the femur needs to be visualized, an AP projection of the proximal femur can be performed by placing a 35- × 43-cm grid lengthwise under the proximal femur and hip. The top of the grid is placed at the level of the ASIS to ensure that the hip joint is included. The central ray is directed to the center of the grid and long axis of the femur (see Fig. 29-2).

Fig. 29-20 Mobile AP femur radiograph showing a fracture of the midshaft with femoral rod placement. Note that the knee joint is included on the image.

Fig. 29-21 Mobile mediolateral left femur. An assistant wearing a lead apron holds and positions the right leg and femur and steadies the grid.

Fig. 29-22 Mobile lateromedial left femur. Note that the grid is placed between the legs and steadied by the patient.

▲ LATERAL PROJECTION*
Mediolateral or lateromedial
Dorsal decubitus position

The femur may not be able to be moved, which presents a challenge to the radiographer. The *mediolateral* projection is generally preferred because more of the proximal femur is demonstrated.

Image receptor: 35 × 43 cm grid lengthwise

Position of patient
- The patient is in the supine position.

Position of part
- Determine whether a mediolateral or lateromedial projection will be performed.
  #### Mediolateral projection
- Visualize the optimum length of the patient's femur by placing the grid in a vertical position next to the lateral aspect of the femur.
- Place the distal edge of the grid low enough to include the patient's knee joint.
- Have the patient, if able, hold the upper corner of the grid for stabilization; otherwise, support the grid firmly in position.
- Support the unaffected leg by using the patient's support (a trapeze bar if present) or a support block.
- Elevate the *unaffected* leg until the femur is nearly vertical. An assistant may need to elevate and hold the leg of a critically ill patient. The assistant may also steady the grid and must wear a lead apron for protection (Fig. 29-21).
  #### Lateromedial projection
- Place the grid next to the medial aspect of the affected femur (between the patient's legs), and ensure that the knee joint is included (Fig. 29-22).
- Ensure that the grid is placed *perpendicular* to the epicondylar plane.
- *Shield gonads.*
- *Respiration:* Suspend.

---

*The nonmobile projection is described in Chapter 6.

Central ray

- Perpendicular to the long axis of the femur, entering at its midpoint
- Ensure that the central ray and grid are aligned to prevent grid cutoff; the central ray is centered to the femur and not to the center of the grid

The thickest portion of the femur (proximal area) must be measured carefully, and an appropriate kVp must be selected to penetrate this area. The computer cannot form an image of any anatomy in this area if penetration does not occur. A light area of the entire proximal femur will result. Positioning the cathode over the proximal femur will improve CR image quality.

Structures shown

This projection demonstrates the distal two thirds of the femur, including the knee joint, without superimposition of the opposite thigh (Fig. 29-23).

EVALUATION CRITERIA

The following should be clearly demonstrated:

- Majority of femur, including knee joint
- Patella in profile
- Superimposition of femoral condyles
- Opposite femur and soft tissue out of area of interest
- Adequate penetration of proximal portion of femur
- Orthopedic appliance, if present

Fig. 29-23 Mobile lateral femur radiographs demonstrating midshaft fractures and femoral rod placement. Note that the knee joints are included on the image. **A,** Mediolateral. **B,** Lateromedial.

Fig. 29-24 Measuring caliper used to hold a 24 × 30 cm (10 × 12 inch) grid in place for mobile lateral cervical spine radiography.

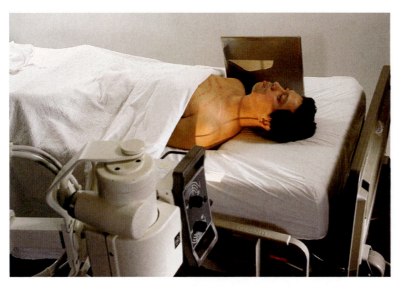

Fig. 29-25 Mobile lateral cervical spine.

♠ LATERAL PROJECTION*
Right or left dorsal decubitus position

Image receptor: 10 × 12 inch (24 × 30 cm) grid lengthwise; may be performed with a non-grid IR on smaller patients

Position of patient
- Position the patient in the supine position with arms extended down along the sides of the body.
- Observe whether a cervical collar or another immobilization device is being used. *Do not remove the device without the consent of the nurse or physician.*

Position of part
- Ensure that the upper torso, cervical spine, and head are not rotated.
- Place the grid lengthwise on the right or left side, parallel to the neck.
- Place the top of the grid approximately 1 inch (2.43 cm) above the external acoustic meatus (EAM) so that the grid is centered to C4 (upper thyroid cartilage).
- Raise the chin slightly. *In the patient with new trauma, suspected fracture, or known fracture of the cervical region, check with the physician before elevating the chin. Improper movement of a patient's head can disrupt a fractured cervical spine.*
- Immobilize the grid in a vertical position. The grid can be immobilized in multiple ways if a holding device is not available. The best method is to use the measuring caliper. Slide the long portion of the caliper under the shoulders of the patient, with the short end of the caliper pointing toward the ceiling and the grid held between the ends of the caliper (Fig. 29-24). Another method is to place pillows or a cushion between the side rail of the bed and the IR, thereby holding the IR next to the patient. Tape also works well in many instances (Fig. 29-25).
- Have the patient relax the shoulders and reach for the feet, if possible.
- *Shield gonads.*
- *Respiration:* Full expiration to obtain maximum depression of the shoulders.

---

*The nonmobile projection is described in Chapter 8.

Central ray

- Horizontal and perpendicular to the center of the grid. This should place the central ray at the level of C4 (upper thyroid cartilage).
- Ensure that proper alignment of the central ray and grid is maintained to prevent grid cutoff.
- Because of the great object–to–image-receptor distance (OID), an SID of 60 to 72 inches (158 to 183 cm) is recommended. This also helps demonstrate C7.

DIGITAL RADIOGRAPHY

To ensure that the lower cervical vertebrae are fully penetrated, the kVp must be set to penetrate the C7 area.

Structures shown

This projection demonstrates the seven cervical vertebrae, including the base of the skull and the soft tissues surrounding the neck (Fig. 29-26).

EVALUATION CRITERIA

The following should be clearly demonstrated:

- All seven cervical vertebrae, including interspaces and spinous processes
- Neck extended when possible so that rami of mandible are not overlapping C1 or C2
- C4 in center of grid
- Superimposed posterior margins of each vertebral body

NOTE: It is essential that C6 and C7 be included on the image. To accomplish this, the radiographer should instruct the patient to relax the shoulders toward the feet as much as possible. If the examination involves pulling down on the patient's arms, the radiographer should exercise extreme caution and evaluate the patient's condition carefully to determine whether pulling of the arms can be tolerated. Fractures or injuries of the upper limbs, including the clavicles, must be considered. Furthermore, applying a strong pull to the arms of a patient in a hurried or jerking manner can disrupt a fractured cervical spine. If the lateral projection does not adequately visualize the lower cervical region, the Twining method, sometimes referred to as the "swimmers" position, which eliminates pulling of the arms, may be recommended for individuals who have experienced trauma or have a known cervical fracture. One arm must be placed above the patient's head (see Twining method, Chapter 8).

Fig. 29-26 Mobile lateral cervical spine radiographs performed at the patient's bedside several weeks after trauma. **A,** Entire cervical spine shows slight anterior subluxation of the dens on the body of C2 *(arrow)*. **B,** Entire cervical spine shows a nearly vertical fracture through the body of C5 with slight displacement *(arrow)*. **C,** The first five cervical vertebrae show vertical fractures through posterior aspects of C2 laminae *(arrow)* with 4-mm displacement of the fragments. Earlier radiographs demonstrated that C6 and C7 were unaffected and did not need to be included in this follow-up radiograph.

Fig. 29-27 IR being placed on a special tray for placement below the infant. Numbers along the side of tray correspond with numbers along the side of the bed railing to allow accurate positioning of the IR.

🏿 AP PROJECTION

The chest and abdomen combination described here is typically ordered for neonatal premature infants who are in the neonatal intensive care unit. If a chest or abdomen projection is ordered separately, the radiographer should adjust the central ray and collimator accordingly.

Image receptor: 8 × 10 inch (20 × 24 cm) lengthwise

Position of patient

Position the infant supine in the center of the IR. Some bassinets have a special tray to hold the IR. Positioning numbers along the tray permits accurate placement of the IR (Fig. 29-27). If the IR is directly under the infant, cover it with a soft, warm blanket.

Fig. 29-28 Neonatal intensive care unit bassinet with premature infant. Overhead heating unit *(arrow)* is moved out of the way to accommodate the mobile x-ray machine tube head.

Mobile radiography

Position of part

- *Carefully* position the x-ray tube over the infant (Fig. 29-28).
- Ensure that the chest and abdomen are not rotated.
- Move the infant's arms away from the body or over the head and bring the legs down and away from the abdomen. The arms and legs may have to be held by a nurse, who should wear a lead apron.
- Leave the head of the infant rotated. (See note at end of this section.)
- Adjust the collimators closely to the chest and abdomen (Fig. 29-29).
- *Shield gonads.*
- *Respiration:* Inspiration. The neonatal infant has an extremely fast respiratory rate and cannot hold the breath. Make the best attempt possible to perform the exposure on full inspiration (Fig. 29-30).

Fig. 29-29 Mobile chest and abdomen radiograph of neonate. Note the male gonadal shield. (In actual practice the IR is covered with a soft, warm blanket.)

Fig. 29-30 Radiographs on inspiration and expiration in a neonatal infant. **A,** Left side of chest is shown at full expiration. Note the lack of normal lung markings and the illusion of massive pulmonary disease. The diaphragm is not seen, and the heart appears enlarged. **B,** Repeat radiograph of the same patient performed correctly at full inspiration. The diaphragm may be seen correctly at the level of the tenth posterior rib. The same technical factors were used for both exposures.

(Courtesy Department of Radiology, Rochester General Hospital, Rochester, NY; from Cullinan AM, Cullinan JE: *Producing quality radiographs,* ed 2, Philadelphia, 1994, Lippincott.)

Central ray

• Perpendicular to the midpoint of the chest and abdomen along the midsagittal plane

Structures shown

The anatomy of the entire chest and abdomen is demonstrated (Fig. 29-31).

EVALUATION CRITERIA

The following should be clearly demonstrated:

■ Anatomy from apices to pubic symphysis in the thoracic and abdominal regions
■ No motion
■ No blurring of lungs, diaphragm, and abdominal structures
■ No rotation of patient

NOTE: When performing an AP or lateral projection of the chest, the radiographer should keep the head and neck of the infant straight so that the anatomy in the upper chest and airway is accurately visualized. However, straightening the head of a neonatal infant in the supine position can inadvertently advance an endotracheal tube too far into the trachea. Therefore it is sometimes more important to leave the head of an intubated neonatal patient rotated in the position in which the infant routinely lies to obtain accurate representation of the position of the endotracheal tube on the radiograph.

Fig. 29-31 Mobile AP chest and abdomen radiograph of a neonate. The exposure technique demonstrates the anatomy of the entire chest and abdomen. Note the gonadal shield accurately positioned on this male infant (arrow).

⚜ LATERAL PROJECTION
Dorsal decubitus position

Image receptor: 8 × 10 inch (20 × 24 cm) lengthwise

Most neonatal premature infants cannot be turned on their sides or placed upright for a lateral projection.

Position of patient
- *Carefully* place the x-ray tube on the side of the bassinet.
- Position the infant supine on a radiolucent block covered with a soft, warm blanket. If a radiolucent block is not readily available, an inverted box of tissues works well.

Position of part
- Ensure that the infant's chest and abdomen are centered to the IR and not rotated.
- Move the infant's arms above the head. The arms will have to be held up by a nurse, who should wear a lead apron.
- Place the IR lengthwise and vertical beside the patient and then immobilize it.
- Leave the head of the infant rotated. (See note on p. 260).
- Adjust the collimators closely to the chest and abdomen (Fig. 29-32).
- *Shield gonads.*
- *Respiration:* Inspiration. The neonatal infant has an extremely fast respiratory rate and cannot hold the breath. Make the best attempt possible to perform the exposure on full inspiration.

Fig. 29-32 Mobile lateral chest and abdomen of a neonate in the dorsal decubitus position. The infant is positioned on a raised block with the IR below the block.

Central ray

- Horizontal and perpendicular to the midpoint of the chest and abdomen along the midcoronal plane

Structures shown

This projection demonstrates the anatomy of the entire chest and abdomen, with special attention to the costophrenic angles in the posterior chest. If present, air and fluid levels are visualized (Fig. 29-33).

EVALUATION CRITERIA

The following should be clearly demonstrated:

- Anatomy of chest and abdomen from apices to pubic bone
- No motion
- No blurring of lungs, diaphragm, and abdominal structures
- No rotation of patient
- Air and fluid levels, if present

Selected bibliography

Adler AM, Carlton RR: *Introduction to radiography and patient care,* Philadelphia, 1994, Saunders.

Bontrager KL: *Textbook of radiographic positioning,* ed 4, St Louis, 1997, Mosby.

Bushong SC: *Radiologic science for technologists,* ed 6, St Louis, 1997, Mosby.

Carlton RR, Adler AM: *Principles of radiographic imaging: an art and a science,* ed 2, Albany, NY, 1996, Delmar.

Cullinan AM, Cullinan JE: *Producing quality radiographs,* ed 2, Philadelphia, 1994, Lippincott.

Drafke MW: *Trauma and mobile radiography,* Philadelphia, 1990, FA Davis.

Ehrlich RA, McClosky ED: *Patient care in radiography,* ed 4, St Louis, 1997, Mosby.

Gray JE et al: *Quality control in diagnostic imaging,* Rockville, Md, 1983, Aspen.

Hall-Rollins J, Winters R: Mobile chest radiography: improving image quality, *Radiolog Technol* 71:5, 2000.

Kowalczyk N, Donnet K: *Introductory patient care for the imaging professional,* ed 2, St Louis, 1998, Mosby.

Statkiewicz-Sherer MA, Visconti PJ, Ritenour ER: *Radiation protection in medical radiography,* St Louis, 1998, Mosby.

Thompson MA et al: *Principles of imaging science and protection,* Philadelphia, 1994, Saunders.

Torres LS: *Basic medical techniques and patient care in imaging technology,* Philadelphia, 1997, Lippincott.

Fig. 29-33 Mobile lateral chest and abdomen radiograph of a neonate in the dorsal decubitus position. The exposure technique demonstrates the anatomy of the entire chest and abdomen.

30

SURGICAL RADIOGRAPHY

KARI J. WETTERLIN

JOEL A. PERMAR

Fluoroscopic image of cervical
spine in lateral projection showing plate and screws used to
fuse vertebrae.

Surgical radiology is a dynamic experience. The challenges a radiographer encounters in the surgical suite are unique. Knowing the machinery and its capabilities and limitations is most important; in that regard, the radiographer can enter any operating room (OR) case, whether routine or extraordinary, and, with good communication, be able to perform all tasks well. An understanding of common procedures and familiarity with equipment enables the radiographer to perform most mobile examinations ordered by the physician. Surgical radiography can be a challenging and exciting environment for the radiographer but can also be intimidating and stressful. Surgical radiology requires educated personnel familiar with specific equipment routinely used during common surgical procedures. It requires expertise in teamwork. Preparedness and familiarity with equipment are key. Standard health and safety protocols must be followed to avoid contamination and ensure patient safety. These are the basics, and the pieces come together in surgical radiology in distinctive ways.

This chapter focuses on the most common procedures performed in the surgical area. The basic principles of mobile imaging are detailed, and helpful suggestions are provided for successful completion of the examinations. This chapter is not intended to cover every possible combination of examinations or situations that a radiographer may encounter but rather to provide an overview of the surgical setting, as well as a summary of common examinations. The scope of radiologic examinations in a surgical setting is vast and may differ greatly among health care facilities (Box 30-1). Therefore the goals of this chapter are to (1) provide an overview of the surgical setting and explain the role of the radiographer as a vital member of the surgical team, (2) assist the radiographer in developing an understanding of the imaging equipment used in surgical situations, and (3) present common radiographic procedures performed in the OR.

The Surgical Team

At no other time will the patient be so well attended as during the surgical procedure. A surgeon, one or two assistants, a surgical technologist, an anesthesia provider, a circulating nurse, and various support staff surround the patient. These individuals, each with specific functions to perform, form the OR team. This team literally has the patient's life in its hands. The OR team has been described as a symphony orchestra, with each person an integral entity in unison and harmony with his or her colleagues for the successful accomplishment of the expected outcomes. The OR team is subdivided, according to the functions of its members, into sterile and nonsterile teams.

BOX 30-1

Scope of surgical radiography

Surgical fluoroscopic procedures
- Abdomen: cholangiogram
- Chest-line placement: bronchoscopy
- C-spine: anterior cervical discectomy and fusion
- Lumbar spine
- Hip: cannulated hip screws or hip pinning, decompression hip screw
- Femoral and tibial nailing
- Extremity fluoroscopy
- Humerus: shoulder in beach chair position
- Transsphenoidal resection of pituitary tumor
- Femoral/tibial arteriogram

Mobile surgical radiography procedures
- Localization examinations of cervical, thoracic, and lumbar spine
- Mobile extremity examinations in the operating room

STERILE TEAM MEMBERS

Sterile team members scrub their hands and arms, don a sterile gown and gloves over proper surgical attire, and enter the sterile field. The sterile field is the area of the OR that immediately surrounds and is specially prepared for the patient. To establish a sterile field, all items necessary for the surgical procedure are sterilized. After this process the scrubbed and sterile team members function within this limited area and handle only sterile items (Fig. 30-1). The sterile team consists of the following members:

- Surgeon: The surgeon is a licensed physician who is specially trained and qualified by knowledge and experience to perform surgical procedures. The surgeon's responsibilities include preoperative diagnosis and care, selection and performance of the surgical procedure, and postoperative management of care. The surgeon assumes full responsibility for all medical acts of judgment and for the management of the surgical patient.

- Surgical Assistant: The first assistant is a qualified surgeon or resident in an accredited surgical educational program. The assistant should be capable of assuming responsibility for performing the procedure for the primary surgeon. Assistants help to maintain visibility of the surgical site, control bleeding, close wounds, and apply dressings. The assistant's role varies depending on the institution, as well as with the type of procedure or surgical specialty.

- Physician Assistant: The physician assistant is a nonphysician allied health practitioner who is qualified by academic and clinical training to perform designated procedures in the OR and in other areas of surgical patient care.

- Certified Surgical Technologist (CST): The CST is responsible for maintaining the integrity, safety, and efficiency of the sterile field throughout the surgical procedure. The CST prepares and arranges instruments and supplies and assists the surgical procedure by providing the required sterile instruments and supplies. In some institutions a licensed practical nurse (LPN) or registered nurse (RN) may assume this role.

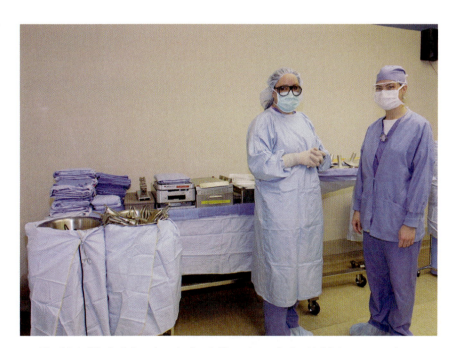

Fig. 30-1 OR staff showing sterile *(left)* and nonsterile *(right)* team members.

NONSTERILE TEAM MEMBERS

Nonsterile team members do not enter the sterile field; they function outside and around it. They assume responsibility for maintaining sterile techniques during the surgical procedure, but they handle supplies and equipment that are not considered sterile. Following the principles of aseptic technique, they keep the sterile team supplied, provide direct patient care, and respond to any requests that may arise during the surgical procedure.

- Anesthesia Provider: The anesthesia provider is an MD (anesthesiologist) or certified RN anesthetist who specializes in the art and science of administering anesthetics. Choosing and applying appropriate agents and suitable techniques of administration, monitoring physiologic functions, maintaining fluid and electrolyte balance, and performing blood replacements are essential responsibilities of the anesthesia provider during the surgical procedure.

- Circulator: The circulator is preferably an RN. The circulator monitors and coordinates all activities within the OR, provides supplies to the CST during the surgical procedure, and manages the care of the patient.
- Radiographers: The radiographer's role in the OR is to provide intraoperative imaging in a variety of examinations and with various types of equipment.
- Others: The OR team may also include biomedical technicians, monitoring technologists, and individuals specialized in equipment or monitoring devices necessary during the surgical procedure.

Proper Surgical Attire

Surgical attire protocols may change from institution to institution but should be available for review, understood, and followed by all staff. Although some small variances in protocol exist among institutions, there are common standards.

Large amounts of bacteria are present in the nose and mouth, on the skin, and on the attire of personnel who enter the restricted areas of the surgical setting. Proper facility design and surgical attire regulations are important ways of preventing transportation of microorganisms into surgical settings, where they may infect patients' open wounds. Infection control practices also involve personal measures including personal fitness for work, skin disinfection (patient and personnel), preparation of personnel hands, surgical attire, and personal technique (surgical conscience). Daily body cleanliness and clean, dandruff-free hair help prevent superficial wound infections.

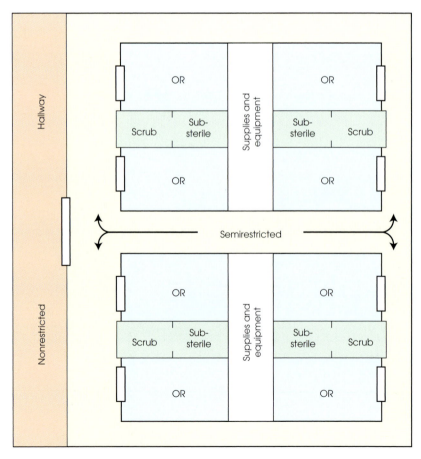

Fig. 30-2 Operating suite layout showing restricted, nonrestricted, and semirestricted areas. Operating rooms (OR) are "restricted."

Operating Room Attire

The OR should have specific written policies and procedures for proper attire to be worn within the semirestricted and restricted areas of the OR suite. The dress code should include aspects of personal hygiene important to environmental control. Protocol is strictly monitored so that everyone conforms to established policy.

Street clothes should never be worn within semirestricted or restricted areas of the surgical suite (Fig. 30-2). Clean, fresh attire should be donned at the beginning of each shift in the OR suite and as needed if the attire becomes wet or grossly soiled. Soiled surgical attire should be changed to reduce the potential of cross-infection. Bloodstained or soiled attire including shoe covers is unattractive and can also be a source of cross-infection or contamination. Soiled attire is not worn outside of the OR suite, and steps should be taken to remove soiled clothing immediately on exiting. OR attire should not be hung in a locker for wearing a second time. Underclothing should be clean and totally covered by the scrub suit (Fig. 30-3). Other aspects of proper attire include the following:

- Protective eyewear: OSHA regulations require eyewear to be worn when contamination from blood or body fluids is possible.
- Masks: Masks should be worn at all times in the OR but are not necessary in all semirestricted areas.
- Shoe covers: Shoe covers should be worn when contamination from blood or body fluids can be reasonably anticipated. Shoe covers should be changed whenever they become torn, soiled, or wet and should be removed before leaving the surgical area.
- Caps: Caps should be worn to cover and contain hair at all times in the restricted and semirestricted areas of the OR suite. Hoods are also available to cover hair, such as facial hair, that cannot be contained by a cap and mask.
- Gloves: Gloves should be worn when contact with blood or body substances is anticipated.
- Radiation badge and proper identification should be worn at all times.

PERSONAL HYGIENE

A person with an acute infection, such as a cold, open cold sore, or sore throat, is known to be a carrier of transmittable conditions and should not be permitted within the OR suite. Daily body cleanliness and clean hair are also important because good personal hygiene helps to prevent transportation of microbial fallout that can cause open wound infections.

Fig. 30-3 Properly attired radiographers with protective eyewear.

The Dance of the Operating Room

The concepts of sterile and aseptic technique date back to Hippocrates, who boiled wine and water to pour into open wounds in an attempt to prevent infection. Galen changed the technique a bit and began boiling the instruments instead, and shortly thereafter Semmelweis noted a dramatic decline in postoperative infection by having the staff wash their hands and change gowns between surgical procedures.

Maintaining the sterile field in an operating suite can be like a well-choreographed dance when the team works well together. Certain moves and rules must be followed. Proper adherence to aseptic technique eliminates or minimizes modes and sources of contamination. Basic principles must be observed during the surgical procedure to provide the patient with a well-defined margin of safety. Everyone who cares for patients must carry out effective hospital and OR infection control programs. Infection control involves a wide variety of concepts including methods of environmental sanitation and maintenance of facilities; cleanliness of the air and equipment in the suite; cleanliness of the skin and apparel of patients, surgeons, and personnel; sterility of surgical equipment; strict aseptic technique; and careful observance of procedural rules and regulations.

Up to 10,000 microbial particles can be shed from the skin per minute. Therefore nonsterile team members should not reach over a sterile field. When working over the sterile field (e.g., performing a posteroanterior [PA] lumbar spine), the sterile field should be covered with a sterile drape to protect the field (Fig. 30-4). Only after the sterile cover is in place can the technologist move the radiographic equipment into position over the sterile field. A sterile team member should fold over the sterile drape on itself, and then a nonsterile team member should carefully remove the covering drape, being careful not to compromise the sterile field. If a sterile field is compromised, the OR staff should be notified immediately.

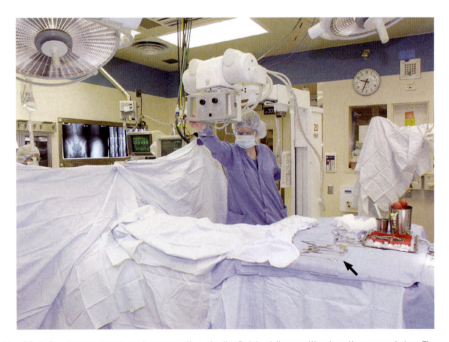

Fig. 30-4 Radiographer leaning over the sterile field while positioning the x-ray tube. The sterile incision site over which the radiographer works is properly covered to maintain a sterile field. Note the sterile instruments in the foreground *(arrow)*. The radiographer should never move radiographic equipment over uncovered sterile instruments or an uncovered surgical site.

Communication is of utmost importance. As a result of the surgical sterile field, the radiographer is unable to help position the image receptor (IR) or the patient. Therefore good, professional communication is essential while using sound, basic knowledge of anatomy and positioning. The radiographer may have to instruct the surgeon or resident on the proper position to best visualize the desired portion of the anatomy. For example, a surgeon or resident may not be aware of the exact rotation and foot flexion required to achieve a proper mortise view of the ankle.

PROPER IMAGE RECEPTOR HANDLING IN THE STERILE FIELD

To maintain proper universal precautions, the radiographer must follow specific steps when handling an IR in the OR.

Surgical technologist (CST) taking the IR: The CST will hold a sterile IR cover open toward the radiographer. The radiographer should hold one end of the IR while placing the other end of the IR into the sterile IR cover. The CST will grasp the IR and wrap the protective cover securely (Fig. 30-5).

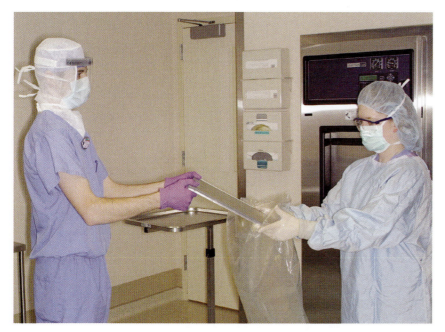

Fig. 30-5 Radiographer and CST place the IR into the sterile drape.

A

B

Fig. 30-6 A, Radiographer correctly removes the IR from the now-contaminated bag to a clean table, being careful not to brush contaminants from bag onto self or others. **B,** Radiographer disposes of the bag and removes contaminated gloves before handling the IR.

Radiographer accepting the IR after exposure: After the exposure is made, the radiographer will need to retrieve the IR. The radiographer must be wearing gloves to accept a covered IR that has been in the sterile field or under an open incision. The protective cover is possibly contaminated with blood or body fluids and should be treated accordingly. The radiographer should grasp the IR, open the protective cover carefully away from himself or herself or others so as not to spread blood or body fluids, and then slide the IR out of the cover (Fig. 30-6). The radiographer should dispose of the IR cover in a proper receptacle and remember to remove the gloves before handling the IR or any other equipment because the gloves are now considered contaminated. If contamination of the IR occurs, the radiographer should use hospital-approved disinfectant for cleaning before leaving the OR (Box 30-2).

ENEMIES OF THE STERILE FIELD

Lengthy or complex procedures increase the chance of sterile field contamination. Physical limitations, such as crowding, poor lighting, and staffing levels, are also a consideration. The floor is always considered contaminated. Therefore the radiographer should avoid placing IRs, lead aprons, and shields on the floor.

BOX 30-2

Principles of aseptic techniques

- Only sterile items are used within the sterile field.

- Only sterile persons handle sterile items or touch sterile areas.

- Nonsterile persons touch only unsterile items or areas.

- Movement within or around a sterile field must not contaminate the sterile field.

- Items of doubtful sterility must be considered unsterile.

- When a sterile barrier is permeated, it must be considered contaminated.

- Sterile gowns are considered sterile in front from the shoulder to the level of the sterile field, and at the sleeves from the elbow to the cuff.

- Tables are sterile only at table level.

- Radiographers should not walk between two sterile fields if at all possible.

- Radiographers should avoid turning their backs toward the sterile field in compromised spaces.

- Watch the front of clothing when it is necessary to be next to the patient.

- Be aware of machinery close to the sterile field including lead aprons hanging from the portable machine that may swing toward the sterile field.

- Secure the lead apron if wearing it next to the sterile field. The apron can easily slip forward when raising one's arms up to position the tube. A properly worn apron does not compromise the sterile field or jeopardize proper body mechanics.

- When positioning an IR under the OR table, the radiographer should not lift the sterile drapes above table level because this would compromise the sterile field.

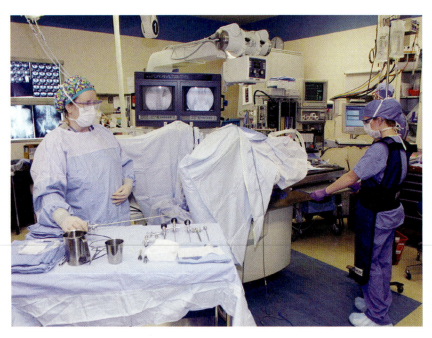

Fig. 30-7 In-room urologic radiographic equipment used for retrograde ureterograms.

Fig. 30-8 C-arm radiographic/fluoroscopic system used in the OR.

Equipment

The radiographer must be well acquainted with the radiologic equipment. Some procedures may seldom occur. The radiographer need not fear a rare procedure if good communication and equipment knowledge are in place. IR holders enable the radiographer to perform cross-table projections on numerous cases and eliminate the unnecessary exposure of personnel who may volunteer to hold the IR. In mobile radiography, exposure times may increase for larger patients and a holder eliminates the chance of motion from hand-held situations.

Some operating suites, such as those used for stereotactic or urologic cases, have dedicated radiologic equipment (Fig. 30-7). However, a majority of the radiographic examinations in the OR are performed with mobile equipment.

Mobile image machines are not as sophisticated as larger stationary machines in the radiology department. Mobile fluoroscopic units, many times referred to as *C-arms* because of their shape (Fig. 30-8), are commonplace in the surgical suite. Mobile radiography is also widely used in the OR.

Cleaning of the Equipment

The x-ray equipment should be cleaned after each surgical case. If at all possible, the radiographer should clean the mobile image machine, including the base, in the OR suite, especially when the equipment is obviously contaminated with blood or surgical scrub solution. Cleaning within the OR helps reduce the possibility of cross contamination. The x-ray equipment must be cleaned with a hospital-approved cleaning solution. Cleaning solutions should not be sprayed in the OR suite during the surgical procedure. If cleaning is necessary during the surgical procedure, opening the cleaning container and pouring the solution on a rag for use prevents possible contamination from scattered spray. Gloves should always be worn during cleaning. The underside of the image machine should be checked to make sure contaminants that might have splashed up from the floor are removed. Cleaning the equipment after an isolation case is necessary to prevent the spread of contaminants. All less-used equipment should undergo a thorough cleaning at least once a week and just before being taken into the OR.

Radiation Exposure Considerations

Radiation protection for the radiographer, others in the immediate area, and the patient is of paramount importance when mobile fluoroscopic examinations are performed. The radiographer should wear a lead apron and stand as far away from the patient, x-ray tube, and useful beam as the procedure, OR, and exposure cable allow. The single most effective means of radiation protection is *distance.* The recommended *minimal* distance is 6 feet (2 m). When possible, the radiographer should stand at a right angle (90 degrees) to the primary beam and the object being radiographed. The least amount of scatter radiation occurs at this position. The greatest amount of scatter radiation occurs on the tube side of the fluoroscopic machine. Therefore it is recommended that the x-ray tube always be placed *under the patient* (Fig. 30-9). Because of the significant amount of exposure to the facial and neck region, the x-ray tube should never be placed above the patient unless absolutely necessary.

The OR may have signs posted outside the room warning of radiation in use, or "lead aprons required when entering this room." Lead protection should be provided for individuals who are unable to leave the room.

The patient's gonads should be shielded with appropriate radiation protection devices during examinations in which shielding will not interfere with imaging of the anatomy that must be demonstrated. Remember, when using fluoroscopic equipment with the tube *under* the table, shielding should be placed under the patient. In addition, the source-to-skin distance (SSD) should not be less than 12 inches (30 cm).

Fluoroscopic Procedures for the Operating Room

OPERATIVE (IMMEDIATE) CHOLANGIOGRAPHY

Operative cholangiography, introduced by Mirizzi in 1932, is carried out during biliary tract surgery. After the bile has been drained, and in the absence of obstruction, this technique permits the major intrahepatic ducts and the extrahepatic ducts to be filled with contrast medium.

The value of operative cholangiography is such that it has become an integral part of biliary tract surgery. It is used to investigate the patency of the bile ducts and the functional status of the sphincter of the hepatopancreatic ampulla to reveal the presence of calculi that cannot be detected by palpation and to demonstrate such conditions as small intraluminal neoplasms and stricture or dilation of the ducts. When the pancreatic duct shares a common channel with the distal common bile duct before emptying into the duodenum, it is sometimes seen on operative cholangiograms because it has been partially filled by reflux.

After exposing, draining, and exploring the biliary tract, and frequently after excising the gallbladder, the surgeon injects the contrast medium. This solution is usually introduced into the common bile duct through a needle; small catheter; or, after cholecystectomy, through an inlaying T tube. When the latter route is used, the procedure is referred to as *delayed operative* or *operative T-tube cholangiography.*

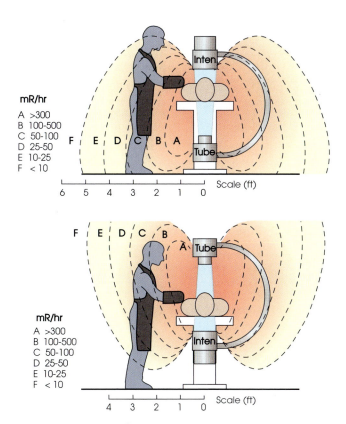

mR/hr
A >300
B 100-500
C 50-100
D 25-50
E 10-25
F < 10

Fig. 30-9 Radiation safety with the C-arm. In the upper image, less radiation reaches the facial and neck region when the x-ray tube is *under the patient.* This is the recommended position of the C-arm. Note that in the lower image there is a greater amount of radiation reaching the facial and neck regions.

(From Giese RA, Hunter DW: Personnel exposure during fluoroscopy, *Postgrad Radiol* 8:162, 1988.)

A,

B,

Position of patient

The patient is supine with the abdomen exposed. In laparoscopic cases, such as cholecystectomy, the abdomen is distended because air is injected into the abdominal cavity to allow adequate room for maneuvering of the camera and instruments. The radiographer should make sure no obstacles will impede the movement of the C-arm (Fig. 30-10).

NOTE: The radiographer should shield pregnant patients. The central ray comes from under the table, so the lead shield should be placed under the patient and placed so as not to obscure any pertinent anatomy.

Position of C-arm

Center the C-arm in the PA projection over the right side of the abdomen below the rib line. The patient may be tilted to the left or in the Trendelenburg position to aid in the flow of contrast to the complete biliary system. The C-arm should be tilted or canted until the PA projection is achieved. The C-arm may also have to be rotated to ensure that the spine does not obscure the biliary system. Once the position is obtained, the surgeon injects contrast into the duct system under fluoroscopy. The radiographer should do the following:

- Provide radiation protection for all persons in the room.
- Bring an adequate number of IRs for immediate processing of all images.
- Remember that examination is optimal with suspended respiration, but due to the length of time it may take for contrast to fill all ducts, respiration may be continued throughout the examination.

Fig. 30-10 A, C-arm in correct position for an abdominal cholangiogram. Assistant surgeon checks the syringe for air bubbles before handing it to surgeon for injection. Note that the radiographer positioned the fluoroscopic image intensifier *(arrows)* carefully to avoid hitting laparoscopic instruments protruding from the patient's abdomen.
B, Surgeon standing behind a sterile, draped lead shield injecting contrast media for an operative cholangiogram.

Structures shown

This examination shows the biliary system full of contrast including a portion of the cystic duct, the branches of the hepatic duct, the common bile duct, and often the pancreatic duct.

- Biliary system should be completely filled with contrast (Fig. 30-11).
- No extravasation of contrast occurs at the injection site.
- Biliary system should not be obscured by any extraneous anatomy or instrumentation.
- Prompt emptying of contrast into the duodenum occurs.
- Proper radiographic technique is maintained.
- Sterile field is maintained.

Fig. 30-11 Hard copy images of anatomy visualized during a cholangiogram using fluoroscopy. **A,** Intraoperative cholangiogram. **B,** Intraoperative cholangiogram showing the pancreatic duct *(arrow)*.

Fluoroscopic procedures for the operating room

CHEST (LINE PLACEMENT, BRONCHOSCOPY)

Position of patient

The patient is supine with the arms secured at his or her sides. The radiographer should be certain there are no bars or supports in the table that will obscure the view of the chest. Allow room under the table for the C-arm to maneuver.

Position of C-arm

The C-arm should be covered with a sterile drape before entering the field. The C-arm will enter the sterile field perpendicular to the patient and in position for a PA projection. If the surgeon prefers, the radiographer can reverse or invert the image to obtain anatomic position. Radiation protection should be provided for all persons in the room.

- Line placement: Find the point of insertion and follow the catheter to its end. This examination is done to ensure there are no kinks in the catheter and to show it is in proper position. A number of catheters may be used in the OR. They are usually inserted to deliver medicines to chronically ill patients.
- Rigid and flexible bronchoscopy: may be done to perform biopsies, place stents, or dilate the bronchi.

Structures shown

Structures shown include all anatomy of the chest cavity including the heart, lung fields, and ribs and any instrumentation that may be introduced during the procedure. These may include catheters, guide wires, bronchoscopes, stent devices, dilatation balloons, or biopsy instruments.

EVALUATION CRITERIA

- Pertinent parts of the chest are distinguished easily (Fig. 30-12).
- Proper radiographic technique and contrast are maintained on the monitor.
- Image on monitor is in true anatomic position or per the physician's preference.
- Sterile technique is maintained.

Fig. 30-12 Patient and C-arm in position for a Hickman catheter placement. Introduction of the catheter begins in the upper thorax and is completed with the catheter in the heart.

C-SPINE (ACDF)

Position of patient

The patient is supine with the chin elevated and the neck in flexion. The patient's arms will be at his or her sides and may be pulled in traction to help keep the shoulders from obscuring the spine.

Position of C-arm

PA projection

Cover the C-arm with sterile drape. Enter the sterile field perpendicular to the patient. Tilt the C-arm 15 degrees cephalad and center the beam over the C-spine. Raise the C-arm to allow the surgeon to work if necessary. Make sure the spine is in the center of the monitor and the top of spine and skull are at the top of the screen with no rotation.

Lateral projection

Rotate the C-arm under the table into lateral position with the beam parallel to the floor. Angle the C-arm either cephalad or caudal to obtain a true lateral view. Raise or lower the C-arm to bring the spine into the center of the field of view. Rotate the image on the monitor to the same plane as the patient with the spine parallel with the floor. Cases in which a PA projection is not necessary may opt to have the C-arm positioned in "rainbow" fashion or arched over the patient (Fig. 30-13).

- Be certain there are no obstacles under the table that impede movement of the C-arm.
- The C-arm is often positioned before the patient is draped. In this case the surgical team drapes the C-arm into the sterile field. Make sure the C-arm can be moved out of the way without disturbing any instrumentation.

Structures shown

These positions show the affected area of the C-spine, as well as any hardware that may be introduced (Fig. 30-14). Because this surgery is most often performed to repair physiologic defects, abnormalities (e.g., osteophytes, degenerated disk spaces, subluxation) may be visible, especially in the lateral view.

EVALUATION CRITERIA

- ■ C-spine and its affected part are in the center of the monitor to maintain proper radiographic technique.
- ■ Image is rotated in the same plane as patient.
- ■ PA projection should show spinous processes in the center of spinous bodies.
- ■ Lateral projection should show the bodies in profile and the interarticular facets aligned.
- ■ Sterile field is maintained.

Fig. 30-13 C-arm placed in "rainbow" position for cervical procedures.

Fig. 30-14 Fluoroscopic image of cervical spine in lateral projection showing plate and screws used to fuse vertebrae.

LUMBAR SPINE

Position of patient

The patient is prone and positioned on chest rolls or a frame to flex the spine. His or her arms are placed on arm boards and located by the head of the table to bring them out of the field of view.

Position of C-arm

AP projection

Cover the C-arm with a sterile drape. The C-arm enters the field perpendicular to the patient. Center the beam in the AP projection over the affected area of the spine. Raise the C-arm to leave enough room between the IR and the patient so that the surgeon can work without being obstructed (Fig. 30-15). Be certain there is nothing in or under the table to impair the view of the spine.

A

B

C

Fig. 30-15 **A,** C-arm correctly placed in the rainbow position for lateral lumbar procedures. The rainbow position is used especially for larger patients in which the table or size of the patient would not allow enough elevation of the C-arm to include the lumbar spine. **B,** C-arm positioned under the table. **C,** C-arm positioned for AP projection of the lumbar spine.

Lateral projection

- Rotate the C-arm under the table into lateral position. Raise or lower the C-arm to bring the spine into the center of the monitor. The C-arm may need to be angled cephalad or caudal to obtain true lateral projection. Rotate the image on the monitor until the image is in same plane as the patient. The C-arm may be arched over the patient for the lateral projection, especially on hypersthenic patients because rotating the C-arm under the table would not allow a great enough height to visualize the lumbar region.
- The surgical team will place sterile drapes over both ends of the C-arm when they drape the patient.

Structures shown

These projections show the affected area of the spine, which includes the bodies, disk spaces, spinous processes, lamina, pedicles, and facets. When the case is completed there will be hardware in the spine, such as rods, plates, and screws, to hold the spine in alignment. A bone graft or interbody fusion device may also exist in the disk space to fuse the bones together (Fig. 30-16).

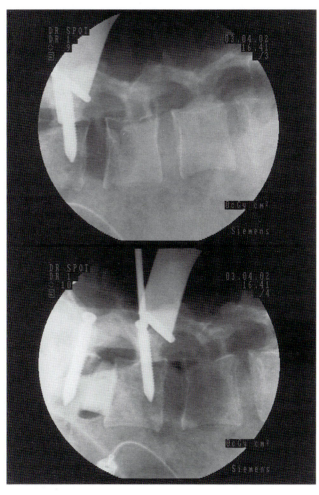

Fig. 30-16 Fluoroscopic hard copy lateral projection image of the lumbar spine with instrumentation.

Fig. 30-17 AP projection fluoroscopic images during laparoscopic lumbar fusion.

HIP (CANNULATED HIP SCREWS OR HIP PINNING)

Position of patient

The patient is supine with the legs abducted and the affected leg held in traction. The patient's arm on the affected side is crossed over the body to be kept out of the field of view.

- These procedures are often done using an isolation drape or "shower curtain." In these cases it is not necessary to cover the C-arm with a sterile drape; however, a nonsterile bag over the tube is recommended to prevent Betadine staining of the C-arm.
- The radiographer is positioned between the patient's legs to make sure the patient is covered completely for privacy.

Position of C-arm

Position the C-arm between the patient's legs and center the beam over the affected hip (Fig. 30-18). To obtain the lateral projection, rotate the C-arm under the leg and table to a lateral position (Fig. 30-19). Do not dislodge any instrumentation when rotating the C-arm.

Fig. 30-18 C-arm positioned for PA projection of the hip.

Fig. 30-19 C-arm properly positioned for lateral projection of the hip. After preliminary images are obtained, the hip is prepared for incision and the C-arm is sterile draped.

- Before the procedure, the surgeon will manipulate the leg under fluoroscopy to reduce the fracture (Fig. 30-20).
- The C-arm may have to be manipulated to achieve projections and may not be in true PA or lateral projection. Note the position of the C-arm on PA and lateral projections to return to this angle when necessary.
- When hardware is in the hip, rotate the C-arm under fluoroscopy to ensure that no hardware is in the hip joint space.

Fig. 30-20 PA projection of the hip with fracture of the femoral neck.

Structures shown

This examination shows all parts of the proximal femur and hip joint including the acetabular rim, femoral head and neck, and greater and lesser trochanters. Hardware may include cannulated screws or pins running parallel with the femoral neck used to reduce the fracture (Fig. 30-21).

- Hip is centered on monitor and in correct plane.
- Lateral side of femur and acetabular rim must be visualized to determine a starting point and to ensure no hardware enters the joint.
- Lesser trochanter is visible in profile on PA projection. Greater trochanter lies behind the femoral neck and shaft in lateral view.
- Proper radiographic technique is maintained.
- Sterile field is maintained.
- Radiation protection is provided.

A   B

Fig. 30-21 PA projection **(A)** and lateral projection **(B)** fluoroscopic hard copy images of a hip fracture reduction.

FEMUR NAIL

Position of patient and C-arm

During this procedure a rod is inserted into the intramedullary (IM) canal to reduce a fracture of the shaft of the femur (Fig. 30-22). This rod or nail can be introduced either antegrade through the greater trochanter or retrograde through the popliteal notch.

Antegrade femoral nailing

During antegrade nailing the patient is either supine or in the lateral position. In the supine position the affected leg will most likely be in traction to help reduce the fracture. The legs will be abducted, and the unaffected leg will be flexed at the knee and hip and raised to allow the C-arm enough room to enter the sterile field. The patient's arm on the injured side is draped across the chest to keep it from obstructing the surgeon. With the patient in lateral position, the affected leg is extended forward to clear the opposite leg. If the patient is supine, the C-arm is positioned between the patient's legs, parallel to the unaffected leg, and centered over the hip. The C-arm may have to be rotated forward or backward to obtain a true PA projection. Rotate the C-arm under the table for a lateral projection.

Antegrade with the patient in the lateral position requires the radiographer to enter the sterile field and rotate the C-arm under the table to find a PA projection of the femur. Lateral projection is achieved with the tube starting in a true PA projection, rotating the C-arm forward 10 to 15 degrees, and tilting it 5 to 10 degrees cephalad.

Fig. 30-22 Image of a midshaft femoral fracture with guide rod being inserted to align the fracture.

Retrograde femoral nailing

During the retrograde femoral nailing, the patient is supine with the injured leg exposed and the knee flexed and supported with a bump. This position allows the surgeon access to the popliteal notch without injuring the patella.

The sterile field is entered with the C-arm perpendicular to the patient. Tilt the C-arm cephalad to account for the flexed knee and to find PA projection. The C-arm is rotated under the table for lateral position (Fig. 30-23).

Method

• Instruments or hardware may protrude from the operation site. Be certain to avoid disturbing these instruments or hardware or allowing them to puncture a sterile drape.
• Center the C-arm over the fracture site during canal reaming to ensure that the fracture remains reduced (Fig. 30-24).
• The table must allow for movement of the C-arm from the knee to the hip.
• Allow enough room between the patient and C-arm for the surgeon to work.

Screws will be inserted into the femur and through the nail to fix the nail in place. When lining up the screw holes in the nail, the hole should be perfectly round and not oblong. Center the screw hole on the monitor. The magnification feature may be used to give the surgeon a better view. The C-arm may need to be tilted or rotated to obtain perfect circles. The surgeon will also manipulate the leg to help align the screw holes. Once the screws are inserted, check the length of the screws by placing the C-arm in PA projection. Screws should not protrude excessively from the cortical bone (Fig. 30-25).

A

B

Fig. 30-23 A, C-arm positioned between patient's legs for a PA projection during femoral nailing. *Arrow* is pointing to the femur. **B,** C-arm rotated under femur *(arrow)* for a lateral projection.

Fig. 30-24 Image of femur fracture during canal reaming.

Structures shown

All parts of the femur including the greater and lesser trochanters, the femoral neck, shaft, and condyles are seen in the PA and lateral positions. Different instrumentation will be in the IM canal beginning with a guide rod that is used to help reduce the fracture and provide a means for the canal reamers to pass through the fracture site (Fig. 30-26). After reduction, the nail and screws are seen.

Fig. 30-25 PA projection of proximal screw in a femoral nail.

Fig. 30-26 PA projection of a femur fracture reduced with guide rod and distal interlocking screws inserted.

Fluoroscopic procedures for the operating room

285

TIBIA (NAIL)

Position of patient

The patient is supine with the affected leg exposed. The knee is flexed to allow access to the tibial tuberosity without injuring the patella. The injured leg is on the opposite side of the table so that the C-arm does not interfere with the surgical team.

Position of C-arm

Cover the C-arm with a sterile drape. Move the C-arm into the field perpendicular to the patient. Center the beam over the leg and tilt the tube to match the angle of the leg (Fig. 30-27). No obstructions should be under the table to avoid interfering with the C-arm movement. Rotate the C-arm under the table and into the lateral position, making certain not to disturb any instrumentation protruding from the operative site. Center the leg on the monitor by raising or lowering the C-arm. The surgeon will manipulate the leg, and the radiographer will tilt or rotate the C-arm to obtain round holes (Figs. 30-28 and 30-29). Use the magnification feature to enlarge the image if necessary. Advance the C-arm until its tube side is far enough from the injured leg to allow the surgeon to fit the drill and drill bit into the area.

- Along its shaft the tibia is triangular shaped, so when checking the length of the screws the C-arm may have to be rotated forward or back to get a true length.
- Center the beam on the fracture site during canal reaming. Once the leg is in the center of the monitor, turn the wheels of the C-arm horizontally to allow the machine to move longitudinally down the shaft of the leg without moving out of the field of view.

Fig. 30-27 C-arm positioned for tibial nailing. Note that the radiographer tilted the fluoroscopic image intensifier to be parallel with the long axis of the leg.

Fig. 30-28 Image of tibial nail screw holes in incorrect alignment and oblong in shape.

Fig. 30-29 Image of tibial nail screw holes perfectly round and magnified to assist proper alignment.

Structures shown

Structures shown include the tibia and fibula, the tibial shaft along with any fracture, the tibial plateau, tibial tuberosity, distal tibia, and ankle joint (Fig. 30-30). After hardware is inserted, the tibial nail will fill the IM canal, with proximal and distal screws prominent.

Fig. 30-30 A, Improper alignment of distal screw holes. **B,** Screw holes properly aligned with screwdriver over distal screw hole.

Fluoroscopic procedures for the operating room

HUMERUS

Position of patient

The patient is supine or in a reclining or beach chair position (Fig. 30-31). The injured arm may be resting on a Mayo stand with the surgeon's assistant holding the arm to stabilize and align the humerus. The patient should be positioned with the shoulder off the side of the table. This position allows the humerus to be seen in its entirety without being obscured by the table.

Position of C-arm

Cover the C-arm with a sterile drape. Enter the field parallel to, or at a 45-degree angle to, the patient. The assistant will rotate the arm medially with the elbow bent 90 degrees. The C-arm is tilted and rotated to obtain a true lateral projection, depending on the angle of patient position. The arm is held at the elbow to provide support, and the arm is rotated until the hand is pointing upward. The C-arm is tilted to obtain PA projection according to the patient's angle. Center the beam on the humerus.

- When installing a nail or rod into the humerus and trying to locate and center the distal screws, place a sterile drape over the tube or pull the sheets draping the patient over the tube. Only touch the underside of the sheets when placing them over the tube. Raise the tube to magnify the screw holes and to allow the surgeon to work.

Fig. 30-31 C-arm positioned for patient in beach chair position for preliminary imaging.

NOTE: Do not leave any drape over the tube for a long time to prevent unnecessary heat buildup in the tube.

• Be careful not to strike the patient's head with the image intensifier.

Structures shown

This procedure should show all parts of the humerus including the head, neck, greater and lesser tubercles, shaft, and distal portion of the humerus. Also seen are any fractures and the hardware used for repair (Fig. 30-32).

■ Angle of humerus and C-arm coincide to obtain true PA and lateral projections.
■ When nailing the distal screws, holes should be perfectly round to allow screws to pass through the nail.
■ Humerus is in the center of the monitor to maintain radiographic technique.
■ Image is rotated in the same plane as the humerus.
■ Sterile field is maintained, especially with the proximity of possibly nonsterile portions of the tube to the sterile field.
■ Radiation protection is provided for surgical team.

Fig. 30-32 A, Images of a humeral fracture with nails used to reduce the fracture of the humeral head. **B,** Image of a clavicle fracture with plate and screw fixation.

Fluoroscopic procedures for the operating room

TRANSSPHENOIDAL RESECTION OF PITUITARY TUMOR

Position of patient

The patient is supine with the arms down at the sides. The head will either be on the table or off the end of the table and held in a halo. The head will be tilted toward the surgical team slightly, and the chin will be extended upward.

Position of C-arm

The C-arm is placed into position before the procedure begins. The C-arm will enter perpendicular to the patient. Rotate the tube into the lateral position. Tilt and rotate the C-arm to obtain true lateral position. Center the beam on the temporal bone to put the sella turcica in the middle of the monitor. The x-ray tube should be positioned closer to the skull to magnify the view of the pituitary region. Lock the machine in place (Fig. 30-33). The C-arm position is demonstrated during the actual procedure in Fig. 30-34.

Fig. 30-33 **A,** C-arm positioned for transsphenoidal tumor removal. **B,** Transsphenoidal tumor removal with scope in place.

Structures shown

The skull is shown in lateral projection with concentration on the area of the pituitary gland. The sella turcica, base of the skull, orbits, maxillary sinuses, and portions of the C-spine and mandible are also seen.

EVALUATION CRITERIA

- True lateral view of the skull is shown with the sella turcica in the center of the monitor.
- Orbits, sphenoid wings, and maxillary sinuses are superimposed.
- Proper radiographic technique is maintained.
- Surgical team should maintain sterile field when the machine is draped into the sterile field.
- Image of the skull should be in the same plane as patient.

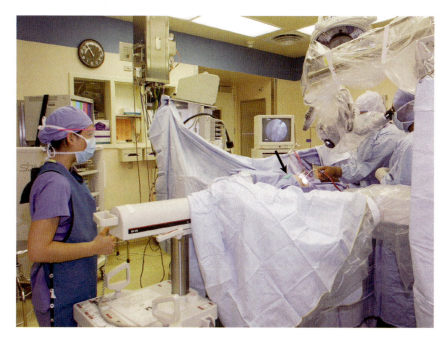

Fig. 30-34 C-arm sterile draped and positioned for transsphenoidal tumor removal. Patient's head is indicated by arrow.

FEMORAL/TIBIAL ARTERIOGRAM

Position of patient

The patient is supine with the affected leg exposed from the groin area to the foot. There should be enough room under the table to allow the C-arm to move from the hip to the foot. The leg may be rotated medially or laterally to keep the femur or tibia from obscuring any vasculature (Fig. 30-35).

Position of C-arm

Cover the C-arm with a sterile drape and enter the field perpendicular to the patient. Once the leg is in the center of the monitor, turn the wheels of the C-arm horizontally to allow the machine to move to the left or right without taking the leg out of the field of view. Use the subtraction or road-mapping feature to remove all structures except the contrast that is injected into the artery (Fig. 30-36). This feature shows any stenoses or injuries to the artery.

Fig. 30-35 Subtraction image of a surgical femoral artery angiogram with stenosis (arrow).

Structures shown

The bones of the leg are seen before subtraction. After contrast is introduced the femoral artery and its branches are seen, and, following the contrast down the leg, the popliteal and tibial arteries are seen. The contrast images show any pathologic defects in the arterial structures.

EVALUATION CRITERIA

- All pertinent vasculature must be shown without being obscured by the table or bones of the leg.
- Integrity of the mask image should be maintained by not moving the leg or the C-arm during subtraction or road mapping.
- Proper radiographic technique is maintained.
- Sterile field is maintained.
- Radiation protection is provided for surgical team.

Fig. 30-36 Subtraction image of a surgical femoral artery angiogram after balloon angioplasty.

Mobile Radiography Procedures for the Operating Room
CERVICAL SPINE

Image receptor: 10 × 12 inch grid IR crosswise

Position of patient

The patient is upright, prone, or supine. In the upright and prone positions the patient's head is held in a traction device to align the spine. In the supine position the chin is elevated and held with a strap or tape.

Position of image receptor and portable machine (Fig. 30-37)

- Place the grid IR in the IR holder and cover with a sterile drape.
- Position the IR holder on the opposite side of the patient. The surgical technician will move the sterile back table so that the radiographer does not compromise the sterile field.
- Direct the beam perpendicular to the IR and parallel to the floor.
- The beam enters perpendicular to the IR to eliminate grid cut-off.
- Raise or lower the tube and IR to center on the C-spine.

Structures shown

- Cervical spine in lateral projection (Fig. 30-38).
- Degenerative or pathologic defects, such as osteophytes, fractures, or subluxation.
- Radiograph may be taken at the beginning of the case to verify the correct portion of spine to be repaired. Instruments will be placed to designate the level of the spine (Fig. 30-39).

- Entire spine is on the radiograph.
- Spine is in the center of the radiograph and is not rotated.
- Proper radiographic technique is used.
- Radiation protection is provided for surgical team.
- All hardware that may be used should be included.
- Grid cut-off is absent.

Fig. 30-37 Mobile radiographic machine *(arrow)* in position for an upright lateral cervical spine. A surgical clamp, which is attached to the spinous process of interest, extends from the incision site. The IR draped and in the holder *(double arrow)* is centered to the patient.

Fig. 30-38 Lateral cervical spine radiograph (patient in sitting position for surgery) showing a localization marker in place on the spinous process of C6.

Fig. 30-39 Lateral projection of the cervical spine with patient supine. This was done to verify the correct position of instruments before continuing surgery. Often a spinal needle is placed in the disk space to show position.

THORACIC OR LUMBAR SPINE

Image receptor: 35 × 43 cm grid IR crosswise

Position of patient

The patient is prone or supine with the arms placed up by the head. The chest and abdomen are supported by a frame or chest roll to flex the spine into anatomic position. A radiograph may be done to verify that the surgeon is working on the correct vertebra or to show the position of hardware (Fig. 30-40).

Lateral projection

Place grid IR in IR holder and cover with a sterile drape. Position the holder next to the patient and move the IR up or down to center on the lumbar spine. Direct the beam perpendicular to the IR and parallel to the floor (Fig. 30-41). Respiration should be suspended during exposure.

PA projection

For the PA radiograph, slide film in the slot under the table and center on the spine. Cover field with sterile drape. Center the beam to the IR and perpendicular to the long axis of the spine.

Structures shown

- The lumbar spine in PA and lateral projections.
- Vertebral bodies, spinous processes, facets, and lamina.
- Hardware to repair any defects. Bone grafts or interbody fusion devices may be used.
- Instrumentation is often seen on radiograph.
- PA projection may be obscured by the patient support.

EVALUATION CRITERIA

- Spine is in the center of the radiograph and in true PA or lateral projection.
- Spine bodies are seen without any rotation.
- All hardware used must be seen on radiograph.
- All unnecessary instrumentation is removed to avoid obscuring spine.
- Proper radiographic technique is used.
- Radiation protection is provided for surgical team.

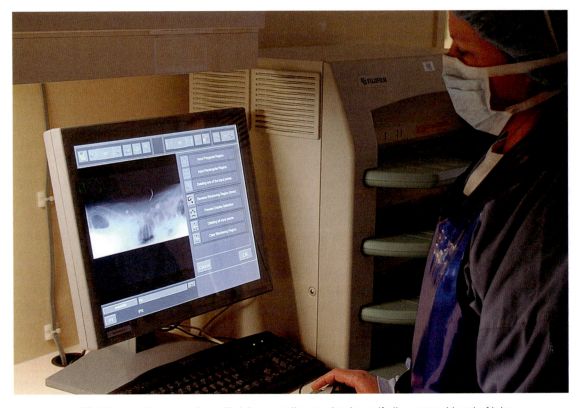

Fig. 30-40 Lateral lumbar spine with intraoperative marker to verify the correct level of interest. CR allows postprocessing adjustments.

A

B

Fig. 30-41 **A,** Mobile x-ray machine correctly positioned for cross-table lateral lumbar spine. **B,** Radiographer positioning mobile unit intraoperatively for lateral lumbar spine procedure.

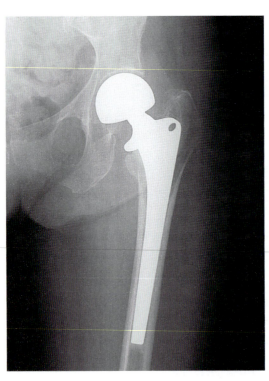

Fig. 30-42 PA projection of the hip with joint replacement.

EXTREMITY EXAMINATIONS

Image receptor: Choose the appropriate-size IR to include all appropriate anatomy and hardware.

Position of patient

The patient is supine, prone, reclining, or in the beach chair position.

Portable machines approach perpendicular to the patient. Institutions may cover the tube or sterile field, or both, with a sterile drape. Angle the tube to match the IR or desired projection. The surgeon may choose to hold the patient's limb in position during the exposure. To reduce exposure to the surgeon, positioning aids, such as sterile towels, sponges, or mallets, may be used.

Fig. 30-43 Image of an ankle fracture with an external fixator in place. The external fixator will hold the foot and leg in place until the tibia heals.

Fig. 30-44 AP lateral image of the foot with antibiotic beads in the talar space. Antibiotic beads are placed at the site of infection to promote healing.

The surgeon may also cover the field with a cloth sterile drape rather than a plastic sterile drape. If so, the surgeon will mark the location of the part to ensure proper centering. Lighting may also need to be adjusted for better visualization of the field. For cross-table examinations the beam is directed perpendicular to the film and parallel to the floor. Center the beam to the IR and raise or lower the tube to the center of the part.

Structures shown

- All pertinent anatomy in correct alignment
- Hardware including plates, wires, pins, screws, external fixation, and joint replacement components used to repair fractures or degenerative problems (Figs. 30-42 through 30-47)

Fig. 30-45 AP projection of proximal tibia with a plate and screw fixation used to repair a tibial plateau fracture.

Fig. 30-46 Lateral projection of the elbow with plate and screws used to reduce a forearm fracture.

Fig. 30-47 Internal rotation projection of the shoulder with a plate and screws. Creative patient positioning or tube angulation may be necessary to achieve optimal images on complex comminuted fractures.

EVALUATION CRITERIA

- Complete joint including all hardware is seen on the film.
- Proper radiographic technique is used.
- Sterile field is maintained.
- Radiation protection is provided for surgical team.
- Collimation to include all hardware used.
- No unnecessary instruments are in field.

NOTE: Often to save time or cost, multiple projections are done on one imaging plate. Be careful not to superimpose any of the projections. Many surgeons will request different projections depending on the individual case. For example, when performing a wrist examination, the arm is positioned on one side of the film with the wrist in the AP or PA projection. Center the beam and collimate to the wrist to include all hardware. Once the exposure is complete, the surgeon will move the arm to the other side of the film in the lateral position. Center the beam on the wrist and collimate (Fig. 30-48).

A

B

Fig. 30-48 A, Radiographer positioning a mobile machine for a lateral projection of the wrist. **B,** AP and lateral projections of the wrist on 24 × 30 cm IR. Note fracture of the navicular with fixation screw in place.

Definition of Terms

antisepsis The chemical disinfection of the skin.

asepsis The absence of infection, germs, or elimination of infectious agents.

aseptic technique Principles involved with manipulation of sterile and unsterile items to prevent or minimize microbiologic contamination.

contamination The presence of pathogenic microorganisms.

microbial fallout Microorganisms normally shed from skin that can contaminate sterile surfaces or areas.

restricted area Operating rooms, clean core or sterile storage areas.

semirestricted area Area of peripheral support, such as hallways or corridors leading to restricted areas.

sterile A substance or object that is completely free of living microorganisms and is incapable of producing any form of organism.

strike-through Soaking through of moisture from nonsterile surfaces to sterile surfaces, or vice versa, allowing transportation of bacteria to sterile areas.

teamwork The Association of Surgical Technologists (AST) Standards of Practice Standard I states: Teamwork is essential for perioperative patient care and is contingent on interpersonal skills. Communication is critical to the positive attainment of expected outcomes of care. All team members should work together for the common good of the patient, for the benefit of the patient and the delivery of actions with the health care team, the patient and family, superiors, and peers. Personal integrity and surgical conscience are integrated into every aspect of professional behavior.

unrestricted area Areas in which street clothes are permitted, such as outer hallways, family waiting areas, locker rooms, and employee lounges.

Selected bibliography

Anderson AC: *The radiologic technologist's handbook of surgical procedures,* Philadelphia, 2000, CRC Press.

Fortunato N: *Berry & Kohn's operating room technique,* ed 9, St Louis, 2000, Mosby.

Huth-Meeker M, Rothrock JC: *Alexander's care of the patient in surgery,* ed 10, St Louis, 1995, Mosby.

Huth-Meeker M, Rothrock JC: *Alexander's care of the patient in surgery,* ed 11, St Louis, 1999, Mosby.

Wetterlin KJ: Mobile radiography. In Ballinger PW, Frank ED, editors: *Merrill's atlas of radiographic positions and radiologic procedures,* ed 9, vol 3, St Louis, 1999, Mosby.

31

COMPUTED TOMOGRAPHY

GAYLE K. WRIGHT

Thorax 3D reconstruction from 64-slice CT scanner.

Fundamentals of Computed Tomography

Computed tomography (CT)* is the process of creating a cross-sectional tomographic plane of any part of the body (Fig. 31-1). For CT, a patient is scanned by an x-ray tube rotating about the body part being examined. A detector assembly measures the radiation exiting the patient and feeds back the information, referred to as primary data, to the host computer. Once the computer has compiled and calculated the data according to a preselected *algorithm,* it assembles the data in a *matrix* to form an *axial* image. Each image, or *slice,* is then displayed on a *cathode ray tube* (CRT) in a cross-sectional format.

In the early 1970s CT scanning was only used clinically for imaging of the brain. Furthermore, the first CT scanners were capable of producing only axial images and thus were called *CAT (computed axial tomography)* units by the public; this term is no longer accurate because images can now be created in multiple planes. In the past few decades, dramatic technical advancements have led to the development of CT scanners that can be used to image virtually every structure within the human body. Improvements in scanner design and computer science have produced CT units with new imaging capabilities and reconstruction techniques. Three-dimensional (3D) reconstruction of images of the internal structures is becoming a popular choice for surgical planning, CT angiography, radiation therapy planning, and virtual reality.

CT-guided biopsies and fluid drainage offer an alternative to surgery for some patients. Although the procedures are considered invasive, they offer shorter recovery periods, no exposure to anesthesia, and less risk of infection. CT is also used in radiation oncology for radiation therapy planning. CT scans taken through the treatment field, with the patient in treatment position, have drastically improved the accuracy and quality of radiation therapy.

*Almost all italicized words on the succeeding pages are defined at the end of this chapter.

Computed Tomography and Conventional Radiography

When a conventional x-ray exposure is made, the radiation passes through the patient and produces an image of the body part. Frequently body structures are superimposed (Fig. 31-2). Visualizing specific structures requires the use of contrast media, varied positions, and usually more than one exposure. Localization of masses or foreign bodies requires at least two exposures and a ruler calibrated for magnification.

In the CT examination, a tightly collimated x-ray beam is directed through the patient from many different angles, resulting in an image that represents a cross section of the area scanned. This imaging technique essentially eliminates the superimposition of body structures. The CT technologist controls the method of acquisition, the slice thickness, the reconstruction algorithm, and other factors related to image quality.

Fig. 31-1 CT scanner provides cross-sectional images by rotating about the patient.

Fig. 31-2 Conventional radiograph superimposes anatomy and yields one diagnostic image with fixed density and contrast.

In the digital radiograph of the abdomen shown in Fig. 31-3, high-density bone and low-density gas are seen, but many soft tissue structures, such as the kidneys and intestines, are not clearly identified. Contrast media are needed to visualize these structures. A CT examination of the abdomen would demonstrate all the structures that lie within the slice. In Fig. 31-4, *A*, the liver, stomach, kidneys, spleen, and aorta can be identified. In addition to eliminating superimposition, CT is capable of differentiating among tissues with similar densities. This differentiation of densities is referred to as *contrast resolution*. The improved contrast resolution with CT, when compared with conventional radiography, is due to a reduction in the amount of scattered radiation.

Fig. 31-4, *B* is an axial image of the brain that differentiates the gray matter from the white matter and shows bony structures and cerebrospinal fluid within the ventricles. Because CT can demonstrate subtle differences in various tissues, radiologists are able to diagnose pathologic conditions more accurately than if they were to rely on radiographs alone. Furthermore, because the image is digitized by the computer, numerous image manipulation techniques can be used to enhance and optimize the diagnostic information available to the physician (Fig. 31-5).

A

B

Fig. 31-4 A, Axial image of abdomen demonstrating liver (*L*), stomach (*ST*), spleen (*SP*), aorta (*A*), inferior vena cava (*IVC*), vertebral body of thoracic spine (*VB*), and kidney (*K*). **B,** Axial CT scan of lateral ventricles (*LVah*), septum (*Sep*), and third ventricle (*3V*).

(**B,** From Kelley LL, Petersen CM: *Sectional anatomy for imaging professionals,* St Louis, 1997, Mosby.)

Fig. 31-3 Digital kidney, ureter, and bladder (KUB).

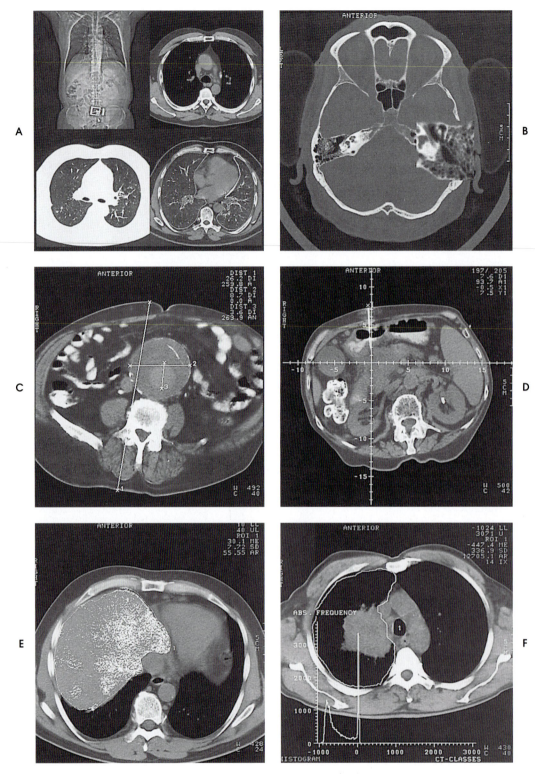

Fig. 31-5 Image manipulation techniques used to enhance diagnostic information in a CT image. **A,** Multiple imaging and windows; **B,** image magnification; **C,** measurement of distances; **D,** superimposition of coordinates on the image; **E,** highlighting; and **F,** histogram.

(Courtesy Siemens Medical Systems, Iselin, NJ.)

Historical Development

CT was first demonstrated successfully in 1970 in England at the Central Research Laboratory of EMI, Ltd. Dr. Godfrey Hounsfield, an engineer for EMI, and Allan Macleod Cormack, a nuclear physicist from Johannesburg, South Africa, are generally given credit for the development of CT. For their research they were awarded the Nobel Prize in medicine and physiology in 1979. After CT was shown to be a useful clinical imaging modality, the first full-scale commercial unit, referred to as a *brain tissue scanner*, was installed in Atkinson Morley's Hospital in 1971. An example of an early dedicated head CT scanner is shown in Fig. 31-6. Physicians recognized its value for providing diagnostic neurologic information, and its use was accepted rapidly. The first CT scanners in the United States were installed in June 1973 at the Mayo Clinic, Rochester, Minn, and later that year at Massachusetts General Hospital, Boston. These early units were also dedicated head CT scanners. In 1974, Dr. Robert S. Ledley of Georgetown University Medical Center, Washington, D.C., developed the first whole-body scanner, which greatly expanded the diagnostic capabilities of CT.

After CT was accepted by physicians as a diagnostic modality, numerous companies in addition to EMI began manufacturing scanners. Although the units differed in the design, the basic principles of operation were the same. CT scanners have been categorized by *generation*, which is a reference to the level of technologic advancement of the tube and detector assembly. There were four recognized generations of CT scanners; however, newer scanners are no longer categorized by generation but by tube and detector movement.

Fig. 31-6 First-generation EMI CT unit: dedicated head scanner.

(Photograph taken at Röntgen Museum, Lennep, Germany.)

The early units, referred to as the *first-generation scanners,* worked by a process known as *translation/rotation.* The tube produced a finely collimated beam, or pencil beam. Depending on the manufacturer, one to three *detectors* were placed opposite the tube for radiation detection. The linear tube movement (translation) was followed by a rotation of 1 degree. Scan time was usually 3 to 5 minutes per scan, which required the patient to hold still for extended periods. Because of the slow scanning and reconstruction time, the use of CT was limited almost exclusively to neurologic examinations. A CT image from a first-generation scanner is shown in Fig. 31-7.

The second-generation scanners were considered a significant improvement over first-generation scanners. The x-ray tube emitted a fan-shaped beam that was measured by approximately 30 detectors placed closely together in a detector array. All subsequent generations would use the fan beam geometry. Tube and detector movement was still translation/rotation, but the rotation was 10 degrees between each translation. These changes improved overall image quality and decreased scan time to about 20 seconds for a single slice. However, the time required to complete one CT examination remained relatively long.

The third generation of scanners introduced a *rotate/rotate movement* in which both the x-ray tube and detector array rotate simultaneously around the patient. An increase in the number of detectors (more than 750) and their arrangement in a "curved" detector array considerably improved image quality (Fig. 31-8). Scan times were decreased to 1 to 10 seconds per slice, which made the CT examination much easier for patients and helped decrease motion artifact. Advancements in computer technology also decreased image reconstruction time, substantially reducing examination time.

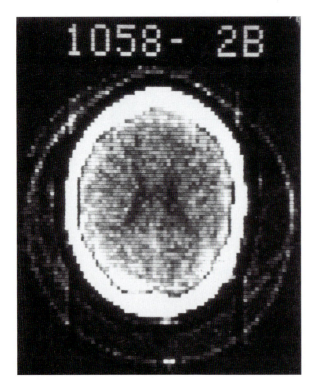

Fig. 31-7 Axial brain image from the first CT scanner in operation in the United States: Mayo Clinic, Rochester, Minn. The 80 × 80 matrix produced a noisy image. The examination was performed in July 1973.

Fig. 31-8 Rotate/rotate movement: tube and detector movement of a third-generation scanner.

The fourth-generation scanners introduced the *rotate-only movement* in which the tube rotated about the patient, but the detectors were in fixed positions, forming a complete circle within the gantry (Fig. 31-9). The use of stationary detectors required greater numbers of detectors to be installed in a scanner. Fourth-generation scanners tended to yield a higher patient dose per scan than previous generations of CT scanners.

In contemporary CT scanners, both third- and fourth-generation designs incorporate the latest technologic advances and produce similar image quality.

Technical Aspects

The axial images acquired by CT scanning provide information about the positional relationships and tissue characteristics of structures within the section of interest. The computer performs a series of steps to generate one axial image. With the patient and gantry perpendicular to each other, the tube rotates around the patient, irradiating the area of interest. For every position of the x-ray tube, the detectors measure the transmitted x-ray values, convert them into an electric signal, and relay the signal to the computer. The measured x-ray transmission values are called *projections (scan profiles)* or *raw data.* Once collected, the electric signals are digitized, a process that assigns a whole number to each signal. The value of each number is directly proportional to the strength of the signal.

The digital image is an array of numbers arranged in a grid of rows and columns called a *matrix.* A single square, or picture element, within the matrix is called a *pixel.* The slice thickness gives the pixel an added dimension called the *volume element,* or *voxel.* Each pixel in the image corresponds to the volume of tissue in the body section being imaged. The voxel volume is a product of the pixel area and slice thickness (Fig. 31-10). The *field of view* (FOV) determines the amount of data to be displayed on the monitor.

Each pixel within the matrix is assigned a number that is related to the linear attenuation coefficient of the tissue within each voxel. These numbers are called *CT numbers* or *Hounsfield units.* CT numbers are defined as a relative comparison of x-ray attenuation of a voxel of tissue to an equal volume of water. Water is used as reference material because it is abundant in the body and has a uniform density; therefore water is assigned an arbitrary value of 0. Tissues that are denser than water are given positive CT numbers, whereas tissues with less density than water are assigned negative CT numbers. The scale of CT numbers ranges from −1000 for air to +14,000 for dense bone. Average CT numbers for various tissues are listed in Table 31-1.

For displaying the digital image on the CRT, each pixel within the image is assigned a level of gray. The gray level assigned to each pixel corresponds to the CT number for that pixel.

Fig. 31-9 Rotate-only movement: tube movement with stationary detectors of a fourth-generation scanner.

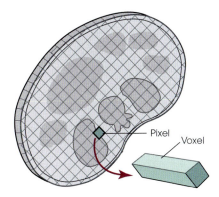

Fig. 31-10 A CT image is composed of a matrix of pixels, with each pixel representing a volume of tissue (voxel).

TABLE 31-1

Average Hounsfield units (HU) for selected substances

Substance	HU
Air	−1000
Lungs	−250 to −850
Fat	−100
Orbit	−25
Water	0
Cyst	−5 to +10
Fluid	0 to +25
Tumor	+25 to +100
Blood (fluid)	+20 to +50
Blood (clotted)	+50 to +75
Blood (old)	+10 to +15
Brain	+20 to +40
Muscle	+35 to +50
Gallbladder	+5 to +30
Liver	+40 to +70
Aorta	+35 to +50
Bone	+150 to +1000
Metal	+2000 to +4000

System Components

The three major components of the CT scanner are shown in Fig. 31-11. Because each component has several subsystems, only a brief description of their main functions is provided in the following sections.

COMPUTER

The computer provides the link between the CT technologist and the other components of the imaging system. The computer system used in CT has four basic functions: control of data acquisition, image reconstruction, storage of image data, and image display.

Data acquisition is the method by which the patient is scanned. The technologist must select among numerous parameters, such as scanning in the conventional or helical mode, before the initiation of each scan. During implementation of the *data acquisition system* (DAS), the computer is involved in sequencing the generation of x-rays, turning the detectors on and off at appropriate intervals, transferring data, and monitoring the system operation.

The *reconstruction* of a CT image depends on the millions of mathematic operations required to digitize and recon-struct the raw data. This image reconstruction is accomplished using an array processor that acts as a specialized computer to perform mathematic calculations rapidly and efficiently, thus freeing the host computer for other activities. Currently, CT units can acquire scans in less than 1 second and require only a few seconds more for image reconstruction.

The *host computer* in CT has limited storage capacity, so image data can be stored only temporarily. Therefore other storage mechanisms are necessary to allow for long-term *data storage* and *retrieval*. After reconstruction, the CT image data can be transferred to another storage medium such as magnetic tapes or optical disks. This allows CT studies to be removed from the limited memory of the host computer and stored independently, a process termed *archiving*.

The reconstructed images are displayed on a CRT or video monitor. At this point the technologist or physician can communicate with the host computer to view specific images, post images on a scout, and/or implement image manipulation techniques such as zoom, control contrast and brightness, and image analysis techniques.

GANTRY AND TABLE

The *gantry* is a circular device that houses the x-ray tube, DAS, and detector array. Newer CT units also house the continuous *slip ring* and high-voltage generator in the gantry. The structures housed in the gantry collect the necessary attenuation measurements to be sent to the computer for image reconstruction.

The x-ray tube used in CT is similar in design to the tubes used in conventional radiography, but it is specially designed to handle and dissipate excessive heat units created during a CT examination. Most CT x-ray tubes use a rotating anode to increase heat dissipation. Many CT x-ray tubes can handle around 2.1 million heat units (MHU), whereas advanced CT units can tolerate 4 to 5 MHU.

The detectors in CT function as image receptors. A detector measures the amount of radiation transmitted through the body and then converts the measurement into an electric signal proportional to the radiation intensity. The two basic detector types used in CT are scintillation (solid-state) and ionization (xenon gas) detectors.

The gantry can be tilted forward or backward up to 30 degrees to compensate for body part angulation. The opening within the center of the gantry is termed the *aperture*. Most apertures are about 28 inches (71.1 cm) wide to accommodate a variety of patient sizes as the patient table advances through it.

Fig. 31-11 Components of a CT scanner: *1*, Computer and operator's console; *2*, gantry; *3*, patient table.

(Courtesy GE Medical Systems, Waukesha, Wis.)

For certain head studies, such as those of facial bones, sinuses, or the sella turcica, a combination of patient positioning and gantry angulation results in a *direct coronal* image of the body part being scanned. Fig. 31-12, *A* demonstrates a typical direct coronal image of C1-C2. In comparison, a computer-reconstructed coronal image created from axial scans through the body part is shown in Fig. 31-12, *B*. Overall image resolution and quality are lost in the reconstructed image as compared with the direct coronal image.

The *table* is an automated device linked to the computer and gantry. It is designed to move in increments *(index)* after every scan according to the scan program. The table is an extremely important part of a CT scanner. Indexing must be accurate and reliable, especially when thin slices (1 or 2 mm) are taken through the area of interest. Most CT tables can be programmed to move in or out of the gantry, depending on the examination protocol and the patient.

CT tables are made of wood or low-density carbon composite, both of which support the patient without causing image artifacts. The table must be very strong and rigid to handle patient weight and at the same time maintain consistent indexing. All CT tables have a maximum patient weight limit; this limit varies by manufacturer from 300 to 600 lb (136 to 272 kg). Exceeding the weight limit can cause inaccurate indexing, damage to the table motor, and even possible breakage of the tabletop, which could cause serious injury to the patient.

Accessory devices can be attached to the table for a variety of uses. A special device called a *cradle* is used for head CT examinations. The head cradle helps hold the head still; because the device extends beyond the tabletop, it minimizes artifacts or attenuation from the table while the brain is being scanned. It can also be used in positioning the patient for direct coronal images.

Fig. 31-12 **A,** Direct coronal image of C1-C2. **B,** Computed-reconstructed images of C1-C2. **C,** Axial image for coronal reconstruction.

(Courtesy Siemens Medical Systems, Iselin, NJ.)

OPERATOR'S CONSOLE

The *operator's console* (Fig. 31-13) is the point from which the technologist controls the scanner. A typical console is equipped with a keyboard for entering patient data and a graphic monitor for viewing the images. Other input devices, such as a touch display screen and a computer mouse, may also be used. The operator's console allows the technologist to control and monitor numerous scan parameters. Radiographic technique factors, slice thickness, table index, and reconstruction algorithm are some of the scan parameters that are selected at the operator's console.

Before starting an examination, the technologist must enter the patient information. Therefore a keyboard is still necessary for some functions. Usually the first scan program selected is the scout program from which the radiographer plans the sequence of axial scans. An example of a typical scout image is seen in Fig. 31-3. The operator's console is also the location of the CRT, where image manipulation takes place. Most scanners display the image on the CRT in a 1024 matrix interpolated by the computer from the 512 reconstructed images.

OTHER COMPONENTS

Display monitor

For the CT image to be displayed on a CRT monitor in a recognizable form, the digital CT data must be converted into a *gray-scale image*. This process is achieved by the conversion of each digital CT number in the matrix to an analog voltage. The brightness values of the gray-scale image correspond to the pixels and CT numbers of the digital data they represent.

Fig. 31-13 Console with display monitors, keyboards, and workstation for 3D image manipulation.

(Courtesy Marconi Medical Systems, Inc., Highland Heights, Ohio.)

Because of the digital nature of the CT image data, image manipulation can be performed to enhance the appearance of the image. One of the most common image processing techniques is called *windowing,* or *gray-level mapping.* This technique allows the technologist to alter the contrast of the displayed image by adjusting the window width and window level. The *window width* is the range of CT numbers that are used to map signals into shades of gray. Basically, the window width determines the number of gray levels to be displayed in the image. A narrow window width means that there are fewer shades of gray, resulting in higher contrast. Likewise, a wide window width results in more shades of gray in the image, or a longer gray scale. The *window level* determines the midpoint of the range of gray levels to be displayed on the monitor. It is used to set the center

CT number within the range of gray levels being used to display the image. The window level should be set to the CT number of the tissue of interest, and the window width should be set with a range of values that will optimize the contrast between the tissues in the image. Fig. 31-14 shows an axial image seen in two different windows: a standard abdomen window and a bone window adjusted for the spine.

The gray level of any image can be adjusted on the CRT to compensate for differences in patient size and tissue densities or to display the image as desired for the examination protocol. Examples of typical window width and level settings are listed in Table 31-2. These settings are averages and usually vary by machine. It is important to note that the level, although an average, is approximately the same as the CT numbers expected for the tissue densities.

TABLE 31-2
Typical window settings

CT examination	Width	Center (level)
Brain	190	50
Skull	3500	500
Orbits	1200	50
Abdomen	400	35
Liver	175	45
Mediastinum	325	50
Lung	2000	−500
Spinal cord	400	50
Spine	2200	400

Fig. 31-14 A, Abdominal image, soft tissue window. **B,** Abdominal image, bone window.

Multiplanar reconstruction

Another advantage of the digital nature of the CT image is the ability to reconstruct the axial images into coronal, sagittal, or oblique body planes without additional radiation to the patient. Image reconstruction in a variety of planes is accomplished by stacking multiple contiguous axial images, creating a volume of data. Because the CT numbers of the image data within the volume are already known, a sectional image can be generated in any desired plane by selecting a particular plane of data. This postprocessing technique is termed *multiplanar reconstruction* (MPR). A sagittal reconstruction of data obtained from axial images is shown in Fig. 31-15, *A.* A coronal reconstruction is seen in Fig. 31-15, *B.*

One of the most important functions of the operator's console is to produce hard copies of axial images in the form of film. The most commonly used filming devices are the matrix camera and the laser printer. The matrix camera once was the standard imaging device used in CT. Now the laser printer is the preferred device for imaging, and it should be docked directly to a processor whenever possible.

Diagnostic Applications

The original CT studies were used primarily for diagnosing neurologic disorders. As scanner technology advanced, the range of applications was extended to other areas of the body. The most commonly requested procedures involve the head, chest, and abdomen. CT is the examination of choice for head trauma; it clearly demonstrates skull fractures and associated subdural hematomas. CT examinations of the head are one of the first tests performed on patients being evaluated for stroke or cerebrovascular accident (CVA) where evidence of hemorrhage must be ruled out. CT imaging of the central nervous system can demon-

A

B

Fig. 31-15 A, Computer-reconstructed sagittal image. **B,** Computer-reconstructed coronal image.

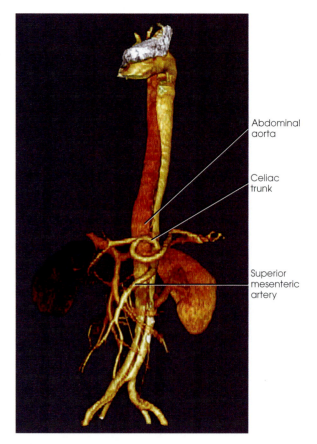

Fig. 31-16 Aortic dissection in color, rendered three dimensionally.

Abdominal aorta

Celiac trunk

Superior mesenteric artery

strate infarctions, hemorrhage, disk herniations, craniofacial and spinal fractures, and tumors and other cancers. CT imaging of the body excels at demonstrating soft tissue structures within the chest, abdomen, and pelvis. Among the abnormalities demonstrated in this region are metastatic lesions, aneurysms, abscesses, and fluid collections from blunt trauma (Fig. 31-16).

CT is also used for numerous interventional procedures such as abscess drainage, tissue biopsy, and cyst aspiration. In addition, CT is being used during both radiofrequency (RF) ablations and cryoablations of tumors. Fig. 31-17 demonstrates a number of structures and pathologic conditions identified by CT.

For any procedure a protocol is required to maximize the amount of diagnostic information available. Specific examination protocols vary according to the needs of different medical facilities and physicians.

Fig. 31-17 A, Abdominal image demonstrating transverse colon *(TC)* with air-fluid levels; the liver *(L)*, pancreas *(P)*, spleen *(SP)*, kidney *(K)*, portal vein *(PV)*, celiac trunk *(CT)*, and splenic veins *(SV)* are demonstrated with contrast medium. Surgical clips are seen in posterior liver. **B,** Abdominal image demonstrating extremely large ovarian cyst *(arrows)*. **C,** Brain image demonstrating parietooccipital mass *(arrow)* with characteristic IV contrast ring enhancement *(arrowhead)*. **D,** Image of L3 postmyelogram demonstrating contrast in thecal sac *(arrow)*.

Contrast Media

Contrast media is used in CT examinations to help distinguish normal anatomy from pathology and to make various disease processes more visible. Contrast can be administered intravenously, orally, or rectally. Generally, the intravenous (IV) contrast media are the same as those used for excretory urograms. Many facilities use nonionic contrast material for these studies, despite the relatively high cost, because of the low incidence of reaction and known safety factors associated with nonionic contrast. IV contrast media are useful for demonstrating tumors within the head; Fig. 31-18 shows a brain scan with and without contrast. The anterior lesion is evident in the unenhanced scan; in the enhanced scan, the tumor demonstrates characteristic ring enhancement typical of tumors seen in CT scans. IV contrast media is also used to visualize vascular structures in the body.

IV contrast should be used only with approval of the radiologist and after careful consideration of patient history. Many CT examinations can be performed without IV contrast if necessary; however, the amount of diagnostic information available can be limited.

Oral contrast media must be used for imaging the abdomen. When given orally, the contrast material in the gastrointestinal tract helps differentiate between loops of bowel and other structures within the abdomen. An oral contrast medium is generally a 2% barium mixture. The low concentration prevents contrast artifacts but allows good visualization of the stomach and intestinal tract. An iodinated contrast material such as oral Hypaque can be used, but it must be mixed at low concentrations to prevent contrast artifacts. Rectal contrast is often requested as part of an abdominal or a pelvic protocol. Usually mixed in the same concentration as the oral contrast, the rectal contrast material is useful for demonstrating the distal colon relative to the bladder and other structures of the pelvic cavity.

Factors Affecting Image Quality

In CT, the technologist has access to numerous scan parameters that can have a dramatic effect on image quality. The four main factors contributing to image quality are spatial resolution, contrast resolution, noise, and artifacts.

SPATIAL RESOLUTION

Spatial resolution describes the amount of blurring in an image. The scan parameters that affect spatial resolution include focal spot size, slice thickness, display FOV, matrix, and reconstruction algorithm. The detector aperture width is the most significant geometric factor that contributes to spatial resolution. The spatial resolution in CT is not as good as in conventional radiography.

Fig. 31-18   A, Brain image without IV contrast demonstrating lesion *(arrow)*. **B,** Brain image with IV contrast.

CONTRAST RESOLUTION

Contrast resolution is the ability to differentiate between small differences in density within the image. Currently, tissues with density differences of less than 0.5% can be distinguished with CT. The scan parameters that affect contrast resolution are slice thickness, reconstruction algorithm, image display, and x-ray beam energy. The size of the patient and the detector sensitivity also have a direct effect on contrast resolution.

NOISE

The most common cause of *noise* in CT is *quantum noise.* This type of noise arises from the random variation in photon detection. Noise in a CT image primarily affects contrast resolution. As noise increases in an image, contrast resolution decreases. Noise gives an image a grainy quality or a mottled appearance. Among the scan parameters that influence noise are matrix size, slice thickness, x-ray beam energy, and reconstruction algorithm. Scattered radiation and patient size also contribute to the noise of an image.

ARTIFACTS

Metallic objects, such as dental fillings, pacemakers, and artificial joints, can cause starburst or *streak artifacts,* which can obscure diagnostic information. Dense residual barium from fluoroscopy examinations can cause *artifacts* similar to those caused by metallic objects. Many CT departments do not perform a patient's CT examination until several days after barium studies to allow the body to eliminate the residual barium from the area of interest. Large differences in tissue densities of adjoining structures can cause artifacts that detract from image quality. Bone–soft-tissue interfaces, such as occur with the skull and brain, often cause streak or shadow artifacts on CT images; these artifacts are referred to as *beam hardening* (Fig. 31-19).

OTHER FACTORS
Patient factors

Patient factors also contribute to the quality of an image. If a patient cannot or will not hold still, the scan will likely be nondiagnostic. Body size also can have an effect on image quality. Large patients attenuate more radiation than small patients; this can increase image noise, detracting from overall image quality. An increase in milliampere-seconds (mAs) is usually required to compensate for large body size. Unfortunately, this increase results in a higher radiation dose to the patient. Image quality factors under technologist control include slice thickness, *scan time, scan diameter,* and patient instructions. Slice thickness is usually dictated by image *protocol.* As in tomography, the thinner the slice thickness, the better the image-recorded detail. Thin-section CT scans, often referred to as *high-resolution scans,* are used to better demonstrate structures (Fig. 31-20).

As in conventional radiography, patient instructions are a critical part of a diagnostic examination. Explaining the procedure fully in terms that the patient can understand will increase the level of compliance from almost any patient.

Fig. 31-19 Streaking through the posterior fossa representing beam-hardening artifact. Normal appearance of the brain; *1,* sphenoidal sinus; *2,* trigeminal ganglion; *3,* fourth ventricle; *4,* temporal lobe; *5,* pons; *6,* middle cerebellar peduncle; *7,* cerebellar hemisphere.

Fig. 31-20 High-resolution 1-mm slice using edge enhancement algorithm, demonstrating nodule in left lung *(arrow).*

Scan times

Scan times are usually preselected by the computer as part of the scan program, but they can be altered by the technologist. When selecting a scan time, the technologist must take into account possible patient motion such as inadvertent body movements, breathing, or peristalsis. A good guideline is to choose a scan time that will minimize patient motion and at the same time provide a quality diagnostic image. When it is necessary to scan an uncooperative patient quickly, using the shortest scan time possible may allow the technologist to complete the examination, although the quality of the images obtained will likely be somewhat compromised.

Scan diameter

The image that appears on the CRT depends on the *scan diameter,* also called scan FOV. The technologist can adjust the scan diameter to include the entire cross section of the body part being scanned or to include only a specified region within the part. The anatomy displayed is often referred to as the display FOV. Like scan time, scan diameter is usually preselected by the computer as part of a scan program, but it can also be adjusted as necessary by the technologist. For most head, chest, and abdomen examinations, the selected scan diameter includes all anatomy of the body part to just outside the skin borders. Certain examinations may require the scan diameter to be reduced to include specific anatomy such as the sella turcica, sinuses, one lung, mediastinal vessels, suprarenal glands, one kidney, or the prostate.

Special Features
DYNAMIC SCANNING

One of the advantages of CT is that data can be obtained for image reconstruction by the computer. The scanner can be programmed to scan through an area rapidly. In this situation raw data are saved, but image reconstruction after each scan is bypassed to shorten scan time.

Dynamic scanning is based on the principle that after contrast administration, different structures enhance at different rates. Dynamic scanning can consist of rapid sequential scanning at the same level to observe contrast filling within a structure, such as is performed when looking for an aortic aneurysm. Another form of dynamic scanning is incremental dynamic scanning, which consists of rapid serial scanning at consecutive levels during the bolus injection of a contrast medium.

Fig. 31-21 Continuous gantry rotation combined with continuous table rotation, forming a spiral path of data.

SPIRAL/HELICAL CT

Spiral CT or *helical* CT are terms used to describe the newest method of data acquisition in CT. During spiral CT, the gantry is rotating continuously while the table moves through the gantry aperture at the same time. The continuous gantry rotation combined with the continuous table movement forms the spiral path from which raw data are obtained (Fig. 31-21). Slip-ring technology has made continuous rotation of the x-ray tube possible by eliminating the cables between the gantry and the generators.

One of the unique features of spiral CT is that it scans a volume of tissue rather than a group of individual slices. This method makes it extremely useful for the detection of small lesions because an arbitrary slice can be reconstructed along any position within the volume of raw data. In addition, because a volume of tissue is scanned in a single breath, respiratory motion can be minimized. For a volume scan of the chest such as that shown in Fig. 31-22, the patient was instructed to hold the breath, and a tissue volume of 24 mm was obtained in a 5-second spiral scan.

Two of the resultant images demonstrate a small lung nodule without breathing interference of *image misregistration;* a 3D reconstruction of the lung clearly shows the pathologic condition. Spiral CT is also used to scan noncooperative or combative patients, patients who cannot tolerate lying down for long periods of time, and patients who will not hold still, such as pediatric patients or trauma patients. In some examinations, the use of spiral CT may decrease the amount of contrast medium necessary to visualize structures; this makes the examination both safer and more cost effective.

A

B

C

Fig. 31-22 A and **B,** Spiral images of lung demonstrating lung nodule and associated vasculature. **C,** 3D reconstruction of lung nodule *(arrow)* after spiral scan.

(Courtesy Siemens Medical Systems, Iselin, NJ.)

MULTI-SLICE SPIRAL/HELICAL CT

Multi-slice helical CT (MSHCT) systems have detectors arrays containing multiple rows of elements along the z axis compared with the single row of detectors in conventional spiral CT. For example, in a "four-row" scanner the detector array is connected to four data acquisition systems that generate four channels of data (Fig. 31-23). This type of detector array would allow a scan four times faster than the conventional single row spiral/helical scanner. The latest technology of detector arrays has 64 rows of elements.

These types of scanners are referred to as *volume CT (VCT)* systems because covering entire body sections is easily accomplished in a single breath-hold. Cardiac imaging using VCT is a rapidly growing component of CT imaging. The advantages of MSHCT include isotropic viewing, longer anatomic coverage, multiphase studies, faster examination times, and improved spatial resolution. The advancement of VCT, with increasing larger detector arrays, promises to provide new and unique clinical opportunities in diagnostic medicine.

CT ANGIOGRAPHY

CT angiography (CTA) is an application of spiral CT that uses 3D imaging techniques. With CTA the vascular system can be viewed in three dimensions. The three basic steps required to generate CTA images are as follows:

1. Choice of parameters for IV administration of the *bolus* of contrast medium (i.e., injection rate, injection duration, and delay between bolus initiation and the start of the scan sequence)
2. Choice of spiral parameters to maximize the contrast in the target vessel (i.e., *scan duration,* collimation, and *table speed*)
3. Reconstruction of two-dimensional (2D) image data into 3D image data

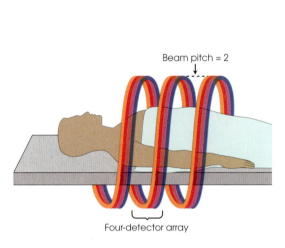

Fig. 31-23 A four-detector array with a beam pitch of 2.0 covers eight times the tissue volume of a single-slice spiral CT.

Fig. 31-24 Color CT angiography of the circle of Willis.

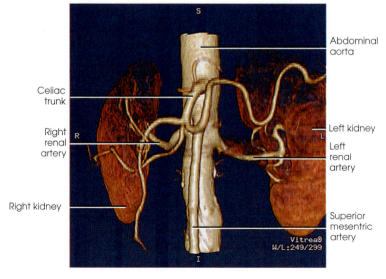

Fig. 31-25 Color CT angiography of the renal vessels in 3D format.

CTA has several advantages over conventional angiography. CTA uses spiral technology; therefore an arbitrary image within the volume of data can be retrospectively reconstructed without exposing the patient to additional IV contrast medium or radiation. Furthermore, during postprocessing of the image data, overlying structures can be eliminated so that only the vascular anatomy is reconstructed. Finally, because CTA is an IV procedure that does not require arterial puncture, only minimal postprocedure observation is necessary.

Currently, CTA is replacing angiography as a diagnostic tool for some studies. This is especially true in those departments using multi-row detectors that allow significantly faster scanning. Fig. 31-24 demonstrates the vessels of the brain, whereas Fig. 31-25 highlights the renal vessels in a 3D format. The heart and coronary vessels are visualized in Fig. 31-26 as well as a graft in Fig. 31-27.

Fig. 31-26 Color 3D cardiac CTA.

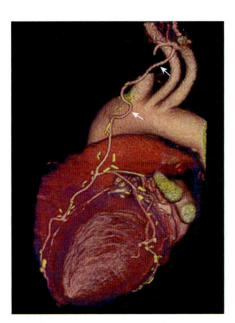

Fig. 31-27 Color 3D cardiac CTA with graft (arrows).

THREE-DIMENSIONAL IMAGING

A rapidly expanding area of CT is 3D imaging. This is a *postprocessing* technique that is applied to the raw data to create realistic images of the surface anatomy to be visualized.

The introduction of advanced computers and faster software programs has dramatically increased the applications of 3D imaging. The common techniques used in creating 3D images include *maximum intensity projection* (MIP), *shaded surface display* (SSD), and *volume rendering* (VR). All techniques use three initial steps to create the 3D images from the original CT data.

1. Construction of a volume of 3D data from the original 2D CT image data. This same process is used in MPR.
2. *Segmentation* to crop or edit the target objects from the reconstructed data. This step eliminates unwanted information from the CT data.
3. *Rendering* or *shading* to provide depth perception to the final image.

Maximum intensity projection

The MIP technique consists of reconstructing the brightest pixels from a stack of 2D or 3D image data into a 3D image. The data are rotated on an arbitrary axis, and an imaginary ray is passed through the data in specific increments. The brightest pixel found along each ray is then *mapped* into a gray-scale image. The MIP technique is commonly used for CTA.

Fig. 31-28 3D images. **A,** Lumbar spine. **B,** Bony orbits.

(Courtesy Marconi Medical Systems, Inc., Highland Heights, Ohio.)

Shaded surface display

An SSD image provides a 3D image of a particular structure's surface. Once the original 2D data are reconstructed into 3D information, the different tissue types within the image need to be separated. This process, called *segmentation,* can be performed by drawing a line around the tissue of interest or, more commonly, by setting *threshold values.* A threshold value can be set for a particular CT number; the result is that any pixel having an equal or higher CT number than the threshold value will be selected for the 3D image. Once the threshold value is set and the data are reconstructed into a 3D image, a shading technique is applied. The shading or rendering technique provides depth perception in the reconstructed image.

Volume rendering

Volume rendering techniques incorporate the entire volume of data into a 3D image by summing the contributions of each voxel along a line from the viewer's eye through the data set. This results in a 3D image in which the dynamic range throughout the image is preserved. Rather than being limited to surface data, a VR image can display a wide range of tissues that will accurately depict the anatomic relationships between vasculature and viscera. Because VR incorporates and processes the entire data set, much

more powerful computers are required to reconstruct 3D VR images at a reasonable speed.

Referring physicians and surgeons use 3D images to clinically correlate CT images to the actual anatomic contours of their patients (Fig. 31-28). These reconstructions are especially useful in surgical procedures. 3D reconstructions are often requested as part of patient evaluation after trauma and for presurgical planning. Fig. 31-29 provides examples of the three common 3D rendering techniques.

Fig. 31-29 Common 3D rendering techniques used in CT.

(Courtesy Elscint, Hackensack, NJ.)

Special features

323

RADIATION TREATMENT PLANNING

Radiation therapy has been used for nearly as long as radiology has been in existence. The introduction of CT has had a major impact on radiation treatment planning. The use of spiral CT in conjunction with MPR provides a 3D approach to radiation treatment planning. This method helps the dosimetrist plan treatment so that the radiation dose to the target is maximized and the dose to normal tissue is minimized. The 3D simulation software offers the following: volumetric, high-precision localization; calculation of the geometric center of the defined target; patient marking systems; and virtual simulators capable of producing digitally reconstructed radiographs in *real time*. With the new, specially designed software, a single CT simulation procedure can replace a total of three procedures (one conventional CT and two conventional simulations) for radiation treatment planning (Fig. 31-30).

If the CT system is being used for radiation treatment planning, the standard curved couch should not be used. Instead, a flat board should be placed on the couch. In this way the actual therapy delivery can be simulated more accurately. Fig. 31-31 demonstrates the external skin markers and structures that will be in the beam's path.

Fig. 31-30 A, Therapy planning using CT. **B,** Color-coded CT therapy plan.

QUALITY CONTROL

The goal of any quality assurance program in CT is to ensure that the system is producing the best possible image quality with the minimum radiation dose to the patient. A CT system is a complex combination of sensitive and expensive equipment that requires systematic monitoring for performance and image quality. Most CT systems require weekly or biweekly preventive maintenance to ensure proper operation.

Preventive maintenance is usually performed by a service engineer from the manufacturer or a private company.

Increasingly, however, the technologist is being assigned the responsibility of performing and documenting routine quality assurance tests. Many technologists routinely perform daily test scans on a water phantom to measure the consistency of the CT numbers and to record the standard deviation. As data are recorded over time, the CT scanner's current operating condition, as well as its performance over longer time periods, can be evaluated. Many units are also capable of *air calibrations,* which do not require the water phantom and can be performed between patients for unit self-calibration.

A CT phantom is typically multisectioned and is constructed from plastic cylinders, with each section filled with test objects designed to measure the performance of specific parameters. Some phantoms are designed to allow numerous parameters to be evaluated with a single scan. The recommended quality assurance tests for evaluating routine performance include the following: contrast scale and mean CT number of water, high-contrast resolution, low-contrast resolution, laser light accuracy, noise and uniformity, slice thickness, and patient dose.

Special features

Fig. 31-31 Patient in prone position for radiation treatment planning. Radiopaque markers *(arrows)* demonstrate location of treatment field skin marks: tumor *(T),* heart *(H),* liver *(L),* right lung *(RL),* and left lung *(LL).*

Computed Tomography and Radiation Dose

Calculating the radiation dose received during CT examinations presents a unique set of circumstances. Typically, radiation received during radiologic examinations comes from a fixed source with delivery to the patient in one or two planes (e.g. AP and lateral views). These exposure parameters typically produce a much higher entrance skin dose than the exit skin dose, which creates a large dose gradient across the patient. In contrast, CT exposures (helical/spiral) come from an essentially continuous source that rotates 360 degrees around the patient.

This results in a radially symmetric radiation dose gradient within the patient.

Measurements of CT dose are typically performed using a circular CT dosimetry phantom that is made of polymethyl methacrylate (PMMA) with implanted thermoluminescent dosimeters (TLDs). The TLDs are positioned 1 cm below the surface around the periphery of the phantom and at the center (isocenter). The typical phantom sizes are 32 cm for body calculations and 16 cm for head calculations. For a single axial scan location (one full rotation of the tube, no table movement), the typical dose for the body phantom is 20 mGy at the periphery and 10 mGy at the isocenter. The typical dose for the head phantom is higher at 40 mGy at the

periphery and 40 mGy at the isocenter. See Fig. 31-32 for the body and Fig. 31-33 for the head. This indicates that dose is size dependent (e.g., dose is different depending on head scan or body scan and whether patient is pediatric or adult).

Another component of dose to the patient is distribution of absorbed dose along the length of the patient from one single scan (full rotation at one table location). The radiation dose profile (Fig. 31-34) is not limited just to the slice location; the "tails" of the dose profile contribute to the absorbed dose outside of the primary beam. The size of the contribution to dose from the adjacent sections is directly related to the spacing of the slices and the width and shape of the radiation profile.

Fig. 31-32 CT dose profile for body.

(From McNitt-Gray MF: AAPM/RSNA physics tutorial for residents: topics in CT. Radiation dose in CT, *Radiographics* 22:1541, 2002.)

Fig. 31-34 Single-slice CT dose profile.

Fig. 31-33 CT dose profile for head.

(From McNitt-Gray MF: AAPM/RSNA physics tutorial for residents: topics in CT. Radiation dose in CT, *Radiographics* 22:1541, 2002.)

The method used first to describe dose as a result of multiple scan locations was the *multiple scan average dose* (MSAD). MSAD described average dose resulting from scans over an interval length on the patient. The next to follow was the *computed tomography dose index* (CTDI), which was calculated using a normalized beam width and a standard of 14 contiguous axial slices. This method required a dose profile measured with TLDs or film, neither of which was convenient. To overcome the measurement limitations, another dose index, the $CTDI_{100}$, was developed. This allowed profile calculations along the full length (100 mm) of a pencil ionization chamber and did not require nominal section widths. To provide a weighted average of the center and peripheral contributions, $CTDI_w$ was created. The final descriptor is $CTDI_{vol}$, which accounts for the helical pitch or axial scan spacing that is used for a specific protocol. The most common reporting method of dose reporting on the present scanners is the *dose-length product* (DLP). This is the $CTDI_{vol}$ multiplied by the length of the scan (cm). It is reported in mGy/cm.

ESTIMATING EFFECTIVE DOSE

Effective dose takes into account where the radiation dose is being absorbed (e.g., which tissue/organ has absorbed the radiation). The weighting factors are set for each radiosensitive organ by the International Commission on Radiological Protection (ICRP) (available at www.ICRP.org). Effective dose is measured in sieverts (Sv) or rems (100 rem = 1 Sv). The effective dose is determined by multiplying the DLP by a region-specific conversion factor. The conversion factors for chest imaging are 0.017 mSv/mGy.cm, pelvis is 0.019 mSv/mGy.cm, and head is 0.0023 mSv/mGy.cm. Note that the conversion factor for head scans is considerably less because there are fewer radiosensitive organs that are irradiated. (Example: The DLP for a given chest examination is 375 mGy, the resulting estimated effective dose is 375 multiplied by 0.017 which equals 6.4 mSv.)

FACTORS THAT AFFECT DOSE

The factors that directly influence the radiation dose to the patient are beam energy (kVp), tube current (mA), rotation or exposure time (seconds), section or slice thickness (beam collimation), object thickness and attenuation (size of patient, pediatric versus adult), pitch and/or section spacing (table distance traveled in one 360-degree rotation), dose reduction techniques (mA modulation), and distance from the tube to isocenter.

Beam collimation (slice thickness) varies in single-detector scanners and multi-detector scanners. Beam collimation for single-detector systems has minimal effect on dose; however, this is not the case for multi-detector scanners. These scanners have multiple ways to scan and reconstruct images. For example, a multi-detector scanner can perform axial scans of 4 × 1.25 mm (5 mm beam width, 1.25 mm slice reconstruction), 4 × 2.5 mm (10 mm beam width, 2.25 mm slice reconstruction), and 4 × 5.0 mm (20 mm beam width, 5.0 mm slice reconstruction). When all other parameters are kept constant, there are significant differences in dose. Beam collimation, not reconstruction thickness, a difference, in some cases 55% in the head phantom and 65% in the body phantom when comparing single- vs. multi-detector scanners. See Table 31-3 for single detector imaging and Table 31-4 for multi-detector imaging dose charts.

Patient size must be considered carefully when setting up scan parameters. The small adult or pediatric patient absorbs less of the entrance radiation than larger patients. This results in the exit radiation dose of higher intensity, which results in a more uniform dose distribution. The distribution is nearly equal at all locations in a 16-cm phantom, a factor of 2 times greater. The larger patient has a much lower exit radiation dose, which lowers the total dose distribution in a 32-cm phantom.

TABLE 31-3
Single-detector doses

Collimation (mm)	$CTDI_w$ head phantom (mGy)	$CTDI_w$ body phantom (mGy)
1	46	20
3	42	19
5	40	18
7	40	18
10	40	18

$CTDI_w$, Computed tomography dose index$_w$.

TABLE 31-4
Multi-detector doses

Collimation (mm)	Total beam width (mm)	$CTDI_w$ head phantom (mGy)	$CTDI_w$ body phantom (mGy)
4 × 1.25	5	63	34
2 × 2.5	5	63	34
1 × 5	5	63	34
4 × 2.5	10	47	25
2 × 5	10	47	25
4 × 5	10	47	21

$CTDI_w$, Computed tomography dose index$_w$.

Comparison of Computed Tomography and Magnetic Resonance Imaging

As CT was developing and advancing into a significant diagnostic modality, magnetic resonance imaging (MRI) was also progressing. Like CT, MRI was first used to image the brain; whole-body scans were developed shortly afterward. As MRI advanced and the quality of the images improved, it became apparent that MRI images exhibited better low-contrast resolution than CT images. Brain soft tissue detail is not demonstrated as well with CT as with MRI performed at approximately the same level (Fig. 31-35).

The initial introduction of MRI raised concerns that CT scanners would become obsolete. However, each modality has been found to have unique capabilities. Thus CT and MRI are useful for different clinical applications. As previously mentioned, CT does not demonstrate soft tissue as well as MRI; however, CT demonstrates bony structures better than MRI.

Patients often have ferrous metal within their bodies. Such patients cannot always be scanned by MRI. CT is one option for these patients. The CT scanner does not affect metal in a patient, but metal can cause artifacts on CT images when the metal lies within the scan plane.

Many patients (especially pediatric and trauma patients) are extremely claustrophobic, combative, or uncooperative. CT is useful for scanning these patients quickly and easily because of the small gantry, relatively large aperture, and short scan times.

Because equipment costs are lower and a greater number of procedures can be accomplished per day, CT can often be a less costly examination than MRI. Physicians have found that CT and MRI can be complementary examinations. In many situations, both examinations are ordered to provide as much diagnostic information as possible.

A   B

Fig. 31-35 A, Axial CT scan of lateral ventricles *(LVah)*. **B,** Axial MR scan of corpus callosum.

(From Kelley LL, Petersen CM: *Sectional anatomy for imaging professionals,* St Louis, 1997, Mosby.)

The Future

In the last 5 years, CT has significantly increased its diagnostic capabilities. The development of multi-row detectors was central to the advancement of CT as a discipline. With the rapid advancements in technology, the CT technologist has an increased responsibility to understand contrast dynamics and the spiral scan parameters of pitch, collimation, scan timing, and table speed.

Advances in computing power and design have provided workstations that can generate 3D models in 30 seconds or less, rotate the models along any axis, and display the models with varying parameters (Fig. 31-36). Digital subtraction CT, multimodality image superimposition, and translucent shading of soft tissue structures are some of the new applications coming from technologic advancements. Soon, CT will provide image data sets that will allow physicians to manipulate the anatomy on virtual reality and other graphics platforms. Multi-energy detectors as well as 128- and 256-row detectors are in development. As the higher-quality images increase the accuracy of diagnosis and treatment, patient care will be improved. Because of the superb diagnostic information and cost-effectiveness that CT provides, this imaging modality will continue to be a highly respected diagnostic tool.

Fig. 31-36 Full-body 3D reconstruction from 64-row CT scanner.

Definition of Terms

air calibration Scan of air in gantry; based on a known value of -1000 for air, the scanner will calibrate itself according to this density value relative to the actual density value measured.

algorithm Mathematic formula designed for computers to carry out complex calculations required for image reconstruction; designed for enhancement of soft tissue, bone, and edge resolution.

aperture Opening of the gantry through which patient passes during scan.

archiving Storage of CT images on long-term storage device such as cassette tape, magnetic tape, or optical disk.

artifact Distortion or error in image that is unrelated to subject being studied.

attenuation Coefficient CT number assigned to measured remnant radiation intensity after attenuation by tissue density.

axial Describes plane of image as presented by CT scan; same as *transverse.*

bolus Preset amount of radiopaque contrast medium injected rapidly per IV administration to visualize high-flow vascular structures, usually in conjunction with dynamic scan; most often injected using a pressure injector.

cathode ray tube (CRT) Electronic monitor used for image display or scan protocol display; resolution of a CRT depends on lines per inch; the greater the lines per inch, the better the resolution.

computed tomography (CT) X-ray tube and detector assembly rotating 360 degrees about a specified area of the body; also called CAT (computed axial tomography) scan.

computed tomography dose index (CTDI) Radiation dose descriptor calculated with normalized beam widths for 14 contiguous sections/slices.

computed tomography dose index$_{100}$ (CTDI$_{100}$) Radiation dose descriptor calculated with the full length of a 100-mm pencil ionization chamber. Measures larger scan distances than the CTDI, but only one location is calculated.

computed tomography dose index$_{vol}$ (CTDI$_{vol}$) Radiation dose descriptor that takes into account the parameters that are related to a specific imaging protocol. Considers helical pitch or axial scan spacing in its calculation. More accurate measure of dose per protocol.

computed tomography dose index$_w$ (CTDI$_w$) Radiation dose descriptor that provides a weighted average of the center and peripheral contributions to dose within the scan plane. More accurate than the CTDI$_{100}$ due to calculations from more than one location.

CT angiography Use of volumetric CT scanning with spiral technique to acquire image data that are reconstructed into 3D CT angiograms.

CT number Arbitrary number assigned by computer to indicate relative density of a given tissue; CT number varies proportionately with tissue density; high CT numbers indicate dense tissue, and low CT numbers indicate less dense tissue. All CT numbers are based on the density of water, which is assigned a CT number of 0. Also referred to as a *Hounsfield unit.*

contrast resolution Ability of a CT scanner to demonstrate different tissue densities.

data acquisition system (DAS) Part of detector assembly that converts analog signals to digital signals that can be used by the CT computer.

detector Electronic component used for radiation detection; made of either high-density photoreactive crystals or pressurized stable gases.

detector assembly Electronic component of CT scanner that measures remnant radiation exiting the patient, converting the radiation to an analog signal proportionate to the radiation intensity measured.

direct coronal Describes the position used to obtain images in coronal plane; used for head scans to provide images at right angles to axial images; patient is positioned prone for direct coronal images and supine for reverse coronal images.

dose length product (DLP) Commonly reported dose descriptor on CT scanners. Calculated by multiplying the CTDI$_{vol}$ by the length of the scan (cm). DLP = CTDI$_{vol}$ × scan length.

dynamic scanning Process by which raw data are obtained by continuous scanning; images are not reconstructed but are saved for later reconstruction; most often used for visualization of high-flow vascular structures; can be used to scan a noncooperative patient rapidly.

field of view (FOV) Area of anatomy displayed by the CRT; can be adjusted to include entire body section or a specific part of the patient anatomy being scanned.

gantry Part of CT scanner that houses x-ray tube, cooling system, detector assembly, and DAS; often referred to as the "doughnut" by patients.

generation Description of significant levels of technologic development of CT scanners; specifically related to tube/detector movement.

gray-scale image Analog image whereby each pixel in the image corresponds to a particular shade of gray.

helical CT Relatively new data acquisition method that combines continuous gantry rotation with continuous table movement to form a helical path of scan data; also called *spiral CT.*

high-resolution scans Use of scanning parameters that enhance contrast resolution of an image, such as thin slices, high matrices, high-spatial frequency algorithms, and small-display FOV.

host computer Primary link between system operator and other components of imaging system.

Hounsfield unit (HU) Number used to describe average density of tissue; term is used interchangeably with *CT number;* named in honor of Sir Godfrey Hounsfield, the man generally given credit for development of the first clinically viable CT scanner.

image misregistration Image distortion caused by combination of table indexing and respiration; table moves in specified increments, but patient movement during respiration may cause anatomy to be scanned more than once or not at all.

index Table movement; also referred to as *table increments.*

mapping Assignment of appropriate gray level to each pixel in an image.

matrix Mathematical formula for calculation made up of individual cells for number assignment; CT matrix stores a CT number relative to the tissue density at that location; each cell or "address" stores one CT number for image reconstruction.

maximum intensity projection (MIP) Reconstruction of brightest pixels from stack of image data into a 3D image.

multiplanar reconstruction (MPR) Postprocessing technique applied to stacks of axial image data that can then be reconstructed into other orientations or imaging planes.

multiple scan average dose (MSAD) Dose descriptor that calculates the average dose resulting from a series of scans over an interval length of scans.

noise Random variation of CT numbers about some mean value within a uniform object; noise produces a grainy appearance in the image.

partial volume averaging Calculated linear attenuation coefficient for a pixel that is a weighted average of all densities in the pixel; the assigned CT number and ultimately the pixel appearance are affected by the average of the different densities measured within that pixel.

pixel (picture element) One individual cell surface within an image matrix used for CRT image display.

postprocessing techniques Specialized reconstruction techniques that are applied to CT images to display the anatomic structures from different perspectives.

primary data CT number assigned to the matrix by the computer; the information required to reconstruct an image.

protocol Instructions for CT examination specifying slice thickness, table increments, contrast administration, scan diameter, and any other requirements specified by the radiologist.

quantum noise Any noise in the image that is a result of random variation in the number of x-ray photons detected.

real time Ability to process or reconstruct incoming data in a matter of milliseconds.

reconstruction Process of creating a digital image from raw data.

region of interest (ROI) Measurement of CT numbers within a specified area for evaluation of average tissue density.

rendering Process of changing the shading of a 3D image; commonly used to increase depth perception of an image.

retrieval Reconstruction of images stored on long-term device; can be done for extra film copies or when films are lost.

scan Actual rotation of x-ray tube about the patient; used as a generic reference to one slice or an entire examination.

scan diameter Also referred to as the *zoom* or *focal plane* of a CT scan; predetermined by the radiographer to include the anatomic area of interest; determines FOV.

scan duration Amount of time used to scan an entire volume during a single spiral scan.

scan time X-ray exposure time in seconds.

segmentation Method of cropping or editing target objects from image data.

shaded surface display (SSD) Process used to generate 3D images that show the surface of a 3D object.

shading Postprocessing technique used in 3D reconstructions to separate tissues of interest by applying a threshold value to isolate the structure of interest.

slice One scan through a selected body part; also referred to as a *cut;* slice thickness can vary from 1 mm to 1 cm, depending on the examination.

slip ring Low-voltage electrical contacts within the gantry designed to allow continuous rotation of an x-ray tube without the use of cables connecting internal and external components.

spatial resolution Ability of a CT scanner to demonstrate small objects within the body plane being scanned.

spiral CT Relatively new data acquisition method that combines a continuous gantry rotation with a continuous table movement to form a spiral path of scan data; also called *helical CT.*

streak artifact Artifact created by high-density objects that result in an arc of straight lines projecting across the FOV from a common point.

system noise Inherent property of a CT scanner; the difference between the measured CT number of a given tissue and the known value for that tissue; most often evaluated through the use of water phantom scans.

table increments Specific amount of table travel between scans; can be varied to move at any specified increment; most protocols specify from 1 mm to 20 cm, depending on type of examination; also referred to as *indexing.*

table speed Longitudinal distance traveled by the table during one revolution of the x-ray tube.

threshold value CT number used in defining the corresponding anatomy that will comprise a 3D object; any pixels within a 3D volume having the threshold value (CT number) or higher will be selected for the 3D model.

useful patient dose Radiation dose received by the patient that is actually detected and converted into an image.

voxel (volume element) Individual pixel with the associated volume of tissue based on the slice thickness.

window Arbitrary numbers used for image display based on various shades of gray; window width controls the overall gray level and affects image contrast; window level (center) controls subtle gray images within a certain width range and ultimately affects the brightness and overall density of an image.

Selected bibliography

Adachi H, Nagai J: *Three-dimensional CT angiography,* Boston, 1995, Little, Brown.

Berland L: *Practical CT: technology and techniques,* New York, 1987, Raven Press.

Bushberg et al: *The essential physics of medical imaging,* Baltimore, 1994, Williams & Wilkins.

Bushong: *Radiologic science for technologists: physics, biology, and protection,* ed 8, St Louis, 2004, Mosby.

Fishman EK, Jeffrey RB: *Spiral CT: principles, techniques, and clinical applications,* New York, 1995, Raven Press.

Haaga JR et al: *Computed tomography of the whole body,* ed 2, vols I and II, St Louis, 1988, Mosby.

Hendee WR: *The physical principles of computed tomography,* Boston, 1983, Little, Brown.

Kalender WA: *Computed tomography: fundamentals, system technology, image quality, applications,* ed 2, New York, 2006, Wiley-VCH.

Marshall, C: *The physical basis of computed tomography,* St Louis, 1982, Warren H. Green.

Morgan C: *Basic principles of computed tomography,* Baltimore, 1983, University Park Press.

Seeram E: *Computed tomography: physical principles, clinical applications, and quality control,* ed 2, St Louis, 2001, Saunders.

Sprawls P: *Physical principles of medical imaging,* Rockville, Md, 1987, Aspen.

Wegener O: *Whole body computed tomography,* ed 2, Malden, Mass, 1992, Blackwell.

Zeman R et al: *Helical/spiral CT: a practical approach,* New York, 1995, McGraw-Hill.

32

TOMOGRAPHY

AP tomogram of C1-C3 demonstrating complete fracture at base of dens *(arrow)*.

Historical Development

Since its inception in the 1890s, radiography has faced the problem of trying to record three-dimensional body structures accurately as two-dimensional images. This unavoidably results in the superimposition of structures, which often obscures important diagnostic information. One attempt to overcome this problem is the use of right-angle images. Over the years many other techniques have been developed that partially circumvent the problem of superimposition, such as multiple radiographs, stereoscopic images, and subtraction techniques in angiography.

The partial or complete elimination of obscuring shadows by the effect of motion on shadow formation is a common technique used in radiography. This effect is frequently used with conventional projections. For example, in conjunction with a long exposure time, breathing motion is used to reduce rib and pulmonary shadows to a background blur on frontal images of the sternum and lateral radiographs of the thoracic spine.

Body-section radiography (or more appropriately, *tomography*) is a term used to designate a radiographic technique by which most of the problems of superimposed images are overcome. *Tomography** is the term used to designate the technique

---

*Almost all italicized words on the succeeding pages are defined at the end of the chapter.

whereby a predetermined plane of the body is demonstrated in focus on the radiograph. Other body structures above or below the plane of interest are eliminated from the image or are rendered as a low-density blur caused by motion.

The origin of tomography cannot be attributed to any one person; in fact, tomography was developed by several gifted individuals experimenting in different countries at about the same time without any knowledge of each other's work. In 1921 Dr. André-Edmund-Marie Bocage, a French dermatologist, described in an application for a patent many of the principles used in modern tomographic equipment. Many other early investigators made significant contributions to the field of tomography. Each of these pioneers applied a different name to a particular device or process of body-section radiography. Bocage (1922) termed the result of his process *moving film roentgenograms;* the Italian Vallebona (1930) chose the term *stratigraphy;* and the Dutch physician Ziedses des Plantes (1932), who made several significant contributions, called his process *planigraphy.* The term *tomography* came from the German investigator Grossman, as does the *Grossman principle,* which is discussed later.

Tomography was invented in the United States in 1928 by Jean Kieffer, a radiographer who developed the special radio-

graphic technique to demonstrate a form of tuberculosis that he had. His process was termed *laminagraphy* by another American, J. Robert Andrews, who assisted Kieffer in the construction of his first tomographic device, the laminagraph.[1]

A great deal of confusion arose over the many different names given to the general process of body-section radiography. To eliminate this confusion, the International Commission of Radiological Units and Standards appointed a committee in 1962 to select a single term to represent all of the processes. *Tomography* is the term the committee chose, and this term is now recognized throughout the medical community as the single appropriate term for all forms of *body-section radiography.*[2]

Physical Principles

The physical principles of tomography are discussed in detail in all of the physics and imaging-related textbooks. Because the primary purpose of this atlas is to present radiographic positions, projections, and procedures, the physical principles previously discussed in this text have been removed. See the sixth through ninth editions of this atlas for the previously contained physical principles.

---

[1]Littleton JT: *Tomography: physical principles and clinical applications,* Baltimore, 1976, Williams & Wilkins.
[2]Vallebona A, Bistolfi F: *Modern thin-section tomography,* Springfield, Ill, 1973, Charles C. Thomas.

Clinical Applications

Tomography is a proven diagnostic tool that can be of significant value when a definitive diagnosis cannot be made from conventional radiographs. This is because tomography can remove confusing shadows from the point of interest. Tomography may be used in any part of the body but is most effective in areas of high contrast, such as bone and lung. Body-section radiography is used to demonstrate and evaluate a number of different pathologic processes, traumatic injuries, and congenital abnormalities. A basic familiarization with the clinical applications of tomography helps the tomographer to be more effective. Some of the major clinical applications of tomography are described in the following sections. However, this versatile technique has other applications as well.

PATHOLOGIC PROCESSES IN SOFT TISSUES

Tomography is frequently used to demonstrate and evaluate benign processes and malignant neoplasms in the lungs. Benign lesions and malignancies cannot always be differentiated with conventional chest radiography. However, tomography is capable of defining the location, size, shape, and marginal contours of a lesion.

Benign lesions characteristically have smooth, well-marginated contours and frequently contain bits of calcium. The presence of calcium in a chest lesion usually confirms it as being benign. The benign lesions most commonly found in the lungs are granulomas, which form as a tissue reaction to a chronic infectious process that has healed.

Conversely, carcinogenic neoplasms characteristically have ill-defined margins that feather or streak into the surrounding tissue and rarely contain calcium (Fig. 32-1). Lung cancers may originate in the lung, in which case the neoplasm is termed a *primary malignancy*. Bronchogenic carcinoma is an example of a *primary malignancy* that may develop in the chest. Lung cancers may develop as the result of the spread of cancer from another area of the body to the lungs. These malignancies are termed *secondary*, or *metastatic, tumors*. Breast cancer, testicular cancer, and other malignancies may metastasize to the lungs.

When an apparent solitary nodule is noted on a conventional chest radiograph, the presence or exclusion of other lesions may be determined with general tomographic surveys of both lungs. These "whole-lung" or "full-lung" tomograms are used to exclude the possibility of metastatic disease from other organs. Frequently these lesions cannot be visualized by conventional radiographic techniques, and tomography is one means of identifying these occult nodules. Demonstration of the number of tumors and their location, size, and relationship to other pulmonary structures is crucial to the physician's plan of treatment and the prognosis for the patient. Reexamination by tomography may be performed at a later date to check on the progress of the disease and the effectiveness of the therapy.

A

B

C

Fig. 32-1 A, PA chest radiograph demonstrating ill-defined density *(arrow)* in right upper chest. **B** and **C,** Collimated AP tomograms of patient in **A,** demonstrating lesion in posterior chest plane with ill-defined margins that feather or streak into surrounding lung tissue, characteristic of a malignant chest lesion.

PULMONARY HILA

Neoplasms involving the pulmonary hila are effectively evaluated by tomography, which can determine if and to what degree the individual bronchi are patent or obstructed. This partial or complete obstruction may occur when a neoplasm develops within the bronchus and bulges into the bronchial airspace when a tumor grows adjacent to the bronchus. As the lesion grows, it may press against the bronchus, reducing the size of the lumen and thus restricting or obstructing airflow to that part of the lung. Pneumonia, atelectasis, and other inflammatory or reactive changes that may occur with the obstruction may further hinder conventional imaging of this area. Demonstration of bronchial patency through a density is strong evidence that the lesion is inflammatory and not malignant (Fig. 32-2).

SOFT TISSUE LESIONS AFFECTING BONY STRUCTURES

Tomography is also used to demonstrate and evaluate soft tissue neoplasms in the presence of bony structures. Because of the high density of bone and the relatively low density of soft tissue neoplasms, the actual lesion usually cannot be demonstrated, but the bony destruction caused by the tumor may be demonstrated with great clarity.

For example, neoplasms involving the pituitary gland (e.g., pituitary adenoma) usually cause bony changes or destruction of the floor of the sella turcica, which indicates the presence of a pituitary adenoma. In addition to showing destruction caused by the tumor, tomography can demonstrate bony septations in the sphenoidal sinus, which aids the surgeon in removal of the tumor (Fig. 32-3).

Fig. 32-2 Normal bronchotomogram through midplane of hilum. **A,** Linear tomogram. **B,** Trispiral tomogram demonstrating the hilar structures more clearly: *1,* trachea; *2,* carina; *3,* left main bronchus; *4,* right main bronchus; *5,* intermediate bronchus; *6,* right upper lobe bronchus; *7,* right lower lobe bronchus; *8,* left lower lobe bronchus; *9,* left upper lobe bronchus.

Fig. 32-3 Tomograms through midplane of sella turcica demonstrating destruction of floor *(arrows)* caused by a pituitary adenoma. **A,** Lateral tomogram. **B,** AP tomogram.

LESIONS IN BONE

Subtle changes that may occur as a result of a pathologic process in bone tissue may be noted on conventional radiographs, but in many instances only tomography can determine the true nature and extent of the involvement (Fig. 32-4). Pathologic processes involving bony structures are normally characterized by bone destruction and changes in bone tissue or surface margins. More specifically, in tomography an attempt is made to identify the extent of bone destruction; the status of the cor-

tex of the bone (i.e., whether destruction extends through the cortical bone); the presence of any periosteal reaction to the lesion, changes in the bone matrix, or new bone formation; and the status of the zone between diseased and normal bone.

Destruction or other alterations of bone may result from a multitude of benign or malignant processes that manifest themselves in different ways. Some benign processes, such as osteomyelitis, are characterized by areas of bone destruction, whereas others, such as osteomas, appear

as abnormal growths of bone from bone tissue. Some processes may exhibit a combination of bone destruction and new growth, as occurs in Paget's disease and rheumatoid arthritis.

Malignant neoplasms in bone tissue may occur in the form of primary lesions or secondary lesions resulting from the metastatic spread of cancer from another area of the body. Some forms of cancer occurring in bone exhibit areas of both destruction and new growth, whereas others exhibit only areas of extensive destruction.

Fig. 32-4 A, PA wrist radiograph demonstrating healing fracture *(white arrow)* of scaphoid bone and increased density *(black arrow)* of proximal end. **B** through **D,** Tomograms at 3-mm intervals demonstrating fracture site *(white arrows)* with dense area *(black arrows)* of sclerotic bone at proximal end of scaphoid bone, consistent with aseptic necrosis.

FRACTURES

The three major clinical applications for tomography when dealing with known and suspected fractures are (1) identification and evaluation of occult fractures, (2) better evaluation of known fractures, and (3) evaluation of the healing process of fractures.

Occult fractures

If a fracture is suspected clinically but cannot be ruled out or identified by conventional imaging techniques, tomography may be indicated. Tomography is often used when fractures are suspected in areas of complex bone structures, such as the cervical spine. The cervical spine projects a myriad of confusing shadows, often hiding fracture lines and making an accurate diagnosis impossible. Tomography can identify and evaluate these occult fractures (Fig. 32-5). Knowledge of these fractures can be crucial to the plan of treatment and the prognosis for the patient.

The skull is another area that frequently requires tomographic evaluation for occult fractures. The skull has many complicated bone structures that often make identification and evaluation of fractures extremely difficult without the use of tomography. The facial nerve canal that courses through the temporal bone is just one of many areas that are difficult to evaluate for fractures without tomography. Blowout fractures of the orbital floor also frequently require tomographic evaluation because of the difficulty in identifying and evaluating fractures and fragments of the thin bones comprising the floor and medial wall of the orbit (Fig. 32-6).

Known fractures

Tomography may also be used to evaluate known fractures with greater efficiency than is possible with conventional radiography. In some instances a fracture may be visualized on a conventional radiograph, but because of the complex nature of the fracture or superimposition of shadows from adjacent structures, the fracture site cannot be adequately evaluated without the use of tomography. This is often the case in hip fractures involving the acetabulum. In acetabular fractures, portions of the acetabulum are often broken into many fragments that may be difficult to identify. With tomography the fragments and any possible femoral fracture can be evaluated before an attempt is made to reduce the fracture.

Fig. 32-5 AP tomogram of C1-C3 demonstrating complete fracture at base of dens *(arrow)*.

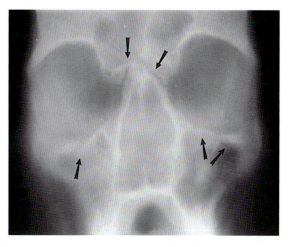

Fig. 32-6 Frontal tomogram using reverse Caldwell method, demonstrating multiple facial fractures *(arrows)*.

Healing fractures

Tomography may also be used to evaluate the healing process of fractures when conventional imaging techniques prove inadequate because of overlying shadows of fixation devices, adjacent structures, or bone callus. In these situations, tomography may be essential to assess whether the bone is healing properly throughout the fracture site. Tomography also can identify areas of incomplete healing in the fracture (Fig. 32-7).

ABDOMINAL STRUCTURES

Because of the relatively homogeneous densities of abdominal structures, both radiographic and tomographic imaging of this area are most effectively performed in conjunction with the use of contrast materials. Zonography is usually preferred for tomographic evaluation of these organs. As previously stated, zonography produces focal plane images of greater contrast than is possible with thin-section tomography. This increased level of contrast aids in visualization of the relatively low-density organs of the abdomen. The extensive blurring of remote structures that occurs with wide-angle tomography is not necessary in the abdomen because relatively few high-density structures exist in this area to compromise the zonographic imaging of the abdominal structures. Thick sections of organs are depicted with each zonogram, and entire organs can be demonstrated in a small number of tomographic sections.

A circular motion with an exposure angle of 8 or 10 degrees is recommended for use in the abdomen. Occasionally, an angle of 15 degrees may be necessary to eliminate bowel-gas shadows if the smaller angle does not provide adequate effacement (blurring) of the bowel.

Fig. 32-7 A, AP distal tibia radiograph demonstrating questionable complete union of fractures. **B,** AP tomogram of same patient as in **A,** demonstrating incomplete union of longitudinal fracture *(arrow)*. **C** and **D,** Tomograms demonstrating incomplete union of oblique fractures *(arrows)* through shaft of tibia of same patient as in **A** and **B. C,** Tomogram obtained 0.5 cm to **B. D,** Tomogram obtained ⅜ inch (1 cm) posterior to **B.**

Zonography using a linear movement is not recommended because it does not provide adequate blurring of structures outside the focal plane. If a linear movement is employed, an exposure angle of 15 degrees should be used to provide adequate blurring. Linear tomography does not produce accurate focal plane images because of the incomplete blurring effect of structures oriented parallel to the tube movement. Although the possibility of false image formation exists with circular tomography, the image of the focal plane is far more accurate than with linear tomography. Linear tomograms are higher in contrast than circular tomograms, but this is actually a result of the linear streaking caused by the incomplete blurring characteristics of linear motion. Circular motion, on the other hand, pro-duces an accurate focal plane image with slightly less but even contrast.

The most common tomographic examinations of the abdomen are of the kidneys and biliary tract. These examinations are normally performed with contrast material.

Renal tomography

Many institutions include tomography of the kidneys as part of the intravenous urography (IVU) procedure (Fig. 32-8). The tomograms are usually taken immediately after bolus injection of the contrast material. At this time the kidney is entering the nephrogram phase of the IVU, in which the nephrons of the kidney begin to absorb the contrast material, causing the parenchyma of the kidney to become somewhat radiopaque. Zonography may then be used to demonstrate lesions in the kidney that may have been overlooked with conventional radiography.

Another typical renal tomographic examination is the nephrotomogram. The major difference between this and the IVU is the method of introduction of the contrast material. In nephrotomography the contrast material is drip-infused throughout the examination instead of introduced in a single bolus injection. This method allows for a considerably longer nephrographic effect because the nephrons opacify the kidney as they continuously absorb and excrete the contrast material.

Fig. 32-8 **A,** IVU, AP abdomen radiograph. Bowel shadows obscure kidneys. **B,** AP tomogram of same patient as in **A,** obtained through midplane of kidneys using 8-degree circular motion. Bowel shadows are absent, and compared with **C,** visualization of kidneys is improved. **C,** AP tomogram of same patients as in **A** and **B** and at same levels as in **B,** but employing 20-degree linear motion. Note linear streaking and loss of detail of collecting systems and kidney borders.

Basic Principles of Positioning

Rarely in conventional radiography does one single radiographic image contain all the diagnostic information necessary to make an accurate diagnosis. This is also true in tomography; one series of tomograms in a single plane usually does not contain enough information to make an accurate diagnosis. As in radiography, two or more image planes are usually required for most tomographic examinations. For bilateral structures such as the internal acoustic canals, only one radiograph may be used. In such cases tomograms of the contralateral side are obtained for comparison.

Many fundamental radiographic body positions are used in tomography. The AP and lateral projections are basic to most tomographic examinations. Occasionally a special oblique projection may be necessary for optimal visualization of the part under investigation. The radiographer should observe the following positioning guidelines:

- In tomography, orient the structures either parallel or perpendicular to the tomographic plane. For example, when evaluating structures in the base of the skull, position the patient's head for a basal projection so that the base of the skull is oriented parallel to the section plane. This parallel position not only produces images that are more anatomically correct but also reduces the total number of tomograms necessary to cover the area of interest. If the base of the skull is not parallel but is slightly oblique, more tomograms are required to evaluate the area of interest adequately. This also pertains to other areas of the body in which large, relatively flat surfaces occur, such as in long bones.
- When producing tomograms of long bones, such as the femur, adjust the long axis of the bone to be parallel to the tomographic plane.

- For some structures, such as the sella turcica, use a perpendicular orientation for tomography. Because the presence of a pituitary adenoma usually affects the floor of the sella, orient the floor perpendicular to the section plane. AP and lateral radiographs are routinely used; for both images, the floor remains perpendicular to the tomographic plane.

Very few areas in radiology place greater demand on the knowledge and ability of the radiographer than the field of tomography. The tomographer must possess a strong background and understanding of anatomy and the spatial relationships of the structures of the body (see Chapter 26). The tomographic radiographer must know where certain structures of the general body parts are located, the best way to position those structures for tomographic examination, the depth at which particular structures are located, and the way the tomographic image should appear. On many occasions, even experienced tomographers must rely heavily on the knowledge and instruction of the radiologist monitoring the examination. The radiographer and radiologist should work together closely because no two tomographic examinations are exactly alike and each patient must be considered individually. The radiographer should observe the following guidelines when assisting with the tomographic examination:

- Provide the radiologist with an adequate clinical history of the patient. If this information is not provided on the examination requisition, obtain it by studying the patient's medical records or interviewing the patient.
- Review and discuss this clinical information and any pertinent radiographs with the radiologist before beginning the examination. After reviewing the information, the radiologist and radiographer can then determine the area of interest, the optimum position, the size of the field of exposure, the type of blurring motion and exposure angle

to be used, the separation intervals between tomographic sections, and the parameters for the fulcrum height. The most complex motion available should be used whenever possible.

- Complete all equipment preparation before positioning the patient. This reduces the amount of time that the patient is required to maintain an often uncomfortable position.
- Briefly and simply explain the procedure to the patient, and offer a rough estimate of the expected length of the examination. Many patients are under the mistaken impression that the procedure consists of a few radiographs taken in a matter of minutes and that they will then be permitted to leave. They are not aware that they will be required to maintain a certain position throughout the procedure. The patient who knows what to expect will be better able to cooperate throughout the lengthy examination.
- Ensure the patient's comfort, which is extremely important. The use of a suitable table pad is recommended for tomographic examinations. A table pad that is 1½ inches (3.8 cm) thick adds an insignificant amount to the overall patient thickness and greatly increases the patient's comfort. If uncomfortable, even the most cooperative patient will be unable to hold still for the examination.
- When necessary, use angle sponges and foam blocks to help the patient maintain the correct position. Do not, however, use foam sponges in tomographic examinations of the head. Section intervals of 1 or 2 mm are often employed in this area, and foam sponges do not give sufficiently firm support to the head. With little change in pressure the head may move, drastically altering the desired focal plane levels. Use folded towels to support the head if necessary; they offer greater resistance to any downward pressure.

Immobilization Techniques

The most effective immobilization technique is the radiographer's instructions to the patient. No amount of physical restraint can keep patients from moving if they do not fully understand the importance of holding still from the first preliminary image to the end of the tomographic series. The radiographer should observe the following guidelines:

- Because suspension of respiration is mandatory in examinations of the chest and abdomen, give explicit breathing instructions to the patient for examinations of these areas.
- In chest tomography, instruct the patient to take a consistent, uniform deep breath for each tomogram. Caution the patient not to strain to take in the maximum breath because the patient may have difficulty in holding the breath during the exposure. Tell the patient to take a moderately deep breath that can be comfortably held for the duration of the tomographic exposure. This not only allows for optimum inflation of the lungs but also provides consistency between the focal plane levels throughout the tomographic series. Consistency in inspirations is vitally important if the area of interest is located near the diaphragm. Slight variations in the amount of air taken in may result in obscuring of the area of interest by the elevated diaphragm. Suspension of respiration is also necessary to prevent blurring of structures by the breathing motion.
- Have the patient suspend respiration in the expiratory phase in examinations of the abdomen to elevate the diaphragm and visualize more of the abdomen. As in chest tomography, the suspension of respiration assists in maintaining consistency in tissue planes and reduces motion artifacts.

- Use suspended respiration techniques in tomographic examinations of the head if necessary. Unwanted motion of the head may occur when obese patients or patients with large breasts are positioned in the right anterior oblique (RAO) body position for lateral skull tomography. This problem may be resolved by having the patient suspend respiration during the exposure or by turning the patient over into a left posterior oblique (LPO) body position.
- Mark the entrance point of the central ray on the patient's skin. If the patient moves, this mark can be used as a reference point for repositioning, eliminating the need to take another scout image to recheck the position. If the mark is made with a grease pencil, it can easily be removed after the examination.
- When performing tomographic examination of the skull in the lateral position, place a small midline mark on the patient's nasion to assist measuring for the midline tomogram and to recheck the position between the scout image and the actual tomographic series. By ensuring that this mark is still at the same level from the tabletop, the interpupillary line is still perpendicular to the tabletop, and the central ray is still entering at the reference mark, the correct position can be maintained throughout the examination.

Scout Tomograms

Three preliminary tomograms are usually taken to locate the correct levels for the tomographic series. One tomogram is taken at the level presumed to be at the middle of the structure or area to be examined. The other two scout tomograms are taken at levels higher and lower than this midline tomogram. The separation interval between these tomograms depends on the thickness of the structure. Tomograms of small structures, such as those found in the skull, may be made at 5-mm or 1-cm intervals for the preliminary images. After the correct planes have been determined, the tomographic series is taken at smaller intervals. When the total depth of the area of interest is several centimeters thick, the separation interval for these scout tomograms is increased to $\frac{3}{4}$ inch (1.9 cm) or more. Table 32-1 includes separation intervals for the preliminary tomograms and tomographic series. The following guidelines are observed:

- Use external landmarks as reference points to assist in determining the proper fulcrum level.
- In some cases, such as chest lesions that can be identified on PA and lateral chest radiographs, take measurements from these radiographs to aid in the selection of the scout tomogram levels. For example, to determine the proper level for AP tomography of a chest lesion, measure the distance on the conventional lateral chest radiograph from the posterior chest wall to the middle of the lesion. Add this distance to the thickness of the table pad. Ensure that a scout tomogram taken at this fulcrum height is in the middle of the lesion.
- Use a similar process for tomography in the lateral position, taking the measurements from the AP chest radiograph.
- If the area of interest is not localized on the scout images, take a plain radiograph using the same centering as for the preliminary tomograms. This confirms that the area of interest is actually in the collimated field of interest and recentering is not required.

TABLE 32-1

Positioning for tomography

Examination part	Projection	Central ray position	Preliminary tomographic levels	Separation intervals	Comments
Sella turcica	AP	Glabella	1.5, 2.5, and 3.5 cm anterior to tragus	2 mm	Shield eyes
	Lateral	2.5 cm anterior and superior to tragus	21, 0, and 1 cm to midline of skull	2 mm	Place water bag under patient's chin for support
Middle ear (internal acoustic canal, facial nerve canal)	AP	Midpoint between inner and outer canthi	−0.5, 0, and 0.5 mm to tip of tragus	1 or 2 mm	Shield eyes
	Lateral	5 mm posterior and superior to external acoustic canal	At level of outer canthus and 1 and 2 cm medial	1 or 2 mm	Place water bag under patient's chin for support
Paranasal sinuses (general survey) and orbital floors	Reverse Caldwell	Intersection of midsagittal plane and infraorbital rims	22, 0, and 2 cm to level of outer canthus	3-5 mm	Infraorbitomeatal line should be perpendicular to tabletop
	Lateral	2 cm posterior to outer canthus	23 and 3 cm to midline of skull	3-5 mm	Place water bag under patient's chin for support
Base of skull	Submento-vertex	Midpoint between angles of mandible	21, 0, and 1 cm	2 or 3 mm	Orbitomeatal line should be parallel to tabletop
Cervical spine	AP	To vertebral body/bodies of interest	0, 22, and 24 cm to external acoustic meatus	3 or 5 mm	
	Lateral	To vertebral body/bodies of interest	22, 0, and 2 cm from midline of back	3 or 5 mm	Place water bag under patient's chin for support and two or more on neck to equalize density for entire cervical spine
Thoracic spine	AP	To vertebral body/bodies of interest	3, 5, and 7 cm from tabletop	5 mm	Flex knees slightly to straighten spine
	Lateral	To vertebral body/bodies of interest	22 and 2 cm from midline of back	5 mm	Flex knees, and place sponge against patient's back for support

TABLE 32-1

Positioning for tomography—cont'd

Examination part	Projection	Central ray position	Preliminary tomographic levels	Separation intervals	Comments
Lumbar spine	AP	To vertebral body/bodies of interest	4, 7, and 10 cm from tabletop	5 mm	Flex knees slightly to straighten spine
	Lateral	To vertebral body/bodies of interest	22, 0, and 2 cm from midline of back	5 mm	Flex knees and place sponge against patient's back for support
Hip	AP	Head of femur	22, 0, and 2 cm for greater trochanter	5 mm	Place water bag over area of greater trochanter to equalize density to hip
	Lateral (frog leg)	Head of femur	5, 7, and 9 cm from tabletop	5 mm	Place water bag over area of femoral neck to equalize density
Limbs	AP and lateral	At area of interest	5 mm to 1.5 cm, depending on size of limb	2-5 mm	Adjust limb to be parallel to tabletop
Chest (whole lung and hila)	AP	9-12 cm below sternal notch	10, 11, and 12 cm above tabletop	1 cm	Use through filter (80-90 kVp)
	Lateral	Midchest at level of pulmonary hila	25, 0, and 15 cm from midline of back	1 cm	Place sponge against patient's back for support
Chest (localized lesion)	AP and lateral	Measure distance to lesion from chest wall on plain radiographs, and center at this point on patient	Measure distance to lesion on lateral chest image and thickness of table pad; 22, 0, and 12 cm from measurement	2, 3, or 5 cm	Use low kVp (50-65) for high contrast
Nephrotomogram	AP	Midpoint between xiphoid process and top of iliac crests	7 cm for small patient; 9 cm for average patient; 11 cm for large patient	1 cm	Use 8-10 degrees of circular movement or 15-20 degrees of linear movement
Intravenous cholangiogram	AP oblique, 20-degree right posterior oblique	10 cm lateral to lumbar spine	10, 12, and 14 cm for small patient; 12, 14, and 16 cm for average patient; 13, 16, and 19 cm for large patient	5 mm-1 cm	Use 8-10 degrees of circular movement or 15-20 degrees of linear movement

Scout tomograms

General Rules for Tomography

The following rules are essential:

- Know the anatomy involved.
- Position the patient as precisely as possible.
- Use proper immobilization techniques.
- Use a small focal spot for tomography of the head and neck and limbs.
- Use a large focal spot for other areas of the body where fine recorded detail is not crucial.
- Use low kVp when high contrast is desired.
- Use high kVp when contrast differences between structures must be reduced; for example, whole-lung tomography requires a high kVp—80 to 90 kVp—in conjunction with a trough filter.
- When necessary, use water or flour bags to absorb primary or secondary radiation. For example, in lateral cervical spine tomography, place the bags on the upper cervical spine area to reduce the density difference between the spine and dense shoulders. Collimate the beam as tightly as possible to reduce patient exposure and improve contrast.
- Shield the patient, especially the eyes, in examinations of the skull and upper cervical spine.
- Use the proper blurring motion. In general, use the most complex blurring motion available. If zonography is required, use a circular motion. If only linear motion is available, take care to orient the part correctly to the direction of the tube.

- Mark each tomogram with the correct layer height. This may be done by directly exposing lead numbers on each tomogram or by marking each tomogram after it is processed. Another technique is to shift vertically the right or left marker used on each successive image. If the level of the first image is known, the correct level for each successive image can be determined. If multiple tomograms are taken on one image receptor, follow the same shift sequence to avoid confusion in marking the layer heights.

TOMOGRAPHY OF THE SKULL

Strict immobilization techniques must be used for any tomographic examination of the skull. Reference points should be marked on the patient for rechecking of the position.

The basic skull positions are outlined in the following sections and are to be used in conjunction with Table 32-1.

AP projection

- Adjust the patient's head to align the orbitomeatal line (OML) and the midsagittal plane perpendicular to the tabletop.
- Ensure that the distances from the tabletop to each tragus (the tonguelike projection of the ear just in front of the external acoustic meatus) are equal; this indicates that the head is positioned perfectly.

AP projection: reverse Caldwell method

- Position the infraorbitomeatal line (IOML) and the midsagittal plane perpendicular to the tabletop.
- Ensure that the tragi are equidistant from the tabletop.

Lateral projection

- Position the midsagittal plane parallel to the tabletop.
- Ensure that the interpupillary line is perpendicular to the tabletop.
- Check that the OML is approximately parallel to the lower border of the image receptor.

TOMOGRAPHY OF OTHER BODY PARTS

Standard radiographic projections (AP, lateral, and oblique) are used for most areas of the body. The same general rules of tomography apply to all areas. In general the projection that best demonstrates the area of interest in a conventional radiograph is usually the best for tomography. Selected tomograms are shown in Figs. 32-9 to 32-14.

Information on panoramic tomography, which is used to demonstrate the entire mandible and temporomandibular joint using one tomographic type of exposure, is provided in Chapter 21 of this atlas.

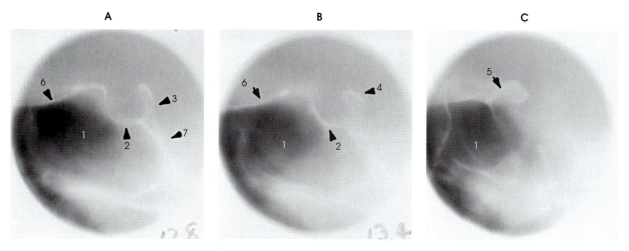

Fig. 32-9 Lateral sella turcica. **A,** Tomogram through midplane of sella. **B,** Tomogram 5 mm lateral to **A. C,** Tomogram ⅜ inch (1 cm) lateral to **A.** *1,* Sphenoidal sinus; *2,* floor of sella; *3,* dorsum sellae; *4,* posterior clinoid process; *5,* anterior clinoid process; *6,* planum sphenoidale; *7,* clivus.

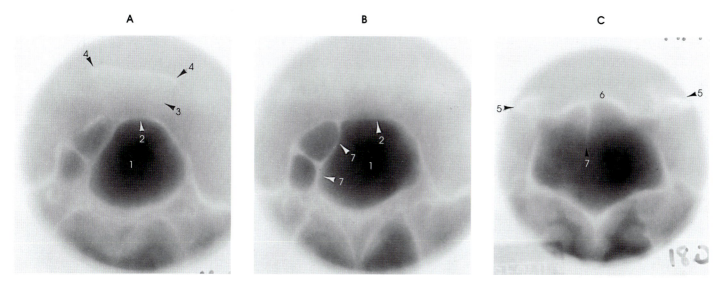

Fig. 32-10 AP tomograms of sella turcica. **A,** Tomogram in posterior plane of sella turcica. **B,** Tomogram ⅜ inch (1 cm) anterior to **A,** demonstrating floor of sella. **C,** Tomogram 2 cm anterior to **A,** demonstrating anterior clinoid processes. *1,* Sphenoidal sinus; *2,* floor of sella; *3,* dorsum sellae; *4,* posterior clinoid processes; *5,* anterior clinoid processes; *6,* planum sphenoidale; *7,* septations of sphenoidal sinus.

A   B   C

D   E   F

Fig. 32-11 AP tomograms of middle ear. Longitudinal linear **(A)**, transverse linear **(B)**, and trispiral **(C)** motion are at same posterior level of middle ear. Note improved visualization of structures with trispiral motion. AP tomograms anterior to level of **C** by 2 mm **(D)**, 4 mm **(E)**, and 6 mm **(F)**. *1*, External acoustic canal; *2*, internal acoustic canal; *3*, ossicular mass including malleus, incus, and lateral and superior semicircular canals; *4*, acoustic ossicles; *5*, vestibule; *6*, fenestra vestibuli; *7*, fenestra cochlea; *8*, cochlea; *9*, cochlea portion of facial nerve canal; *10*, carotid canal.

Fig. 32-12 AP lumbar spine showing suspected fracture *(arrow)* of L2 (see Fig. 32-13).

Fig. 32-13 AP tomograms further delineating fracture site shown in AP radiograph in Fig. 32-12. **A,** Tomogram through anterior plane of vertebral body, demonstrating wedging of vertebral body of L2 *(arrows)*. **B,** AP tomogram 2 cm posterior to **A** through lane of pedicles. Fracture line extends through right pedicle *(white arrow)* and vertebral body *(black arrow)*. **C,** AP tomogram 3 cm posterior to **A,** demonstrating displacement of fracture *(arrow)*. **D,** AP tomogram 4 cm posterior to **A,** demonstrating displaced fracture *(arrow)* of superior articular process of L3.

A　　　　　　　　B

C　　　　　　　　D

Fig. 32-14 AP tomograms of hip with fixation device at same level, comparing different blurring motions: **A,** trispiral; **B,** circular; **C,** longitudinal linear; **D,** oblique linear.

Conclusion

Tomography has changed dramatically since the early days of Bocage and des Plantes. Their crude devices bear little resemblance to today's modern tomographic machines. Tomography has been widely accepted as an extremely useful diagnostic tool. Linear tomographic machines can now usually be found in even the smallest hospitals. Many large hospitals have one or more linear units in addition to a pluridirectional machine.

Computed tomography (CT) and magnetic resonance imaging (MRI) have certainly proved themselves as extremely valuable diagnostic tools, and in most cases their images are far superior to those of conventional tomography. However, in many instances tomography can provide sufficient information for an accurate diagnosis at a cost far less than that of the more sophisticated imaging modalities. Furthermore, most MRI and CT scanners are extremely busy, and many cannot handle the high workload. Conventional tomography can often answer diagnostic questions satisfactorily or at least screen patients for further evaluation by the other, more sophisticated imaging modalities.

Although many equipment manufacturers still market a variety of x-ray machines capable of performing linear tomography, the more expensive, complex motion tomography units have been dropped from their product lines. In this era of cost containment, most health care facilities can ill afford to dedicate a piece of radiographic equipment solely for conventional tomography. Equipment manufacturers have taken note of this and have responded accordingly. Most equipment companies now offer a variety of tomographic options to their line of radiographic, fluoroscopic, and fixed radiographic units.

"Add-on" tomography devices of the twenty-first century look nothing like their crude predecessors, with their long metal bar attachments with sliding sleeves and thumbscrews to adjust fulcrum heights. The new units are simple to connect and usually provide push-button control for adjusting amplitude and layer height. Some of these devices do not even have a mechanical linkage but rather use microprocessor-controlled motorized drive units for the tube and Bucky, or other image receptor, trays to impart their motion. Although the linear tomographic images produced by these units do not quite compare with those produced by pluridirectional units, they are often considered quite acceptable. In this cost-conscious era, tomography will likely remain for many years a valuable diagnostic imaging tool for both small and large hospitals.

Definition of Terms

adjustable fulcrum Tomographic fulcrum that is either raised or lowered to achieve the desired fulcrum height (see *planigraphic principle*).

body-section radiography See *tomography*.

complex tomographic motion See *pluridirectional tomographic motion*.

exposure angle Degree of arc angulation described by the movement of the x-ray tube and cassette during a tomographic motion.

fixed fulcrum Tomographic fulcrum remains at a fixed height (see *Grossman principle*).

focal plane Plane of tissue that is in focus on a tomogram.

fulcrum Point of axis of rotation for a tomographic motion.

Grossman principle Tomographic principle in which the fulcrum or axis of rotation remains at a fixed height; the focal plane level is changed by raising or lowering the tabletop through this fixed point to the desired height.

laminagraphy See *tomography*.

linear tomographic motion Basic tomographic movement that occurs when x-ray tube and cassette movement occurs with the longitudinal axis of the tomographic table.

moving film roentgenogram See *tomography*.

phantom images False tomographic images that appear but do not represent an actual object or structure within the focal plane; these images are created by the incomplete blurring or the fusion of the blurred margins of some structures characteristic to the type of tomographic motion used.

planigraphic principle Tomographic principle in which the fulcrum, or axis of rotation, is raised or lowered to alter the level of the focal plane; the tabletop height remains constant.

planigraphy Synonymous with *tomography*.

pluridirectional tomographic motion Tomographic motion in many different directions.

section thickness Tomographic plane that is in maximum focus.

stratigraphy Synonym for *tomography*.

tomographic angle See *exposure angle*.

tomography Radiographic technique that depicts a single plane of tissue by blurring images of structures above and below the plane of interest.

unidirectional tomographic motion Tomographic motion in only a linear direction.

zonography Tomography that uses exposure angles of 10 degrees or less to depict thick sections or zones of tissue.

Selected bibliography

Andrews JR: Planigraphy. I. Introduction and history, *AJR* 36:575, 1936.

Berrett A: *Modern thin-section tomography*, Springfield, Ill, 1973, Charles C. Thomas.

Bocage AEM: French patent no. 536464, 1922.

Bosniak MA: Nephrotomography: a relatively unappreciated but extremely valuable diagnostic tool, *Radiology* 113:313, 1974.

Chasen MH et al: Tomography of the pulmonary hila: anatomical reassessment of the conventional 55 posterior oblique view, *Radiology* 149:365, 1983.

Durizch ML: *Technical aspects of tomography*, Baltimore, 1978, Williams & Wilkins.

Ho C, Sartoris DJ, Resnick D: Conventional tomography in musculoskeletal trauma, *Radiol Clin North Am* 27:929, 1989.

Holder JC et al: Metrizamide myelography with complex motion tomography, *Radiology* 145:201, 1982.

Kieffer J: United States patent, 1934.

Littleton JT: *Tomography: physical principles and clinical applications*, Baltimore, 1976, Williams & Wilkins.

Littleton JT et al: Adjustable- versus fixed-fulcrum tomographic systems, *AJR* 117:910, 1973.

Littleton JT et al: Linear vs. pluridirectional tomography of the chest: correlative radiographic anatomic study, *AJR* 134:241, 1980.

Maravilla KR et al: Digital tomosynthesis: technique for electronic reconstructive tomography, *AJR* 141:497, 1983.

Older RA et al: Importance of routine vascular nephrotomography in excretory urography, *Radiology* 136:282, 1980.

Potter GD et al: Tomography of the optic canal, *AJR* 106:530, 1969.

Sone S et al: Digital image processing to remove blur from linear tomography of the lung, *Acta Radiol* 32:421, 1991.

Stanson AW et al: Routine tomography of the temporomandibular joint, *Radiol Clin North Am* 14:105, 1976.

Valvasori GE: Laminagraphy of the ear: normal roentgenographic anatomy, *AJR* 89:1155, 1963.

33

MAGNETIC RESONANCE IMAGING

LUANN J. CULBRETH

Coronal MRI scan of the brain in a patient with a meningioma arising from the tentorium cere-belli. The precontrast T1-weighted image shows an inhomogeneous area of abnormality (*black arrows*), with mass effect elevat-ing the right lateral ventricle (*R*) and midline shift of the third ven-tricle (*V*). Artifact (*A*) from metal in skull from previous surgery.

Principles of Magnetic Resonance Imaging

*Magnetic resonance imaging** (MRI) has generated a great deal of interest among medical workers and the general public because it is an examination technique that provides both anatomic and physiologic information noninvasively. Like computed tomography (CT) (see Chapter 31), MRI is a computer-based cross-sectional imaging modality. However, the physical principles of MRI are totally different from those of CT and conventional radiography in that no x-rays are used to generate the MRI image. Indeed, no ionizing radiation of any kind is used in MRI. Instead, MRI creates images of structures through the interactions of magnetic fields and radio waves with tissues.

MRI was originally called *nuclear magnetic resonance* (NMR), with the word "nuclear" indicating that the non-radioactive atomic nucleus played an important role in the technique; however, this term has since been disassociated from MRI because of public apprehension about nuclear energy and nuclear weapons—neither of which is associated with MRI in any way (unless by coincidence a nuclear power plant is supplying electricity to an MRI unit). In addition, some forms of MRI do not involve the atomic nucleus and may, in the future, be used for imaging under the "magnetic resonance" umbrella.

---

*Almost all italicized words on the succeeding pages are defined at the end of this chapter.

Comparison of Magnetic Resonance Imaging and Conventional Radiography

Because MRI provides sectional images, it serves as a useful adjunct to conventional x-ray techniques. On a radiograph, all body structures exposed to the x-ray beam are superimposed into one "flat" image. In many instances, multiple projections or contrast agents are required to clearly distinguish one anatomic structure or organ from another. Sectional imaging techniques such as ultrasonography, CT, and MRI more easily separate the various organs because there is no superimposition of structures. However, multiple slices (cross sections) are required to cover a single area of the body.

In addition to problems with overlapping structures, conventional radiography is relatively limited in its ability to distinguish types of tissue. In radiographic techniques, *contrast* (the ability to discriminate two different substances) depends on differences in x-ray *attenuation* within the object and the ability of the recording medium (e.g., film) to detect these differences.

Radiographs cannot detect small attenuation changes. In general, conventional radiographs can distinguish only air, fat, soft tissue, bone, and metal because of the considerable difference in attenuation with each group. Most organs, such as the liver and kidneys, cannot be separated by differences in x-ray attenuation alone unless the differences are magnified through the use of contrast agents.

CT is much more sensitive to small changes in x-ray attenuation than is plain-film radiography. Thus CT can distinguish the liver from the kidneys on the basis of their different x-ray attenuation, as well as by position.

Like CT, MRI can resolve relatively small contrast differences among tissues. However, these tissue differences are unlike the differences in x-ray attenuation and the exiting radiation that produces the image. Contrast in MRI depends on the interaction of matter with electromagnetic forces other than x-rays.

Historical Development

The basic principle of MRI (discussed more fully in the next section) is that protons in certain atomic nuclei, if placed in a magnetic field, can be stimulated by (absorb energy from) radio waves of the correct frequency. After this stimulation the protons relax while energy is induced into a receiver antenna (the MRI signal), which is then digitized into a viewable image. *Relaxation times* represent the rates of signal decay and the return of protons to equilibrium.

Separate research groups headed by Bloch and Purcell first discovered the properties of magnetic resonance in the 1940s. Their work led to the use of MRI *spectroscopy* for the analysis of complex molecular structures and dynamic chemical processes. In 1952, Bloch and Purcell were jointly awarded the Nobel Prize in physics, and spectroscopic MRI is still in use today.

Nearly 20 years after the properties of MRI were discovered, Damadian showed that the relaxation time of water in a tumor differed from the relaxation time of water in normal tissue. This finding suggested that images of the body might be obtained by producing maps of relaxation rates. In 1973, Paul Lauterbur published the first cross-sectional images of objects obtained with MRI techniques. These first images were crude, and only large objects could be distinguished. Peter Mansfield further showed how the signals could be mathematically analyzed, which made it possible to develop a useful imaging technique. Mansfield also showed how extremely fast imaging could be achieved. Since that time, MRI technology has developed so much that tiny structures can be imaged rapidly with increased resolution and contrast.

In 2003, the Nobel Prize in Physiology or Medicine was jointly awarded to Lauterbur and Mansfield for their discoveries in MRI.

Physical Principles

SIGNAL PRODUCTION

The structure of an atom is often compared with that of the solar system, with the sun representing the central atomic *nucleus.* The planets orbiting the sun represent the electrons circling around the *nucleus.* MRI depends on the properties of the nucleus. Currently, most MRI scanners use the element hydrogen, the nucleus of which is a single proton, to generate a *signal.* Hydrogen nuclei are the strongest nuclear magnets on a per-nucleus basis; thus they create the strongest MRI signal. Also, hydrogen is the most common element in the body, which is another reason that it creates the strongest signal. Strong signals are important to produce satisfactory images.

Many atomic nuclei have magnetic properties, which means they act like tiny bar magnets (Fig. 33-1). Normally the magnetic protons point in random directions in the human body, as shown in Fig. 33-2. However, if the body is placed in a strong, uniform magnetic field, the nuclei attempt to line up with the direction of the magnetic field, much as iron filings line up with the field of a toy magnet. The word *attempt* is appropriate because the protons do not line up precisely with the external field but at an angle to the field, and they rotate about the direction of the magnetic field in a manner similar to the wobbling of a spinning top. This wobbling motion, depicted in Fig. 33-3, is called *precession*

and occurs at a specific *frequency* (rate) for a given atom's nucleus in a magnetic field of a specific strength. These precessing protons can absorb energy if they are exposed to *radiofrequency* (RF) pulses, which are very fast bursts of radio waves, provided that the radio waves and nuclear precession are of the same frequency. This absorption of energy occurs through the process of *resonance.*

The resonant frequency varies depending on the field strength of the MRI scanner. For example, at a field strength of 1.5 *tesla,* the frequency is approximately 63 MHz; at 1 tesla, the frequency is approximately 42 MHz; at 0.5 tesla, the frequency is approximately 21 MHz; and at 0.2 tesla, the frequency is approximately 8 MHz.

Before exposure to the RF pulse, the bulk of the hydrogen protons are oriented with the direction of the magnetic field. This causes the tissues to be magnetized in the longitudinal direction, which is also parallel to the magnetic field. When the RF pulse is applied and the protons absorb the energy, the result is a reorientation of the bulk of the tissue magnetization into a plane perpendicular to the main field. This is known as the *transverse plane.* The magnetization in the transverse plane also precesses at the same resonant frequency. The precessing transverse magnetization in the tissues then creates an electrical current in the receiving *antenna.* This follows Faraday's law of induction, in which a moving magnetic field induces electrical

current in a coil of wire. The electrical current in this application is measured as the MRI signal, which is much like the broadcasting radio waves that induce current in a car radio antenna.

The MRI signal is picked up by a sensitive antenna, amplified, and processed by a computer to produce a sectional image of the body. This image, like the image produced by a CT scanner, is an electronic image that can be viewed on a computer monitor and adjusted to produce the most information. If desired, the image can be printed for further study.

Many other nuclei in the body are potential candidates for use in imaging. Nuclei from elements such as phosphorus and sodium may provide more useful or diagnostic information than hydrogen nuclei, particularly in efforts to understand the metabolism of normal and abnormal tissues. Metabolic changes may prove to be more sensitive and specific in detecting abnormalities than the more physical and structural changes recognized by hydrogen-imaging MRI or by CT. However, the MRI signal from nonhydrogen nuclei is weak, imaging requires more elaborate equipment, and to date anatomic detail produced with sodium and phosphorus MRI is less complete than that produced with hydrogen MRI. Nonhydrogen nuclei may be of particular importance for combined imaging and spectroscopy, in which small volumes of tissue may be analyzed for chemical content.

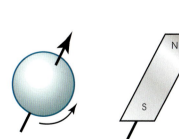

Fig. 33-1 A proton with magnetic properties can be compared with a tiny bar magnet. The curved arrow indicates that a proton spins on its own axis; this motion is different from that of precession.

Fig. 33-2 In the absence of a strong magnetic field, the protons *(arrows)* point in random directions and cannot be used for imaging.

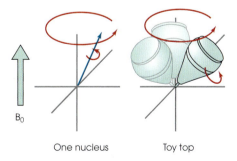

Fig. 33-3 Precession. Both the protons *(arrow)* and the toy top spin on their own axes. Both also rotate *(curved arrows)* around the direction of an external force in a wobbling motion called *precession.* Precessing protons can absorb energy through resonance. B_0 represents the external magnetic field acting on the nucleus. The toy top precesses under the influence of gravity.

SIGNIFICANCE OF THE SIGNAL

Conventional radiographic techniques, including CT, produce images based on a single property of tissue: x-ray attenuation or density. MR images are more complex because they contain information about three properties of tissue: nuclear density, relaxation rates, and flow phenomena. Each property contributes to the overall strength of the MRI signal. Computer processing converts signal strength to a shade of gray on the image. Strong signals are represented by white in the image, and weak signals are represented by black.

One determinant of signal strength is the number of precessing nuclei (spin density) in a given volume of tissue. The signal produced by the excited nuclei is proportional to the number of nuclei present. Therefore signal strength depends on the nuclear concentration, or density. Because the hydrogen nucleus is a single proton, its nuclear concentration is often referred to as *proton density*. Most soft tissues, including fat, have a similar number of protons per unit volume; therefore the use of proton density characteristics alone poorly separates most tissues. However, some tissues have few hydrogen nuclei per unit of volume; examples include the cortex of bone and air in the lungs. These have a weak signal as a result of low proton density and can be easily distinguished from other tissues.

MRI signal intensity also depends on the relaxation times of the nuclei. One component of *relaxation* is the release of energy by the excited protons, which occurs at different rates in different tissues. Excited nuclei relax through two processes. The process of nuclei releasing their excess energy to the general environment or lattice (the arrangement of atoms in a substance) is called *spin-lattice relaxation*. The rate of this relaxation process is measured in milliseconds and is labeled as T1. *Spin-spin relaxation* is the release of energy by excited nuclei through interaction among themselves. The rate of this process is also measured in milliseconds but is labeled as T2.

The rates of relaxation (T1 and T2) of a hydrogen nucleus depend on the chemical environment in which the nucleus is located. Chemical environment differs among tissues. For example, the chemical environment of a hydrogen nucleus in the spleen differs from that of a hydrogen nucleus in the liver. Therefore the relaxation rates of these nuclei differ, and the MRI signals created by these nuclei differ. The different relaxation rates in the liver and spleen result in different signal intensities and appearances on the image, enabling the viewer to discriminate between the two organs. Similarly, fat can be separated from muscle and many tissues can be distinguished from others, based on the relaxation rates of

their nuclei. Indeed, the most important factor in tissue discrimination is the relaxation time.

The signals produced by MRI techniques contain a combination of proton density and T1 and T2 information. However, it is possible to obtain images weighted toward any one of these three parameters by stimulating the nuclei with certain specific radio-wave *pulse sequences*. In most imaging sequences, a short T1 (fast spin-lattice relaxation rate) produces a high MRI signal on T1-weighted images. Conversely, a long T2 (slow spin-spin relaxation rate) generates a high signal on T2-weighted images.

The final property that influences image appearance is flow. For complex physical reasons, moving substances usually have weak MRI signals. (With some specialized pulse sequences, the reverse may be true; see the discussion of magnetic resonance angiography [MRA] later in the chapter.) With standard pulse sequences, flowing blood in vessels produces a low signal and thus is easily discriminated from surrounding stationary tissues without the need for the contrast agents required by regular radiographic techniques. Stagnant blood, such as an acute blood clot, typically has a high MRI signal in most imaging schemes as a result of its short T1 and long T2. The flow sequences of MRI may facilitate the assessment of vessel patency or the determination of the rate of blood flow through vessels (Fig. 33-4).

Fig. 33-4 Axial 1.5-tesla T1-weighted MRI scan through the upper chest. Lungs (L) have low signal as a result of low proton density. Fat (F) has high signal because of its short T1 relaxation rate. Moving blood in vessels (V) has low signal from the flow phenomenon. Hilar tumor (arrow) is easily identified, outlined against the low signal intensity of the lung and the vessels.

Equipment

Like CT, MRI requires a patient area (magnet room), a computer room, and an operator's console. A separate diagnostic workstation is optional.

CONSOLE

The operator's console is used to control the computer. The computer initiates the appropriate radio-wave transmissions and then receives and analyzes the data. Images are viewed on the operator's console to ensure that the proper part of the patient is being evaluated (Fig. 33-5). Images may be printed, most often on special medical film using a laser or multi-image camera.

The independent diagnostic workstation may be used to perform the same functions as those of the operator's console, depending on system configuration. However, usually only the operator's console can control the actual imaging process.

COMPUTER ROOM

The computer room houses the electronics necessary for transmitting the radio-wave pulse sequences and for receiving and analyzing the MRI signal. The *raw data* and the computer-constructed images can be stored on a computer disk temporarily but are usually transferred to a magnetic tape or an optical disk for permanent storage and retrieval.

Fig. 33-5 Operator's console. This device controls the imaging process and allows visualization of images.

(Courtesy General Electric Medical Systems, Milwaukee, Wis.)

MAGNET ROOM

The magnet is the major component of the MRI system in the scanning room. This magnet must be large enough to surround the patient and any antennas that are required for radio-wave transmission and reception. Antennas are typically wound in the shape of a positioning device for a particular body part. These are commonly referred to as *coils*. The patient is usually placed within the coil. Surface coils are placed directly on the patient and are used in the imaging of superficial structures. However, the patient and coil must still be within the magnet to be exposed to the proper magnetic field for imaging. The patient lies on the table and is advanced into the imaging magnetic field (Fig. 33-6).

Various magnet types and strengths may be used to provide the strong uniform magnetic field required for imaging.

Resistive magnets are simple but large electromagnets consisting of coils of wire.

A magnetic field is produced by passing an electric current through the wire coils. High magnetic fields are produced by passing a large amount of current through a large number of coils. The electrical resistance of the wire produces heat and limits the maximum magnetic field strength of resistive magnets. The heat produced is conducted away from the magnet by a cooling system.

Superconductive (cryogenic) magnets are also electromagnets. However, their wire loops are cooled to very low temperatures with liquid helium to reduce electrical resistance. This permits higher magnetic field strengths than those produced by resistive magnets.

Permanent magnets are a third source for producing the magnetic field. A permanent magnet has a constant field that does not require additional electricity or cooling. The early permanent magnets were extremely heavy, even when compared with the massive superconductive and resistive units. Because of their weight, these magnets were difficult to place for clinical use. With improvements in technology, permanent magnets have become more competitive with the other magnet types. For example, the magnetic field of permanent magnets does not extend as far away from the magnet (*fringe field*) as do the magnetic fields of other types of magnets. Fringe fields are a problem because of their effect on nearby electronic equipment.

Various MRI systems operate at different magnetic field strengths. The choice of optimum field strength for imaging is controversial. Magnetic field strength is measured in tesla or *gauss* (G). Most MRI has been performed with field strengths ranging from 0.2 to 1.5 tesla. Resistive systems generally do not exceed 0.15 tesla, and permanent magnet systems do not exceed 0.3 tesla. Higher field strengths require superconductive technology. However, the U.S. Food and Drug Administration (FDA) currently limits clinical MRI systems to a maximum field strength of up to 3.0 tesla. Most research has concluded that field strengths in this range do not produce any substantial harmful effects.

Regardless of magnet type, MRI units remain relatively difficult to install in hospitals. Current units are quite heavy—up to 10 tons for resistive and superconductive magnets and approximately 100 tons for some permanent magnets. Some institutional structures cannot support these weights without reinforcement. In addition, choosing a location for an MRI unit can be difficult because of fringe fields. With resistive and superconductive magnets, the fringe field extends in all directions and thus may interfere with nearby electronic or computer equipment, such as television monitors and computer tapes. In addition, metal objects moving near the magnetic fringe field, such as automobiles or elevators, may cause ripples in the field, similar to the ripples caused by a pebble thrown into a pond. These ripples can be carried into the center of the magnet, where they distort the field and ruin the images. Thus MRI sites must be located far enough away from moving metal objects. Efforts continue to be made to find more ways to shield the magnetic fringe field to prevent its extension beyond the patient area.

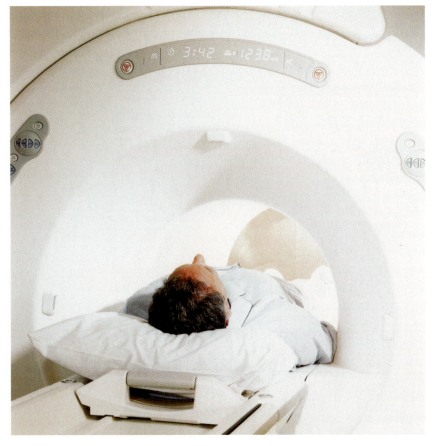

Fig. 33-6 Patient prepared for MRI.

(Courtesy General Electric Medical Systems, Milwaukee, Wis.)

Stray radio waves present another difficulty in the placement of MRI units. The radio waves used in MRI may be the same as those used for other nearby radio applications. Stray radio waves can be picked up by the MRI antenna coils and interfere with normal image production. Many MRI facilities require specially constructed rooms to shield the antenna from outside radio interference, thus adding to the cost of the installation.

Over the last several years, specialty units have become available for limited applications. One example of this is an extremity MRI scanner (Fig. 33-7). This unit is designed so that the patient can sit comfortably in a chair while having an extremity or musculoskeletal joint imaged. These units are lightweight, approximately 1500 pounds, and take up less space than do conventional MRI scanners, and they produce good image quality (Fig. 33-8).

Fig. 33-7 Extremity MRI scanner, 1.0 tesla.

(Courtesy ONI Medical Systems, Inc., Wilmington, Mass.)

Fig. 33-8 Coronal MRI of the knee obtained with extremity MRI scanner.

(Courtesy ONI Medical Systems, Inc., Wilmington, Mass.)

Safety of Magnetic Resonance Imaging

MRI is generally considered safe. It is often preferred over CT for the imaging of children because it does not use ionizing radiation, which has known potential adverse health effects. The young and growing child's body is thought to be more susceptible to the effects of ionizing radiation. Nevertheless, a number of potential safety issues concerning MRI must be raised, some related to potential direct effects on the patient from the imaging environment, and others related to indirect hazards.

Opinions differ about the safety of the varying magnetic and RF fields to which the patient is directly exposed. Many studies in which experimental animal and cell culture systems were exposed to these fields over long periods have reported no adverse effects, whereas others have reported changes in cell cultures and embryos. Some energy is deposited in the patient during imaging and is dissipated in the body as heat. The resulting changes appear to be less than the levels considered clinically significant, even in areas of the body with poor heat dissipation, such as the lens of the eye. The significance of direct short-term exposure (i.e., exposure of a patient) and long-term exposure (i.e., exposure of an employee who works with MRI) is not clear. No clear association of MRI with adverse effects in humans has been proven, but research is continuing.

A number of hazards related to MRI have, however, been well documented. Objects containing magnetic metals (e.g., iron, nickel, cobalt) in various combinations may be attracted to the imaging magnet with sufficient force to injure patients or personnel who may be interposed between them. Scissors, oxygen tanks, and patient gurneys are among the many items that have been drawn into the magnetic field at MRI sites. Metallic implants within patients or personnel can become dislodged within the body and cause injury if they are in delicate locations. Examples include intracranial aneurysm clips, auditory implants, and metallic foreign bodies in the eye. On the other hand, long-standing, firmly bound surgical clips, such as those from a cholecystectomy, do not pose problems. Electronic equipment can malfunction when exposed to strong magnetic fields. The most critical items in this category are cardiac pacemakers and the similar automatic implantable cardiac defibrillators. Therefore patients, visitors, and personnel should be screened to ensure that they do not have metallic objects on or in their bodies that could be adversely affected by exposure to strong magnetic fields.

Patients have received local burns from wires, such as electrocardiographic (ECG) leads, and other monitoring devices touching their skin during MRI examinations. These injuries have resulted from electrical burns caused by currents induced in the wires or thermal burns caused by heating of the wires. Such burns can be prevented by checking wires for frayed insulation, ensuring that no wire loops are within the magnetic field, and placing additional insulation between the patient and any wires exiting the MRI system.

The varying magnetic forces in an MRI unit act on the machine itself, causing knocking or banging sounds. These noises can be loud enough to produce temporary or permanent hearing damage. The use of earplugs or nonmagnetic headphones can be helpful in preventing auditory complications and are highly recommended to be used by each patient being scanned.

Claustrophobia can be a significant impediment to MRI in up to 10% of patients (Fig. 33-9). Patient education is perhaps most important in preventing this problem, but tranquilizers, appropriate lighting and air movement within the magnet bore, and mirrors or prisms that enable a patient to look out of the imager may be helpful. Claustrophobia can also be prevented by having a family member or friend accompany the patient and be present in the room during the scan.

In superconductive magnet systems, rapid venting of the supercooled liquid gases (helium) from the magnet or its storage containers into the surrounding room space is a rare but potential hazard because the relative concentration of oxygen in the air could be reduced to unsafe levels. Unconsciousness or asphyxiation could result. Oxygen monitoring devices in the magnet or cryogen storage room can signal personnel when the oxygen concentration falls too low. Personnel may then evacuate the area and activate ventilation systems to exchange the escaped gas for fresh air.

Fig. 33-9 Patient inside a superconducting 1.5-tesla magnet. Some patients cannot be scanned because of claustrophobia.

(Courtesy General Electric Medical Systems, Milwaukee, Wis.)

Fig. 33-10 Two images (different patients) from a 1.5-tesla superconductive MRI scanner, showing excellent resolution of images. **A,** This image shows remarkable anatomic detail in a midsagittal image of the head. Normal folds *(F)* on the inner surface of the brain are identified. *CC,* Corpus callosum; *CL,* cerebellum; *B,* brainstem; *V,* ventricle; *A,* air in sinuses. **B,** This coronal image of the pelvis shows anatomic relationships of the prostate *(P),* which is enlarged and elevating the bladder *(B).* Hips *(H)* and acetabula *(A)* are also shown. A loop of the sigmoid *(S)* colon is on top of the bladder. This degree of resolution in coronal or sagittal images would be difficult to obtain by reformatting a series of transverse CT slices.

Examination Protocols

IMAGING PARAMETERS

The availability of many adjustable parameters makes MRI a complex imaging technique. Knowledge of the patient's clinical condition or probable disease is important in choosing the proper technique and in imaging the correct area of the body.

The operator may choose to obtain MR images in sagittal, coronal, transverse, or oblique planes. These are independently acquired images with equal resolution in any plane (Fig. 33-10). In contrast, data can be obtained only in the transverse plane with CT. Sagittal and coronal CT images can then be generated by reformatting the data from a series of transverse slices, usually with a loss of resolution.

Another MRI technique, especially when a large number of thin slices and/or multiple imaging planes are desired, is three-dimensional (3D) imaging. In this technique, MRI data are collected simultaneously from a 3D block of tissue rather than from a series of slices. Special data collection techniques and subsequent computer analysis allow the images from the single imaging sequence to be displayed in any plane (Fig. 33-11).

Fig. 33-11 Single slice from a 3D acquisition of the knee on a 1.5-tesla MRI unit. Data from an entire volume within the imaging coil are obtained concurrently. The data may then be reconstructed into thin slices in any plane, such as the sagittal image shown here. This imaging sequence shows hyaline cartilage *(arrowheads)* as a fairly high signal intensity rim overlying the bone. Meniscal fibrocartilage *(arrows)* has low signal intensity. High signal intensity from joint fluid in a tear *(curved arrow)* within the posterior meniscus is visualized.

Slice thickness is important in the visualization of pathology. More MRI signal is available from a thicker slice than a thinner slice, so thicker slices may provide images that are less grainy. However, small pathologic lesions may be hidden by the surrounding tissues in the thicker slices. Therefore slice thickness may need to be adjusted based on the type of lesion under investigation.

Another important MRI parameter is overall imaging time. As imaging time (per slice) is lengthened, more MRI signal is available for analysis. Image quality thus improves with increased signal. However, fewer patients can be imaged when extended data acquisitions are performed. In addition, patient motion increases with prolonged imaging times; as a result, image quality is reduced.

The imaging sequence is a crucial parameter in MRI. Depending on the choice of pulse sequence, the resulting images may be more strongly weighted toward proton density, T1, or T2 information. Depending on the relative emphasis given to these factors, normal anatomy (Fig. 33-12) or a pathologic lesion (Fig. 33-13) may be easily recognized or difficult to see. It is not unusual for a lesion to stand out dramatically when one pulse sequence is used yet be nearly invisible (same MRI signal as surrounding normal tissue) with a different pulse sequence. Considerable research continues to determine the optimum pulse sequences for scanning various patient problems.

Although varying the timing parameters of an individual pulse sequence can alter the relative weighting of information received, certain classes of pulse sequences tend to emphasize information about proton density, T1, T2, and even flow. *Spin echo* sequences are the classic imaging sequences usually used with timing parameters to yield T1-weighted images, but they can also provide proton density–weighted images and T2-

Fig. 33-12 Coronal 1.5-tesla images through a normal brain. **A,** The T1-weighted image shows relatively low differentiation of gray matter *(G)* and white matter *(W)* within the brain. **B,** The heavily T2-weighted image shows improved differentiation between gray and white matter. CSF around the brain *(arrows)* and within the ventricles *(V)* also changes in appearance with change in pulse sequence (low signal on T1-weighted image); fat *(F)* normally shows high signal intensity, whereas on the T2-weighted image, the signal intensity of fat is less than that of CSF.

weighted images. *Inversion recovery* is a sequence that accentuates T1 information but can also provide a special result in that the timing parameters can be chosen to minimize signal intensity in a particular tissue. Fat is usually the tissue chosen to have its intensity minimized, and so-called *fat-suppressed images* can be useful when the high signal from extensive fat overwhelms small signal intensity differences in the tissues of interest. Additional techniques to suppress the signal from fat and/or fluid have been developed for pulse sequences other than inversion recovery.

Standard imaging sequences such as spin echo and inversion recovery are rela-tively time consuming and slow patient "throughput," or productivity regarding the number of procedures per unit of time. Therefore MRI engineers and physicists have developed faster pulse sequences to speed up examinations. The oldest and most common type of faster imaging sequence is the *gradient echo* pulse sequence. In the early 1990s, a fast spin-echo pulse sequence, known as *rapid acquisition recalled echo,* was created. In recent years an even faster sequence, called *echo planar imaging,* has been implemented. Some imaging sequences are short enough that imaging can be accomplished during a breath hold. Many of the fast pulse sequences are sensitive to flow and may be used to provide images of blood vessels. (See the discussion of MRA later in this chapter.)

POSITIONING

Patient positioning for MRI is usually straightforward. In general, the patient lies supine on a table that is subsequently advanced into the magnetic field. As previously discussed, it is important to ensure that the patient has no contraindications to MRI, such as a cardiac pacemaker or intracranial aneurysm clips. As previously noted, claustrophobia may be a problem for some patients because the imaging area is tunnel shaped in most MRI system configurations (see Fig. 33-9).

Fig. 33-13 Axial MRI scans using two different pulse sequences in a child with a medullo-blastoma. **A,** The T1-weighted image shows that limited contrast exists between the tumor (*T*) and normal brain. **B,** The lesion becomes dramatically more obvious using the pulse sequence of the T2-weighted image. Choice of pulse sequence is critical. These images also demonstrate how the lack of bone artifact makes MRI superior to CT for the imaging of posterior fossa lesions.

COILS

The *coils* used for MRI are necessary for both transmitting the RF pulse and receiving the MR signal (as described earlier in Signal Production). Some coils can both transmit and receive (transceiver coils), whereas others may only receive the signal (receiver coils).

The body part to be examined determines the shape of the antenna coil that is used for imaging (Figs. 33-14 and 33-15). Most coils are round or oval in shape, and the body part to be examined is inserted into the coil's open center. Some coils, rather than encircling the body part, are placed directly on the patient over the area of interest. These surface coils are best for the imaging of thin body parts, such as the limbs, or superficial portions of a larger body structure, such as the orbit within the head or the spine within the torso. Another form of receiver coil is the endocavitary coil, which is designed to fit within a body cavity such as the rectum. This enables a receiver coil to be placed close to some internal organs that may be distant from surface coils applied to the exterior body. Endocavitary coils also may be used to image the wall of the cavity itself (Fig. 33-16).

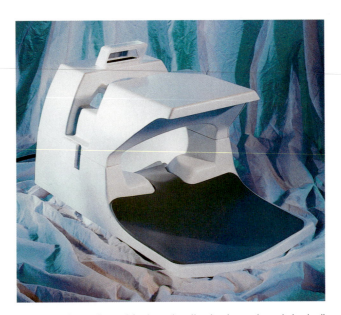

Fig. 33-14 A neurovascular coil used for imaging the brain and neck, including the blood vessels as seen in Figs. 33-31 and 33-32.

(Courtesy General Electric Medical Systems.)

Fig. 33-15 Examples of coils used for MRI. *Upper shelf, left to right:* breast coil, knee and foot/ankle coil. *Lower shelf, left to right:* wrist coil, head coil.

PATIENT MONITORING

Although most MRI sites are constructed so that the operator can see the patient during imaging, the visibility is often limited; thus the patient is relatively isolated within the MRI room (see Fig. 33-9). At most sites, intercoms are used for verbal communication with the patient, and some units have "panic buttons" with which the patient may summon assistance. However, these devices may be insufficient to monitor the health status of a sedated, anesthetized, or unresponsive patient. MRI-compatible devices now exist to monitor multiple physiologic parameters such as heart rate, respiratory rate, blood pressure, and oxygen concentration in the blood. Typically, leads from probes placed on the patient extend to the operator's room, where the data are displayed on a monitor (see Fig. 33-5). Local policy and patient condition dictate which physiologic parameters are monitored.

Fig. 33-16 Axial image of the prostate obtained with an endorectal coil. The mixed signal intensity in the inner gland region (*I*) of the prostate results from benign prostatic hyperplasia. The high-intensity outer gland (*O*) is interrupted by a low intensity region representing prostatic carcinoma (*T*). The close proximity of the endorectal coil to the area of the desired imaging improves resolution. *V,* Signal void from rectum (coil itself is not imaged); *W,* rectal wall.

CONTRAST MEDIA

Contrast agents that widen the signal differences in MR images between various normal and abnormal structures are the subjects of a continuing research and development. A good orally administered agent for identifying bowel loops in MRI scans has not yet been identified. In CT scanning, the use of high-attenuation, orally administered contrast medium allows clear differentiation of the bowel from surrounding lower-attenuation structures. However, in MRI scans, the bowel may lie adjacent to normal or pathologic structures of low, medium, and high signal intensity, and these intensities may change as images of varying T1 and T2 weighting are obtained. It is difficult to develop an agent that provides good contrast between the bowel and all other structures under these circumstances. Air, water, fatty liquids (e.g., mineral oil), dilute iron solutions (e.g., Geritol), gadolinium compounds designed for intravenous (IV) use, barium sulfate, kaolin (a clay), and a variety of miscellaneous agents have all been used—none with complete success.

At this time, the only IV MRI contrast agents approved in the United States for routine clinical use in the whole body are gadolinium-containing compounds.

Gadolinium is a metal with *paramagnetic* effects. Pharmacologically, an intravenously administered gadolinium compound acts in a manner similar to radiographic iodinated IV agents: it distributes through the vascular system, its major route of excretion is the urine, and it respects the blood-brain barrier (i.e., it does not leak out from the blood vessels into the brain substance unless the barrier has been damaged by a pathologic process). Gadolinium compounds have lower toxicity and fewer side effects than the IV iodinated contrast media used in radiography and CT.

Gadolinium compounds are used most commonly in evaluation of the CNS. The most important clinical action of gadolinium compounds is the shortening of T1. In T1-weighted images, this provides a high-signal, high-contrast focus in areas where gadolinium has accumulated by leaking through the broken blood-brain barrier into the brain substance (Fig. 33-17). Furthermore, in gadolinium-enhanced T1-weighted images, brain tumors or metastases are better distinguished from their surrounding edema than in routine T2-weighted images. Gadolinium improves the visualization of small tumors or tumors that have a signal intensity similar to that of a normal brain, such as meningiomas. IV injections

of gadolinium also have been used in dynamic imaging studies of body organs such as the liver and kidneys, similar to techniques using standard radiographic iodinated agents in CT.

A number of novel contrast agents for MRI are under development, but many of them are not yet approved for routine clinical use. An iron oxide mixture (Feridex) is the only *superparamagnetic* contrast agent currently available. This contrast agent is used to detect and diagnose liver lesions.

Contrast media currently in development include agents that are specifically designed to enhance the blood. Imaging using these agents may allow estimates of tissue perfusion and ischemia. Enhancement of heart muscle could assist in differentiating healthy, ischemic, or infarcted myocardial tissue. Contrast agents selectively taken up in the liver may improve the detection of liver tumors or metastases. Selective enhancement of lymph nodes may allow tumor involvement to be detected directly, obviating the need to rely on crude size criteria for abnormality. The production of contrast agents with an affinity for specific tumors may also be possible. Radioactive-labeled antibodies against tumors are available for use in nuclear medicine, and appropriately labeled antibodies could carry paramagnetic compounds to tumor sites.

A

B

C

Fig. 33-17 Use of IV-administered gadolinium contrast medium for lesion enhancement in coronal images of the brain. **A,** T1-weighted sequence. Two brain metastases *(arrowheads)* are identified as focal areas of low signal. **B,** Image obtained using similar parameters after IV administration of gadolinium contrast material. Previously seen metastases are more conspicuous, and additional metastases are visualized *(arrowheads)*. **C,** T2-weighted image. High signal areas *(arrowheads)* represent metastases and surrounding edema; focal lesion size and precise location are more difficult to identify. Additional high signal intensity areas on T2-weighted image represent edema from focal lesions seen on other slices in the gadolinium-enhanced series.

GATING

Gated imaging is another technique for improving image quality in areas of the body in which involuntary patient motion is a problem. A patient can hold the head still for prolonged data acquisition, but the heartbeat and breathing cannot be suspended for the several minutes required for standard MRI studies. Even fast pulse sequences are susceptible to motion *artifact* from the beating heart. This is a problem when images of the chest or upper abdomen are desired. If special techniques are not used, part of the MRI signal may be obtained when the heart is contracted (systole) and part when the heart is relaxed (diastole). When information is combined into one image, the heart appears blurred. This problem is analogous to photographing a moving subject with a long shutter speed. Similar problems in MRI occur with the different phases of respiration.

Gating techniques are used to organize the signal so that only the signal received during a specific part of the cardiac or respiratory cycle is used for image production (Fig. 33-18). Gated images may be obtained in one of two ways. In one technique of cardiac gating, the imaging pulse sequence is initiated by the heartbeat (usually monitored by an ECG). Thus the data collection phase of the pulse sequence occurs at the same point in the cardiac cycle. Another method is to obtain data throughout the cardiac cycle but record the point in the cycle at which each group of data was obtained. After enough data are collected, the data are reorganized so that all data recorded within a certain portion of the cardiac cycle are collated together; for example, data collected during the first eighth of the cycle, second eighth of the cycle, and so on. Each grouping of data can be combined into a single image, producing multiple images at different times in the cycle.

The gating techniques are analogous to obtaining high-quality pictures of eight children on a spinning merry-go-round with a video camera in which the image from a single frame is of insufficient quality. If an image of only one of the children is desired, one video frame could be shot each time the child came into the video viewfinder. Later, all the frames could be combined into one high-quality image. This is equivalent to the first gating technique. Alternately, if pictures of all the children are desired, the video camera could be run continuously, with documentation of which frames have which child in them. Later, all the frames showing the first child could be matched, all the frames showing the second child could be matched, and so forth. The result would be eight pictures, each showing one of the children. This is equivalent to the second gating technique.

Fig. 33-18 Gated images of the heart in different phases of the cardiac cycle. Imaging was obtained continuously, with incoming data subdivided into various portions of the cardiac cycle. **A,** Left ventricular outflow tract. **B,** Short axis images. Anatomy demonstrated includes the aorta (*A*), left ventricle (*LV*), left ventricular wall (*LVW*), pulmonary artery (*PA*), right ventricle (*RV*), and sternal wires resulting in MR signal void (*S*).

OTHER CONSIDERATIONS

When MRI was introduced, quite long imaging times were required to obtain enough information to reconstruct the sectional images. For most routine imaging this remains the standard. With advances in technology, however, it has become possible to quickly (within seconds) obtain enough data to reconstruct an image by using special fast-imaging pulse sequences. These fast-imaging pulse sequences are becoming more popular for specialized applications such as the obtainment of a dynamic series of images after IV administration of contrast agents. In many such sequences, fluid has a high signal intensity. This can produce a myelogram-like effect in studies of the spine or an arthrogram-like effect in evaluation of joint fluid (see Fig. 33-11). Quality assurance is important in a complex technology such as MRI. Calibration

of the unit is generally performed by service personnel. However, routine scanning of phantoms by the technologist can be useful for detecting any problems that may develop.

Clinical Applications
CENTRAL NERVOUS SYSTEM

MRI is superior to CT for imaging the posterior fossa, which is the portion of the brain that includes the cerebellum and brainstem. Artifact from the dense bone of the surrounding skull obscures this area in CT. This area is artifact-free with MRI because there is little MRI signal from bone (see Fig. 33-13).

In general the absence of bone artifact with MRI is a distinct advantage over CT. However, the inability to image calcified structures can be a disadvantage when the lesion is more easily recognized because of its calcium content. Calcified granulo-

mas of the lung or calcifications in certain other tumors are more difficult to detect with MRI than with CT.

MRI plays an increasing role in the routine examination of the brain. Because of the more natural contrast among tissues with MRI than with CT, the differentiation of gray matter from white matter in the brain is better with MRI (see Fig. 33-12). This enables MRI to be more sensitive than CT in detecting white matter disease such as multiple sclerosis.

Primary and metastatic brain tumors, pituitary tumors, and acoustic neuromas (tumors of the eighth cranial nerve) are generally better demonstrated by MRI than by CT. The use of gadolinium-based contrast agents has improved the ability of MRI to identify meningiomas (Fig. 33-19). MRI can detect cerebral infarction earlier than CT, but both tests provide similar information in subacute and chronic strokes.

Fig. 33-19 Coronal MRI scan of the brain in a patient with a meningioma arising from the tentorium cerebelli. **A,** The precontrast T1-weighted image shows an inhomogeneous area of abnormality *(black arrows),* with mass effect elevating the right lateral ventricle *(R)* and midline shift of the third ventricle *(V).* **B,** This image was obtained at the same level after gadolinium enhancement. Active tumor *(T)* demonstrates high signal intensity, and the area of necrosis *(N)* does not enhance. Additional spread of tumor toward the ventricle *(arrows)* is visualized only after contrast enhancement. Choroid plexus *(white arrowhead)* enhances. Note that cerebrospinal fluid in the ventricles does not enhance. *(A),* Artifact from metal in skull defect from previous surgery.

MRI has been successfully used to image the spinal cord. The absence of bone artifact allows excellent visualization of the contents of the neural canal. In addition, the technique can separate the spinal cord from the surrounding cerebrospinal fluid (CSF) without the use of the contrast agents (as required for CT) injected directly into the CSF during radiographic myelography (Fig. 33-20). MRI is sensitive in detecting spinal cord tumors and cystic changes of the spine (syringomyelia). MRI is also valuable in the detection of degenerated and herniated vertebral disks (Fig. 33-21).

Fig. 33-20 Sagittal T2-weighted MRI scan through the upper cervical spine and brainstem. The high signal from CSF *(F)* outlines the normal brainstem *(B)*, cerebellum *(C)*, and spinal cord *(S)*, giving a myelogram-like effect without the use of contrast agents.

Fig. 33-21 Sagittal T2-weighted image of the lumbar spine. The spinal canal is filled with high-signal-intensity CSF *(F)* except for low-signal-intensity linear nerve roots running within the spinal canal. Normal vertebral disks have a high-signal-intensity nucleus pulposus *(N)*. Desiccated disks *(D)* show low-signal-intensity. At L4-L5, note the herniated disk *(arrow)* protruding into the spinal canal and compressing the nerve roots.

CHEST

The chest would seem to be an ideal area for MRI examination because of its anatomy. The lungs have low signal as a result of low proton density, and the flowing blood in the great vessels of the chest also has a low MRI signal when standard pulse sequences are used. The heart muscle is well outlined by the lung and moving blood within the chambers. Furthermore, examination of the mediastinum is potentially fruitful because the normal structures of blood vessels and airways are of low signal. Any tumors of the mediastinum are easily seen as areas of MRI signal standing out against the normal low-signal surroundings (see Fig. 33-4). In addition, the ability of MRI to image in multiple planes may be helpful in evaluating tumor spread in the thoracic inlet, chest wall, or brachial plexus region (Fig. 33-22).

Nonetheless, difficulties with chest imaging remain because of cardiac and respiratory motion. Cardiac gating has markedly improved visualization of the heart with demonstration of septal defects and the cardiac valve leaflets. This is of great value in the study of congenital heart disease. Evaluation of the heart muscle for ischemia or infarction may require MRI contrast agents. Respiratory gating should help chest images.

In 1991, the FDA approved MRI as a supplemental imaging tool, in addition to mammography, to help diagnose breast cancer. Although many improvements in breast imaging have been made since that time, breast MRI still remains a complicated imaging procedure. Currently, standards for breast MRI do not exist as they do for mammography (Fig. 33-23).

A

B

Fig. 33-22 MRI chest images in a patient with extensive mesothelioma. **A,** Image shows axial proton density–weighted image through the middle mediastinum. Because of flow void phenomenon, the ascending and descending aorta (A) and pulmonary artery (P) are well visualized. Extensive rind of tumor (T) is visualized. **B,** This sagittal, fast-sequence image was obtained with breath holding. Although this is a somewhat more noisy image, the lack of motion artifact allows evaluation of the diaphragm. A thin line of diaphragm and fluid (arrows) is intact between the liver (L) and tumor (T), indicating that the tumor has not invaded through the diaphragm. Some pleural fluid (F) is visualized around the tumor in the pleural space.

Fig. 33-23 MRI breast image. A 38-year-old female with complex breast disease. MRI shows enhancing nodule.

ABDOMEN

Respiratory and cardiac motion also detract from upper abdominal images. Again, gating should be of assistance. Evidence exists that MRI is more sensitive than CT in detecting primary and metastatic tumors of the liver (Fig. 33-24). The suprarenals, kidneys, and retroperitoneal structures such as lymph nodes are seen well with MRI. However, limited evidence exists that MRI is superior to CT for abdominal imaging, particularly general screening for abnormalities. Visualization of the normal pancreas has been difficult with MRI.

MRI has some ability to predict the histologic diagnosis of certain abnormalities. For example, hepatic hemangiomas (common benign tumors of the liver) have a distinctive MRI appearance that can be helpful in ruling out other causes of hepatic masses. Patterns of enhancement with gadolinium-based contrast agents can assist in evaluating various tumors (Fig. 33-25).

Fig. 33-24 Axial, heavily T2-weighted MRI scan through the liver in a patient with hemangiocarcinoma. The multiple lesions of this tumor have virtually replaced the entire liver. No contrast agents were required to demonstrate these multiple liver lesions.

Fig. 33-25 Axial, fast-sequence MRI of the central abdomen in a patient with a pancreatic islet cell tumor after gadolinium injection. Enhancement of the rim of the mass *(R)* indicates necrosis *(N)* in a central portion of mass that does not enhance. Also well visualized is the relationship of the mass to vessels, such as compression *(arrowhead)* of left renal vein. *A,* Aorta; *I,* inferior vena cava; *K,* kidney; *L,* lower tip of liver.

PELVIS

Respiratory motion has little effect on the structures in the pelvis. As a result, these structures can be better visualized than those in the upper abdomen. The ability of MRI to image in the coronal and sagittal planes is helpful in examining the curved surfaces in the pelvis. For example, bladder tumors are shown well, including those at the dome and base of the bladder that can be difficult to evaluate in the transverse dimension. In the prostate (see Fig. 33-16) and female genital tract (Fig. 33-26), MRI is useful in detecting neoplasm and its spread.

MUSCULOSKELETAL SYSTEM

MRI produces excellent images of the limbs because involuntary motion is not a problem and MRI contrast among the soft tissues is excellent. The lack of bone artifact in MRI permits excellent visualization of the bone marrow (Fig. 33-27). In plain-film radiography and occasionally in CT, dense cortical bone is often hidden in the marrow space. However, as previously stated, calcium within tumors is better visualized with CT because of the lower MRI signal from calcium.

A

B

Fig. 33-26 T2-weighted images through the pelvis of a woman. **A,** Axial image. **B,** Sagittal image. Both images show solid (S) and cystic (C) components of a large ovarian tumor. The relationship to the uterus (U) and bladder (B) is also shown well using multiple imaging planes.

Fig. 33-27 Coronal MRI scan of the wrist using a surface coil to improve visualization of superficial structures. Marrow within the carpal bones (C), radius (R), and ulna (U) has high signal as a result of its fat content. A thin black line of low-signal cortex (arrows) surrounds the marrow cavity of each bone, and trabecular bone can be seen as low signal detail interspersed within marrow.

Overall, the ability to image in multiple planes, along with excellent visualization of soft tissues and bone marrow, has rapidly expanded the role of MRI in musculoskeletal imaging. MRI is particularly valuable for the study of joints, and it is replacing arthrography and, to a lesser extent, arthroscopy in the evaluation of the injured knee (see Fig. 33-11), ankle, and shoulder. Small joints also are well evaluated with MRI. Local staging of soft tissue and bone tumors is best accomplished with MRI (Fig. 33-28). Early detection of ischemic necrosis of bone is another strength of MRI (Fig. 33-29).

A

B

C

Fig. 33-28 Coronal and axial images of the arm obtained with T1 weighting. **A,** Image obtained before contrast administration. **B** and **C,** Images obtained after IV gadolinium injection. Little contrast between neurofibroma (*T*) and normal tissue is seen before enhancement; the tumor is markedly enhanced after gadolinium injection. The location of the tumor is evident before contrast injection, only because the palpable mass is marked externally with vitamin E capsules *(arrowheads).* The relationship of the tumor to muscles and bone is evident in the coronal and axial sections.

Fig. 33-29 Coronal T1-weighted image of the ankle. The bone marrow demonstrates high signal intensity because of fat. A focal area *(N)* of devascularization at the dome of the talus *(T)* shows low signal intensity. However, the overlying bony cortex and cartilage are intact. *C,* Calcaneus; *F,* fibula; *S,* tibia.

Fig. 33-30 Contrast-enhanced MRA of the abdominal aorta *(arrow)*, showing the renal arteries *(arrowheads)* and iliac bifurcations *(broken arrow)*.

Fig. 33-31 Contrast-enhanced MRA showing the carotid arteries *(arrows)* from the aortic arch *(arrowhead)* to the circle of Willis *(broken arrow)*.

VESSELS

The contrast between soft tissue structures and the typical low signal of flowing blood using standard pulse sequences gives MRI the ability to visualize thrombosis within major vessels such as the venae cavae or the tumor invasion of these vessels. Vascular anomalies, dissections, and coarctations also can be well evaluated by MRI. Special pulse sequences using standard gadolinium-based contrast agents now allow MRI visualization of moving blood within the vascular system (Fig. 33-30). These noninvasive, angiogram-like images of the vessels (magnetic resonance angiograms) improve the visualization of vascular lesions.

The carotid arteries in the neck (Fig. 33-31) and their intracranial branches (Fig. 33-32) can be studied for aneurysms, arteriovenous malformations, plaques, stenoses, and occlusions. Small arteries in the peripheral vascular system also can be studied. Flow studies of the thoracic and abdominal vessels are more difficult, but specialized fast sequences permit cardiac gated images to be obtained during a single breath hold. Typical uses include evaluation of the thoracic aorta for dissections, the abdominal aorta for aneurysms, and the renal arteries for stenoses.

Two common techniques to obtain images of flowing blood are time-of-flight and phase-contrast MRA. Using either of these techniques, magnetic resonance angiograms can be obtained in two-dimensional (obtaining a series of slices) or 3D images. In time-of-flight imaging, a special pulse sequence is used that suppresses the MRI signal from the anatomic area under study (see Fig. 33-31). Consequently, an MRI signal is given only by material that is outside the area of study when the signal-suppressing pulse occurs. Thus incoming blood makes vessels appear bright, whereas stationary tissue signal is suppressed. Phase-contrast imaging takes advantage of the shifts in phase, or orientation, experienced by magnetic nuclei moving through the MRI field (see Fig. 33-32). Special pulse sequences enhance these effects in flowing blood, producing a bright signal in vessels when the unchanging signal from stationary tissue is subtracted.

Gadolinium-based contrast agents also can be useful in MRA studies. Many MRA schemes use fast pulse sequences to reduce overall imaging time, particularly with 3D vascular imaging. For better contrast in images obtained with fast sequences, a gadolinium-based intravascular contrast agent may be injected to shorten the T1 of blood in order to increase its signal intensity.

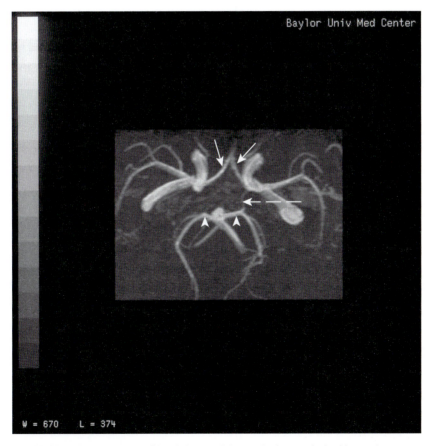

Fig. 33-32 MR angiogram of the intracranial vessels demonstrated in a submentovertex projection showing the left and right anterior cerebral arteries *(arrows).* Also shown are the posterior cerebral arteries *(arrowheads),* which join the posterior communicating artery *(broken arrow)* to form the circle of Willis. Note that only one posterior communicating artery is seen.

DIFFUSION AND PERFUSION

The sensitivity of MRI to motion can be both a handicap and a potential source of information. For example, motion artifacts interfere with upper abdominal images that are affected by heart and diaphragmatic motion, yet flow-sensitive pulse sequences can image flowing blood in blood vessels.

Specialized techniques that can image the *diffusion* and *perfusion* of molecules within matter are currently under investigation. Molecules of water undergo random motion within tissues, but the rate of this diffusion is affected by cellular membranes and macromolecules, as well as by temperature. Molecules also move slowly through tissues with the perfusion of blood into the small capillary vessels. Tissues have structure, and this structure affects both the rates of diffusion and perfusion and their direction; in other words, diffusion and perfusion are not entirely random in a structured tissue. These microscopic motions can be detected by specialized MRI pulse sequences that can image their rate and direction. Diffusion and perfusion motion differ among tissue types. For example, diffusion patterns of gray matter in the brain differ from the diffusion patterns in more directionally oriented fiber tracts of white matter. For technical reasons, most diffusion and perfusion imaging research has focused on the CNS.

Diffusion and perfusion imaging can produce clinically significant images that may help in the understanding of white matter degenerative diseases (e.g., multiple sclerosis, ischemia, infarction), the development of possible therapies to return blood flow to underperfused brain tissue, and the characterization of brain tumors. Similar applications for the rest of the body may be developed if technical difficulties, particularly those related to patient motion such as breathing, can be overcome.

Spectroscopy

With MRI it is generally assumed that each nucleus in a specific small area in space is exposed to the same magnetic field and thus precesses at a particular frequency and releases energy of that frequency. If the magnetic field varies across the imaging volume in a known way, frequency can be used as one determinant of the location from which a signal is originating. A one-to-one relationship between frequency and location is an integral part of creating the image in MRI. In actuality, however, each nucleus in a small area in space does not detect precisely the same magnetic field. The externally imposed field is the same, but the magnetic environments of the nuclei differ depending on the magnetic effects of other nearby atoms. These differences in frequencies are small and generally do not affect the image significantly; each signal is still placed in the correct position in the image. In magnetic resonance spectroscopy, a detailed graph of signal strength against frequency is produced instead of an image. The graphs produced are called *spectra.*

Spectroscopy is essentially a tool for clinical analysis that can determine the relative quantity of chemical substances within a volume of tissue. Because the frequency differences are small and electronic noise is relatively high, large volumes of tissue must be studied to receive enough total signal to produce useful spectra. Nevertheless, it is possible to obtain spectra from organs (e.g., muscle, liver) or large masses to examine normal physiologic changes (e.g., with exercise), chemical alterations in persons with metabolic diseases, or differences in chemical composition between normal tissue and tumors or other pathologic processes (Fig. 33-33). Spectroscopy of the CNS is now widely accepted and routinely used (Fig. 33-34).

Fig. 33-33 Spectra from human muscle before *(red line)* and during *(blue line)* exercise. The thin horizontal lines represent separate baselines for each spectrum. Each peak represents a different chemical species, and the area under the peak down to the baseline indicates the amount of substance present. The inorganic phosphate *(Pi)* peak increases with exercise as energy-rich phosphocreatine *(PCr)* is used to provide energy for muscle contraction.

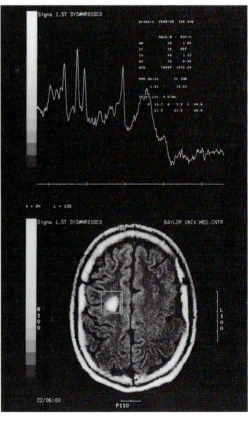

Fig. 33-34 Routine spectroscopy technique in a 31-year-old male patient. The study shows toxoplasmosis with schizencephaly and pachygyria.

Conclusion

MRI is an exciting form of imaging that examines properties of tissue never before visualized. Thousands of publications have attested to the effectiveness of MRI for evaluating various clinical conditions. However, it is more difficult to prove that MRI is clinically superior to all other imaging modalities. Although comparative studies have been completed for some clinical situations, more extensive research is needed for others. In some cases, various imaging modalities are complementary.

MRI is an expensive imaging technology. With the recent increased emphasis on cost constraints, the use of MRI will not expand as quickly as it otherwise might do. MRI will also have to compete with other modalities for an imaging "niche." Nevertheless, MRI is clearly the technique of choice in many clinical situations. MRI applications continue to increase, in part because of the extreme flexibility of this imaging modality. New pulse sequences can be programmed into the computer, and new contrast agents are under development; both provide new information about anatomy and pathology. Thus despite cost constraints, the depth and breadth of the role of MRI in diagnostic imaging continue to increase.

Definition of Terms

antenna Device for transmitting or receiving radio waves.

artifact Spurious finding in or distortion of an image.

attenuation Reduction in energy or amount of a beam of radiation when it passes through tissue or other substances.

coil Single or multiple loops of wire (or another electrical conductor such as tubing) designed to produce a magnetic field from current flowing through the wire or to detect a changing magnetic field by voltage induced in the wire.

contrast Degree of difference between two substances in some parameter, with the parameter varying depending on the technique used; for example, attenuation in radiographic techniques or signal strength in MRI.

cryogenic Relating to extremely low temperature (see *superconductive magnet*).

diffusion Spontaneous random motion of molecules in a medium; a natural and continuous process.

echo planar imaging Fast pulse sequence that can be used to create MR images within a few seconds.

fat suppressed images Images in which the fat tissue in the image is made to be of a lower, darker signal intensity than the surrounding structures.

frequency Number of times that a process repeats itself in a given period; for example, the frequency of a radio wave is the number of complete waves per second.

fringe field That portion of the magnetic field extending away from the confines of the magnet that cannot be used for imaging but can affect nearby equipment or personnel.

gating Organizing the data so that the information used to construct the image comes from the same point in the cycle of a repeating motion, such as a heartbeat. The moving object is "frozen" at that phase of its motion, reducing image blurring.

gauss (G) Unit of magnetic field strength (see *tesla*).

gradient echo Fast pulse sequence that is often used with 3D imaging to generate T2-weighted images.

inversion recovery Standard pulse sequence available on most MRI imagers, usually used for T1-weighted images. The name indicates that the direction of longitudinal magnetization is reversed (inverted) before relaxation (recovery) occurs.

magnetic resonance (MR) Process by which certain nuclei, when placed in a magnetic field, can absorb and release energy in the form of radio waves. This technique can be used for chemical analysis or for the production of cross-sectional images of body parts. Computer analysis of the radio-wave data is required.

noise Random contributions to the total signal that arise from stray external radio waves, imperfect electronic apparatus, etc. Noise cannot be eliminated, but it can be minimized; it tends to degrade the image by interfering with accurate measurement of the true MRI signal, similar to the difficulty in maintaining a clear conversation in a noisy room.

nuclear magnetic resonance (NMR) Another name for magnetic resonance; term is not commonly used.

nucleus Central portion of an atom, composed of protons and neutrons.

paramagnetic Referring to materials that alter the magnetic field of nearby nuclei. Paramagnetic substances are not themselves directly imaged by MRI but instead change the signal intensity of the tissue where they localize, thus acting as MRI contrast agents. Paramagnetic agents shorten both the T1 and T2 of the tissues they affect, actions that tend to have opposing effects on signal intensity. In clinical practice, agents are administered in a concentration in which either T1 or T2 shortening predominates (usually the former) to provide high signal on T1-weighted images.

perfusion Flow of blood through the vessels of an organ or anatomic structure; usually refers to blood flow in the small vessels (e.g., capillary perfusion).

permanent magnet Object that produces a magnetic field without requiring an external electricity supply.

precession Rotation of an object around the direction of a force acting on that object. This should not be confused with the axis of rotation of the object itself; for example, a spinning top rotates on its own axis, but it may also precess (wobble) around the direction of the force of gravity that is acting on it.

proton density Measure of proton (i.e., hydrogen, because its nucleus is a single proton) concentration (number of nuclei per given volume). One of the major determinants of MRI signal strength in hydrogen imaging.

pulse See *radiofrequency (RF) pulse.*

pulse sequence Series of radio-wave pulses designed to excite nuclei in such a way that their energy release has varying contributions from proton density, T1, or T2 processes.

radiofrequency (RF) pulse A short burst of radio waves. If the radio waves are of the appropriate frequency, they can give energy to nuclei that are within a magnetic field by the process of *magnetic resonance*. The length of the pulse determines the amount of energy given to the nuclei.

rapid acquisition recalled echo Commonly known as *fast,* or *turbo, spin echo;* a fast pulse sequence used to rapidly create spin-echo–like T2-weighted images.

raw data Information obtained by radio reception of the MRI signal as stored by a computer. Specific computer manipulation of these data is required to construct an image from them.

relaxation Return of excited nuclei to their normal, unexcited state by the release of energy.

relaxation time Measure of the rate at which nuclei, after stimulation, release their extra energy.

resistive magnet Simple electromagnet in which electricity passing through coils of wire produces a magnetic field.

resonance Process of energy absorption by an object that is tuned to absorb energy of a specific frequency only. All other frequencies will not affect the object; for example, if one tuning fork is struck in a room full of tuning forks, only those forks tuned to that identical frequency will vibrate (resonate).

signal In MRI, the induction of current into a receiver coil by the precessing magnetization.

slice Cross-sectional image; can also refer to the thin section of the body from which data are acquired to produce the image.

spectroscopy Science of analyzing the components of an electromagnetic wave, usually after its interaction with some substance (to obtain information about that substance).

spin echo Standard MRI pulse sequence that can provide T1-, T2-, or proton density–weighted images. The name indicates that a declining MRI signal is refocused to gain strength (like an echo) before it is recorded as raw data.

spin-lattice relaxation Release of energy by excited nuclei to their general environment. One of the major determinants of MRI signal strength. T1 is a rate constant measuring spin-lattice relaxation.

spin-spin relaxation Release of energy by excited nuclei as a result of interaction among themselves; one of the major determinants of MRI signal strength. T2 is a rate constant measuring spin-spin relaxation.

superconductive magnet Electromagnet in which the coils of wire are cooled to extremely low temperature so that the resistance to the conduction of electricity is nearly eliminated (superconductive).

superparamagnetic Material that has a greater effect with a magnetic field; it can dramatically decrease the T2 of tissues, causing a total loss of signal by the absorbing structures.

T1 Rate constant measuring spin-lattice relaxation.

T2 Rate constant measuring spin-spin relaxation.

tesla (T) Unit of magnetic field strength; 1 tesla equals 10,000 gauss or 10 kilogauss (other units of magnetic field strength). The earth's magnetic field approximates 0.5 gauss.

transverse plane A plane that extends across the axis of the body from side to side, dividing the body part into upper and lower portions.

Selected bibliography

Axel L, editor: *Glossary of MRI terms,* ed 3, Reston, Va, 1991, American College of Radiology.

Bloch F: Nuclear induction, *Physiol Rev* 70:460, 1946.

Bushong SC: *MRI physical and biological principles,* ed 3, St Louis, 2003, Mosby.

Damadian R: Tumor detection by nuclear magnetic resonance, *Science* 171:1151, 1971.

Elster AD: *Questions and answers in MRI,* ed 2, St Louis, 2001, Mosby.

Kelley LL, Petersen CM: *Sectional anatomy for imaging professionals,* St Louis, 1997, Mosby.

Purcell EM et al: Resonance absorption by nuclear magnetic moments in a solid, *Physiol Rev* 69:37, 1946.

Shellock FG: *Magnetic resonance procedures: health effects and safety,* Boca Raton, Fla, 2001, CRC Press.

Shellock FG: *Reference manual for magnetic resonance safety, implants, and devices,* Los Angeles, 2005, Biomedical Research Publishing Group.

Woodward P: *MRI for technologists,* ed 2, New York, 2001, McGraw-Hill.

34

DIAGNOSTIC ULTRASOUND

SANDRA L. HAGEN-ANSERT

Three-dimensional reconstruction of the fetal face showing a cleft lip.

Principles of Diagnostic Ultrasound

Diagnostic ultrasound,[*] sometimes called *diagnostic medical sonography, sonography, ultrasonography, vascular sonography,* or *echocardiography,* has become a clinically valuable imaging technique over the past 4 decades. Ultrasound differs from diagnostic radiography in that it uses nonionizing, high-frequency sound waves to generate an image of a particular soft tissue structure in the body. Reflections from soft tissue interfaces of homogeneous, fluid-filled, or solid organs, tumor masses, and muscles located within the body may be imaged with ultrasound.

The blood flow velocities within a vessel may be calculated with the *Doppler* technique. *Pulsed-wave* (PW), *continuous-wave* (CW), and *color-flow Doppler* techniques have been shown to be clinically useful in determining not only the direction of blood flow within vessels but also the flow resistance, turbulence, or *regurgitation* of blood within the vessel or cardiac chamber.

Diagnostic ultrasound has many advantages over other imaging techniques. One advantage is its mobility because the ultrasound system may be moved easily into the surgical suite, emergency department, neonatal nursery, or intensive care unit. The ultrasound system may also be wheeled into a van to provide services for small hospitals and clinics that may not have the patient load to employ a full-time sonographer. Ultrasound is more cost effective than computed tomography (CT), magnetic resonance imaging (MRI), and angiography because ultrasound equipment is less expensive and minimal supplies are necessary to run the ultrasound laboratory.

---

[*]Almost all italicized words on the succeeding pages are defined at the end of this chapter.

Ultrasound, once considered a *noninvasive technique,* now includes examinations that involve transvaginal, transrectal, and transesophageal transducers. Intraluminal transducers have provided the cardiovascular surgeons a "window" for viewing the *intima* of the coronary arteries during a cardiac catheterization or as part of an open cardiovascular surgical case. Three- and four-dimensional reconstructions of the ultrasound image have produced exquisite images of fetal anatomy and other anatomic structures within the body. Contrast media have been used by cardiologists to provide improved visualization of the cardiac muscle found in ischemic heart disease. Radiologists are clinically investigating the usefulness of contrast media to enhance tumor invasion in the liver, gallbladder, pancreas, and spleen. Gynecologists have used contrast to investigate the endometrial cavity and fallopian tubes.

CHARACTERISTICS OF THE DIAGNOSTIC MEDICAL SONOGRAPHER

The diagnostic medical sonographer performs ultrasound studies and gathers diagnostic imaging data under the direct or indirect supervision of a physician. The sonographer has the ability to "look" inside abdominal and pelvic organs in the fetus, neonate, pediatric, and adult population. The cardiac sonographer has the ability to image the dynamic function of the heart under normal and stressful conditions.

The sonographer approaches the evaluation of the patient in a manner very different from the radiographer. The principal difference lies in the sonographer's knowledge of detailed anatomy and pathophysiology. An understanding of the three-dimensional anatomy and reconstruction of the sonographic image is necessary for the sonographer to produce an adequate image.

The sonographer must have intellectual curiosity, the ability to conceptualize a two-dimensional image into a three-dimensional visualization, and the perseverance to answer clinical questions because the examination of each patient can present special challenges. This imaging professional needs to have an analytic capability coupled with organization of protocol to obtain high-quality images. Furthermore, the sonographer must enjoy both working with complex equipment and communicating with patients.

Educational opportunities are available for the student interested in sonography and may be found primarily in 2- or 4-year colleges. Sonography is a career in which specialized skills and abilities make a difference. Although many sonographers work in hospitals or clinics, others have found productive careers with ultrasound companies in product design, marketing, research, application specialists, or education. The work in ultrasound provides day-to-day variety and often allows a flexible schedule. Many employment opportunities are available, and salaries are attractive.

Of course, sonography is not a flawless profession. The work may be stressful and demanding, particularly when patient loads are increased and staff members are reduced. The lack of cure for certain diseases may lead to frustration, and daily contact with a high-risk obstetric patient with an abnormal fetus may lead to depression. Job tasks can be physically demanding in the high-volume hospital and clinical outpatient laboratory. Constant manipulation of patients and positioning of the transducer may lead to muscle fatigue and stress-related inflammation problems of the wrist, arm, and shoulder if proper care is not taken (Fig. 34-1).

RESOURCE ORGANIZATIONS

Resource organizations devoted exclusively to ultrasound include the American Society of Echocardiography (ASE), the Society of Diagnostic Medical Sonographers (SDMS), the American Institute of Ultrasound in Medicine (AIUM), the Society of Radiologists in Ultrasound (SRU), and the Society of Vascular Technology (SVT).

Historical Development

The development of *sonar* was the precursor to medical ultrasound. Sonar equipment was initially constructed for the defense efforts during World War II to detect the presence of submarines. Various investigators later proved that ultrasound had a valid contribution to make in medicine.

In 1947 Dussick positioned two transducers on opposite sides of the head to measure ultrasound transmission profiles. He also discovered that tumors and other intracranial lesions could be detected by this technique. In the early 1950s Dussick, with Heuter, Bolt, and Ballantyne, continued to use *through-transmission* techniques and computer analysis to diagnose brain lesions in the intact skull. However, they discontinued their studies after concluding that the technique was too complicated for routine clinical use.

In the late 1940s Douglas Howry (a radiologist), John Wild (a diagnostician interested in tissue characterization), and George Ludwig (interested in reflections from gallstones) independently demonstrated that when ultrasound waves generated by a piezoelectric crystal transducer were transmitted into the human body, these waves would be returned to the transducer from tissue interfaces of different *acoustic impedances*. At this time, research efforts were directed toward transforming naval sonar equipment into a clinically useful diagnostic tool.

In 1948 Howry developed the first ultrasound scanner, consisting of a cattle watering tank with a wooden rail anchored along the side. The transducer carriage moved along the rail in a horizontal plane, while the object to be scanned and the transducer were positioned inside the water tank. (An early ultrasound scanner is shown on the title page of this chapter.)

Echocardiographic techniques were developed by Hertz and Edler in 1954 in Sweden. These investigators were able to distinguish normal heart valve motion from the thickened, calcified valve motion seen in patients with rheumatic heart disease. Then in 1957 an early obstetric contact-compound scanner was built by Tom Brown and Ian Donald in Scotland. This scanner was used primarily to evaluate the location of the placenta and to determine the gestational age of the fetus.

Further developments have resulted in the real-time ultrasound instrumentation used in hospitals and clinics today. High-frequency transducers with improved *resolution* now allow the sonographer to accumulate several images per second at a rate of up to 30 frames per second. Diagnostic ultrasound as used in clinical medicine has not been associated with any harmful biologic effects and is generally accepted as a safe modality.

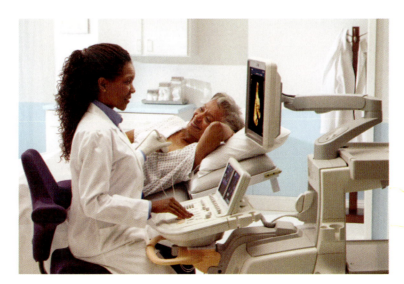

Fig. 34-1 Sonographer performing an ultrasound examination.

(Courtesy Philips Medical Systems.)

Physical Principles
PROPERTIES OF SOUND WAVES

An *acoustic wave* is a propagation of energy that moves back and forth or vibrates at a steady rate. Sound waves are mechanical oscillations that are transmitted by particles in a gas, liquid, or solid medium. Generated by an external source, ultrasound is the transmission of high-frequency mechanical vibrations greater than 20 kHz through a medium.

Ultrasound refers to sound waves beyond the audible range (16,000 to 20,000 cycles/sec). Diagnostic applications of ultrasound use frequencies of 1 to 10 million cycles/sec (1 to 10 MHz). The ultrasound beam is produced from a transducer by the piezoelectric effect. The Curie brothers described the *piezoelectric effect* in 1880, when they observed that when certain crystals, such as quartz, undergo mechanical deformation a potential difference develops across the two surfaces of the crystals.

Acoustic impedance

The *ultrasound* wave is similar to a light beam in that it may be *focused, refracted, reflected,* or *scattered* at interfaces between different media. At the junction of two media of different acoustic properties, an ultrasound beam may be reflected, depending on the difference in acoustic impedance between the two media and the angle at which the beam hits the interface (Fig. 34-2).

Velocity of sound

The *velocity of sound* in a *medium* is determined by the *density* and elastic properties of the medium. The velocity of sound differs greatly among air, bone, and soft tissue but varies only slightly from one soft tissue to another. Sound transmission is impeded by air-filled structures, such as the lungs and stomach, or by gas-filled structures, such as the bowel. However, sound is *attenuated* through most bony structures.

TRANSDUCER SELECTION

In ultrasound, transducers are used to generate the ultrasonic energy. The major component of an ultrasound transducer is the piezoelectric element. The piezoelectric materials are capable of converting one form of energy into another. Transducer designs differ according to the application for which it is used. A *curved linear array transducer* has a narrow rectangular surface with a slight convex curve. Multiple elements within the transducer are pulsed sequentially to produce an image. This type of transducer is used for larger surface areas, such as the abdomen or with an obstetrical patient. The superficial areas (breast, thyroid, scrotum, and limbs) use a smaller linear array transducer with a flat surface for better contact. The cardiac studies are performed with a small-faced, sector-phased array transducer.

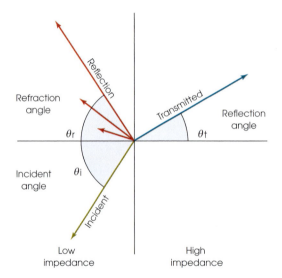

Fig. 34-2 Relationship among incident, reflected, and transmitted waves.

Transducers also have different frequencies ranging from a low frequency of 1 MHz to higher frequencies of 12 to 20 MHz. A good rule to remember is that the smaller the object to be imaged, the higher the transducer frequency. The higher frequency provides better resolution but does not contain enough strength to penetrate deep structures. An example would be found in an abdominal study: An adult patient would require a curved array transducer with a 3 to 4 MHz frequency, whereas a child would require a smaller curved array with a 5 to 7 MHz frequency transducer. A premature infant may require a tiny sector 12 MHz transducer to fit into the soft spot on the anterior fontanelle (Fig. 34-3).

REAL-TIME IMAGING, DOPPLER EFFECT, AND COLOR-FLOW DOPPLER

Real-time imaging is the presentation of multiple image frames per second over selected areas of the body. The transducer may be composed of several elements that can be electronically focused and fired in rapid sequence to produce a real-time image. Thus structures are visible as they change position in time. With this dynamic imaging it is possible to see, for example, pulsatile vascular and cardiac structures, diaphragm motion, and peristalsis in the bowel and stomach.

The *Doppler effect* refers to a change in frequency when the motion of laminar or turbulent flow is detected within a vascular structure. *Color-flow Doppler* is a technique that assigns a color scale to the change in frequency or Doppler shift. Generally, red signifies a shift toward the transducer, whereas blue signifies a shift away from the transducer.

Anatomic Relationships and Landmarks

The ability of the sonographer to understand anatomy as it relates to the *sectional, coronal,* and *oblique planes* is critical to the performance of a high-quality sonogram (see Chapter 26). Normal anatomy varies in size and position, and the sonographer must be able to demonstrate these findings on the sonogram. To complete this task, the sonographer must have a thorough understanding of anatomic relationships and their variations.

Fig. 34-3 Examples of the variety of ultrasound transducers.

(Courtesy Philips Medical Systems.)

Fig. 34-4 Transverse scan of the right lobe of the liver showing multiple hypoechoic areas with a central-core echo pattern suggestive of metastatic disease *(m)* from adenocarcinoma of the colon. The gallbladder *(GB)* is shown along the upper right border.

Clinical Applications
CHARACTERISTICS OF THE SONOGRAPHIC IMAGE

The sonographer must be able to analyze a mass to determine if its borders are smooth, irregular, poorly defined, thin, or thick to further define its characteristics. Once a mass is suspected, the sonographer must evaluate its acoustic properties to determine if it is *heterogeneous, homogeneous, hypoechoic, hyperechoic, isoechoic,* or *anechoic.* A hypoechoic lesion is characterized by low-level echoes with a good posterior border (Fig. 34-4). A hyperechoic mass may represent a tumor, thrombus, or calcification; the lesion presents with bright *echo* reflectors and possibly shadowing beyond it (Fig. 34-5). An isoechoic mass shows nearly the

Fig. 34-5 Sagittal scan of the right upper quadrant showing the liver *(L)* and the anechoic gallbladder with a large echogenic focus (gallstone, *St*) causing a large acoustic shadow posterior to its border *(arrows).*

Fig. 34-6 Sagittal image of the echogenic kidney as compared with the liver parenchyma *(L)*. A small amount of ascites in Morison's pouch *(arrows)* separates the inferior border of the liver from the anterior border of the kidney. The renal cortex *(C)* and medulla *(M)* are isoechoic to one another without a distinguishable border. A small echogenic renal stone *(St)* is found in the lower pole with an acoustic shadow posterior.

same texture pattern as the surrounding parenchyma with no significant change in the through transmission (Fig. 34-6). An anechoic mass shows no internal echoes, has smooth walls, and displays increased through transmission (Fig. 34-7).

A mass that shows characteristics of more than one pattern is considered complex. Examples include an abscess, a necrotic tumor with hemorrhage, a decomposing thrombus, a cyst with septations, or an abscess (Fig. 34-8).

Once a mass has been localized, ultrasound may aid the clinician in the aspiration or biopsy procedure. The sonographer may locate the site of the lesion, calculate its depth, and determine the direction and angulation of needle placement for the procedure.

Fig. 34-7 Sagittal image of the cirrhotic liver *(L)* surrounded by anechoic ascitic fluid *(f)*. The right kidney is well seen posterior to the liver *(K)*.

Fig. 34-8 Transverse scan of a patient with acute cholecystic disease shows a complex mass in the area *(arrows)* of the gallbladder. *L,* Liver.

ABDOMEN AND RETROPERITONEUM

The upper abdominal ultrasound examination generally includes a survey of the abdominal cavity from the diaphragm to the level of the umbilicus. Specific protocols are followed to image the texture, borders, anatomic relationships, and blood flow patterns within the liver, biliary system, pancreas, spleen, vascular structures, retroperitoneum, and kidneys. Patients may be examined in the supine, decubitus, upright, or prone positions.

Air and gas in the abdominal cavity may obstruct the ultrasound beam. Consequently, the upper abdominal ultrasound examination is best performed after a patient has been fasting for at least 6 hours. Fasting also allows the gallbladder and bile duct to be distended for adequate visualization. Specific images of the abdominal cavity are obtained from the dome of the liver to the inferior border of the kidneys, with the vascular structures serving as the primary landmarks for the abdominal organs. Scanning is performed in the transverse, oblique, sagittal, coronal, and *subcostal* planes (Figs. 34-9 and 34-10).

Fig. 34-9 A, Transverse sonogram of the right upper quadrant over the right lobe of the liver. **B,** Line drawing of the gross anatomic section. **C,** Gross anatomic section at approximately the same level as **A.**

A

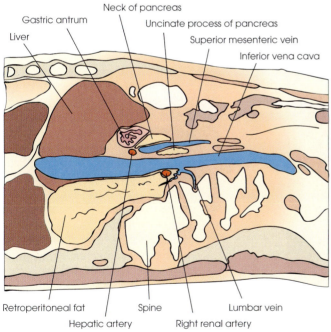

B

Gastric antrum
Neck of pancreas
Liver
Uncinate process of pancreas
Superior mesenteric vein
Inferior vena cava

Retroperitoneal fat
Spine
Lumbar vein
Hepatic artery
Right renal artery

C

Fig. 34-10 A, Sagittal sonogram of the right upper quadrant over the medial segment of the left lobe of the liver *(L),* the hepatic vein *(hv),* and the inferior vena cava *(IVC).* **B,** Line drawing of the gross anatomic section. **C,** Gross anatomic section at approximately the same level as **A.**

The left upper quadrant may be obscured secondary to air in the stomach or gas in the overlying bowel, making it difficult to image the spleen, left kidney, tail of the pancreas, and suprarenal area. The patient position may be rotated to the decubitus position to provide a better "window" to image these structures, or a liquid, such as degassed water, tomato juice, or ultrasound contrast material, may be given to dilate the stomach and fill the duodenum in an effort to improve visualization of the structures in the left upper quadrant.

The sonographer must have an understanding of the patient's clinical history and symptoms to produce an adequate survey of the abdominal cavity. The normal sonographic patterns of all the abdominal organs and vascular structures must be adequately imaged to detect any pathologic condition that may require further investigation. Although ultrasound cannot diagnose the specific pathology of a lesion, the clinical picture may lead to a more specific differential diagnosis to rule out infection, diffuse disease, hematoma, tumor, or an infiltrative process.

Liver and spleen

The liver and spleen are evaluated to assess the size and homogeneity of the parenchymal tissues. The texture of these organs is normally uniform (homogeneous) throughout with the exception of the vascular structures that enter the hilus and branch into the surrounding tissue (Fig. 34-11). Abnormalities in this texture pattern enable the sonographer to determine whether the organ has any of the following: fat infiltration, abscess, hematoma, cystic displacement, diffuse disease, or tumor invasion (Fig. 34-12). The presence or absence of vascular structures within the hepatosplenic organs helps the sonographer determine whether portal hypertension, thrombosis, or diffuse disease is present. The combined use of color-flow and Doppler helps to determine the direction of vascular flow or the presence of thrombus within the portal system or hepatic veins.

Fig. 34-11 A, Normal transverse scan of the liver. Note the homogeneous liver texture with anechoic vascular structures representing the portal and hepatic veins and the inferior vena cava. **B,** Transverse scan of the middle hepatic vein as it empties into the inferior vena cava with spontaneous blood flow. **C,** Three-dimensional image of the hepatic vasculature.

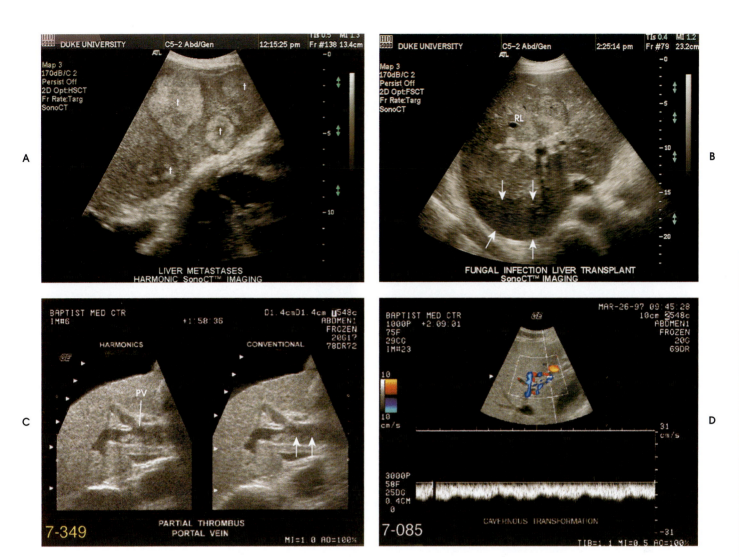

Fig. 34-12 A, Multiple hyperechoic and "bull's-eye" tumors *(t)* within the liver represent metastatic disease. **B,** Inhomogeneity is shown along the posterior right lobe of the liver *(RL)* representing a fungal infection *(arrows)* in this liver transplant patient. **C,** Echoes within the prominent portal vein *(PV)* represent thrombus *(arrows)* secondary to portal hypertension. **D,** Portal hypertension may lead to cavernous transformation of the portal veins.

Fig. 34-13 Transverse scan over the epigastric region of the abdomen demonstrating a normal pancreas *(arrows)*. The left lobe of the liver *(L)* is seen anterior to the pancreas. The aorta *(AO)*, inferior vena cava *(IVC)*, superior mesenteric artery *(SMA)*, and superior mesenteric vein *(SMV)* are the posterior borders.

Pancreas

The pancreas is a retroperitoneal gland. Its head lies in the curve of the duodenum, and its body and tail lie posterior to the antrum of the stomach. The texture of the pancreas varies, depending on the amount of fat that is interspersed throughout its islets of Langerhans. The aorta, inferior vena cava, superior mesenteric artery, and vein serve as the posterior landmarks for the pancreas (Fig. 34-13). Ultrasound examination of the pancreas can demonstrate inflammation (acute or chronic), tumor, abscess, or retroperitoneal bleed (Fig. 34-14).

```
GE MEDICAL SYSTEMS          7cm7cm @546L
IM#4                        MW  ABDMEN1
                                FROZEN
                                43G43
                                66DR66

GE

CHRONIC PANCREATITIS
                        MI=0.4 AO=100%
```

Fig. 34-14 Transverse scan over the pancreas area showing bright, echogenic reflections *(arrows)* that represent chronic, fibrotic pancreatitis. The dilated pancreatic duct is seen *(arrowheads)*.

Biliary system

On ultrasound examination the gallbladder and bile ducts are seen just inferior to the right lobe of the liver and anterior to the right kidney. The intrahepatic bile duct runs slightly anterior to the portal vein as it drains bile from the liver into the storage cistern (gallbladder) via the cystic duct. Bile is released into the common bile duct, where it joins the pancreatic duct secretions to drain into the duodenum at a small raised area called the *duodenal papilla*. The biliary system is evaluated with ultrasound to assess size and wall thickness and to detect sludge, stones, polyps, or other masses (Fig. 34-15).

Fig. 34-15 A, Longitudinal scan of the enlarged gallbladder filled with echogenic sludge *(S)*. The wall of the gallbladder is thickened secondary to acute cholecystitis *(arrows)*. **B,** A patient with HIV shows a distended gallbladder *(GB)* with echogenic sludge *(S)* representing cholangiopathy. **C,** The large gallstone *(St)* within the gallbladder is echogenic with an acoustic shadow posterior *(arrowheads)*. **D,** This prominent gallbladder is distended because of a small echogenic stone *(arrow)* lodged in the distal cystic duct *(arrowhead)*.

Fig. 34-16 Sagittal scan of the right kidney (RK), as it lies posterior to the inferior border of the right lobe of the liver (L).

Kidneys

The kidneys rest on the posterior surface of the abdominal cavity in an oblique plane lateral to the psoas muscles (Fig. 34-16). The large right lobe of the liver causes the right kidney to be slightly lower than the left kidney. The renal vascularity may be imaged with color Doppler as the patient is rolled into a slight decubitus position). The kidneys are assessed for size; dilation of calyces structures (hydronephrosis); or abnormal texture pattern secondary to a cyst, a tumor, an abscess, an infarct, a hematoma, or an infiltrative process (Fig. 34-17). Ultrasound is also useful for denoting the exact location and depth of the lower pole of the kidney; the urologist can then use this information in performing a renal biopsy. The transplanted kidney is placed in the iliac fossa, just superficial to the muscle layer. Ultrasound is useful in measuring the size of the transplanted kidney, imaging the organ's texture to detect abnormal patterns that may suggest rejection, or evaluating the transplant recipient for hydronephrosis. Fluid collections (i.e., lymphocele, seroma, abscess, hematoma) that surround the renal transplant may also be evaluated with ultrasound. The anterior and posterior pararenal spaces may be evaluated for the presence of abnormal fluid or ascites, hematoma, or tumor invasion.

Fig. 34-17 In hydronephrosis of the kidney, the dilated pyelocaliceal system appears as a separation of the renal sinus echoes by fluid-filled areas that conform anatomically to the infundibula, calyces (C), and pelvis (P).

SUPERFICIAL STRUCTURES

Superficial structures, such as the thyroid, breast, scrotum, and penis, are imaged well with ultrasound using high-frequency transducers. Routine ultrasound examination demonstrates minute structures, such as the lactiferous ducts within the breast and the spermatic cord within the testes. In conjunction with mammography, ultrasound can characterize the texture of a breast mass to determine whether the mass is fluid-filled, complex, or solid (Fig. 34-18). Pathologic hypoechoic and hyperechoic areas within the scrotal structures (e.g., cyst, spermatocele, carcinoma, hydrocele, torsion) may be demonstrated with high-resolution ultrasound instrumentation (Fig. 34-19). Real-time evaluation of the thyroid gland may demonstrate enlargement with inhomogeneous texture (goiter), a solid mass with a halo surrounding its border (adenoma), or a solid mass with poorly defined borders (carcinoma) (Fig. 34-20).

A

B

C

Fig. 34-18 A, A simple cyst (C) within the breast is shown with well-defined borders, increased through transmission and no internal echoes. **B,** Fibrocystic breast disease (C) is demonstrated with several anechoic lesions within the breast. **C,** The fibroadenoma (f) has well-defined borders and may have some increased transmission; however, the internal echo pattern is solid and homogeneous.

Fig. 34-19 Longitudinal scan of the scrotum shows the homogeneous teste *(ts)* with a complex echo pattern superior to the testes that represents a spermatocele *(sp).*

Fig. 34-20 A large complex-solid mass *(arrows)* is shown within the thyroid gland *(T).*

NEONATAL NEUROSONOGRAPHY

The premature infant is susceptible to intracranial hemorrhage during the stress of delivery and the struggle to survive. The internal anatomy of the neonatal brain may be well imaged through the coronal suture with high-frequency ultrasound. Structures including the ventricular system, septum pellucidum, corpus callosum, choroid plexus, posterior fossa, vermis, and cerebrum are visualized with detailed resolution (Fig. 34-21). The infant may be examined in the special-care nursery using petite transducers that adapt to the neonatal skull.

Sonography is the preferred clinical diagnostic tool to evaluate the premature infant for intracranial hemorrhage, infection, or shunt drainage for ventriculomegaly (Fig. 34-22). Other pathologic conditions that ultrasound examination can detect within the neonatal skull include meningomyelocele, Arnold-Chiari deformity, hydrocephalus or ventriculomegaly, Dandy-Walker deformity, agenesis of the corpus callosum, and arteriovenous malformation.

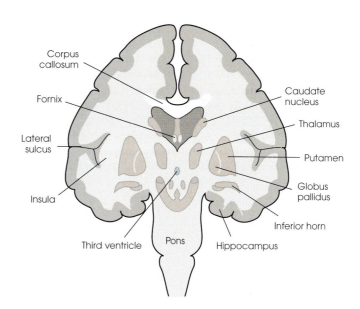

Fig. 34-21 Coronal line drawing of the neonatal head shows the development of the corpus callosum, ventricular system, thalamus, and pons.

Fig. 34-22 Posterior coronal image of an 8-day-old premature infant with a bilateral grade III bleed. The ventricles are slightly dilated, and a subependymal bleed *(arrow)* extends into the ventricular cavity.

GYNECOLOGIC APPLICATIONS
Anatomic features of the pelvis

The pelvis is divided into the greater and lesser pelvic cavity, with the pelvic brim being the circumference of a plane dividing the two cavities. The greater pelvic cavity, or "false" pelvis, is superior to the pelvic brim and is bounded on each side by the ileum. The lesser pelvic cavity, or "true" pelvis, is caudal to the pelvic brim.

The walls of the pelvic cavity are formed by several muscles collectively called the *pelvic diaphragm.* These muscles include the levator ani, piriformis, and coccygeus muscles.

The female peritoneal cavity extends inferiorly into the lesser pelvis and is bounded by the peritoneum, which covers the rectum, bladder, and uterus. In the female the peritoneum descends from the anterior abdominal wall to the level of the pubic bone onto the superior surface of the bladder (Fig. 34-23). It then passes from the bladder to the uterus to form the vesicouterine pouch. The rectouterine pouch, or pouch of Douglas, lies between the uterus and the rectum. Free fluid accumulates in this area before it moves cephalad to fill the gutters of the abdominal cavity.

Fig. 34-23 Sagittal line drawing of the female pelvis.

Sonography of the female pelvis

A complete transabdominal examination of the female pelvis includes visualization of the distended urinary bladder, uterus, cervix, endometrial canal, vagina, ovaries, and supporting pelvic musculature. The full bladder helps to push the small bowel superiorly out of the pelvic cavity, flattens the body of the uterus, and serves as a *sonic window* to image the pelvic structures (Fig. 34-24). The rectum and other bowel structures may also be seen and must be distinguished from the normal pelvic structures. The sonographer may distinguish the bowel by watching for peristalsis or changes in fluid patterns throughout the examination. The fallopian tubes and broad ligaments are usually seen only when the patient presents with excessive free fluid or ascites within the pelvic cavity.

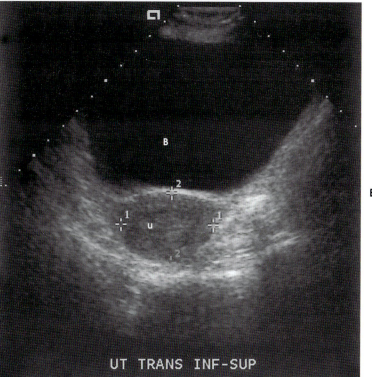

Fig. 34-24 A, Normal sagittal sonogram of the midline of the pelvic cavity. The distended urinary bladder (*B*) is shown anterior to the uterus (*u*). The endometrium appears as the bright linear echo within the uterus (*crossbars*). The myometrium is the homogeneous smooth echo tissue surrounding the endometrium of the uterus. The cervix (*c*) and vagina (*v*) are well seen. **B,** Transverse image of the distended urinary bladder anterior to the uterus (*crossbars*).

Endovaginal ultrasound has now become the preferred procedure for imaging the endometrium, myometrium, and ovaries. A high-frequency transducer is inserted into the vagina to image the uterus, cervix, fallopian tubes, ovaries, and adnexal area in coronal and sagittal planes (Fig. 34-25).

Sonography of the pelvis is clinically useful for imaging normal anatomy, identifying the size of ovarian follicles as part of an infertility workup, measuring endometrial thickness, evaluating the texture of the myometrium, determining if a pregnancy is intrauterine or extrauterine, detecting tumors or abscess formations, and localizing an intrauterine contraceptive device (Fig. 34-26).

Distinct echo patterns of an enlarged uterus allow the sonographer to distinguish a leiomyoma from endometriosis or from a gestational sac. The sonographer can identify the characteristic patterns of a pelvic mass to distinguish whether it is cystic, solid, or complex. The ultrasound interpretation, correlated with the patient's history and clinical symptoms, helps to provide a differential diagnosis for the clinician.

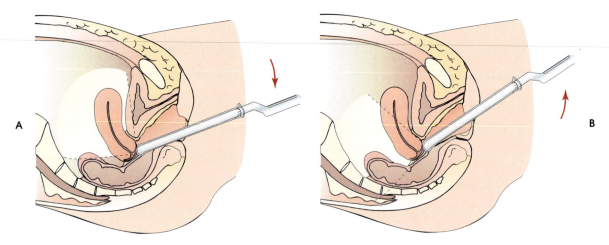

Fig. 34-25 A, Transvaginal sagittal scan with anterior angulation to better visualize the fundus of a normal anteflexed uterus. **B,** Transvaginal sagittal scan with posterior angulation to better visualize the cervix and rectouterine recess.

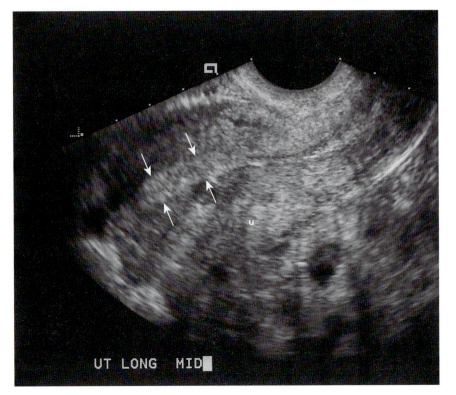

Fig. 34-26 Transvaginal midline sagittal image of the uterus. The endometrium is seen as an echogenic line *(arrows)* in the central part of the uterus *(u)*. The endometrium thickens after ovulation occurs.

Sonography of the follicles within the ovary has been used to follow infertile women to monitor the correct time to receive fertility medication. A large follicular cyst may be an indication that the egg is ready for stimulation with high doses of human chorionic gonadotropin (hCG) and subsequent fertilization.

In postoperative patients with a fever of unknown origin, sonography may play a role in excluding abscess formation that may form in the cul-de-sac, peripheral margins, or gutters of the abdomen or perirenal space.

OBSTETRIC APPLICATIONS

The pregnant woman is the ideal candidate for an ultrasound examination. The amniotic fluid enhances the sound penetration to differentiate fetal anatomy, umbilical cord, placenta, and amniotic membranes within the uterine cavity. *Endovaginal ultrasound* is the procedure of choice during the first trimester of pregnancy to delineate the gestational sac with the embryo, yolk sac, chorion, and amniotic cavities. The gestational sac may be visualized as early as 4 weeks from the date of conception with endovaginal ultrasound (Figs. 34-27 and 34-28). The embryo, heartbeat, and site of the placenta may be seen at 5 weeks of gestation.

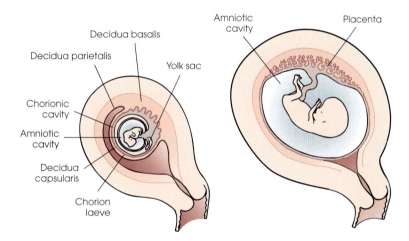

Fig. 34-27 First-trimester representation of the developing embryo and yolk sac within the amniotic and chorionic cavities of the uterus.

Fig. 34-28 A, Transabdominal sonograms of a first-trimester pregnancy demonstrating the distended urinary bladder (B), gestational sac *(large arrow),* and embryo *(small arrow).* **B,** Small yolk sac *(small arrow).* **C,** Beginning of the placenta *(P)* and embryo *(small arrows).*

Fig. 34-29 Three-dimensional reconstruction of the fetal face showing a cleft lip.

The beginning of the second trimester (13 to 28 weeks of gestation) allows the sonographer to image the detailed anatomy of the fetus (Fig. 34-29). Structures such as the brain, face, limbs, neck, abdominal wall, liver, gallbladder, kidneys, stomach, pancreas, bowel, heart, lungs, and bladder may be seen with high-resolution transducers (Fig. 34-30). Heart motion, fetal size and position, and number of fetuses may be easily assessed with sonography. Serial examinations provide information relevant to normal or abnormal growth of the fetus and placenta.

The location and homogeneity of the placenta may be accurately defined in a patient who, presenting with clinical signs of pain and bleeding, may be diagnosed with placenta previa or abruptio placentae. With ultrasound the lower extent of the placenta may be seen in relation to the cervical os to determine whether placenta previa is present. The sonographer may provide support to the perinatologist by helping to localize the position of

Fig. 34-30 A, The placenta is anterior to the fetal head (*H*) with the umbilical cord, umbilical arteries (*UA*), and umbilical vein (*UV*). **B,** The fetal abdomen at the level of the liver (*L*), umbilical vein (*v*), and cord insertion (*u*). **C,** Cross section of the fetal pelvis at the level of the bladder (*b*) and hypogastric arteries (*a*).

the placenta and fetus in amniocentesis, chorionic villus sampling, fetal blood sampling, or cord transfusion procedures. Color-flow Doppler has been useful in defining the vascularity of the placenta in difficult cases, such as placenta previa or placenta accreta. Color-flow Doppler is also useful to evaluate the umbilical cord for the number of vessels, the twist of the cord, the length, thickness, or other abnormalities (Figs. 34-31 and 34-32).

A patient who presents with a uterus larger than expected for the weeks of gestation may be scheduled for an ultrasound examination to assess fetal growth and fluid accumulation. The examination can also assess the patient for the presence of multiple gestations, the development of a hydatidiform mole, or the growth of a fibroid or extrauterine mass secondary to the pregnancy.

Fig. 34-31 **A,** Color Doppler demonstrates the normal umbilical cord with two arteries *(red)* and one vein *(blue)* in a leftward twist. The color flow within the artery shows helical flow patterns of blue/yellow/red. **B,** Color Doppler demonstrates a two-vessel cord with the absence of one umbilical artery and no twist.

Fig. 34-32 Color Doppler demonstrates that the cord *(C)* wrapped around the fetal neck *(N)* is referred to as a nuchal cord.

Diagnostic ultrasound

NORMAL VENTRICLES

Coronal

Transverse

Transverse

Fig. 34-33 Schematic of the normal fetal head: *LV*, Lateral ventricle; *CSP*, cavum septum pellucidum; *TV*, third ventricle; *CP*, choroid plexus; *FH*, frontal horn; *Th*, thalamus; *OH*, occipital horn.

The fetal *biparietal diameter* (BPD) (measurement taken perpendicular to the falx of the midline of the skull) may be measured after the twelfth week of gestation. Along with the fetal abdomen, femur, and head circumference, the BPD is useful in monitoring fetal growth by serial evaluations and measurements (Figs. 34-33 and 34-34).

Ultrasound is helpful for defining both normal and abnormal development of anatomy. A detailed ultrasound examination can assess complications of pregnancy, such as neural tube defects, skeletal or limb anomalies, cardiac defects, gastrointestinal and genitourinary defects, and head anomalies (Figs. 34-35 and 34-36).

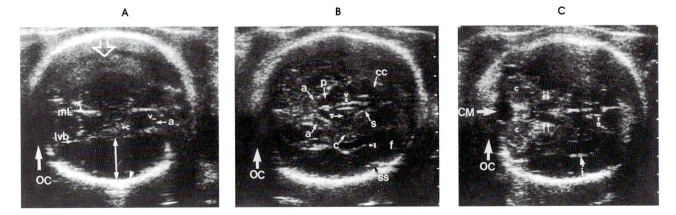

Fig. 34-34 **A,** Anatomic depiction at the ventricular level at 27 weeks of gestation. The open arrow points to a reverberation artifact in the proximal cranial hemisphere. The double-ended arrows point to fetal brain tissue. *OC*, Occiput; *mL*, interhemispheric fissure/falx; *lvb*, lateral ventricular border; *c*, choroid plexus; *v*, ventricular cavity; *a*, anterior chamber of the ventricle. Note the lateral ventricular border, which appears to lie less than halfway between the interhemispheric fissure and inner skull table *(arrowhead)*. **B,** Anatomic depiction at the thalamic level in a 31-week fetus: *T*, thalamus; *p*, cerebral peduncles; *v*, third ventricle; *s*, cavum septum pellucidum; *cc*, area of corpus callosum; *I*, insula; *c*, choroid plexus; *a*, ambient cisterns; *f*, frontal lobe; *ss*, subarachnoid space; *OC*, occiput. **C,** Anatomic depiction at the skull base in a 31-week fetus. The double arrows indicate the cerebral peduncles. *c*, Cerebellum; *CM*, cisternal magna; *i*, insula; *s*, cavum septum pellucidum; *OC*, occiput.

Fig. 34-35 A, Longitudinal image of the fetal kidney in a third-trimester fetus showing the renal cortex *(c)*, renal pelvis *(r)*, and pyramids *(p)*. The kidney is marginated by the renal capsule, which is highly visible later in pregnancy because of perirenal fat *(b, bowel)*. **B,** Sagittal image of the fluid-filled bladder *(b)* in the pelvis. The stomach *(s)* is shown in the upper abdomen with the liver *(L)*; the heart *(h)* is above the diaphragm *(arrows)*.

Fig. 34-36 Sagittal **(A)** and transverse **(B)** images of bilateral hydronephrosis *(h)* in the fetal kidneys. *lt,* Left; *s,* spine.

Fig. 34-37 Longitudinal image of the carotid artery and the bifurcation *(arrow)*.

VASCULAR APPLICATIONS

The use of ultrasound and color-flow Doppler has enhanced the ability to image peripheral vascular structures in the body. The common carotid artery with its internal and external branches and the vertebral artery are well seen with high-frequency ultrasound (Fig. 34-37). The detection of plaque formation, thrombus, obstruction, or stenosis is documented with both color and spectral Doppler waveforms (Fig. 34-38).

The ultrasound assists good visualization of the common femoral artery and vein and their branches as they extend into the calf. Thrombus within a distended venous structure is identified when the sonographer is unable to compress the vein with the transducer. Color-flow Doppler is also useful for denoting an absence of flow within a vessel. Arterial and venous structures may be reliably mapped using the ultrasound vascular mapping technique.

Ultrasound is also useful for imaging the patency of other vascular structures, such as the jugular vein, subclavian artery and vein, brachial artery and vein, and radial grafts.

Fig. 34-38 A, Longitudinal image of the carotid artery with a high-grade stenosis at the bifurcation *(arrow)*. **B,** Color Doppler and spectral waveform demonstrates increased flow velocity in the stenotic external carotid artery.

Cardiologic Applications

Real-time echocardiography of the fetal, neonatal, pediatric, and adult heart has proven to be a tremendous diagnostic aid for the cardiologist and internist. A complete two-dimensional study of the heart uses real-time color-flow Doppler with pulsed and continuous wave Doppler spectral tracings. With echocardiography, it is possible to image cardiac anatomy in detail including the four chambers of the heart; four heart valves (mitral, tricuspid, aortic, and pulmonic); interventricular and interatrial septa; muscular wall of the ventricles; papillary muscles; and chordae tendineae cordis. Difficult cases can be imaged using a transesophageal technique in which the transducer is passed from the mouth, through the esophagus, to the orifice of the stomach. This high-frequency transducer uses the "window" of the stomach and esophagus to exquisitely image intracardiac structures.

PROCEDURE FOR ECHOCARDIOGRAPHY

The echocardiographic examination begins with the patient in a left lateral decubitus position. This position allows the heart to move away from the sternum and fall closer to the chest wall, thereby providing a better cardiac "window," or open area, for the sonographer to image.

The transducer is placed in the third, fourth, or fifth intercostal space to the left of the sternum. The protocol for a complete echocardiographic examination includes images in the long axis, short axis, apical, and suprasternal windows (Fig. 34-39).

CARDIAC PATHOLOGY

Echocardiography is used to evaluate many cardiac conditions. Atherosclerosis or previous rheumatic fever may lead to scarring, calcification, and thickening of the valve leaflets. With these conditions, valve tissue destruction continues, causing stenosis and regurgitation of the leaflets and subsequent chamber enlargement.

The effects of subbacterial endocarditis can also be evaluated with echocardiography. With this infectious process, multiple small vegetations form on the endocardial surface of the valve leaflets. This causes the leaflets to tear or thicken, with resultant severe regurgitation into subsequent cardiac chambers. The echocardiogram of a patient with congestive cardiomyopathy shows generalized four-chamber enlargement, valve regurgitation, and the threat of thrombus formation along the nonfunctioning ventricular wall. The pericardial sac surrounds the ventricles and right atrium and may fill with fluid, impairing normal cardiac function.

The analysis of ventricular function and the serial evaluation of patients after a myocardial infarction are accomplished with two-dimensional echocardiography and, in some cases, stress dobutamine echocardiography.

Complications of myocardial infarction may include rupture of the ventricular septum, development of a left ventricular aneurysm in the weakest area of the wall, or coagulation of thrombus in the akinetic or immobile apex of the left ventricle (Fig. 34-40).

Congenital heart lesions

Echocardiography has been used to diagnose congenital lesions of the heart in fetuses, neonates, and young children. The cardiac sonographer is able to assess abnormalities of the four cardiac valves, determine the size of the cardiac chambers, assess the interatrial and interventricular septum for the presence of shunt flow, and identify the continuity of the aorta and pulmonary artery with the ventricular chambers to look for abnormal attachment relationships.

The premature infant has an improved chance of survival if the correct diagnosis is made early. If the neonate is cyanotic, congenital heart disease or respiratory failure may be rapidly diagnosed with echocardiography. Critical cyanotic disease in the premature infant may include hypoplastic left heart syndrome, transposition of the great vessels with pulmonary atresia, or severe tetralogy of Fallot.

Parasternal long axis

RV
Ao
S
MV
LA
LV

Ant
Inf — Sup
Post

Parasternal short axis: aortic valve level

RV
TV
PV
RA
PA
LA

Ant
R — L
Post

Parasternal short axis: mitral valve level

RV
LV
S
MV

Ant
R — L
Post

**Parasternal short axis:
left ventricle, papillary muscle level**

RV
LV
S

Ant
R — L
Post

Apical four chamber

Inf
R — L
Sup

RV
LV
RA
LA

Apical five chamber

Inf
R — L
Sup

RV
LV
RA
LA
Ao

Subcostal four chamber

Ant
Sup — Inf
Post

RV
RA
LA
LV

Fig. 34-39 A, Parasternal long-axis drawing: *RV,* right ventricle; *Ao,* aorta; *LV,* left ventricle; *LA,* left atrium; *S,* septum; *MV,* mitral valve. **B,** Parasternal short-axis drawings at various levels. Aortic valve level: *RA,* right atrium; *LA,* left atrium; *TV,* tricuspid valve; *RV,* right ventricle; *PV,* pulmonic valve; *PA,* pulmonary artery. Mitral valve level: *RV,* right ventricle; *S,* septum; *LV,* left ventricle; *MV,* mitral valve. Left ventricle, papillary muscle level: *RV,* right ventricle; *S,* septum; *LV,* left ventricle. **C,** Apical four-chamber image: *RV,* right ventricle; *LV,* left ventricle; *RA,* right atrium; *LA,* left atrium. Apical five-chamber image: *RA,* right atrium; *RV,* right ventricle; *LV,* left ventricle; *LA,* left atrium; *Ao,* aorta. **D,** Subcostal four-chamber image: *RA,* right atrium; *RV,* right ventricle; *LA,* left atrium; *LV,* left ventricle.

Conclusion

The contribution of diagnostic ultrasound to clinical medicine has been assisted by technologic advances in instrumentation and transducer design, increased ability to process the returned echo information, and improved methodology for the three-dimensional reconstruction of images. The development of high-frequency *endovaginal, endorectal,* and *transesophageal transducers* with endoscopic imaging has aided the visualization of previously difficult areas. Improved computer capabilities and advances in teleradiography have enabled the sonographer to obtain more information and process multiple data points to obtain a comprehensive report from the ultrasound study. Color-flow Doppler has made it possible for the sonographer to distinguish the direction and velocity of arterial and venous blood flow from vascular and other pathologic structures in the body. Furthermore, Doppler has allowed the sonographer to determine the exact area of obstruction or leakage present and to determine precisely the degree of turbulence within a vessel or cardiac chamber.

Modifications in transducer design have improved resolution in superficial structures, muscles, and tendons. Advancements in equipment and transducer design have also improved the results of ultrasound examinations in neonates and children. Increased sensitivity allows the sonographer to define the texture of organs and glands with more detail and greater tissue differentiation. The improvements in resolution have aided the visualization of small cleft palate defects, abnormal development of fingers and toes, and small spinal defects. The ability to image the detail of the fetal heart has assisted the early diagnosis of congenital heart disease.

Advanced research and development of the computer analysis and tissue characterization of echo reflections should further contribute to the total diagnostic approach using ultrasound. Various abdominal contrast agents continue to be investigated to improve visualization of the stomach, pancreas, and small and large intestines. Cardiac contrast agents are already being used to improve the visualization of viable myocardial tissue within the heart. Furthermore, saline and other contrast agents are being injected into the endometrial cavity to outline the lining of the endometrium for the purpose of distinguishing polyps and other lesions from the endometrial stripe.

Ultrasound has rapidly emerged as a powerful, noninvasive, high-yield clinical diagnostic examination for various applications in medicine. Expected advancements include further developments in transducer design, image resolution, tissue characterization applications, color-flow sensitivity, and four-dimensional reconstruction of images.

Fig. 34-40 Apical four-chamber image with a large apical thrombus. This thrombus *(arrows)* is distinguished from an artifact because it is located in a region with abnormal wall motion, is attached to the apical endocardium, has well-defined borders, and moves in the same direction as the apex. *RV,* Right ventricle; *LV,* left ventricle; *RA,* right atrium; *LA,* left atrium.

Definition of Terms

acoustic impedance Ratio of acoustic pressure to particle velocity at any point in the acoustic field.

acoustic shadow Loss of acoustic power of structures lying behind an attenuating or reflecting target.

acoustic wave Mechanical disturbance that propagates through a medium.

a-mode (amplitude) Method of acoustic echo display in which time is represented along the horizontal axis and echo amplitude is displayed along the vertical axis.

anechoic Property of being free of echoes or without echoes.

angle of incidence Angle at which the ultrasound beam strikes an interface with respect to normal (perpendicular) incidence.

attenuation Reduction of acoustic amplitude along propagation pathway as a result of diffraction, absorption, scattering, reflections, or any other process that redirects the signal away from the receiver.

biparietal diameter (BPD) Largest dimension of the fetal head perpendicular to the midsagittal plane; measured by ultrasonic visualization and used to measure fetal development.

B-mode (brightness) Method of acoustic display on an oscilloscope in which the intensity of the echo is represented by modulation of the brightness of the spot and in which the position of the echo is determined from the position of the transducer and the transit time of the acoustic pulse; displayed in the x-y plane.

color-flow Doppler Velocity in each direction is quantified by allocating a pixel to each area; each velocity frequency change is allocated a color.

continuous wave ultrasound Waveform in which the amplitude modulation factor is less than or equal to a small value.

coronal image plane Anatomic term used to describe a plane perpendicular to both the sagittal and transverse planes of the body.

cross-sectional display Display that presents ultrasound interaction echo data from a single plane within a tissue. It is produced by sweeping the ultrasound beam through a given angle, by translating it along a line, or by some combination of linear and angular motions. The depth in the tissue is represented along one coordinate, and the position in the scan is represented by the second coordinate. The plane of the section may be sagittal, coronal, or transverse. The lateral resolution is determined by the beam width of the transducers.

Doppler effect Shift in frequency or wavelength, depending on the conditions of observation; caused by relative motions among the sources, receivers, and medium.

Doppler ultrasound Application of the Doppler effect to ultrasound to detect movement of a reflecting boundary relative to the source, resulting in a change of the wavelength of the reflected wave.

dynamic imaging Imaging of an object in motion at a frame rate sufficient to cause no significant blurring of any one image and at a repetition rate sufficient to adequately represent the movement pattern. This is frequently referred to as *imaging at a real-time (frame) rate*.

echo Reflection of acoustic energy received from scattering elements or a specular reflector.

echogenic Refers to a medium that contains echo-producing structures.

endometrium Refers to the inner layer of the uterine canal.

endorectal transducer High-frequency transducer that can be inserted into the rectum to visualize the bladder and prostate gland.

endovaginal transducer High-frequency transducer (and decreased penetration) that can be inserted into the vagina to obtain high-resolution images of the pelvic structures.

focus To concentrate the sound beam into a smaller beam area than would exist without focusing.

frequency Number of cycles per unit of time, usually expressed in Hertz (Hz) or megahertz (MHz; a million cycles per second).

hard copy Method of image recording in which data are stored on paper, film, or other recording material.

heterogenous Having a mixed composition.

homogeneous Having a uniform composition.

hyperechoic Producing more echoes than normal.

hypoechoic Producing fewer echoes than normal.

intima Refers to the inner layer of the vessel; the middle layer is the media and the outer layer is the adventitia.

ischemia Refers to an area of the cardiac myocardium that has been damaged by disruption of the blood supply by the coronary arteries.

isoechoic Having a texture nearly the same as that of the surrounding parenchyma.

M-mode (motion) Method in which tissue depth is displayed along one axis and time is displayed along the second axis.

myometrium The thick middle layer of the uterine wall.

noninvasive technique A procedure that does not require the skin to be broken or an organ or cavity to be entered (e.g., taking the pulse).

oblique plane A slanting direction or any variation that is not starting at a right angle to any axis.

parenchyma The outer margin of the organ that is closest to the capsule.

piezoelectric effect Conversion of pressure to electrical voltage or conversion of electrical voltage to mechanical pressure.

pulse wave ultrasound Sound waves produced in pulse form by applying electrical pulses to the transducer.

real-time imaging Imaging with a real-time display whose output keeps pace with changes in input.

reflection Acoustic energy reflected from a structure with a discontinuity in the characteristic acoustic impedance along the propagation path.

refraction Phenomenon of bending wave fronts as the acoustic energy propagates from the medium of one acoustic velocity to a second medium of differing acoustic velocity.

regurgitation Occurs when blood leaks from one high pressure chamber to a chamber of lower pressure.

resolution Measure of the ability to display two closely spaced structures as discrete targets.

retroperitoneal cavity The area posterior to the peritoneal cavity that contains the aorta, inferior vena cava, pancreas, part of the duodenum and colon, kidneys and adrenal glands.

scan Technique for moving an acoustic beam to produce an image for which both the transducer and display movements are synchronized.

scattering Diffusion or redirection of sound in several directions on encountering a particle suspension or rough surface.

sectional plane Plane corresponding to transverse or sagittal plane.

sonar Instrument used to discover objects under the water and to show their location.

sonic window Sonographer's ability to visualize a particular area. For example, the full urinary bladder is a good sonic window to image the uterus and ovaries in a transabdominal scan. The intercostal margins may be a good sonic window to image the liver parenchyma.

through-transmission Process of imaging by transmitting the sound field through the specimen and picking up the transmitted energy on a far surface or a receiving transducer.

transducer Device that converts energy from one form to another.

ultrasound Sound with a frequency greater than 20 kHz.

velocity of sound Speed with direction of motion specified.

wave Acoustic wave is a mechanical disturbance that propagates through a medium.

Selected bibliography

Callen PW: *Ultrasonography in obstetrics and gynecology,* ed 3, Philadelphia, 1998, Saunders.

Curry RA, Tempkin BB: *Ultrasonography: an introduction to normal structure and functional anatomy,* Philadelphia, 2004, Saunders.

Golderg BB, Kurtz AB: *Atlas of ultrasound measurements,* Chicago, 1990, Mosby.

Hagen-Ansert SL: *Abdominal ultrasound study guide and exam review,* St Louis, 1996, Mosby.

Hagen-Ansert SL: *Textbook of diagnostic ultrasonography,* vols I and II, ed 6, St Louis, 2006, Mosby.

Hall R: *The ultrasound handbook,* Philadelphia, 1999, JB Lippincott.

Henningsen C: *Clinical guide to ultrasonography,* St Louis, 2005, Mosby.

Kurtz AB, Middleton WD: *Ultrasound: the requisites,* St Louis, 1996, Mosby.

Nyberg DA, Mahony BS, Pretorious DH: *Diagnostic ultrasound of fetal anomalies: text and atlas,* Chicago, 1990, Mosby.

Oh JK, Seward JB, Tajik AJ: *The echo manual,* ed 2, Boston, 1999, Little, Brown.

Rumack CM, Wilson SR, Charboneau JW: *Diagnostic ultrasound,* ed 3, St Louis, 2005, Mosby.

Zagzebski J: *Essentials of ultrasound physics,* St Louis, 1996, Mosby.

Zweibel WJ, editor: *Introduction to vascular ultrasonography,* New York, 1993, Grune & Stratton.

35

NUCLEAR MEDICINE

NANCY L. HOCKERT

ELTON A. MOSMAN

PET scan performed using ^{18}F-FDG in a patient with a left lung mass. The scan shows a large FDG avid mass in the left lower lobe.

Principles of Nuclear Medicine

Nuclear medicine is a medical specialty that focuses on the use of radioactive materials called *radiopharmaceuticals**** for diagnosis, therapy, and medical research. Unlike radiologic procedures, which determine the presence of disease based on structural appearance, nuclear medicine studies determine the cause of a medical problem based on organ or tissue *function* (physiology).

In a nuclear medicine test, the radioactive material, or *tracer,* is generally introduced into the body by injection, swallowing, or inhalation. Different tracers are used to study different parts of the body. Tracers are selected that localize in specific organs or tissues. The amount of radioactive tracer material is selected carefully to provide the lowest amount of radiation exposure to the patient and still ensure a satisfactory examination or therapeutic goal. Radioactive tracers produce *gamma-ray* emissions from within the organ being studied. A special piece of equipment, known as a *gamma* or *scintillation camera,* is used to transform these emissions into images that provide information about the function (primarily) and anatomy of the organ or system being studied.

*Almost all italicized words on the succeeding pages are defined at the end of this chapter.

Nuclear medicine tests are performed by a team of specially educated professionals: a nuclear medicine physician, a specialist with extensive education in the basic and clinical science of medicine who is licensed to use radioactive materials; a nuclear medicine technologist who performs the tests and is educated in the theory and practice of nuclear medicine procedures; a physicist who is experienced in the technology of nuclear medicine and the care of the equipment, including computers; and a pharmacist or specially prepared technologist who is qualified to prepare the necessary radioactive pharmaceuticals.

Positron emission tomography (PET) is a noninvasive nuclear imaging technique that involves the administration of a positron-emitting radioactive molecule and subsequent imaging of the distribution and kinetics of the radioactive material as it moves into and out of tissues. PET imaging of the heart, brain, lungs, or other organs is possible if an appropriate radiopharmaceutical, also called a *radiotracer* or *radiolabeled molecule,* can be synthesized and administered to the patient.

Three important factors distinguish PET from all radiologic procedures and from other nuclear imaging procedures. First, the results of the data acquisition and analysis techniques yield an image related to a particular physiologic parameter such as blood flow or metabolism. The ensuing image is aptly called a *functional* or *parametric image.* Second, the images are created by the simultaneous detection of a pair of *annihilation* radiation photons that result from *positron* decay (Fig. 35-1). The third factor that distinguishes PET is the chemical and biologic form of the radiopharmaceutical. The radiotracer is specifically chosen for its similarity to naturally occurring biochemical constituents of the human body. Because extremely small amounts of the radiopharmaceutical are administered, equilibrium conditions within the body are not altered. If, for instance, the radiopharmaceutical is a form of sugar, it will behave very much like the natural sugar used by the body. The kinetics or the movement of the radiotracer such as sugar within the body is followed by using the PET scanner to acquire many images that measure the distribution of the *radioactivity concentration* as a function of time. From this measurement the local tissue metabolism of the sugar may be deduced by converting a temporal sequence of images into a single parametric image that indicates tissue glucose utilization or, more simply, tissue metabolism.

Fig. 35-1 A, PET relies on the simultaneous detection of a pair of annihilation radiations emitted from the body. **B,** In contrast, CT depends on the detection of x-rays transmitted through the body.

Historical Development

John Dalton is considered the father of the modern theory of *atoms* and molecules. In 1803, this English schoolteacher stated that all atoms of a given element are chemically identical, are unchanged by chemical reaction, and combine in a ratio of simple numbers. Dalton measured atomic weights in reference to hydrogen, to which he assigned the value of 1 (the atomic number of this element).

The discovery of x-rays by Wilhelm Conrad Roentgen in 1895 was a great contribution to physics and the care of the sick. A few months later, another physicist, Henri Becquerel, discovered naturally occurring radioactive substances. In 1898, Marie Curie discovered two new elements in the uranium ore pitchblende. Curie named these trace elements *polonium* (after her homeland, Poland) and *radium.* Curie also coined the terms *radioactive* and *radioactivity.*

In 1923, Georg de Hevesy, often called the "father of nuclear medicine," developed the tracer principle. He coined the term "radioindicator" and extended his studies from inorganic to organic chemistry. The first radioindicators were naturally occurring substances such as radium and radon. The invention of the *cyclotron* by Ernest Lawrence in 1931 made it possible for de Hevesy to expand his studies to a broader spectrum of biologic processes by using phosphorus-32, sodium-22, and other cyclotron-produced (manmade) radioactive tracers.

Radioactive elements began to be produced in *nuclear reactors* developed by Enrico Fermi and his colleagues in 1946. The nuclear reactor greatly extended the ability of the cyclotron to produce radioactive tracers. A key development was the introduction of the *gamma camera* by Hal Anger in 1958. In the early 1960s David Edwards and Roy Kuhl made the next advance in nuclear medicine with the development of a crude single photon emission computed tomography (SPECT) camera known as the MARK IV. With this new technology, it was possible to create three-dimensional (3D) images of organ function instead of the two-dimensional (2D) images created previously. It was not until the early 1980s, when computers became fast enough to successfully acquire and process all of the information, that SPECT imaging would need to become standard practice.

With the development of more suitable *scintillators,* such as sodium iodide (NaI), and more sophisticated nuclear counting electronics, positron coincidence localization became possible. F.W. Wrenn demonstrated the use of positron-emitting radioisotopes for the localization of brain tumors in 1951. G.L. Brownell further developed instrumentation for similar studies. The next major advance came in 1967, when G. Hounsfield demonstrated the clinical use of computed tomography (CT). The mathematics of PET image *reconstruction* is very similar to that used for CT reconstruction techniques. Instead of x-rays from a point source traversing the body and being detected by a single or multiple detectors as in CT, PET imaging uses two opposing detectors to simultaneously count pairs of 0.511-MeV photons that originate from a single positron-electron annihilation event.

From 1967 through 1974, significant developments occurred in computer technology, scintillator materials, and *photomultiplier tube* (PMT) design. In 1975, the first closed-ring transverse positron tomograph was built for PET imaging by M.M. Ter-Pogossian and M.E. Phelps.

Developments now continue on two fronts that have accelerated the use of PET. First, scientists are approaching the theoretical limits (1 to 2 mm) of PET scanner resolution by employing smaller, more efficient scintillators and PMTs. Microprocessors tune and adjust the entire ring of *detectors* that surround the patient. Each ring in the PET tomograph may contain as many as 1000 detectors. Furthermore, the tomograph may be composed of 30 to 60 rings of detectors. The second major area of development is in the design of new radiopharmaceuticals. Agents are being developed to measure blood flow, metabolism, protein synthesis, lipid content, receptor binding, and many other physiologic parameters and processes.

During the mid-1980s, PET was used predominantly as a research tool; however, by the early 1990s, clinical PET centers had been established and PET was routinely used for diagnostic procedures on the brain, heart, and tumors. The middle to late 1990s saw the development of 3D PET systems that eliminated the use of interdetector *septa.* This allowed the injected dose of the radiopharmaceutical to be reduced by approximately sixfold to tenfold.

One of the first organs to be examined by nuclear medicine studies using *external radiation detectors* was the thyroid. In the 1940s, investigators found that the rate of incorporation of radioactive iodine by the thyroid gland was greatly increased in hyperthyroidism (overproduction of thyroid hormones) and greatly decreased in hypothyroidism (underproduction of thyroid hormones). Over the years tracers and instruments were developed to allow almost every major organ of the body to be studied by application of the tracer principle. Images subsequently were made of structures such as the liver, spleen, brain, and kidneys. Today the emphasis of nuclear medicine studies is more on function and chemistry than anatomic structure. In PET, new image reconstruction methods have been developed to better characterize the distribution of annihilation photons from these 3D systems. Beginning in 2000, major nuclear medicine camera manufacturers developed combined PET and CT systems that can simultaneously acquire PET functional images and CT anatomic images. Both modalities are co-registered or exactly matched in size and position. The success of these camera systems led to the development of combined SPECT and CT systems as well. Significant benefits are expected for diagnosing metastatic disease because precise localization of tumor size and tumor function can be determined. Rapid enhancements and developments are anticipated throughout the next several years with this technology.

Comparison with Other Modalities

PET is predominantly used to measure human cellular, organ, or system function. In other words, a parameter that characterizes a particular aspect of human physiology is determined from the measurement of the radioactivity emitted by a radiopharmaceutical in a given volume of tissue. In contrast, conventional radiography measures the structure, size, and position of organs or human anatomy by determining x-ray transmission through a given volume of tissue. X-ray attenuation by structures interposed between the x-ray source and the radiographic image receptor provides the contrast necessary to visualize an organ. CT creates cross-sectional images by computer reconstruction of multiple x-ray transmissions (see Chapter 31). The characteristics of PET and other imaging modalities are compared in Table 35-1.

Radionuclides used for conventional nuclear medicine include ^{99m}Tc (technetium), ^{123}I (iodine), ^{131}I (iodine), ^{111}In (indium), ^{201}Tl (thallium), and ^{67}Ga (gallium). Labeled compounds with these high atomic weight radionuclides often do not mimic the physiologic properties of natural substances because of their size, mass, and distinctly different chemical properties.

Thus compounds labeled with conventional nuclear medicine radionuclides are poor radioactive *analogs* for natural substances. Imaging studies with these agents are qualitative and emphasize nonbiochemical properties. The elements hydrogen, carbon, nitrogen, and oxygen are the predominant constituents of natural compounds found in the body. They have low atomic weight radioactive counterparts of ^{11}C (carbon), ^{13}N (nitrogen), and ^{15}O (oxygen). Furthermore, these positron-emitting radionuclides can directly replace their stable isotopes in substrates, metabolites, drugs, and other biologically active compounds without disrupting normal biochemical properties. In addition, ^{18}F can replace hydrogen in many molecules, thereby providing an even greater assortment of biologic analogs that are useful PET radiopharmaceuticals.

SPECT employs nuclear imaging techniques to determine tissue function. Because SPECT employs collimators and lower-energy photons, it is less sensitive (by 10^1 to 10^5) and less accurate than PET. In general, PET resolution is better than SPECT resolution by a factor of 2 to 10. PET easily accounts for photon loss through attenuation by performing a *transmission scan*. This is difficult to achieve and not routinely done with SPECT imaging; however, newly designed SPECT instrumentation that couples a low-output x-ray CT to the gamma camera for the collection of attenuation information is now being used in select sites to correct for gamma attenuation. Software approaches are also being investigated that assign known *attenuation coefficient*s for specific tissues to *segmented regions* of images for analytic attenuation correction of SPECT data.

The differences between the various imaging modalities can be highlighted using a study of brain blood flow as an example. Without an intact circulatory system, an intravenously injected radiopharmaceutical cannot make its way into the brain for distribution throughout that organ's capillary network and ultimately diffusing into cells that are well perfused. For radiographic procedures such as CT, structures within the brain may well be intact but there may be impaired or limited blood flow to and through major vessels within the brain. Under these circumstances, the CT scan may appear almost normal despite reduced blood flow

TABLE 35-1

Comparison of imaging modalities

Modality information	Positron emission tomography	Single photon emission computer tomography	Magnetic resonance imaging	Computed tomography
Measures	Physiology	Physiology	Anatomy (physiology*)	Anatomy
Resolution	3-5 mm	8-10 mm	0.5-1 mm	1-1.5 mm
Technique	Positron annihilation	Gamma emission	Nuclear magnetic resonance	Absorption of x-rays
Harmful effects	Radiation exposure	Radiation exposure	None known	Radiation exposure
Use	Research and clinical	Clinical	Clinical (research*)	Clinical
Number of examinations per day	4-12	5-10	10-15	15-20

*Secondary function.

to the brain. If the circulatory system at the level of the capillaries is not intact, a PET scan can be performed but no perfusion information is obtained because the radioactive water used to measure blood flow is not transported through the capillaries and diffused into the brain cells.

The image-enhancing contrast agents used in many radiographic studies may cause a toxic reaction. The x-ray dose to the patient in these radiographic studies is greater than the radiation dose in nuclear imaging studies. The radiopharmaceuticals used in PET studies are similar to the body's own biochemical constituents and are administered in very small amounts. Biochemical compatibility of the tracers with the body minimizes the risks to the patient because the tracers are not toxic. Trace amounts minimize alteration of the body's *homeostasis*.

An imaging technique that augments both CT and PET is *magnetic resonance imaging* (MRI) (see Chapter 33). Images obtained with PET and MRI are shown in Fig. 35-2. MRI is used primarily to measure anatomy or morphology. Unlike CT, which derives its greatest image contrast from varying tissue densities (bone from soft tissue), MRI better differentiates tissues by their proton content and the degree to which the protons are bound in lattice structures. The tightly bound protons of bone make it virtually transparent to MRI.

It is important to note that CT, MRI, and other anatomic imaging modalities provide complementary information to nuclear medicine imaging and PET. These imaging modalities benefit from *image co-registration* with CT and MRI by pinpointing physiologic function from precise anatomic locations. Greater emphasis is being placed on multimodality image co-registration between PET, CT, SPECT, and MRI for brain research and for tumor localization throughout the body (Fig. 35-3). Nearly all new PET imaging systems are fused with a CT scanner for attenuation and anatomic positioning information. Newer SPECT imaging systems are also incorporating CT technology for the same purposes.

Fig. 35-2 Co-registered MRI and PET scans. The arrows indicate an abnormality on the anatomic image (**A,** MRI scan) and the functional image (**B,** PET scan). The ^{18}F-FDG PET image depicts hypometabolic area of seizure focus *(arrow)* in a patient diagnosed with epilepsy.

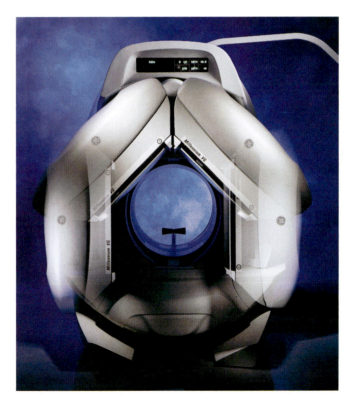

Fig. 35-3 Combined SPECT/CT camera for a blending of imaging function and form.

(Courtesy General Electric.)

Physical Principles of Nuclear Medicine

An understanding of radioactivity must precede an attempt to grasp the principles of nuclear medicine and how images are created using radioactive compounds. The term *radiation* is taken from the Latin word *radii,* which refers to the spokes of a wheel leading out from a central point. The term *radioactivity* is used to describe the radiation of energy in the form of high-speed *alpha* or *beta particles* or waves (gamma rays) from the nucleus of an atom.

BASIC NUCLEAR PHYSICS

The basic components of an atom include the nucleus, which is composed of varying numbers of *protons* and *neutrons,* and the orbiting *electrons,* which revolve around the nucleus in discrete energy levels. Protons have a positive electric charge, electrons have a negative charge, and neutrons are electrically neutral. Both protons and neutrons have masses nearly 2000 times the mass of the electron; therefore the nucleus comprises most of the mass of an atom. The Bohr atomic model (Fig. 35-4) can describe this configuration. The total number of protons, neutrons, and electrons in an atom determines its characteristics, including its stability.

The term *nuclide* is used to describe an atomic species with a particular arrangement of protons and neutrons in the nucleus. Elements with the same number of protons but a different number of neutrons are referred to as *isotopes.* Isotopes have the same chemical properties as one another because the total number of protons and electrons is the same. They differ simply in the total number of neutrons contained in the nucleus. The neutron-to-proton ratio in the nucleus determines the stability of the atom. At certain ratios, atoms may be unstable, and a process known as spontaneous *decay* can occur as the atom attempts to regain stability. Energy is released in various ways during this decay, or return to *ground state.*

Radionuclides decay by the emission of alpha, beta, and gamma radiation. Most radionuclides reach ground state through various decay processes, including alpha, beta, or positron emission and *electron capture,* as well as several other methods. These decay methods determine the type of particles or gamma rays given off in the decay.

To better explain this process, investigators have created decay schemes to show the details of how a *parent* nuclide decays to its *daughter* or ground state (Fig. 35-5, *A*). Decay schemes are unique for each radionuclide and identify the type of decay, the energy associated with each process, the probability of a particular decay process, and the rate of change into the ground state element, commonly known as the *half-life* of the radionuclide.

Radioactive decay is considered a purely random and spontaneous process that can be mathematically defined by complex equations and represented by average decay rates. The term *half-life* ($T\frac{1}{2}$) is used to describe the time it takes for a quantity of a particular radionuclide to decay to one half of its original activity. This radioactive decay is a measure of the physical time it takes to reach one half of the original number of atoms through spontaneous disintegration. The rate of decay has an exponential function, which can be plotted on a linear scale (see Fig. 35-5, *B*). If plotted on a semilogarithmic scale, the decay rate would be represented

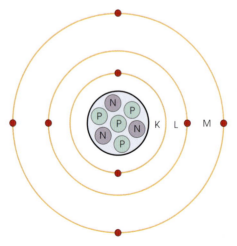

Fig. 35-4 Diagram of Bohr atom containing a single nucleus of protons *(P)* and neutrons *(N)* with surrounding orbital electrons of varying energy levels (*K, L, M,* etc.).

as a straight line. Radionuclide half-lives range from milliseconds to years. The half-lives of most radionuclides used in nuclear medicine range from several hours to several days.

NUCLEAR PHARMACY

The radionuclides used in nuclear medicine are produced in reactors, or *particle accelerators*. Naturally occurring radionuclides have very long half-lives (i.e., thousands of years). These natural radionuclides are unsuitable for nuclear medicine imaging because of both limited availability and the high absorbed dose the patient would receive. Thus the radionuclides for nuclear medicine are produced in a particle accelerator through nuclear reactions created between a specific target chemical and high-speed charged particles. The number of protons in the target nuclei is changed when the nuclei are bombarded by the high-speed charged particles, and a new element or radionuclide is produced. Radionuclides can be created in nuclear reactors either by inserting a target element into the reactor core where it is irradiated or by separating and collecting the *fission* products.

The most commonly used radionuclide in nuclear medicine is technetium-99 (^{99m}Tc), which is produced in a generator system. This system makes available desirable short-lived radionuclides—the *daughters*—which are formed by the decay of relatively longer-lived radionuclides—the *parents*. The generator system uses molybdenum-99 as the parent. ^{99}Mo has a half-life of 66.7 hours and decays (86%) to a daughter product known as *metastable* technetium (^{99m}Tc). Because technetium and molybdenum are chemically different, they can easily be separated through an ion-exchange column. ^{99m}Tc exhibits nearly ideal characteristics for use in nuclear medicine examinations, including a relatively short physical half-life of 6.04 hours and a high-yield (98.6%), 140-keV, low-energy, gamma photon (see Fig. 35-5, *A*).

Because radiopharmaceuticals are administered to patients, they need to be sterile and *pyrogen free*. They also need to undergo all of the quality control measures required of conventional drugs. A radiopharmaceutical generally has two components: a *radionuclide* and a *pharmaceutical*. The pharmaceutical is chosen on the basis of its preferential localization or participation in the physiologic function of a given organ. A radionuclide is tagged to a pharmaceutical. After the radiopharmaceutical is administered, the target organ is localized and the radiation emitted from it can be detected by imaging instruments, or gamma cameras.

The following characteristics are desirable in an imaging radiopharmaceutical:
- Ease of production and ready availability
- Low cost
- Lowest possible radiation dose
- Primary photon energy between 100 and 400 keV
- Physical half-life greater than the time required to prepare the material for injection
- Effective half-life longer than the examination time
- Suitable chemical forms for rapid localization
- Different uptake in the structure to be detected than in the surrounding tissue
- Low toxicity in the chemical form administered to the patient
- Stability or near-stability

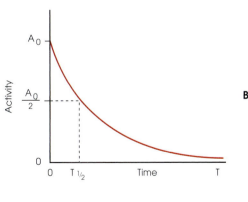

Fig. 35-5 A, Decay scheme illustrating the method by which radioactive molybdenum (^{99}Mo) decays to radioactive technetium (^{99m}Tc), one of the most commonly used radiopharmaceuticals in nuclear medicine. **B,** Graphic representation showing the rate of physical decay of a radionuclide. The y (vertical) axis represents the amount of radioactivity, and the x (horizontal) axis represents the time at which a specific amount of activity has decreased to one half of its initial value. Every radionuclide has an associated half-life that is representative of its rate of decay.

^{99m}Tc can be bound to biologically active compounds or drugs to create a radiopharmaceutical that localizes in a specific organ system or structure when the radionuclide is administered intravenously or orally. A commonly used radiopharmaceutical is ^{99m}Tc tagged to a macroaggregated albumin (MAA). After IV injection, this substance follows the pathway of blood flow to the lungs, where it is distributed throughout and trapped in the small pulmonary capillaries (Fig. 35-6). Blood clots along the pathway prevent this radiopharmaceutical from distributing in the area beyond the clot. As a result, the image shows a void or clear area, often described as *photopenia* or a *cold spot*. More than 30 different radiopharmaceuticals are used in nuclear medicine (Table 35-2).

Radiopharmaceutical doses vary depending on the radionuclide used, the examination to be performed, and the size of the patient. The measure of radioactivity is expressed as either the *becquerel* (Bq), which corresponds to the decay rate, expressed as one disintegration per second, or as the *curie* (Ci), which equals 3.73×10^{10} disintegrations per second, relative to the number of decaying atoms in 1 g of radium.

POSTERIOR   RPO   RT. LATERAL   LPO

PERFUSION LUNG SCAN

LT. LATERAL   ANTERIOR

DIACAM

MATRIX: 128 x 128

DOSE: 3 mCi 99mTc-MAA

COUNTS: 500K / VIEW

Hx: 46 YEAR OLD FEMALE
HISTORY OF SHORTNESS OF BREATH

Dx: NORMAL LUNG STUDY

Fig. 35-6 Normal perfusion lung scan using 3 mCi of ^{99m}Tc tagged to a macroaggregated albumin (*^{99m}Tc MAA*) on a large field-of-view gamma camera approximately 5 minutes after injection of the radiopharmaceutical. *LPO*, Left posterior oblique; *LT*, left; *RPO*, right posterior oblique; *RT*, right.

(Courtesy Siemens Medical Systems, Iselin, NJ.)

TABLE 35-2

Radiopharmaceuticals used in nuclear medicine

Radionuclide	Symbol	Physical half-life	Chemical form	Diagnostic use
Chromium	^{51}Cr	27.8 days	Sodium chromate	Red blood cell volume and survival
			Albumin	Gastrointestinal protein loss
Cobalt	^{57}Co	270 days	Cyanocobalamin (vitamin B_{12})	Vitamin B_{12} absorption
Fluorine	^{18}F	110 minutes	Fluorodeoxyglucose	Oncology and myocardial hibernation
Gallium	^{67}Ga	77 hours	Gallium citrate	Inflammatory process and tumor imaging
Indium	^{111}In	67.4 hours	DTPA	Cerebrospinal fluid imaging
			Ibritumomab tiuxetan	Localization of tumor
			OctreoScan (pentetreotide)	Neuroendocrine tumors
			ProstaScint (capromab-pendetide)	Prostate cancer
			Oxine	White blood cell/abscess imaging
Iodine	^{123}I	13.3 hours	Sodium iodide	Thyroid function and imaging
			Human serum albumin	Plasma volume
	^{131}I	8 days	Sodium iodide	Thyroid function, imaging, and therapy
			Hippurate	Renal function
Nitrogen	^{13}N	10 minutes	Ammonia	Myocardial perfusion
Rubidium	^{82}Rb	75 seconds	Rubidium chloride	Cardiovascular imaging
Technetium	^{99m}Tc	6 hours	Sodium pertechnetate	Imaging of brain, thyroid, scrotum, salivary glands, renal perfusion, and pericardial effusion; evaluation of left-to-right cardiac shunts
			Sulfur colloid	Imaging of liver and spleen and renal transplants, lymphoscintigraphy
			Macroaggregated albumin	Lung imaging
			Sestamibi	Cardiovascular imaging, myocardial perfusion
			DTPA	Brain and renal imaging
			DMSA	Renal imaging
			MAG_3	Renal imaging
			Diphosphonate	Bone imaging
			Pyrophosphate	Bone and myocardial imaging
			Red blood cells	Cardiac function imaging
			HMPAO	Functional brain imaging and white blood cell/abscess imaging
			Iminodiacetic derivations	Liver function imaging
			Neurolite (Bicisate)	Brain imaging
			Myoview (Tetrofosmin)	Myocardial perfusion
			CEA-scan (Arcitumomab)	Gastrointestinal tract
			Cardiolite (Sestamibi)	Myocardial perfusion
			Apcitide (AcuTect)	Acute venous thrombosis
Thallium	^{201}Tl	73.5 hours	Thallous chloride	Myocardial imaging
Xenon	^{133}Xe	5.3 days	Xenon gas	Lung ventilation imaging

DMSA, Dimercaptosuccinic acid; *DTPA,* diethylenetriamine pentaacetic acid; *HMPAO,* hexamethylpropyleneamineoxime; *MAG₃,* mertiatide.

Radiation Safety in Nuclear Medicine

The radiation protection requirements in nuclear medicine differ from the general radiation safety measures used for diagnostic radiography. The radionuclides employed in nuclear medicine are in liquid, solid, or gaseous form. Because of the nature of radioactive decay, these radionuclides continuously emit radiation after administration (unlike diagnostic x-rays, which can be turned on and off mechanically). Therefore special precautions are required.

In general, the quantities of radioactive tracers used in nuclear medicine present no significant hazard. Nonetheless, care must be taken to reduce unnecessary exposure. The high concentrations or activities of the radionuclides used in a nuclear pharmacy necessitate the establishment of a designated preparation area that contains isolated ventilation, protective lead or glass shielding for vials and syringes, absorbent material, and gloves. The handling and administering of diagnostic doses to patients warrants the use of gloves and a lead syringe shield, especially effective for reduction of exposure to hands and fingers during patient injection, at all times (Fig. 35-7).

Any radioactive material that is spilled continues to emit radiation and therefore must immediately be cleaned up and contained. Because radioactive material that contacts the skin can be absorbed and may not be easily washed off, it is very important to wear protective gloves when handling radiopharmaceuticals.

Technologists and nuclear pharmacists are required to wear appropriate radiation monitoring (dosimetry) devices, such as film badges and thermoluminescent dosimetry (TLD) rings, to monitor radiation exposure to the body and hands. The ALARA (*as low as reasonably achievable*) program applies to all nuclear medicine personnel.

Fig. 35-7 A, Area in a radiopharmacy in which doses of radiopharmaceuticals are prepared in a clean and protected environment. **B,** Nuclear medicine technologist administering a radiopharmaceutical intravenously using appropriate radiation safety precautions, including gloves and a syringe shield.

Instrumentation in Nuclear Medicine

MODERN-DAY GAMMA CAMERA

The term *scintillate* means to emit light photons. Becquerel discovered that ionizing radiation caused certain materials to glow. A *scintillation detector* is a sensitive element used to detect ionizing radiation by observing the emission of light photons induced in a material. When a light-sensitive device is affixed to this material, the flash of light can be changed into small electrical impulses. The electrical impulses are then amplified so that they may be sorted and counted to determine the amount and nature of radiation striking the scintillating materials. Scintillation detectors were used in the development of the first-generation nuclear medicine scanner, the *rectilinear scanner,* which was built in 1950.

Scanners have evolved into complex imaging systems known today as *gamma cameras* (because they detect gamma rays). These cameras are still scintilla- tion detectors that use a thallium-acti- vated sodium iodide crystal to detect and transform radioactive emissions into light photons. Through a complex process, these light photons are amplified and their locations are electronically recorded to produce an image that is displayed as a hard copy or on computer output systems. Scintillation cameras with single or multiple crystals are used today. The gamma camera has many components that work together to produce an image (Fig. 35-8).

Fig. 35-8 Typical gamma camera system, which includes complex computers and electronic mechanical components for acquiring, processing, displaying, and analyzing nuclear medicine images.

Collimator

Located at the face of the detector, where photons from radioactive sources first enter the camera, is a *collimator*. The collimator is used to separate gamma rays and keep scattered rays from entering the scintillation crystal. *Resolution* and *sensitivity* are terms used to describe the physical characteristics of collimators. Collimator sensitivity is determined by the fraction of photons that are actually transmitted through the collimator and strike the face of the camera crystal. Spatial resolution is the capability of a system to produce an image in which the small details are observable.

Collimators are usually made of a material with a high atomic number, such as lead, which absorbs scattered gamma rays. Different collimators are used for different types of examinations, depending on photon energy and the desired level of sensitivity and resolution.

Crystal and light pipe

The scintillation crystals commonly used in gamma cameras are made of sodium iodide with trace quantities of thallium added to increase light production. This crystal composition is effective for stopping most common gamma rays emitted from the radiopharmaceuticals used in nuclear medicine.

The thickness of the crystal varies from ¼ inch to ½ inch (0.6 to 1.3 cm). Thicker crystals are better for imaging radiopharmaceuticals with higher energies (more than 180 keV) but have decreased resolution. Thinner crystals provide improved resolution but cannot efficiently image photons with a higher kiloelectron voltage.

A *light pipe* may be used to attach the crystal to the *photomultiplier tubes* (PMTs). The light pipe is a disk of optically transparent material that helps direct photons from the crystal into the PMTs.

Detector electronics

An array of PMTs is attached to the back of the crystal or light pipe. Inside the detector are PMTs used to detect and convert light photons emitted from the crystal into an electronic signal that amplifies the original photon signal by a factor of as much as 10^7. A typical gamma camera detector head contains 80 to 100 PMTs.

The PMTs send the detected signal through a series of processing steps, which include determining the location (x, y) of the original photon and its amplitude or energy (z). The x and y values are determined by where the photon strikes the crystal. Electronic circuitry known as a *pulse height analyzer* is used to eliminate the z signals that are not within a desired preset energy range for a particular radionuclide. This helps reduce scattered lower energy, unwanted photons ("noise") that generally would degrade resolution of the image. Once the information has been processed, the signals are transmitted to the display system, which includes a cathode ray tube and a film imaging system or computer to record the image.

A

B

D

Cortical Analysis			
	Left Kidney	Right Kidney	Bladder
Appearance time in collecting system	2.7 min	2.7 min	3.8 min
Time to peak	2.7 min	2.5 min	
20 min counts / peak counts	21.7 %	21.2 %	
T 3/4 clearance	4.0 min	4.2 min	
T 1/2 clearance	6.5 min	6.7 min	

Lt   Rt

C

RENAL PERFUSION STUDY

DIAMONDS-Aorta   CROSS-Left Kidney   SQUARES-Right Kidney

CORTICAL ANALYSIS

CROSS-Left Kidney   SQUARES-Right Kidney

E

Fig. 35-9 A, Posterior renal blood flow in an adult patient using 10 mCi of ^{99m}Tc with DTPA imaged at 3 seconds per frame. The image in the lower right corner is a blood-pool image taken immediately after the initial flow sequence. Together the images demonstrate normal renal blood flow to both kidneys. **B,** Normal, sequential dynamic 20-minute ^{99m}Tc with mertiatide (MAG₃) images. **C,** Renal arterial perfusion curves showing minor renal blood flow asymmetry. **D,** Renal cortical analysis curves showing rapid uptake and prompt parenchymal clearance. **E,** Quantitative renal cortical analysis indices showing normal values.

Multihead gamma camera systems

The standard gamma camera is a single detector that can be moved in various positions around the patient. Gamma camera systems may include as many as three detectors (heads). Dual-head gamma camera systems allow simultaneous anterior and posterior imaging and may be used for whole-body bone or tumor imaging. Triple-head systems may be used for brain and heart studies. Although these systems are primarily suited for SPECT, they can also provide multiplanar images (see Imaging Methods later in this chapter).

COMPUTERS

Computers have become an integral part of the nuclear medicine imaging system. Computer systems are used to acquire and process data from gamma cameras. They allow data to be collected over a specific time frame or to a specified number of counts; the data can then be analyzed to determine functional changes occurring over time (Fig. 35-9, *A* and *B*). A common example is the renal study, in which the radiopharmaceutical that is administered is cleared by normally functioning kidneys in about 20 minutes. The computer can collect images of the kidney during this period and analyze the images to determine how effectively the kidneys clear the radiopharmaceutical (see Fig. 35-9, *C* to *E*). The computer also allows the operator to enhance a particular structure by adjusting the contrast and brightness of the image.

Computerization of the nuclear pharmacy operation also has become an important means of record keeping and quality control. Radioactive dosages and dose volumes can be calculated more quickly by computer than by hand. The nuclear pharmacy computer system may be used to provide reminders and keep records as required by the Nuclear Regulatory Commission (NRC), the U.S. Food and Drug Administration (FDA), and individual state regulatory agencies. Computers can also assist in the scheduling of patients, based on dose availability and department policies.

Computers are necessary to acquire and process SPECT images, as is discussed in the next section. SPECT uses a scintillation camera that moves around the patient to obtain images from multiple angles for tomographic image reconstruction. SPECT studies are complex and, like MRI studies, require a great deal of computer processing to create images in transaxial, sagittal, or coronal planes. Rotating 3D images can also be generated from SPECT data (Fig. 35-10, *A*).

A

B

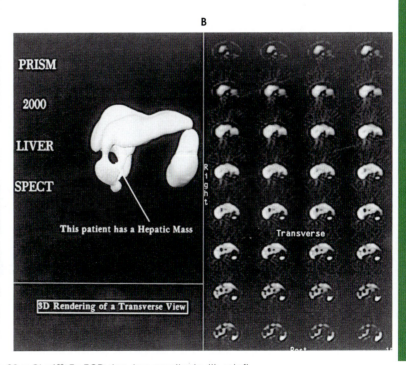

PRISM 2000 LIVER SPECT

This patient has a Hepatic Mass

3D Rendering of a Transverse View

Transverse

Fig. 35-10 A, 3D SPECT brain study using 20 mCi of ^{99m}Tc ECD showing a patient with a left frontal lobe brain infarct *(top).* Baseline and Diamox challenge transaxial, coronal, and sagittal images of the same patient, showing the left frontal lobe brain infarct *(bottom).* **B,** 3D SPECT liver study using 8 mCi of ^{99m}Tc sulfur colloid. A mass is seen on both the 3D image *(left)* and the transaxial images *(right).*

Computer networks are an integral part of the way a department communicates information within and among institutions. In a network, several or many computers are connected so that they all have access to the same files, programs, printers, etc. Networking allows the movement of both image-based and text-based data to any computer or printer in the network. Networking improves the efficiency of a nuclear medicine department. A computer network can serve as a vital component, reducing the time expended on menial tasks while allowing retrieval and transfer of information. Consolidation of all reporting functions in one area eliminates the need for the nuclear medicine physician to travel between departments to read studies. Centralized archiving, printing, and retrieval of the majority of image-based and non–image-based data have increased the efficiency of data analysis, reduced the cost of image hard copy, and permitted more sophisticated analysis of image data than would routinely be possible.

Electronically stored records can decrease reporting turnaround time, physical image storage requirements, and the use of personnel for record maintenance and retrieval. Long-term computerized records can also form the basis for statistical analysis to improve testing methods

and predict disease courses. Most institutions now use some form of picture archiving and communication systems (PACS) to organize all of the imaging that is done. These systems are the foundation of a digital department, allowing for easy transfer, retrieval, and archiving of all imaging done in the nuclear medicine department.

QUANTITATIVE ANALYSIS

Many nuclear medicine procedures require some form of quantitative analysis to provide physicians with numeric results based on and depicting organ function. Specialized software allows computers to collect, process, and analyze functional information obtained from nuclear medicine imaging systems. Cardiac ejection fraction is one of the more common quantitation studies (Fig. 35-11). In this dynamic study of the heart's contractions and expansions, the computer accurately determines the ejection fraction, or the amount of blood pumped out of the left ventricle with each contraction.

Imaging Methods

A wide variety of diagnostic imaging examinations are performed in nuclear medicine. These examinations can be

described on the basis of the imaging method used: static, whole body, dynamic, SPECT, and PET.

STATIC IMAGING

Static imaging is the acquisition of a single image of a particular structure. This image can be thought of as a "snapshot" of the radiopharmaceutical distribution within a part of the body. Examples of static images include lung scans, spot bone scan images, and thyroid images. Static images are usually obtained in various orientations around a particular structure to demonstrate all aspects of that structure. Anterior, posterior, and oblique images are often obtained.

In static imaging, low radiopharmaceutical activity levels are used to minimize radiation exposure to the patients. Because of these low activity levels, images must be acquired for a preset time or a minimum number of counts or radioactive emissions. This time frame may vary from a few seconds to several minutes to acquire 100,000 to more than 1 million counts. Generally, it takes from 30 seconds to 5 minutes to obtain a sufficient number of counts to produce a satisfactory image.

  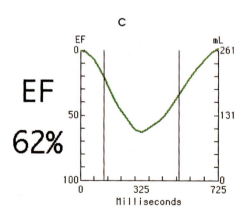

Fig. 35-11 Gated first-pass cardiac study and quantitative results, including the cardiac ejection fraction, of a normal patient. **A,** An anterior image of the left ventricle at end-diastole (relaxed phase), with a region of interest drawn around the left ventricle.
B, Same view showing end-systole (contracted phase). **C,** Curve representing the volume change in the left ventricle of the heart before, during, and after contraction. This volume change is referred to as the ejection fraction (*EF*), with a normal value being approximately 62%.

WHOLE-BODY IMAGING

Whole-body imaging uses a specially designed moving detector system to produce an image of the entire body or a large body section. In this type of imaging, the gamma camera collects data as it passes over the body. Earlier detector systems were smaller and required as many as two or three incremental passes to encompass the entire width of the body.

During the past several years the detector width for whole-body systems has been increased to allow for a single head-to-foot pass that encompasses the entire body from side to side. These systems may also include dual heads for simultaneous anterior and posterior imaging. Whole-body imaging systems are used primarily for whole-body bone scans, whole-body tumor or abscess imaging, and other clinical and research applications (Fig. 35-12).

DYNAMIC IMAGING

Dynamic images display the distribution of a particular radiopharmaceutical over a specific period. A dynamic or "flow" study of a particular structure is generally used to evaluate blood perfusion to the tissue. This can be thought of as a sequential or time-lapse image. Images may be acquired and displayed in time sequences as short as one tenth of a second to longer than 10 minutes per image. Dynamic imaging is commonly used for first-pass cardiac studies, hepatobiliary studies, and gastric emptying studies.

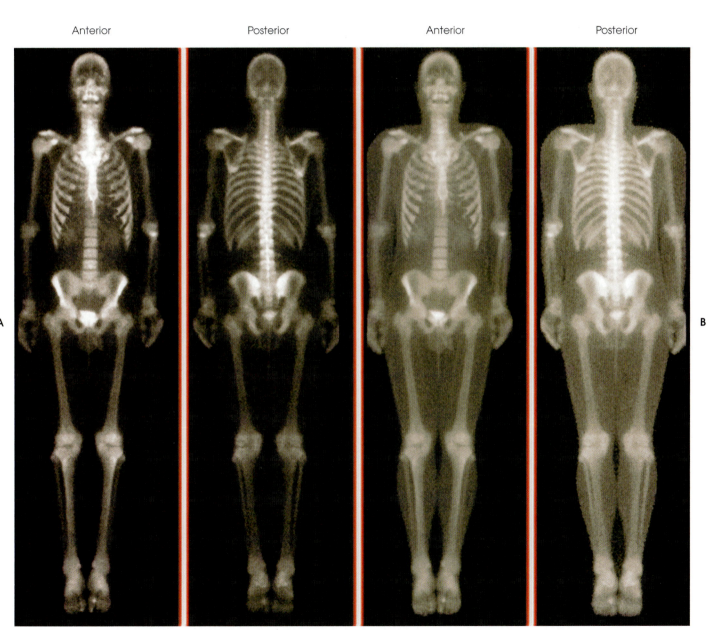

Anterior   Posterior   Anterior   Posterior

A   B

Fig. 35-12 Whole-body scan performed using 25 mCi ^{99m}Tc HDP in a 25-year-old male. The study was normal. **A,** Anterior and posterior whole-body view in a linear gray scale. **B,** Anterior and posterior whole-body view in a square-root gray scale, to enhance soft tissue.

(Courtesy General Electric.)

Imaging methods

A

B

C

Fig. 35-13 SPECT camera systems. **A,** Single-head system. **B,** Dual-headed system. **C,** Triple-headed system.

(**A,** Courtesy General Electric. **B,** Courtesy Siemens Medical Systems, Inc. **C,** Courtesy Marconi Medical Systems.)

SPECT IMAGING

SPECT produces images similar to those obtained by CT or MRI in that a computer creates thin slices through a particular organ. This imaging technique has proved very beneficial for delineating small lesions within tissues, and it can be used on virtually any structure or organ. Improved clinical results with SPECT are due to improved target-to-background ratios. Planar images record and demonstrate all radioactivity emitting from the patient above and below the region of interest, causing degradation of the image. In contrast, SPECT eliminates the unnecessary information.

With SPECT, one to three gamma detectors may be used to produce tomographic images (Fig. 35-13). Tomographic systems are designed to allow the detector heads to rotate as much as 360 degrees around a patient's body to collect "projection" image data. The image data are reconstructed by a computer in several formats, including transaxial, sagittal, coronal, planar, and 3D representations. The computer-generated images allow for the display of thin slices through different planes of an organ or structure, thereby helping to identify small abnormalities.

The most common uses of SPECT include cardiac perfusion, brain, liver (see Fig. 35-10, B), tumor, and bone studies. An example of a SPECT study is the myocardial perfusion thallium study, which is used to identify perfusion defects in the left ventricular wall. Radioactive thallium is injected intravenously while the patient is being physically stressed on a treadmill or is being infused with a vasodilator. The radiopharmaceutical distributes in the heart muscle in the same fashion as blood flowing to the tissue. An initial set of images is acquired immediately after the stress test. A second set is obtained several hours later when the patient is rested (when the thallium has redistributed to viable tissue) to determine whether any blood perfusion defects that were seen on the initial images have resolved. By comparing the two image sets, the physician may be able to tell whether the patient has damaged heart tissue resulting from a myocardial infarction or myocardial ischemia (Fig. 35-14).

Fig. 35-14 Thallium-201 myocardial perfusion study comparing stress and redistribution (resting) images in various planes of the heart (short axis and long axis). A perfusion defect is identified in the stress images but not seen in the redistribution (rest) images. This finding is indicative of ischemia.

COMBINED SPECT AND CT IMAGING

Now a blending of imaging function and form is available. By merging the functional imaging of SPECT with the anatomic landmarks of CT, more powerful diagnostic information is obtainable (Fig. 35-15). This combination will have a significant impact on diagnosing and staging malignant disease and on identifying and localizing metastases. This new technology will be used for both anatomic localization and attenuation correction. Manufacturers report that statistics are demonstrating that adding CT (both for attenuation correction and anatomic definition) changes the patient course of treatment 25% to 30% from what would have been done when using the functional image alone.

Clinical Nuclear Medicine

The term *in vivo* means "within the living body." Because all diagnostic nuclear medicine imaging procedures are based on the distribution of radiopharmaceuticals within the body, they are classified as in vivo examinations.

Patient preparation for nuclear medicine procedures is minimal, with most tests requiring no special preparation. Patients usually remain in their own clothing. However, all metal objects outside or inside the clothing must be removed because they may mimic, or attenuate, pathologic conditions on nuclear medicine imaging. The waiting time between dose administration and imaging varies with each study. After completion of a routine procedure, patients may resume all normal activities.

Following are technical summaries of some of the more commonly performed nuclear medicine procedures. After each procedure summary is a list, by organ or system, of many common studies that may be done in an average nuclear medicine department.

BONE SCINTIGRAPHY

Bone scintigraphy is generally a survey procedure to evaluate patients with malignancies, diffuse musculoskeletal symptoms, abnormal laboratory results, and hereditary or metabolic disorders. Tracer techniques have been used for many years to study the exchange between bone and blood. Radionuclides have played an important role in understanding both normal bone metabolism and the metabolic effects of pathologic involvement of bone. Radiopharmaceuticals used for bone imaging can localize in bone and also in soft tissue structures. Skeletal areas of increased uptake are commonly a result of tumor, infection, or fracture.

Bone scan
Principle

It is not entirely clear how ^{99m}Tc-labeled diphosphonates are incorporated into bone at the molecular level; however, it appears that regional blood flow, osteoblastic activity, and extraction efficiency are the major factors that influence the uptake. In areas in which osteoblastic activity is increased, active hydroxyapatite crystals with large surface areas appear to be the most suitable sites for uptake of the diphosphonate portion of the radiopharmaceutical.

Radiopharmaceutical

The adult dose of 20 mCi (740 MBq) of ^{99m}Tc hydroxymethylene diphosphonate (HDP) or 20 mCi (740 MBq) of ^{99m}Tc methylene diphosphonate (MDP) is injected intravenously. The pediatric dose is adjusted according to the patient's weight.

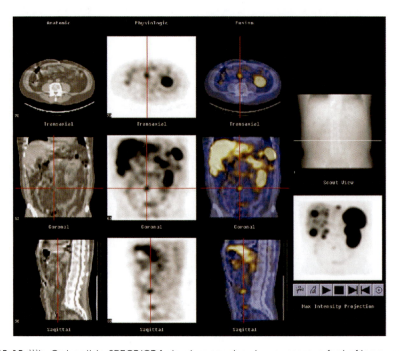

Fig. 35-15 ^{111}In-Octreotide SPECT/CT fusion images showing numerous foci of increased uptake within the liver. This is consistent with the patient's known hepatic metastases. A very small focus of increased uptake is also seen in the inferior abdomen, near midline, anterior to the lumbar spine, and is consistent with nodal metastasis. These findings are indicative of somatostatin-avid hepatic and probable nodal metastases.

Scanning

A routine survey (whole body, spot views, or SPECT) begins about 3 hours after the injection and takes 30 to 60 minutes. A flow study would commence immediately after the injection while extremity imaging may be needed 4 to 5 hours later. The number of camera images acquired depends on the indication for the examination.

Bone (skeletal) studies

Skeletal studies include bone scan, bone marrow scan, and joint scan.

NUCLEAR CARDIOLOGY

Nuclear cardiology has experienced rapid growth in recent years and currently comprises a significant portion of daily nuclear medicine procedures. These noninvasive studies assess cardiac performance, evaluate myocardial perfusion, and measure viability and metabolism. Advances in computers and scintillation camera technology have facilitated the development of a quantitative cardiac evaluation unequaled by any other noninvasive or invasive methods. The stress test is performed with the patient using a treadmill or pharmacologic agent. During the stress test the patient's heart rate, electrocardiogram (ECG), blood pressure, and symptoms are continuously monitored. Some patients cannot exercise because of peripheral vascular disease, neurologic problems, or musculoskeletal abnormalities. In these patients, a pharmacologic intervention can be used in place of the exercise test to alter the blood flow to the heart in a way that simulates exercise, allowing the detection of myocardial ischemia.

Radionuclide angiography
Principle

Gated radionuclide angiography (RNA) can be used to measure left ventricular ejection fraction and evaluate left ventricular regional wall motion. RNA requires that the blood be labeled with an appropriate tracer such as ^{99m}Tc. The technique is based on imaging using a multigated acquisition (MUGA) format. During a gated acquisition the cardiac cycle is divided into 16 to 20 frames. The R-wave of each cycle resets the gate so that each count is added to each frame, until there are adequate count statistics for analysis.

RNA requires simultaneous acquisition of the patient's ECG and images of the left ventricle. The *ejection fraction* (EF) and wall motion analysis are measured at rest.

Radiopharmaceutical

The adult dose is 25 or 30 mCi (1110 MBq) of ^{99m}Tc-labeled red blood cells, depending on whether the test is an EF only or a rest MUGA based on the patient's body surface area (i.e., height and weight). The pediatric dose is adjusted according to the patient's weight.

Scanning

Imaging can begin immediately after the injection and takes about 1 hour. For a rest MUGA, imaging of the heart should be obtained in the anterior, left lateral, and left anterior oblique positions. For an EF-only MUGA, only the left anterior oblique is obtained.

^{201}Tl myocardial perfusion study
Principle

The stress thallium-201 study has high sensitivity (about 90%) and specificity (about 75%) for the diagnosis of coronary artery disease. This study also has been useful for assessing myocardial viability in patients with known coronary artery disease and for evaluating patients after revascularization. At rest, symptoms may not be apparent. ^{201}Tl is an analog of potassium and has a high rate of extraction by the myocardium over a wide range of metabolic and physiologic conditions. ^{201}Tl is distributed in the myocardium in proportion to regional blood flow and myocardial cell viability. Under stress, myocardial ^{201}Tl uptake peaks within 1 minute. ^{201}Tl uptake in the heart ranges from about 1% of the injected dose at rest to about 4% with maximum exercise. Regions of the heart that are infarcted or underperfused at the time of injection appear as areas of decreased activity (photopenia).

Radiopharmaceutical

The adult dose for a stress study is 3 mCi (111 MBq) of ^{201}Tl thallous chloride administered intravenously at peak stress; 1 mCi (37 MBq) of ^{201}Tl is administered intravenously before the delayed study, generally 3 to 4 hours after stress. The adult dose for a rest study is 4 mCi (148 MBq) of ^{201}Tl administered intravenously before the rest study. The minimum dose recommended for pediatric patients is 300 μCi (11.1 MBq) of ^{201}Tl thallous chloride. Whenever possible, ^{99m}Tc sestamibi should be used in place of ^{201}Tl in obese patients so that a higher dose may be administered for clearer imaging results.

Scanning

The images obtained include the anterior planar image of the chest and heart, followed by a 180-degree SPECT study (45 degrees right anterior oblique to 45 degrees left posterior oblique).

^{99m}Tc sestamibi myocardial perfusion study
Principle

Like ^{201}Tl, ^{99m}Tc sestamibi is a cation; however, it has a slightly lower fractional extraction than thallium, particularly at high flow rates. ^{99m}Tc sestamibi has favorable biologic properties for myocardial perfusion imaging. It is used to assess myocardial salvage resulting from therapeutic intervention in acute infarction, to determine the myocardial blood flow during periods of spontaneous chest pain, and to diagnose coronary artery disease in obese patients. A first-pass flow study can be performed with a rest or stress ^{99m}Tc sestamibi myocardial perfusion scan. A first-pass study evaluates heart function (ejection fraction) during the short time (in seconds) that it takes the injected bolus to travel through the left ventricle.

Radiopharmaceutical

The adult dose for the stress study is 25 mCi (925 MBq) for a two-day study and 40 mCi (1480 MBq) for a one-day study of ^{99m}Tc sestamibi administered intravenously at peak stress. The adult dose for rest study is 10 mCi (370 MBq) for a one-day study and 35 mCi (1295 MBq) for a two-day study of ^{99m}Tc sestamibi administered intravenously.

Scanning

SPECT imaging should normally be done 30 to 60 minutes after injection of the dose, for both stress and rest studies. When needed, more delayed images can be obtained for as long as 4 to 6 hours after injection. A 2-day protocol provides optimum image quality, but the 1-day protocol is more convenient for patients, technologists, and physicians.

Cardiovascular studies

Cardiovascular studies include aortic/mitral regurgitant index, cardiac shunt study, dobutamine MUGA, rest MUGA, rest MUGA–ejection fraction only, exercise MUGA, stress testing (myocardial perfusion), ^{201}Tl myocardial perfusion scan, ^{99m}Tc sestamibi first-pass study, ^{99m}Tc sestamibi myocardial perfusion scan, ^{99m}Tc pyrophosphate (PYP) myocardial infarct scan, and rest ^{201}Tl scan with infarct quantitation.

CENTRAL NERVOUS SYSTEM

The central nervous system (CNS) consists of the brain and spinal cord. For patients with diseases of the central or peripheral nervous systems, nuclear medicine techniques can be used to assess the effectiveness of surgery or radiation therapy, document the extent of involvement of the brain by tumors, and determine progression or regression of lesions in response to different forms of treatment. Brain perfusion imaging is useful in the evaluation of patients with stroke, transient ischemia, and other neurologic disorders such as Alzheimer's disease, epilepsy, and Parkinson's disease. Radionuclide cisternography is particularly useful in the diagnosis of CSF leakage after trauma or surgery as well as normal-pressure hydrocephalus. Recent studies indicate that documented lack of cerebral blood flow should be the criterion of choice to confirm brain death when clinical criteria are equivocal, when a complete neurologic examination cannot be performed, or when patients are younger than 1 year.

Brain SPECT study
Principle

Some imaging agents are capable of penetrating the intact blood-brain barrier. After a radiopharmaceutical crosses the *blood-brain barrier*, it becomes trapped inside the brain. The regional uptake and retention of the tracer are related to the regional perfusion. Note that before the imaging agent is injected, the patient is placed in a quiet, darkened area and instructed to close the eyes. These measures are helpful in reducing uptake of the tracer in the visual cortex.

Radiopharmaceutical

The adult dose is 20 mCi (740 MBq) of ^{99m}Tc ethylcysteinate dimer (ECD) or ^{99m}Tc hexamethylpropyleneamine-oxime (HMPAO). The pediatric dose is based on body surface area.

Scanning

Imaging begins 1 hour after ^{99m}Tc ECD injection or ^{99m}Tc HMPAO injection. Tomographic images of the brain are obtained.

Central nervous system studies

CNS studies include brain perfusion imaging–SPECT study, brain imaging–acetazolamide challenge study, CNS shunt patency, CSF imaging–cisternography/ventriculography, ^{201}Tl scan for recurrent brain tumor, and ^{99m}Tc HMPAO scan for determination of brain death.

ENDOCRINE SYSTEM

The endocrine system organs, located throughout the body, secrete hormones into the bloodstream. Hormones have profound effects on overall body function and metabolism. The endocrine system consists of the thyroid, parathyroid, pituitary, and suprarenal glands, the islet cells of the pancreas, and the gonads. Nuclear medicine procedures have played a significant part in the current understanding of the function of the endocrine glands and their role in health and disease. These procedures are useful for monitoring treatment of endocrine disorders, especially in the thyroid gland. Thyroid imaging is performed to evaluate the size, shape, nodularity, and functional status of the thyroid gland. Imaging is used to screen for thyroid cancer and to differentiate hyperthyroidism, nodular goiter, solitary thyroid nodule, and thyroiditis.

Thyroid scan
Principle

^{99m}Tc pertechnetate or ^{123}I can be used to image the thyroid gland. ^{99m}Tc pertechnetate is trapped by the thyroid gland but, unlike iodine-131, is not organified *into* the gland. It offers the advantages of low radiation dose to the patient, no particulate radiation (unlike ^{131}I), and well-resolved images. ^{123}I is organified into the gland. Imaging is used to determine the relative function in different regions within the thyroid, with special emphasis on the function of nodules compared with the rest of the gland. Scanning can also determine the presence and site of thyroid tissue in unusual areas of the body, such as the tongue and anterior chest (ectopic tissue).

Radiopharmaceutical

The adult dose is 5 mCi (185 MBq) of ^{99m}Tc pertechnetate administered intravenously, or 1 mCi ^{123}I administered orally. The pediatric dose is adjusted according to the patient's weight. Uptake may be affected by thyroid medication and by foods or drugs, including some iodine-containing contrast agents used for renal radiographic imaging and CT scanning.

Scanning

Scanning should start 20 minutes after the injection of ^{99m}Tc, or 4 to 24 hours after the administration of ^{123}I. A gamma camera with a pinhole collimator is used to obtain anterior, left oblique, and right anterior oblique thyroid images and a 6-inch (15-cm) anterior neck image. The pinhole collimator is a thick, conical collimator that allows for magnification of the thyroid.

^{131}I thyroid uptake measurement
Principle

Radioiodine is concentrated by the thyroid gland in a manner that reflects the ability of the gland to handle stable dietary iodine. Therefore ^{123}I uptake is used to estimate the function of the thyroid gland by measuring its avidity for administered radioiodine. The higher the uptake of ^{131}I, the more active the thyroid; conversely, the lower the uptake, the less functional the gland. Uptake conventionally is expressed as the percentage of the dose in the thyroid gland at a given time after administration. ^{131}I uptake measurement is of value in distinguishing between thyroiditis (reduced uptake) and Graves' disease or toxic nodular goiter (Plummer's disease), which has an increased uptake. It is also used to determine the appropriateness of a therapeutic dose of ^{131}I in patients with Graves' disease, residual or recurrent thyroid carcinoma, or thyroid remnant after thyroidectomy.

Radiopharmaceutical

All doses of ^{131}I sodium iodide are administered orally. The adult dose for a standard uptake test is 3 to 5 μCi (148 to 222 kBq) of ^{131}I. The pediatric dose is adjusted according to the patient's weight. A standard dose is counted with the thyroid probe, in the morning of the scan, and is used as 100% of maximum counts. The patient's total count is compared with the standard counts to obtain the patient percent uptake.

Measurements are obtained using an uptake probe consisting of a 2 × 2 inch (5 × 5 cm) sodium iodide/photomultiplier tube assembly fitted with a flat-field lead collimator (Fig. 35-16). Uptake readings are acquired at 4 or 6 hours and/or at 24 hours.

Total-body ^{123}I scan
Principle
A total-body ^{123}I (TBI) scan is recommended for locating residual thyroid tissue or recurrent thyroid cancer cells in patients with thyroid carcinoma. Most follicular or papillary thyroid cancers concentrate radioiodine; other types of thyroid cancer do not. A TBI scan is usually performed 1 to 3 months after a thyroidectomy to check for residual normal thyroid tissue as well as metastatic spread of the cancer before ^{131}I ablation therapy. After the residual thyroid tissue has been ablated (destroyed), another ^{123}I TBI scan may be performed to check for residual disease.

Radiopharmaceutical
The adult dose for a total-body ^{123}I scan is generally 5 mCi (185 MBq) of ^{123}I sodium iodide administered orally. Thyrogen may be injected on each of two days before dose administration to allow the patient to remain on their thyroid medications. The pediatric dose is adjusted according to the patient's weight.

Scanning
Total-body imaging begins 24 hours after dose administration. Images are obtained of the anterior and posterior whole body.

Endocrine studies
Endocrine studies include adrenal cortical scan (NP-59), adrenal medullary scan (mIBG), ectopic thyroid scan (^{131}I/^{123}I), thyroid scan (^{99m}Tc pertechnetate), ^{131}I thyroid uptake measurement, ^{123}I thyroid uptake/scan, ^{123}I total body iodine scan, parathyroid scan, indium-111 pentetreotide scan.

GASTROINTESTINAL SYSTEM
The gastrointestinal system, or alimentary canal, consists of the mouth, oropharynx, esophagus, stomach, small bowel, colon, and several accessory organs (salivary glands, pancreas, liver, and gallbladder). The liver is the largest internal organ of the body. The portal venous system brings blood from the stomach, bowel, spleen, and pancreas to the liver.

Liver/spleen scan
Principle
Liver and/or spleen scanning is used to evaluate the liver for functional disease (e.g., cirrhosis, hepatitis, metastatic disease) and to look for residual splenic tissue following splenectomy. Imaging techniques such as ultrasonography, CT, and MRI provide excellent information about the anatomy of the liver, but nuclear medicine studies can assess the *functional* status of this organ. Liver and spleen scintigraphy is also useful for detecting hepatic lesions and evaluating hepatic morphology and function. It is also used to determine whether certain lesions found with other methods may be benign (e.g., focal nodular hyperplasia), thereby obviating the need for biopsy. Uptake of a radiopharmaceutical in the liver, spleen, and bone marrow depends on blood flow and the functional capacity of the phagocytic cells. In normal patients, 80% to 90% of the radiopharmaceutical is localized in the liver, 5% to 10% in the spleen, and the rest in the bone marrow.

Radiopharmaceutical
Adults receive 6 mCi (222 MBq) of ^{99m}Tc sulfur colloid injected intravenously. The pediatric dose is adjusted according to the patient's weight.

Scanning
Images obtained may be planar standard (anterior, posterior, right and left anterior oblique, right and left lateral, right posterior oblique, and a marker view), life-size, or SPECT.

Gastrointestinal studies
Gastrointestinal studies include anorectal angle study, colonic transit study, colorectal/neorectal emptying study, esophageal scintigraphy, gastroesophageal reflux (adults and children) study, gastric emptying study, small-bowel transit study, hepatic artery perfusion scan, hepatobiliary scan, hepatobiliary scan with gallbladder ejection fraction, evaluation of human serum albumin for protein-losing gastroenteropathy, liver/spleen scan, liver hemangioma study, Meckel's diverticulum scan, and salivary gland study.

Fig. 35-16 Uptake probe used for thyroid uptake measurements over the extended neck area.

GENITOURINARY NUCLEAR MEDICINE

Genitourinary nuclear medicine studies are recognized as reliable, noninvasive procedures for evaluating the anatomy and function of the systems in nephrology, urology, and kidney transplantation. These studies can be accomplished with minimum risk of allergic reactions, unpleasant side effects, or excessive radiation exposure to the organs.

Dynamic renal scan
Principle

Renal scanning is used to assess renal perfusion and function, particularly in renal failure and renovascular hypertension and after renal transplantation. ^{99m}Tc mertiatide (MAG_3) is secreted primarily by the proximal renal tubules and is not retained in the parenchyma of normal kidneys.

Radiopharmaceutical

The adult dose is 10 mCi (370 MBq) of ^{99m}Tc MAG_3. The pediatric dose is adjusted according to the patient's weight.

Scanning

Imaging is initiated immediately after the injection. Because radiographic contrast media may interfere with kidney function, renal scanning should be delayed for 24 hours after contrast studies. Images are often taken over the posterior lower back, centered at the level of the twelfth rib. Transplanted kidneys are imaged in the anterior pelvis. Patients need to be well hydrated, determined by a specific gravity test, before all renal studies.

Genitourinary studies

Genitourinary studies include dynamic renal scan, dynamic renal scan with furosemide, dynamic renal scan with captopril, pediatric furosemide renal scan, ^{99m}Tc dimercaptosuccinic acid (DMSA) renal scan, residual urine determination, testicular scan, and voiding cystography.

IN VITRO AND IN VIVO HEMATOLOGIC STUDIES

In vitro and in vivo hematologic studies have been performed in nuclear medicine for many years. Quantitative measurements are made after a radiopharmaceutical has been administered, often at predetermined intervals. The two types of nonimaging nuclear medicine procedures are as follows:

- *In vitro* radioimmunoassay for quantitating biologically important substances in the serum or other body fluids.
- *In vivo* evaluation of physiologic function by administering small tracer amounts of radioactive materials to the patient and subsequently counting specimens of urine, blood, feces, or breath. A wide variety of physiologic events may be measured, including vitamin B_{12} absorption (Schilling test), red cell survival and sequestration, red cell mass, and plasma volume.

Hematologic studies

Hematologic studies include plasma volume measurement, Schilling test, red cell mass, red cell survival, and red cell sequestration.

IMAGING FOR INFECTION

Imaging for infection is another useful nuclear medicine diagnostic tool. Inflammation, infection, and abscess may be found in any organ or tissue and at any location within the body. Imaging procedures such as gallium-67 scans, and ^{111}In-labeled white cell scans are both useful for diagnosis and localization of infection and inflammation.

Infection studies

Infection studies include ^{67}Ga gallium scan, ^{111}In white blood cell scans, ^{99m}Tc HMPAO, and post total hip or knee replacement surgery.

RESPIRATORY IMAGING

Respiratory imaging commonly involves the demonstration of pulmonary perfusion using limited, transient capillary blockade and the assessment of ventilation using an inhaled radioactive gas or aerosol. Lung imaging is most commonly performed to evaluate pulmonary emboli, chronic obstructive pulmonary disease, chronic bronchitis, emphysema, asthma, and lung carcinoma. It is also used for lung transplant evaluation.

^{133}Xe lung ventilation scan
Principle

Lung ventilation scans are used in combination with lung perfusion scans. The gas used for a ventilation study must be absorbed significantly by the lungs and diffuse easily. Xenon-133 has adequate imaging properties, and the body usually absorbs less than 15% of the gas.

Radiopharmaceutical

The adult dose is 15 to 30 mCi (555 to 1110 MBq) of ^{133}Xe gas administered by inhalation.

Scanning

Imaging starts immediately after inhalation of the xenon gas begins in a closed system to which oxygen is added and carbon dioxide is withdrawn. When ^{133}Xe gas is used, the ventilation study must precede the ^{99m}Tc perfusion scan. Posterior and anterior images are obtained for the first breath equilibrium and *washout*. If possible, left and right posterior oblique images should be obtained between the first breath and equilibrium.

^{99m}Tc macroaggregated albumin lung perfusion scan
Radiopharmaceutical

The adult dose is 4 mCi (148 MBq) of ^{99m}Tc MAA. The pediatric dose is adjusted according to the patient's weight.

Scanning

Imaging starts 5 minutes after the injection. Eight images should be obtained: anterior, posterior, right and left lateral, right and left anterior oblique, and right and left posterior oblique. The nuclear medicine physician may need additional images. All patients should have a chest radiograph within 24 hours of the lung scan. The chest radiograph is required for accurate interpretation of the lung scans, to determine the probability for pulmonary embolism.

Respiratory studies

Respiratory studies include ^{99m}Tc diethylenetriamine pentaacetic acid (DTPA) lung aerosol scan, ^{99m}Tc MAA lung perfusion scan, and ^{133}Xe lung ventilation scan.

SENTINEL NODE

Many tumors metastasize via lymphatic channels. Defining the anatomy of nodes that drain a primary tumor site helps guide surgical and radiation treatment for certain tumor sites. Contrast lymphangiography, MRI, and CT are the standard methods to evaluate the status of the lymph nodes. Radionuclide lymphoscintigraphy has been useful in patient studies in whom the channels are relatively inaccessible. This method has been used primarily in patients with truncal melanomas and prostate and breast cancer to map the routes of lymphatic drainage and permit more effective surgical or radiation treatment of draining regional lymph nodes.

Principle

Colloidal particles injected intradermally or subcutaneously adjacent to a tumor site demonstrate a drainage pattern similar to that of the tumor. Colloidal particles in the 10- to 50-nm range appear to be the most effective for this application. The colloidal particles drain into the sentinel lymph node, where they are trapped by phagocytic activity. This aids in the identification of the lymph nodes most likely to be sites of metastatic deposits from the tumor.

Radiopharmaceutical

The adult dose is 100 μCi of ^{99m}Tc sulfur colloid in a volume of 0.1 mL per injection site.

Scanning

Patients with malignant melanoma should be positioned supine or prone on the imaging table. Images are acquired immediately after injection, then every few minutes for the first 15 minutes followed by every 5 minutes for 30 minutes. Additional lateral and oblique views are required after visualization of the sentinel nodes. Breast cancer patients should be positioned supine on the imaging table with the arms extended over the head.

THERAPEUTIC NUCLEAR MEDICINE

The potential that radionuclides have for detecting and treating cancer has been recognized for decades. Radioiodine is a treatment in practically all adults with Graves' disease, except those who are pregnant or breast-feeding. High-dose ^{131}I therapy (30 mCi or more) is used in patients with residual thyroid cancer or thyroid metastases. Phosphorus-32 in the form of sodium phosphate can be used to treat polycythemia, a disease characterized by the increased production of red blood cells. ^{32}P chromic phosphate colloid administered into the peritoneal cavity is useful in the postoperative management of ovarian and endometrial cancers because of its effectiveness in destroying many of the malignant cells remaining in the peritoneum. Skeletal metastases occur in more than 50% of patients with breast, lung, or prostate cancer in the end stages of the disease. Strontium-99 is often useful for managing patients with bone pain from metastases when other treatments have failed.

Therapeutic procedures

Therapeutic procedures include ^{131}I therapy for hyperthyroidism and thyroid cancer, ^{32}P therapy for polycythemia, ^{32}P intraperitoneal therapy, ^{32}P intrapleural therapy, and ^{89}Sr bone therapy.

SPECIAL IMAGING PROCEDURES

Special imaging procedures include dacryoscintigraphy, LeVeen shunt patency test, sentinel node studies for melanoma or breast cancer, and lymphoscintigraphy of the limbs.

TUMOR IMAGING

OctreoScan

^{111}In OctreoScan is a radiolabeled analog of the neuroendocrine peptide somatostatin. It localizes in somatostatin receptor–rich tumors, primarily of neuroendocrine origin. It is currently indicated for the scintigraphic localization of the following tumors: carcinoid, islet cell carcinoma, gastrinoma, motilinoma, pheochromocytoma, small cell carcinoma, medullary thyroid carcinoma, neuroblastoma, paraganglioma, glucagonoma, pituitary adenoma, meningioma, VIPoma, and insulinoma.

Principle

Somatostatin is a neuroregulatory peptide known to localize on many cells of neuroendocrine origin. Cell membrane receptors with a high affinity for somatostatin have been shown to be present in the majority of neuroendocrine tumors including carcinoids, islet cell carcinomas, and gonadotropin hormone (GH)-producing pituitary adenomas. Tumors such as meningiomas, breast carcinomas, astrocytomas, and oat cell carcinomas of the lung have been reported to have a large number of binding sites.

Radiopharmaceutical

The adult dose is 5 to 6 mCi (203.5 MBq) ^{111}In pentetreotide administered intravenously. The pediatric dose is adjusted according to the patient's weight.

Scanning

The patient should be well hydrated before administration of OctreoScan. At 4 hours after injection, anterior and posterior whole-body images should be acquired. At 24 hours, anterior and posterior spot views of the chest and abdomen should be obtained. SPECT imaging is most helpful in the localization of intraabdominal tumors. SPECT/CT can assist in lesion localization. Co-registered images of the liver and spleen are performed with dual-isotope SPECT imaging.

Tumor studies

Tumor studies include ^{67}Ga tumor scan, ^{99m}Tc sestamibi breast scan, ^{111}In ProstaScint (capromab pendetide) scan, ^{99m}Tc CEA gastrointestinal scan, ^{99m}Tc verluma for small cell lung cancer, and ^{111}In OctreoScan.

			F 17	F 18	F 19	F 20
			64.5 s	1.83 h	100%	11 s
	O 14	O 15	O 16	O 17	O 18	O 19
	70.6 s	122.2 s	99.76%	0.04%	0.2%	26.9 s
	N 13	N 14	N 15	N 16		
	9.97 m	99.63%	0.37%	7.13 s		
C 11	C 12	C 13	C 14	C 15		
20.3 m	98.9%	1.1%	5730 y	2.45 s		

Fig. 35-17 Excerpt from *The Chart of the Nuclides* showing the stable elements *(shaded boxes)*, positron emitters (to the left of the stable elements), and beta emitters (to the right of the stable elements). Isotopes farther from their stable counterparts have very short half-lives. The most commonly used PET nuclides are ^{11}C, ^{13}N, ^{15}O, and ^{18}F.

(From Walker FW et al: *The chart of the nuclides*, ed 13, San Jose, Calif, 1984, General Electric Company.)

BOX 35-1

Positron characteristics

Definition: positively charged electron
Origin: neutron-deficient nuclei
Production: accelerators
Nuclide decay: p = n + β⁺neutrino
Positron decay: annihilation to two 0.511-MeV photons
Number: about 240 known
Range: proportional to kinetic energy of β⁺
Routine PET nuclides: ^{11}C, ^{13}N, ^{15}O, ^{18}F, ^{68}Ga, ^{82}Rb

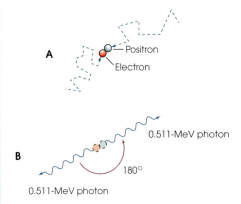

Fig. 35-18 Neutron-deficient nuclei decay by positron emission. A positron is ejected from the nucleus and loses kinetic energy by scattering *(erratic line on A)* until it comes to rest and interacts with a free electron. Two photons of 0.511 MeV (E = m_oc^2) result from the positron and electron annihilation *(wavy line in B)*.

Principles and Facilities in Positron Emission Tomography

This discussion focuses on major concepts of *positrons*, PET, and the equipment used in this type of imaging. PET is a multidisciplinary technique that involves four major processes: radionuclide production, radiopharmaceutical production, data acquisition (PET scanner or tomograph), and a combination of image reconstruction and image processing to create images that depict tissue function.

POSITRONS

Living organisms are composed primarily of compounds that contain the elements hydrogen, carbon, nitrogen, and oxygen. In PET, radiotracers are made by synthesizing compounds with radioactive isotopes of these elements. Chemically the radioactive isotope is indistinguishable from its equivalent stable isotope. Neutron-rich (i.e., having more neutrons than protons) radionuclides emit electrons or beta particles. The effective range or distance traveled for a 1-MeV beta particle (β⁻) in human tissue is only 4 mm. These radionuclides typically do not emit other types of radiation that can be easily measured externally with counters or scintillation detectors. The only radioisotopes of these elements that can be detected outside the body are positron-emitting nuclides. The stable and radioactive nuclides of several elements are depicted in Fig. 35-17.

Positron-emitting radionuclides have a neutron-deficient nucleus (i.e., the *nucleus* contains more protons than neutrons and thus is also called a *proton-rich* nucleus). Positrons (β⁺) are identical in mass to electrons, but they possess positive instead of negative charge. The characteristics of positrons are given in Box 35-1. Positron decay occurs in unstable radioisotopes only if the nucleus possesses excess energy greater than the energy equivalent of two electron rest masses, or a total of 1.022 MeV. Positrons are emitted from the nucleus with high velocity and kinetic energy. They are rapidly slowed by interactions in the surrounding tissues until all of the positron kinetic energy is lost. At this point the positron combines momentarily with an electron. The combination of particles will totally annihilate or disintegrate, and the combined positron-electron mass of 1.022 MeV is transformed into two equal-energy photons of 0.511 MeV, which are emitted at 180 degrees from each other (Fig. 35-18).

These annihilation photons behave like gamma *rays,* have sufficient energy to traverse body tissues with only modest attenuation, and can be detected externally. Because two identical or isoenergetic photons are emitted at exactly 180 degrees from each other, the nearly simultaneous detection of both photons defines a line that passes through the body. The line is located precisely between the two scintillators that detected the photons. A simplified block diagram for a single coincidence circuit is shown in Fig. 35-19. The creation of images from coincidence detection is discussed under Data Acquisition.

The positron annihilation photons from the positron-emitting radionuclides of carbon, nitrogen, and oxygen can be used for external detection. Table 35-3 depicts the positron ranges for three positron energies in tissue, air, and lead. Hydrogen has no positron-emitting radioisotope; however, ^{18}F is a positron (β^+) emitter that is used as a hydrogen substitute in many compounds. This substitution of radioactive fluorine for hydrogen is successfully accomplished because of its small size and strong bond with carbon.

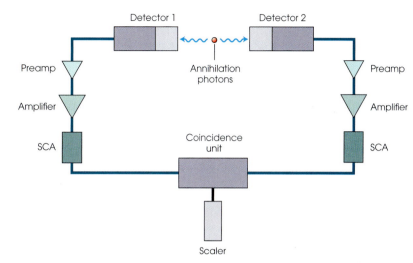

Fig. 35-19 Simplified coincidence electronics for one pair of detectors in a PET tomograph.

TABLE 35-3

Range (R) of positrons (β^+) in centimeters

E(MeV)*	R_{tissue}	R_{air}	R_{lead}
0.5	0.15	127	0.01
1.0	0.38	279	0.03
1.5	0.64	508	0.05

From U.S. Dept. of Health, Education, and Welfare: *Radiological health handbook,* Rockville, Md, 1970, Bureau of Radiological Health.
*The average positron energy is approximately one third the maximum energy (see Fig. 35-21).

RADIONUCLIDE PRODUCTION

Positron-emitting radionuclides are produced when a *nuclear particle accelerator* bombards appropriate nonradioactive *target* atoms with nuclei accelerated to high energies. The high energies are necessary to overcome the electrostatic and nuclear forces of the target nuclei so that a nuclear reaction can take place. An example is the production of ^{15}O. Deuterons, or heavy hydrogen ions (the deuterium atom is stripped of its electron, leaving only the nucleus with one proton and one neutron), are accelerated to approximately 7 MeV. The target material is stable nitrogen gas in the form of an N_2 molecule. The resultant nuclear reaction yields a neutron and an ^{15}O atom, which can be written in the following form: $^{14}N(d,n)^{15}O$. The ^{15}O atom quickly associates with a stable ^{16}O atom that has been intentionally added to the target gas to produce a radioactive ^{15}O-^{16}O molecule in the form of O_2.

The unstable or radioactive ^{15}O atom emits a positron when it decays. This radioactive decay process transforms a proton into a neutron. Hence upon decay the ^{15}O atom becomes a stable ^{15}N atom and the O_2 molecule breaks apart. This process is shown in Fig. 35-20, and the decay schemes for the four routinely produced PET radionuclides are depicted in Fig. 35-21. The common reactions used for the production of positron-emitting forms of carbon, nitrogen, oxygen, and fluorine are given in Table 35-4.

Because of the very short half-lives of the routinely used positron-emitting nuclides of oxygen, nitrogen and carbon, nearby access to a nuclear particle accelerator is necessary to produce sufficient quantities of these radioactive materials. The most common device to achieve nuclide production within reasonable space ($250 ft^2$ [$223 m^2$]) and energy (150 kW) constraints is a compact medical cyclotron (Fig. 35-22). This device is specifically designed for the following: (1) simple operation by the technologist staff, (2) reliable and routine operation with minimal downtime, and (3) computer-controlled automatic operation to reduce overall staffing needs.

Fig. 35-20 Typical radionuclide production sequence. The $^{14}N(d,n)^{15}O$ reaction is used for making ^{15}O-^{16}O molecules. *1,* A deuteron ion is accelerated to high energy (7 MeV) by a cyclotron and impinges on a stable ^{14}N nucleus. *2,* As a result of the nuclear reaction, a neutron is emitted, leaving a radioactive nucleus of ^{15}O. *3,* The ^{15}O atom quickly associates with an ^{16}O atom to form an O_2 molecule. Sometime later, the unstable ^{15}O atom emits a positron. *4,* As a result of positron decay (i.e., positron exits nucleus), the ^{15}O atom is transformed into a stable ^{15}N atom and the O_2 molecule breaks apart.

Fig. 35-21 Decay schemes for ^{11}C, ^{13}N, ^{15}O, and ^{18}F. Each positron emitter decays to a stable nuclide by ejecting a positron from the nucleus. E_{max} represents the maximum energy of the emitted positron. Electron capture is a competitive process with positron decay; hence positron decay is not always 100%.

Nuclear medicine

TABLE 35-4

Most common production reactions and target materials
for the typical nuclides used in positron emission tomography

Nuclide	Half-life	Reaction(s) Proton	Deuteron	Target material
^{11}C	20.4 min	$^{14}N(p,\alpha)^{11}C$		N_2 (gas)
^{13}N	9.97 min	$^{16}O(p,\alpha)^{13}N$		H_2O (liquid)
^{15}O	2.03 min	$^{15}N(p,n)^{15}O$	$^{14}N(d,n)^{15}O$	$N^2 + 1\% O_2$ (gas)
^{18}F	109.8 min	$^{18}O(p,n)^{18}F$		95% $^{18}O - H_2O$ (liquid)
			$^{20}Ne(d,\alpha)^{18}F$	Ne + 0.1% F_2 (gas)

Fig. 35-22 Compact cyclotron (2.2 m high by 1.5 m wide by 1.5 m deep) used for routine production of PET isotopes. The cyclotron can be located in a concrete vault, or it can be self-shielded. Particles are accelerated in vertical orbits and impinge on targets located near the top center of the machine. This is an example of a negative-ion cyclotron.

(Courtesy GE Medical Systems, Milwaukee, Wis.)

RADIOPHARMACEUTICAL PRODUCTION

Radiopharmaceuticals are synthesized from radionuclides derived from the target material. These agents may be simple, like the ^{15}O-^{16}O molecules described earlier, or they may be complex. Regardless of the chemical complexity of the radioactive molecule, all radiopharmaceuticals must be synthesized rapidly. This entails specialized techniques not only to create the labeled substance but also to verify the purity (chemical, radiochemical, and radionuclidic) of the radiotracer.

Two important radiopharmaceuticals are presently used in many PET studies. The simplest is ^{15}O water (^{15}O-H_2O), which is produced continuously from the $^{14}N(d,n)^{15}O$ nuclear reaction or in batches from the $^{15}N(p,n)^{15}O$ nuclear reaction. As previously discussed, the radioactive oxygen quickly combines with a stable ^{16}O atom, which has been added to the stable N_2 target gas, to form an oxygen molecule (O_2). The ^{15}O-^{16}O molecule is reduced over a platinum catalyst with small amounts of stable H_2 and N_2 gas. Radioactive water vapor is produced and collected in sterile saline for injection. A typical bolus injection of ^{15}O-H_2O is approximately 30 to 50 mCi in a volume of 1 to 2 mL of saline for use in a PET scanner that acquires data in 2D and approximately 3 to 8 mCi in the same volume of saline for a PET tomograph of the newer 3D design. A dose of radioactive water can be prepared every 2 to 5 minutes. Radioactive ^{15}O-H_2O is used primarily for the determination of *local cerebral blood flow* (LCBF). PET LCBF images from one subject using two different techniques are shown in Fig. 35-23. Blood flow to tumor, heart, kidney, or other tissues can also be measured using ^{15}O-H_2O.

The most widely used PET radiopharmaceutical for clinical PET imaging is more complex than labeled water and employs ^{18}F-labeled fluoride ions (F-) to form a sugar analog called [^{18}F]-2-fluoro-2-deoxy-D-glucose, or ^{18}F-FDG. This agent is used to determine the *local metabolic rate of glucose utilization* (LMRG) in tumor, brain, heart, or other tissues that use glucose as a metabolic substrate. For example, the glucose obtained from food is metabolized by the brain to provide the adenosine triphosphate necessary for maintaining the membrane potential of neurons within the brain. The metabolism of glucose is proportional to the neural activity of the brain and thus brain metabolism. Radioactive ^{18}F-FDG and glucose enter the same biochemical pathways in the brain. However, unlike glucose, ^{18}F-FDG cannot be completely metabolized in the brain because its metabolism is blocked at the level of fluoro-deoxyglucose-6-phosphate ([^{18}F]-FDG-6-PO_4). Because ^{18}F-FDG follows the glucose pathway into the brain, the concentration of [^{18}F]-FDG-6-PO_4 within the brain cells is proportional to brain tissue metabolism. These pathways for glucose and ^{18}F-FDG are shown schematically in Fig. 35-24.

Fig. 35-23 PET LCBF images. The images in the top row were created using a standard filtered backprojection reconstruction technique. An iterative reconstructive method was used to create the images in the bottom row from the same raw data that were used for the upper images. In all images, dark areas correspond to high brain blood flow. There is about an 8-mm separation between each brain slice within a row.

Fig. 35-24 Glucose compartmental model *(above the dashed line)* compared with the ^{18}F-FDG model *(below the dashed line)*. Note that ^{18}F-FDG does not go to complete storage (glycogen) or metabolism (CO_2 + H_2O) as does glucose. The constants *(K)* refer to reaction rates for moving substances from one compartment to another. Dashed arrow refers to extremely small K value that can usually be neglected.

Injected doses of ^{18}F-FDG range from 5 to 20 mCi with a standard dose being 15-20 mCi. FDG is dissolved in a few milliliters of isotonic saline and is administered intravenously. The total time for FDG production, which includes target irradiation (1 hour to 90 minutes), radiochemical synthesis (30 minutes to 1 hour), and purity certification (15 minutes), is approximately 2 to 3 hours, depending on the exact synthesis method used. Because of the short half-life of most positron-emitting radioisotopes, radiopharmaceutical production must be closely tied to the clinical patient schedule.

DATA ACQUISITION

The positron-electron annihilation photons are detected and counted with a PET scanner or tomograph (Fig. 35-25). The bore width of these scanners is approximately 70 cm, with newer scanners being slightly larger in diameter. The radial field of view (FOV) or the imaging dimension parallel to the detector rings for these scanners is approximately 24 cm (10 inches) and 55 cm (22 inches), respectively (Fig. 35-26). The z-axis or dimension perpendicular to the detector rings is 15 to 50 cm (6 to 20 inches). Typical new scanners have 800 to 1000 detectors per ring. A detector module consists of *BGO scintillators* organized into a matrix (6 × 6, 7 × 8, or 8 × 8) of small rectangular boxes (3 to 6 mm long, 3 to 6 mm wide, and 10 to 30 mm deep), which are coupled to photomultiplier tubes (PMTs). A new scintillator, lutetium orthosilicate (Lu$_2$SiO$_5$:Ce), also known as LSO, has a higher light output (approximately four times that of BGO) and faster photofluorescent decay (approximately 7.5 times that of BGO). Scintillator dimensions are being reduced to improve resolution. Currently, the resolution within the image plane for PET scanners is between 3 and 5 mm full width at half maximum (FWHM). Thus an image of a point source of radioactivity appears to be 3 to 5 mm wide at one half the maximum intensity of the source image. The concept of PET scanner resolution can be explained using a bicycle wheel as an example. In the case of PET, lines drawn between detectors or

Fig. 35-25 Typical whole-body PET scanner. The bed is capable of moving in and out of the scanner to measure the distribution of PET radiopharmaceuticals throughout the body, and it adjusts to a very low position for easy patient access. Sophisticated computer workstations are required to view and analyze data.

(Courtesy GE Medical Systems, Milwaukee, Wis.)

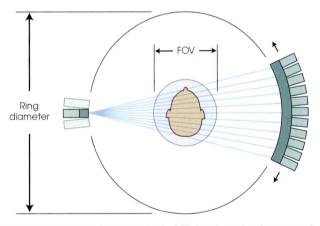

Fig. 35-26 Detector arrangement in neurologic PET ring (head-only scanner). Rays from opposed detector pairs (*lines* between detectors) depict possible coincidence events. The useful field of view (*FOV*) is delineated by the central circle.

rays correspond to the bicycle spokes. The highest density of spokes is located at the hub. At the rim of the wheel, the density of spokes is reduced. The same is true for the density of rays between detectors. That is why the selected radial imaging FOV for these scanners is approximately the middle third of the distance from one detector face to the opposite detector face. Adequate ray density for the best resolution for image reconstruction is achieved only within this FOV. The same holds for the axial or longitudinal dimension (z-axis). Approximately two thirds of the axial FOV contains sufficient ray sampling. By acquiring several axial FOVs, which is achieved by moving the bed through the PET scanner, the amount of data undersampled is significantly reduced. Each axial FOV is overlapped with the next. Therefore sufficient axial sampling is achieved for all but the first and last bed position.

Coincidence counts are collected not only for detector pairs within each ring (direct-plane information), but also between adjacent rings (cross-plane information) as shown in Fig. 35-27. However, not all photons emitted from the patient can be detected. Some of the pairs of 0.511-MeV photons from the positron annihilation impinge on detectors in the tomograph ring and are detected; most do not. The photon pairs are emitted 180 degrees from each other. The emission process is *isotropic,* which means that the annihilation photons are emitted with equal probability in all directions so that only a small fraction of the total number of photons emitted from the patient actually strike the tomograph detectors (Fig. 35-28).

PET scanners originally used ray information only from the nearest adjacent planes. However, with improvements in software reconstruction techniques and the elimination of septa between detector rings, the second, third, fourth, and upward adjacent planes are used to produce 3D PET images. With inclusion of the additional cross-plane information, PET scanner *sensitivity* is greatly increased. Hence, the injected doses of radiopharmaceutical are significantly reduced (50% to 90% less radioactivity given) to yield PET images with a quality equivalent to that of images obtained from the original dose levels used in 2D PET scanners with septa.

When pairs of photons are detected, they are counted as valid events (i.e., true positron annihilation) only if they appear at the detectors within the resolving time

Fig. 35-27 Side-view schematic of a small portion of a multiring (three-ring) PET tomograph. The darker green squares indicate the scintillator-matrix, which is attached to multiple-photocathode PMTs. Solid lines indicate the direct planes, and dashed lines depict the cross planes. The X determined by the pair of cross planes forms a data plane located between direct planes. Improvements in PET scanner instrumentation not only permit cross-plane information between adjacent rings to be acquired but also allow for expansion to the second, third, fourth, and fifth near neighbor rings. This significantly enhances overall scanner sensitivity.

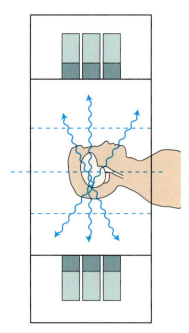

Fig. 35-28 Side view of PET scanner, illustrating possible photon directions. Only 15% of the total number of emitted photons from the patient can be detected in a whole-body tomograph (ring diameter: 100 cm (39 inches)). This is increased to 25% for a head tomograph (ring diameter: 60 cm (24 inches)). For these estimates, the z axis coverage was considered to be 15 cm (6 inches). The actual number of detected coincidences will be less than either the 15% or 25% estimate because the detector efficiency is not 100% (typical efficiency: 30%).

for the coincidence electronics. For many PET tomographs this is typically 8 to 12 nsec. If one photon is detected and no other photon is observed during that time window, the original event is discarded. This is defined as electronic collimation. No conventional lead collimators as needed with SPECT are used in PET scanners. However, thick lead shields absorb annihilation photons created out of the axial FOV before interacting with the PET detectors. These shields help reduce random events and high singles counting events. PET scanners must operate with high sensitivity and as a result scanners must also be able to handle very high count rates with minimum *deadtime* losses.

For PET procedures, data acquisition is not limited to images of tomographic count rates. For example, the creation of *quantitative* parametric images of glucose metabolism requires that the blood concentrations of the radiopharmaceutical be measured. This is accomplished by discrete or continuous arterial sampling, discrete or continuous venous sampling, or *region of interest* (ROI) analysis of a sequential time series of major arterial vessels observed in reconstructed tomographic images. For arterial sampling, an indwelling catheter is placed in the radial artery. Arterial blood pressure forces blood out of the catheter for collection and radioactivity measurement. For venous sampling, blood is withdrawn through an indwelling venous catheter. However, for obtaining *arterialized venous blood,* the patient's hand is heated to between 104° F and 108° F (40° C and 42.2° C). In this situation arterial blood is shunted directly to the venous system. The arterial concentration of radioactivity can then be assessed by measuring the venous radioactivity concentration. If plasma radioactivity measurement is required in discrete samples, the red blood cells are separated from whole blood by centrifugation and the radioactivity concentration within plasma is determined by discrete sample counting in a gamma well counter. Continuous counting is performed on whole blood by directing the blood through a radiation detector via small-bore tubing. A peristaltic pump, a syringe pump, or the subject's arterial blood pressure is used for continuous or discrete blood sampling. For ROI analysis, the arterial blood curve is generated directly from each image of a multiple-frame, time-series PET scan. An ROI is placed around the arterial vessel visualized in the PET images. The average number of counts for the ROI from each frame is plotted against time. Actual blood sampling is not usually required for ROI analysis. However, a single venous (or arterial) blood sample may be taken at times when tracer equilibrium has been established between arterial and venous blood to appropriately position the blood curve on an absolute scale.

A typical set of blood and tissue curves is given in Fig. 35-29. Curves created from plasma data, as well as other information (e.g., nonradioactive plasma glucose level), are supplied to a mathematical model that appropriately describes the physiologic process being measured (i.e., metabolic rate of glucose utilization in tissue). Parametric or functional images are created by applying the model to the original PET image data.

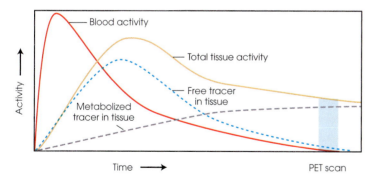

Fig. 35-29 Decay-corrected radioactivity curves for ^{18}F-FDG in tissue and blood (plasma). Injection occurs at the origin. The blood activity rapidly peaks after the injection. The metabolized tracer ((^{18}F)-FDG-6-PO$_4$) slowly accumulates in tissue. Typical static PET scanning occurs after an incorporation time of 40 to 60 minutes (as shown by the shaded box) in which the uptake of ^{18}F-FDG is balanced with the slow washout of the labeled metabolite.

Fig. 35-30 A, Uncorrected image of a phantom homogeneously filled with a water-soluble PET nuclide of ^{68}Ga or ^{18}F. **B,** Attenuation-corrected image of the same phantom. Cross-sectional cuts through the center of each image are shown in the lower panels. The attenuation correction for a phantom with a diameter of 20 cm (8 inches) can be as large as 70% in the center of the object.

Fig. 35-31 A typical PET/CT scanner.

(Courtesy GE Medical Systems, Milwaukee, Wis.)

IMAGE RECONSTRUCTION AND IMAGE PROCESSING

An FOV of 15 to 20 cm (6 to 8 inches in the axial direction) is required to adequately encompass the entire volume of the brain (from the top of the cerebral cortex to the base of the cerebellum) or the entire volume of the heart. Array processors are used to perform the filtered backprojection or maximum likelihood (iterative) reconstruction that converts the raw *sinogram* data into PET images. This technique is similar to that employed for CT image reconstruction. However, faster and less costly desktop computers are replacing array processor technology and thereby greatly simplifying software requirements for image reconstruction.

There are three important corrections that need to be made during the image reconstruction to ensure an accurate and interpretable scan. First, it is very important to note that the disintegration of radionuclides follows Poisson statistics. As a result of this random process, photons from the different annihilation events may strike the tomograph detectors simultaneously. Although these are registered as true events because they occur within the coincidence time window, they degrade the overall image quality. A simple approximation allows for the subtraction of the random events after image acquisition and is based on the individual count rates for each detector and the coincidence resolving time (8 to 12 nsec) of the tomograph electronics.

Second, photons traversing biologic tissues also undergo absorption and scatter. As shown in Fig. 35-30, an attenuation correction is applied to account for those photons that should have been detected but were not. The correction is typically based on a transmission scan acquired under computer control using a radioactive rod or pin source of ^{68}Ge (germanium; 271-day half-life) that circumscribes the portion of the patient's body within the PET scanner. Newer PET/CT scanners use the CT data to more accurately correct for attenuation (Fig. 35-31).

Nuclear medicine

Lastly, count rates from the detectors also need to be corrected for deadtime losses. At high count rates the detector electronics cannot handle every incoming event; therefore some of these events are lost because the electronics are busy processing prior events. Measuring the tomograph response to known input count rates allows empirical formulations for the losses to be determined and applied to the image data. Valid corrections for deadtime losses can approach 100%.

Clinical Positron Emission Tomography

PET is unique in its ability to measure in vivo physiology because its results are quantitative, rapidly repeatable, and validated against those of accurate but much more invasive techniques. It is, however, relatively costly and best used for answering complex questions that involve locating and quantitatively assessing tissue function (Figs. 35-32 and 35-33). Anatomic imaging, such as CT, is often limited in its ability to determine whether found masses are of malignant or benign etiology. Traditional anatomic imaging modalities also have difficulty determining malignancy in small masses or lymph nodes. Because PET is a functional modality, it can often be used to determine malignancy, even in very small nodes or masses.

Patient preparation for PET studies can be detailed and are imperative for optimal images. In most cases the area that is to be examined must be free of metallic objects to avoid creating artifacts on the reconstructed images. This is especially important when using a PET/CT scanner because metallic objects may cause false-positive results in the final images due to attenuation overcorrection in that area. The waiting time between dose administration and imaging varies with each study, as does the total imaging time. After completion of a routine procedure, patients may resume all normal activities.

Following are technical summaries of some of the more commonly performed PET procedures.

A

B

Fig. 35-32 A, PET FDG brain imaging with CT fusion shows a left subcortical resection site consistent with a prior tumor resection. **B,** At the inferior and lateral margins of the resection site, in the adjacent white matter, a hypermetabolic mass is identified. This case represents recurrent high-grade malignancy located in the left periventricular white matter at the frontoparietal junction adjacent to a previous resection site.

Fig. 35-33 PET FDG image with CT fusion demonstrates a large hypermetabolic right lung mass. A large number of PET FDG studies are done for lung cancer because of its high glucose metabolism.

Fig. 35-34 A, PET image to evaluate a patient with a history of melanoma on the scalp. Scan shows no definite evidence for recurrence. **B,** Image 6 months later shows profound and widely disseminated hypermetabolic metastases throughout the body.

FDG WHOLE-BODY TUMOR IMAGING

Clinically, 70% to 80% of PET scans are done to diagnose, stage, or restage cancer (Fig. 35-34), specifically cancer of the lung, breast, colon, lymph system, liver, esophagus, and thyroid. ^{18}F-FDG is the radiopharmaceutical of choice. PET plays an important role in differentiating benign from malignant processes, and it is also used for image-guided biopsy. PET is an important modality for detecting cancer recurrence in patients who have undergone surgery, chemotherapy, and/or radiation treatments. It is also very effective in monitoring therapeutic interventions by rapidly yet noninvasively assessing the metabolic response of the tissues to drugs.

Principle

Although ^{18}F-FDG is currently the prevailing radiopharmaceutical in tumor PET imaging, it was initially developed as a tracer to study the glucose metabolism in the brain. It was not until the late 1980s that successful reports of FDG tumor imaging began to surface. It then became apparent that certain tumors had a much greater uptake of FDG than did surrounding tissues. Tumor cells tend to have a much greater affinity for glucose than those of surrounding tissues due to their higher glucose metabolism. This distinction is paramount in understanding how FDG PET is able to detect metastatic disease.

Although there are many considerations to take into account when doing FDG PET, the most important is in the regulation of the patient's blood glucose. Generally a blood glucose level of less than 150 mg/dL is required for optimal imaging and can be achieved with a 4-hour fast. Patients with high glucose levels generally will have poor FDG uptake due to the already overabundant presence of glucose in their blood. In cases in which the glucose level is less than 150 mg/dL, it is still important to have the patient fasting for approximately 4 hours before the injection of FDG. The reason for this is that postprandially, the insulin response is still strong enough to push the FDG into more soft tissue than is normally seen in a fasting patient. The result is an image that appears to have a low target-to-background ratio. There are many other protocols that various institutions follow to increase FDG uptake by the tumor, including having the patient eat low-carbohydrate meals the day before and the day of the scan.

Radiopharmaceutical

The adult dose of ^{18}F-FDG is 0.214 mCi/kg with a minimum of 15 mCi and a maximum of 20 mCi. Pediatric doses are adjusted according to the patient's weight.

Scanning

^{18}F-FDG studies require a 60- to 90-minute uptake period after injection for incorporation of the radiopharmaceutical into the body. Some protocols suggest that imaging tumors after 90 minutes of FDG incorporation may lead to significantly better signal-to-noise values in the tumor as compared with surrounding tissues. During the uptake phase of the protocol, it is important that the patient be still and relaxed. Any motion, especially in the area of interest, will cause the muscles in that area to accumulate FDG and make interpretation of the images difficult. Therefore no reading, talking on the phone, or other activity is allowed. The patient must also be kept warm. If the patient develops a shiver, muscle uptake can also be increased. Depending on the dose injected and PET scanner sensitivity, approximately 3 to 5 minutes per bed position are required for the emission scan to measure the almost static distribution of ^{18}F-FDG glucose metabolism in tissue. When using a CT for the attenuation map, the total time for a whole-body (generally orbits through proximal femurs) scan is about 30 minutes. When a transmission scan is done instead of the CT for attenuation purposes, the total scan time can be as long as 1 to 2 hours depending on the length of the transmission scan.

FDG WHOLE-BODY TUMOR STUDIES

With new reimbursement policies in effect, most malignant tumors are being imaged with FDG in PET. The most common cancers imaged include lung, colorectal, head and neck, lymphoma, thyroid, esophageal, breast, ovarian, melanoma, testicular, and bladder.

Brain imaging

Because about 25% of the body's total metabolic energy is used by the brain, it provides an excellent gateway for functional imaging of its glucose metabolism using ^{18}F-FDG. In fact, most clinical PET brain imaging is currently done with FDG. The majority of PET brain scanning is done to diagnose or assess brain tumors such as astrocytomas or glioblastomas. When using a PET/CT system, the anatomic information provided by the CT can be especially helpful in determining the effects of therapy. FDG PET can also be used to differentiate necrotic tissue from recurrent disease, diagnose dementia, and monitor cerebrovascular disease. Another use that is proving to be beneficial is using PET imaging in patients with temporal lobe epilepsy.

Principle

The guiding principle in PET brain imaging is that malignant brain tumors have a high glucose metabolism that readily concentrates FDG. PET is also routinely used in monitoring response to therapy. There is normally little FDG uptake in areas of surgical resection or radiation necrosis, whereas viable brain tumor cells will still show an accumulation of FDG.

Radiopharmaceutical

The adult dose of ^{18}F-FDG is 0.214 mCi/kg with a minimum of 15 mCi and a maximum of 20 mCi. Pediatric doses are adjusted according to the patient's weight.

Scanning

Before and after injection with ^{18}F-FDG, the patient should follow the same procedure as though undergoing an FDG

whole-body scan. The main difference is the importance of having no visual or auditory stimulation if possible. The visual cortex has a high rate of glucose metabolism during stimulation, which can make the images more difficult to interpret. Generally the patient is injected with the FDG in a darkened room and is given instructions to remain still and to try to stay awake for a 30-minute uptake period. At the end of this period, the scan is performed in 3D mode, meaning without collimation, with an emission time of 8 minutes. The transmission is generally done for 5 minutes, unless an elliptical or contoured attenuation correction is done. When done on a PET/CT scanner, the CT is used to determine positioning of the brain and for the attenuation map. The time savings of using the CT for the attenuation correction can be very helpful, especially in pediatrics or claustrophobic patients who may have difficulty staying still for any length of time.

Brain studies

Other brain imaging is now being done for Parkinson's disease with ^{18}F-Fluorodopa, which traces dopamine synthesis in the brain. There are also a few ^{15}O radiotracers in use, such as $H_2{}^{15}O$, which are used to quantitatively assess cerebral blood flow.

CARDIAC POSITRON EMISSION TOMOGRAPHY

PET is a highly valuable diagnostic tool in the determination of myocardial viability and coronary flow reserve. Because of its higher temporal and spatial resolution and its built-in attenuation correction, PET is able to offer higher diagnostic accuracy than conventional nuclear medicine techniques. Because PET tracers emit higher-energy gamma rays (511 keV) compared with conventional nuclear tracers (thallium-201 at 80 keV and technetium-99m sestamibi at 140 keV), it is able to more accurately measure tracer uptake in the body. Currently, clinical application of PET imaging in cardiology can be divided into two main categories: detection of myocardial viability and assessment of coronary flow reserve.

Cardiac Viability
Principle

PET imaging for cardiac viability is an invaluable tool in the assessment of viable tissue in the left ventricle. The use of FDG as an indicator of glucose metabolism allows the clinician to assess the likelihood of successful coronary revascularization. Those patients with moderate to severe left ventricle dysfunction yet high myocardial viability are the most likely to benefit from revascularization. Those patients who are found to have minimally viable tissue will not benefit from revascularization and may undergo the procedure needlessly if no noninvasive testing is done. Normal protocols stipulate that patients undergo a resting cardiac perfusion scan prior to a cardiac FDG PET. Traditional patterns of myocardial viability include decreased resting blood perfusion in the presence of enhanced metabolic uptake.

Radiopharmaceutical

The adult dose of ^{18}F-FDG is 0.214 mCi/kg with a minimum of 15 mCi and a maximum of 20 mCi. The ^{13}N-ammonia dose is calibrated to 20 mCi in adult patients.

Scanning

The day of the scan, all patients are to fast and refrain from caffeine and nicotine. Upon arrival, patients will have two intravenous lines placed, one in each arm. One line is for the radiopharmaceutical injection; the other is for the insulin and dextrose infusion. A rest perfusion scan with ^{13}N-ammonia is usually performed first, and the protocol is the same as for the resting portion of the coronary flow reserve (CFR) study. After its completion, the patient will be given intravenous insulin and dextrose in order to prepare the heart for maximal ^{18}F-FDG uptake. When the patient's blood glucose level reaches an optimal level, the FDG is injected. At 30 minutes after injection, the patient is moved onto the scanner and positioned for the transmission scan. A transmission scan of 10 to 15 minutes ensues with a 10- to 15-minute emission scan to follow. Once the scan is completed, patients are fed a light lunch and their blood glucose levels are monitored until they reach normal levels.

Coronary flow reserve
Principle

PET is now commonly used to diagnose coronary artery disease and to assess coronary flow reserve. It is especially helpful in differentiating between stress induced coronary ischemia, and necrosis. These studies are most often done using ^{13}N-ammonia, but the advantages of other radioisotopes such as ^{82}Ru and ^{15}O are making them more common. The advantage of ^{82}Ru is that it is generator produced and acts as a potassium analog, much like ^{201}Tl. Unfortunately, it is expensive and requires a large patient load to make it cost effective. The benefit of ^{15}O is that it is freely diffusible in the myocardium and is independent of metabolism, making it an excellent choice for quantitative studies. It does, however, present other problems because its short half-life, and therefore short imaging time, can lead to grainy images, making it a poor choice for qualitative studies. ^{13}N-ammonia is most common because of its relatively short half-life (10 minutes) and because it is trapped by the myocardium in the glutamine synthesis reaction.

Radiopharmaceutical

^{13}N-ammonia is injected at a dose of approximately 10 to 20 mCi. Because of its 10-minute half-life and because it is cyclotron produced, it can be difficult to obtain an exact dose. This is especially true during the stress portion of the test.

Scanning

Patients are asked to eat a light meal approximately 2 hours before the test and to avoid caffeine and nicotine products for 24 hours before the test. This is because caffeine may affect the adenosine, which is the pharmacologic stress agent of choice for PET CFR studies. In patients with asthma or other contraindications to adenosine, dobutamine may be preferred. The test consists of two portions: the rest imaging and the stress imaging. The rest imaging is initiated by using the transmission scan to locate and position the heart in the center of the field of view. If the imaging is being done on a PET/CT system, this is done using the CT as a scout. Once the heart is centered a transmission scan of 10 to 15 minutes, based on patient girth, is performed for attenuation purposes. Upon completion of the transmission scan, the ^{13}N-ammonia may be injected. The emission scan generally takes 10 to 15 minutes, and it may be done as a gated acquisition if desired. After approximately 50 minutes (five ^{13}N half-lives), the stress study may begin. The stress agent, usually adenosine, is infused for 7 minutes total with the ^{13}N-ammonia injected 3 minutes into the infusion (other stress agents such as dobutamine or dipyridamole may also be used). Emission imaging should commence immediately. If the patient needed to use the restroom or had any movement between the rest and stress image, another transmission image will need to be acquired. Upon completion of the examination, the patient may be discharged and allowed to resume normal activity.

Future of Nuclear Medicine
RADIOIMMUNOTHERAPY

There are currently several radioimmunotherapy protocols that have become clinical in the last 2 years. Monoclonal antibodies specifically designed to localize on the surface of different types of cancer cells can now be tagged with a radioisotope and then imaged. If the monoclonal antibody successfully localizes on the tumor site, the radioisotope may be replaced with a beta-emitting therapeutic radioisotope such as ^{131}I or ^{90}Y. Current studies are looking to treat osteosarcoma with ^{153}Sm-EDTMP and refractory low-grade transformed B-cell non-Hodgkin's lymphoma with ^{90}Y-Zevalin (ibritumomab tiuxetan) or ^{131}I-Bexxar (tositumomab). These studies provide convincing evidence that more diseases may be treatable in the future using radioimmunotherapy.

DUAL-MODALITY IMAGING

Considerable research into the fusion of functional (SPECT and PET) and anatomic (CT) imaging has led to the introduction of dual-modality imaging systems. This is one of the most exciting developments in the field of nuclear medicine. The combined PET/CT camera shown in Fig. 35-31 couples the functional imaging capabilities of PET with the superb anatomic imaging of CT. Images from each modality are coregistered during the acquisition process and in near simultaneity. Because the images can be overlaid one on another, the position of suspected tumors can easily be identified. Suspicious metabolically active areas can now be identified anatomically from the CT information. These features are key to improving the reliability of SPECT and PET interpretation. Furthermore, metabolic and anatomic evaluation after therapy can both be accomplished in one imaging session, which is likely to significantly improve patient acceptance of the procedures. For all these reasons, SPECT/CT and PET/CT are likely to become one of the most useful diagnostic procedures for assessing treatment and evaluation of cancer. This also seems to point in the direction of a broader integration of imaging modalities within the department of radiology.

POSITRON EMISSION TOMOGRAPHY

PET technology is advancing on many fronts. FDG is routinely being produced in distribution centers throughout the United States and Europe. One or more cyclotrons at each distribution site are continuously producing F fluoride for incorporation into FDG. Unit doses are shipped via common commercial carriers, which also include chartered air and special ground couriers from a network of registered pharmacy distribution centers to individual PET centers that do not have cyclotrons. Hence, to become involved in clinical PET imaging no longer requires the high financial commitment to own and operate a nuclear accelerator to produce PET radiopharmaceuticals at a local site.

New radiopharmaceuticals are being developed. However, as the PET radiopharmaceutical distribution centers expand and are able to handle the daily demands of providing FDG to the existing and new PET centers, production of ^{18}F-labeled radiopharmaceuticals specifically for tumor imaging is likely to become available. FDA approval will be required before clinical imaging, but several PET manufacturers and the PET radiopharmaceutical distribution centers are sponsoring drug clinical trials to accelerate the deployment of new and viable clinical PET imaging agents. Radiolabeled choline, thymidine, fluorodopa, estrogen receptors, and numerous other biomolecules are likely candidates for new PET clinical tracers.

Mobile PET units are a reality, as shown in Figs. 35-35 and 35-36. The PET scanner technology has matured to the point that the original frailty of the electronics and detector systems has been eliminated. Robust mobile units travel to community hospitals that need PET imaging but not at the level that necessitates a dedicated in-house PET scanner. By spending 1 or 2 days per week at several different hospitals in smaller communities or rural settings, the mobile PET camera best serves the needs of the oncology patients. The FDG distribution centers are necessary in this scenario because the mobile PET camera unit needs a supply of radiotracer to carry out the PET imaging study. Until the nationwide FDG distribution centers became a reality, as they now are, the use of mobile PET was extremely limited.

Fig. 35-35 Mobile PET coach showing operator on staff stairs and elevator platform in the elevated position. Elevator used to transport patients from ground level to floor level of the PET scanner unit.

(Courtesy Shared PET Imaging, LLC.)

Fig. 35-36 Interior of a mobile coach showing the PET workstation *(foreground)* and PET scanner *(background).*

(Courtesy Shared PET Services, LLC.)

Conclusion

Nuclear medicine technology is a multidisciplinary field in which medicine is linked to quantitative sciences, including chemistry, radiation biology, physics, and computer technology. During the past 100 years, nuclear medicine has expanded to include molecular nuclear medicine, in vivo and in vitro chemistry, and physiology. The spectrum of nuclear medicine technology skills and responsibilities varies. The scope of nuclear medicine technology includes patient care, quality control, diagnostic procedures, computer data acquisition and processing, radiopharmaceuticals, radionuclide therapy, and radiation safety. Many clinical procedures currently are performed in nuclear medicine departments across the country and throughout the world. Nuclear medicine procedures complement other imaging methods in radiology and pathology departments.

The evolution of PET has provided the nuclear medicine department with a complex diagnostic imaging procedure. Consequently, it is both a clinical tool and a research tool. PET requires the multidisciplinary support of the physician, physicist, physiologist, chemist, engineer, software programmer, and radiographer. This imaging procedure allows numerous biologic parameters in the working human body to be examined without disturbing normal-equilibrium physiology. PET measures regional function that cannot be determined by any other means, which includes CT and MRI. Current PET studies of the brain involve the imaging of patients with epilepsy, Huntington's disease, stroke, schizophrenia, brain tumors, Alzheimer's disease, and other disorders of the central nervous system. PET studies of the heart are providing routine diagnostic information on patients with coronary artery disease by identifying viable myocardium for revascularization. But by far the greatest impact PET has made is the ability to identify highly metabolic tumors. PET scanning is critically involved in the determination of the effects of therapeutic drug regimens on tumors and the differentiation of necrosis from viable tumor. Nearly 80% of all PET imaging today is directed at tumor detection and evaluation of therapeutic intervention. Overall, human physiology will become better understood as the technology advances, yielding higher-resolution instruments, new radiopharmaceuticals, and improved analysis of PET data.

The future of nuclear medicine may lie in its unique ability to identify functional or physiologic abnormalities. With the continued development of new radiopharmaceuticals and imaging technology, nuclear medicine will continue to be a unique and valuable tool for diagnosing and treating disease.

Definition of Terms

alpha particle Nucleus of a helium atom, consisting of two protons and two neutrons, having a positive charge of 2.

analog PET radiopharmaceutical biochemically equivalent to a naturally occurring compound in the body.

annihilation Total transformation of matter into energy; occurs after the antimatter positron collides with an electron. Two photons are created; each equals the rest mass of the individual particles.

arterialized venous blood Arterial blood passed directly to the venous system by shunts in the capillary system after surface veins are heated to between 104° F and 108° F (40° C to 42.2° C). Blood gases from the vein under these conditions reflect near arterial levels of Po_2, Pco_2, and pH.

atom Smallest division of an element that exhibits all the properties and characteristics of the element; composed of neutrons, electrons, and protons.

attenuation coefficient Number that represents the statistical reduction in photons that exit a material (N) from the value that entered the material (N_o). The reduced flux is the result of scatter and absorption, which can be expressed in the following equation: $N = N_o e^{-\mu\chi}$, where μ is the attenuation coefficient and χ is the distance traversed by the photons.

becquerel (Bq) Unit of activity in the International System of Units; equal to 1 disintegration per second (dps): 1 Bq = 1 dps.

beta particle Electron whose point of origin is the nucleus; electron originating in the nucleus by way of decay of a neutron into a proton and an electron.

bit Term constructed from the words *bi*nary dig*it* and referring to a single digit of a binary number; for example, the binary of 101 is composed of 3 bits.

BGO scintillator Bismuth germanate ($Bi_4Ge_3O_{12}$) scintillator with an efficiency twice that of sodium iodide. BGO is used in nearly all commercially produced PET scanners.

blood-brain barrier Anatomic and physiologic feature of the brain thought to consist of walls of capillaries in the CNS and surrounding glial membranes. The barrier separates the parenchyma of the central nervous system from blood. The blood-brain barrier prevents or slows the passage of some drugs and other chemical compounds, radioactive ions, and disease-causing organisms such as viruses from the blood into the CNS.

byte Term used to define a group of bits, usually eight, being treated as a unit by the computer.

CM line Canthomeatal line defined by an imaginary line drawn between the lateral canthus of the eye and meatus of the ear.

cold spot Lack of radiation being received or recorded, thus not producing any image and resulting in an area of no, or very light, density. May be caused by disease or artifact.

collimator Shielding device used to limit the angle of entry of radiation; usually made of lead.

curie Standard of measurement for radioactive decay; based on the disintegration of 1 gram of radium at 3.731010 disintegrations per second.

cyclotron Device for accelerating charged particles to high energies using magnetic and oscillating electrostatic fields. As a result, particles move in a spiral path with increasing energy.

daughter Element that results from the radioactive decay of a parent element.

deadtime Time when the system electronics are already processing information from one photon interaction with a detector and cannot accept new events to be processed from other detectors.

decay Radioactive disintegration of the nucleus of an unstable nuclide.

detector Device that is a combination of a scintillator and photomultiplier tube. It is used to detect x-rays and gamma rays.

deuteron Ionized nucleus of heavy hydrogen (deuterium), which contains one proton and one neutron.

dose Measure of the amount of energy deposited in a known mass of tissue from ionizing radiation. *Absorbed dose* is described in units of rads; 1 rad is equal to 10^{-2} joules/kg or 100 ergs/g.

ejection fraction (cardiac) Fraction of the total volume of blood of the left ventricle ejected per contraction.

electron Negatively charged elementary particle that has a specific charge, mass, and spin.

electron capture Radioactive decay process in which a nucleus with an excess of protons brings an electron into the nucleus, creating a neutron out of a proton, thus decreasing the atomic number by 1. The resulting atom is often unstable and gives off a gamma ray to achieve stability.

external radiation detector Instrument used to determine the presence of radioactivity from the exterior.

^{18}F-FDG Radioactive analog of naturally available glucose. It follows the same biochemical pathways as glucose; however, unlike glucose, it is not totally metabolized to carbon dioxide and water.

fission Splitting of a nucleus into two or more parts with the subsequent release of enormous amounts of energy.

functional image See *parametric image*.

gamma camera Device that uses the emission of light from a crystal struck by gamma rays to produce an image of the distribution of radioactive material in a body organ.

gamma ray High-energy, short-wavelength electromagnetic radiation emanating from the nucleus of some nuclides.

ground state State of lowest energy of a system.

half-life (T½) Term used to describe the time elapsed until some physical quantity has decreased to half of its original value.

homeostasis State of equilibrium of the body's internal environment.

image co-registration Computer technique that permits realignment of images that have been acquired from different modalities and therefore have different orientations and magnifications. With realignment, the images possess the same orientation and size. The images can then be overlaid, one on the other, to demonstrate similarities and differences between the images.

in vitro Outside a living organism.

in vivo Within a living organism.

isotope Nuclide of the same element with the same number of protons but a different number of neutrons.

isotropic Referring to uniform emission of radiation or particles in three dimensions.

kinetics Movement of materials into, out of, and through biologic spaces. A mathematic expression is often used to describe and quantify how substances traverse membranes or participate in biochemical reactions.

light pipe A tubelike structure attached to the scintillation crystal to convey the emitted light to the photomultiplier tube.

local cerebral blood flow (LCBF) Description of the parametric image of blood flow through the brain. It is expressed in units of milliliters of blood flow per minute per 100 g of brain tissue.

magnetic resonance imaging (MRI) Technique of nuclear magnetic resonance (NMR) as it is applied to medical imaging. Magnetic resonance is abbreviated *MR*.

metastable Describes the excited state of a nucleus that returns to its ground state by emission of a gamma ray; has a measurable lifetime.

neutron Electrically neutral particle found in the nucleus; has a mass of 1 mass unit.

nuclear particle accelerator Device to produce radioactive material by accelerating ions (electrons, protons, deuterons, etc.) to high energies and projecting them toward stable materials. The list of accelerators includes linac, cyclotron, synchrotron, Van de Graaff accelerator, and betatron.

nuclear reactor Device that under controlled conditions is used for supporting a self-sustained nuclear reaction.

nuclide General term applicable to all atomic forms of an element.

parametric image Image that relates anatomic position (the x and y position on an image) to a physiologic parameter such as blood flow (image intensity or color). It may also be referred to as a *functional image*.

parent Radionuclide that decays to a specific daughter nuclide either directly or as a member of a radioactive series.

particle accelerator Device that provides the energy necessary to enable a nuclear reaction.

pharmaceutical Relating to a medicinal drug.

photomultiplier tube (PMT) Electronic tube that converts light photons to electric pulses.

photopenia See *cold spot.*

pixel (picture element) Smallest indivisible part of an image matrix for display on a computer screen. Typical images may be 128×128, 256×256, or 512×512 pixels.

positron Positively charged particle emitted from neutron-deficient radioactive nuclei.

positron emission tomography (PET) Imaging technique that creates transaxial images of organ physiology from the simultaneous detection of positron annihilation photons.

proton Positively charged particle that is a fundamental component of the nucleus of all atoms. The number of protons in the nucleus of an atom equals the atomic number of the element.

pulse height analyzer Instrument that accepts input from a detector and categorizes the pulses on the basis of signal strength.

pyrogen free Free of a fever-producing agent of bacterial origin.

quantitative Type of PET study in which the final images are not simply distributions of radioactivity but, rather, correspond to units of capillary blood flow, glucose metabolism, receptor density, etc. Studies between individuals and repeat studies in the same individual permit comparison of pixel values on an absolute scale.

radiation Emission of energy; rays of waves.

radioactive Exhibiting the property of spontaneously emitting alpha, beta, and gamma rays by disintegration of the nucleus.

radioactivity Spontaneous disintegration of an unstable atomic nucleus resulting in the emission of ionizing radiation.

radioisotope Synonym for *radioactive isotope*. Any isotope that is unstable undergoes decay with the emission of characteristic radiation.

radionuclide Unstable nucleus that transmutes by way of nuclear decay.

radiopharmaceutical Refers to a radioactive drug used for diagnosis or therapy.

radiotracer Synonym for *radiopharmaceutical*.

ray Imaginary line drawn between a pair of detectors in the PET scanner or between the x-ray source and detector in a CT scanner.

reconstruction Mathematic operation that transforms raw data acquired on a PET tomograph (sinogram) into an image with recognizable features.

rectilinear scanner Early imaging device that passed over the area of interest, moving in or forming a straight line.

region of interest (ROI) Area that circumscribes a desired anatomic location on a PET image. Image-processing systems permit drawing of ROIs on images. The average parametric value is computed for all pixels within the ROI and returned to the radiographer.

resolution Smallest separation of two point sources of radioactivity that can be distinguished for PET or single photon emission computed tomography imaging.

scintillation camera See *gamma camera*.

scintillation detector Device that relies on the emission of light from a crystal subjected to ionizing radiation. The light is detected by a photomultiplier tube and converted to an electronic signal that can be processed further. An array of scintillation detectors are used in a gamma camera.

scintillator Organic or inorganic material that transforms high-energy photons such as x-rays or gamma rays into visible or nearly visible light (ultraviolet) photons for easy measurement.

septa High-density metal collimators that separate adjacent detectors on a ring tomograph to reduce scattered photons from degrading image information.

single photon emission computed tomography (SPECT) A nuclear medicine scanning procedure that measures conventional single photon gamma emissions (^{99m}Tc) with a specially designed rotating gamma camera.

sinogram 2D raw data format that depicts coincidence detectors against possible rays between detectors. For each coincidence event, a specific element of the sinogram matrix is incremented by 1. The sum of all events in the sinogram is the total number of events detected by the PET scanner minus any corrections that have been applied to the sinogram data.

target Device used to contain stable materials and subsequent radioactive materials during bombardment by high-energy nuclei from a cyclotron or other particle accelerator. The term is also applied to the material inside the device, which may be solid, liquid, or gaseous.

tracer A radioactive isotope used to allow a biologic process to be seen. The tracer is introduced into the body, binds with a specific substance, and is followed by a scanner as it passes through various organs or systems in the body.

transmission scan Type of PET scan that is equivalent to a low-resolution CT scan. Attenuation is determined by rotating a rod of radioactive ^{68}Ge around the subject. Photons that traverse the subject either impinge on a detector and are registered as valid counts or are attenuated (absorbed or scattered). The ratio of counts with and without the attenuating tissue in place provides the factors to correct PET scans for the loss of counts from attenuation of the 0.511-MeV photons.

washout The end of the radionuclide procedure, during which time the radioactivity is eliminated from the body.

Selected bibliography

Bares R et al, editors: *Clinical PET*, Dordrecht, The Netherlands, 1996, Kluwer Academic.

Barnes WE, editor: *Basic physics of radiotracers*, vols I and II, Boca Raton, Fla, 1983, CRC Press.

Beckers C et al: *Positron emission tomography in clinical research and clinical diagnosis*, Dordrecht, The Netherlands, 1989, Kluwer Academic.

Bergmann SR, Sobel BE, editors: *Positron emission tomography of the heart*, Mount Kisco, NY, 1992, Futura.

Bernier DR, Christian PE, Langan JK: *Nuclear medicine technology and techniques*, ed 4, St Louis, 1997, Mosby.

Cember H: *Introduction to health physics*, ed 3, New York, 1996, McGraw-Hill.

Chandra R: *Introductory physics of nuclear medicine*, ed 3, Philadelphia, 1987, Lea & Febiger.

Christian PE, Bernier DR, Langan JK: *Nuclear medicine and PET technology and techniques*, ed 5, St Louis, 2004, Mosby.

Early PJ, Sodee DB: *Principles and practice of nuclear medicine*, ed 2, St Louis, 1995, Mosby.

Hendee WR: *The physical principles of computed tomography*, Boston, 1983, Little, Brown.

Hubner KF et al: *Clinical positron emission tomography*, St Louis, 1992, Mosby.

Livingood JJ: *Principles of cyclic particle accelerators*, Princeton, NJ, 1961, D Van Nostrand.

London ED, editor: *Imaging drug action in the brain*, Boca Raton, Fla, 1993, CRC Press.

Matsuzawa T, editor: *Clinical PET in oncology*, River Edge, NJ, 1994, World Scientific.

Myers R et al: *Quantification of brain function using PET*, San Diego, 1996, Academic.

O'Connor MK: *The Mayo Clinic manual of nuclear medicine*, New York, 1996, Churchill-Livingstone.

Phelps ME et al, editors: *Positron emission tomography and autoradiography: principles and applications for the brain and heart*, New York, 1986, Raven.

Riggs DS: *The mathematical approach to physiological problems*, Cambridge, Mass, 1963, Williams & Wilkins.

Ruhlmann J et al: *PET in oncology*, Berlin, 1999, Springer-Verlag.

Saha GB: *Fundamentals of nuclear pharmacy*, ed 3, New York, 1992, Springer-Verlag.

Sandler MP et al: *Diagnostic nuclear medicine*, ed 3, Baltimore, 1996, Williams & Wilkins.

Shapiro J: *Radiation protection*, ed 3, Cambridge, Mass, 1990, Harvard University Press.

Stein E: *Electrocardiographic interpretation (a self-study approach to clinical electrocardiography)*, Philadelphia, 1991, Lea & Febiger.

Steves AM: *Review of nuclear medicine technology*, ed 2, Reston, Va, 1996, Society of Nuclear Medicine.

Steves AM: *Preparation for examinations in nuclear medicine technology*, Reston, Va, 1997, Society of Nuclear Medicine.

Toga AW et al: *Brain mapping: the methods*, San Diego, 1996, Academic.

Wieler HJ, Coleman RE: *PET in clinical oncology*, Darmstadt, 2000, Steinkopff Verlag.

36

BONE DENSITOMETRY

JOANN P. CAUDILL

Dual energy x-ray absorptiometry (DXA) spine scan of the lumbar spine.

Principles of Bone Densitometry

Bone densitometry* is a general term encompassing the art and science of measuring the bone mineral content and density of specific skeletal sites or the whole body. The bone measurement values are used to assess bone strength, diagnose diseases associated with low bone density (especially *osteoporosis*), monitor the effects of therapy for such diseases, and predict risk of future fractures.

Several techniques are available to perform bone densitometry using ionizing radiation or ultrasound. The most versatile and widely used technique is *dual energy x-ray absorptiometry* (DXA) (Fig. 36-1).[1] This technique has the advantages of low radiation dose, wide availability, ease of use, short scan time, high-resolution images, good *precision,* and stable calibration. DXA is the focus of this chapter, but summaries of other techniques are also presented.

---

*Almost all italicized words on the succeeding pages are defined at the end of this chapter.
[1]Gowin W, Felsenberg D: Acronyms in osteodensitometry, *J Clin Densitometry* 1:137, 1998.

Fig. 36-1 A, DXA spine scan being performed on a Hologic model Discovery. **B,** DXA spine scan being performed on a GE Lunar Advance. **C,** DXA whole-body scan being performed on a Norland model XR-46.

(**A,** Courtesy Hologic, Inc., Bedford, Mass; **B,** courtesy GE Lunar Corp., Madison, Wis; **C,** courtesy Norland, Inc., Ft. Atkinson, Wis.)

DUAL X-RAY ABSORPTIOMETRY AND CONVENTIONAL RADIOGRAPHY

The differences between DXA and conventional radiography are as follows:

1. DXA can be conceptualized as a *subtraction technique.* To quantitate *bone mineral density* (BMD) it is necessary to eliminate the contributions of soft tissue and measure the x-ray attenuation of bone alone. This is accomplished by scanning at two different x-ray photon energies (thus the term *dual energy x-ray*) and mathematically manipulating the recorded signal to take advantage of the differing attenuation properties of soft tissue and bone at the two energies. The density of the isolated bone is calculated on the basis of the principle that denser, more mineralized bone attenuates (absorbs) more x-ray. Having adequate amounts of artifact-free soft tissue is essential to help ensure the reliability of the bone density results.

2. The bone density results are computed by proprietary software from the x-ray attenuation pattern striking the detector, not from the scan image. DXA scans provide images only for the purpose of confirming correct positioning of the patient and correct placement of the *regions of interest* (ROI). Therefore the images may not be used for diagnosis, and any medical conditions apparent on the image must be followed up by appropriate diagnostic tests. The referring and interpreting physicians must be skilled in interpreting the clinical and statistical aspects of the numeric density results and relating them to the specific patient.

3. In conventional radiography, x-ray machines from different manufacturers are operated in essentially the same manner and produce identical images. This is not the case with DXA. Three major DXA manufacturers are in the United States (see Fig. 39-1), and technologists must be educated about the specific scanner model in their facility. The numeric bone density results cannot be compared among manufacturers without proper standardization. This chapter presents general scan positioning and analysis information, but the manufacturers' specific procedures must be used when actual scans are performed.

4. The effective radiation dose for DXA is considerably lower than that for conventional radiography. Thus in some states and countries, scanning can be performed by personnel who are not radiologic technologists. The specific personnel requirements vary among states and countries. However, all bone density technologists should be instructed in core competencies including radiation protection, patient care, history taking, basic computer operation, knowledge of scanner quality control, patient positioning, scan acquisition and analysis, and proper record keeping and documentation.

History of Bone Densitometry

Osteoporosis was an undetected and overlooked disease until the 1920s, when the advent of x-ray film methods allowed the detection of markedly decreased density in bones. The first publications indicating an interest in *bone mass* quantification methods appeared in the 1930s, and much of the pioneering work was performed in the field of dentistry. *Radiographic absorptiometry* (RA) involved taking a radiograph of bone with a known standard placed in the field and optically comparing the densities. Interestingly, this technique has again gained popularity, with the comparison now automated by computer methods.

Radiogammetry was introduced in the 1960s, partly in response to the measurements of bone loss performed in astronauts. As bone loss progresses, the thickness of the outer shell of the small tubular bones (e.g., phalanges and metacarpals) decreases and the inner cavity enlarges. By measuring the inner and outer diameters and comparing them, indices of bone loss are established.

In the late 1970s, the emerging technique of computed tomography (CT) (see Chapter 31) was adapted, through the use of specialized software and reference phantoms, for quantitative measurement of the central area of the vertebral body, where early bone loss occurs. This technique, called *quantitative computed tomography* (QCT), is still widely used.

The 1970s and early 1980s brought the first scanners dedicated to bone densitometry. *Single photon absorptiometry* (SPA) (Fig. 36-2) and *dual photon absorptiometry* (DPA) are based on physical principles similar to those for DXA. The SPA approach was not a subtraction technique but relied on a water bath or other medium to eliminate the effects of soft tissue. It found application only in the peripheral skeleton. DPA used photons of two energies and was used to assess sites in the central skeleton (lumbar spine and proximal femur). The radiation source was a highly collimated beam from a radioisotope, usually iodine-125 for SPA and gadolinium-153 for DPA. The intensity of the attenuated beam was measured by a collimated *scintillation counter,* and the bone mineral was then quantified.

The first commercial DXA scanner was introduced in 1987. In this scanner the expensive, rare, and short-lived radioisotope source was replaced with an x-ray tube. Improvements over time have included the choice of *pencil-beam* or *array-beam collimation;* a rotating C-arm to allow supine lateral spine imaging; shorter scan time; improved detection of low bone density; improved image quality; and enhanced computer power, multimedia, and networking capabilities.

Since the late 1990s, renewed attention has been given to smaller, more portable, less complex techniques for measuring the peripheral skeleton. This trend has been driven by the introduction of new therapies for osteoporosis and the resultant need for simple, inexpensive tests to identify persons with osteoporosis who are at increased risk for fracture. However, DXA of the hip and spine is still the most widely accepted method for measuring bone density, and it remains a superior technique for monitoring the effects of therapy.

Fig. 36-2 SPA wrist scan being performed on a Lunar model SP2. This form of bone densitometry is now obsolete.

(Courtesy GE Lunar Corp., Madison, Wis.)

Bone Biology and Remodeling

The skeleton serves several purposes:
- Supports the body and protects vital organs so that movement, communication, and life processes can be carried on
- Manufactures red blood cells
- Stores the minerals that are necessary for life, including calcium and phosphate

The two basic types of bone are *cortical* (or compact) and *trabecular* (or cancellous). Cortical bone forms the dense, compact outer shell of all bones, as well as the shafts of the long bones. It supports weight, resists bending and twisting, and accounts for about 80% of the skeletal mass. Trabecular bone is the delicate, latticework structure within bones that adds strength without excessive weight. It supports compressive loading in the spine, hip, and calcaneus, and it is also found at the ends of long bones, such as the distal radius. The relative amounts of trabecular and cortical bone differ by bone densitometry technique used and anatomic site measured (Table 36-1).

Bone is constantly going through a remodeling process in which old bone is replaced with new bone. With this *bone remodeling* process (Fig. 36-3) the equivalent of a new skeleton is formed about every 7 years. Bone-destroying cells called *osteoclasts* break down and remove old bone, leaving pits. This part of the process is called *resorption*. Bone-building cells called *osteoblasts* (tip: remember "B" for "build") fill the pits with new bone. This process is called *formation*. The comparative rates of resorption and formation determine whether bone mass increases (more formation than resorption), remains stable (equal resorption and formation), or decreases (more resorption than formation).

Osteoclasts and osteoblasts operate as a bone-remodeling unit. A properly functioning bone remodeling cycle is a tightly coupled physiologic process in which resorption equals formation and the net bone mass is maintained. The length of the resorption process is about 1 week compared with a longer formation process of about 3 months. At any point in time, millions of remodeling sites within the body are in different phases of the remodeling cycle or at rest.

TABLE 36-1

Bone densitometry regions of interest: estimated percentage of trabecular and cortical bone and preferred measurement sites

Region of interest	% Trabecular bone	% Cortical bone	Preferred measurement site
AP Spine (by DXA)	66	34	Cushing's disease, corticosteroid use
AP Spine (by QCT)	100		
Femoral neck	25	75	Type II osteoporosis Second choice for hyperparathyroidism
Trochanteric region	50	50	
Calcaneus	95	5	
33% radius	1	99	First choice for hyperparathyroidism
Ultradistal radius	66	34	
Phalanges	40	60	
Whole body	20	80	Pediatrics

Data from Bonnick SL: *Bone densitometry in clinical practice: application and interpretation*, Totowa, NJ, 1998, Humana Press.
DXA, Dual energy x-ray absorptiometry; *QCT,* quantitative computed tomography.

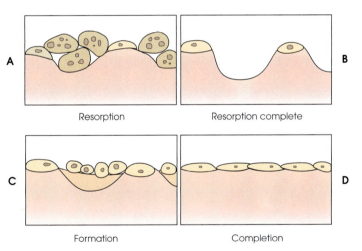

Fig. 36-3 The bone remodeling process. **A,** Osteoclasts break down bone in the process of resorption. **B,** Pits in the bone. **C,** Osteoblasts form new bone. **D,** With equal amounts of resorption and formation, the bone mass is stable.

(From National Osteoporosis Foundation: *Boning up on osteoporosis,* Washington, DC, 1997, The Foundation.)

When the cycle becomes uncoupled, the result is a net loss of bone mass. Some reasons for uncoupling are enhanced osteoclastic recruitment, impaired osteoblastic activity, and an increased number of cycles, which results in shorter time for each cycle. This favors the shorter resorption phase over the longer formation phase.

Bone mass increases in youth until *peak bone mass* is reached at approximately 20 to 30 years of age. This is followed by a stable period in middle age. Then comes a period of decreasing bone mass starting at approximately age 50 in women and approximately age 65 in men. The decrease in bone mass becomes pronounced in women at menopause because of the loss of bone-preserving estrogen. If the peak bone mass is low or the resorption rate is excessive, or both, at menopause, osteoporosis may result (Fig. 36-4).

Fig. 36-4 Trabecular bone obtained from vertebrae. **A,** Normal bone. **B,** Osteoporotic bone. **C,** Severely osteoporotic bone. Note the progressive loss of trabecular continuity resulting from resorptive perforations in the severely osteoporotic subject.

(From Eriksen E: *Bone histomorphometry*, Philadelphia, 1994, Lippincott-Raven.)

Osteoporosis[1]

Osteoporosis is a disease characterized by low bone mass and structural deterioration of bone tissue. This decrease in bone mass and degradation of bone architecture may not support the mechanical stress and loading of normal activity. As a result, the bones are at increased risk for *fragility fractures.* An estimated 10 million Americans have osteoporosis, with 80% (8 million) of those being women. Another 34 million Americans have *osteopenia* or low bone mass, putting them at risk of developing osteoporosis and related fractures. Persons with osteoporosis may experience decreased quality of life from the pain, deformity, and disability of fragility fractures. An increased risk of morbidity and mortality exists, especially from hip fractures. In the United States, annual medical costs for osteoporosis, including hospitalization for osteoporotic hip fractures, were $18 billion in 2002, and the cost is rising.

[1]Appreciation is extended to Pam Johnson, RT(BD), for her work in the preparation of the osteoporosis section.

Many risk factors for osteoporosis have been studied and identified. The following are considered primary risk factors:
- Female sex
- Increased age
- Estrogen deficiency
- Caucasian race
- Low body weight (<127 lb or 58 kg) or low body mass index (BMI) (is weight in kg divided by height in meters squared), or both
- Family history of osteoporosis/fracture
- History of prior fracture as an adult
- Smoking tobacco

Osteoporosis is often overlooked in older men because it is considered a woman's disease. The facts are that 2 million American men have osteoporosis and another 12 million are at risk. This means that 20% of Americans diagnosed with osteoporosis are men. In contrast, men suffer 33% of all hip fractures and one third of these men will not survive 1 year. Clearly, men are at risk for the devastating effects of fragility fracture and would benefit from increased prevention, diagnosis, and treatment of osteoporosis.

The exact cause of osteoporosis is not known, but it is clearly a multifactorial disorder. Major contributors are genetics, metabolic factors regulating internal calcium equilibrium, lifestyle, aging, and menopause. Peak bone mass attained in young adulthood, coupled with the rate of bone loss in older age, determines whether an individual's bone mass becomes low enough to be diagnosed as osteoporosis. Genetic factors are estimated to account for up to 70% of the peak bone mass attained. This is why family history is an important risk factor for osteoporosis and fracture. Calcium equilibrium is maintained by a complex mechanism involving hormones (parathyroid, calcitonin, and vitamin D) controlling key ions (calcium, magnesium, and phosphate) within target tissues (blood, intestine, and bone). Calcium and phosphate enter the blood from the intestine and are stored in bone. The process also occurs in reverse, moving calcium out of the bones for other uses within the body. Nutritional and lifestyle factors can upset the balance and cause too much calcium to move out of bone. In the course of normal aging there is a loss of estrogen at menopause that tends to increase the rate of bone turnover and thereby increase the number of remodeling cycles and shorten the length of each cycle. This allows enough time for the shorter resorption process but cuts short the longer formation process. Various combinations of these factors can result in a net loss of bone mass and thereby increase the risk of osteoporosis and fracture.

Two points are important to note about osteoporosis. First, an older person with a normal rate of bone loss may still develop osteoporosis if his or her peak bone mass was low. Second, it is a common misconception that proper exercise and diet at menopause prevent bone loss associated with the decrease in estrogen. This is not true. Persons concerned about their risk of osteoporosis should consult their physician.

Osteoporosis can be classified as primary or secondary. Importantly, a DXA scan result should not automatically lead to a diagnosis of primary osteoporosis. Secondary causes of systemic or localized disturbances in bone mass must be ruled out before a final diagnosis can be made. Proper choice of treatment should be based on type of osteoporosis and the underlying cause, if secondary osteoporosis is present. The choice of skeletal site to measure depends on the disease process, whether it has a predilection for certain types of bone, and the composition of various skeletal sites (see Table 36-1).

Primary osteoporosis can be *Type I* (postmenopausal) or *Type II* (senile or age related), or both. Type I osteoporosis is caused by bone resorption exceeding bone formation due to estrogen deprivation in women. Type II osteoporosis occurs in aging men and women from a decreased ability to build bone.

Secondary osteoporosis is osteoporosis caused by a heterogeneous group of skeletal disorders resulting in imbalance of bone turnover. Disorder categories include genetic, endocrine and metabolic, hypogonadal, connective tissue, nutritional and gastrointestinal, hematologic, malignancy, and use of certain prescription drugs. Common causes of secondary osteoporosis include *hyperparathyroidism;* gonadal insufficiency (including estrogen deficiency in women and hypogonadism in men); *osteomalacia* (rickets in children); rheumatoid arthritis; anorexia nervosa; gastrectomy; *adult sprue* (hypersensitivity to gluten [wheat protein]); multiple myeloma; and use of corticosteroids, heparin, anticonvulsants, or excessive thyroid hormone treatment.

Several prescription medications arrest bone loss and may increase bone mass. These include traditional estrogen or hormone replacement therapies and the newer bisphosphonates, selective estrogen receptor modulators (SERMs), and calcitonin. Other therapies are in clinical trials and may be available in the future (Table 36-2). The availability of therapies beyond the traditional estrogens has led to the widespread use of DXA to diagnose osteoporosis.

Laboratory tests for *biochemical markers* of bone turnover may be used in conjunction with DXA to determine the need for or the effectiveness of therapy. Problems of poor precision and individual variability have limited their use. Some markers of bone formation found in blood are alkaline phosphatase, osteocalcin, and C- and N-propeptides of type I collagen. Some markers of bone resorption excreted in urine are pyridinium cross-links of collagen, C- and N-telopeptides of collagen, galactosyl hydroxylysine, and hydroxyproline.

TABLE 36-2
Therapies for osteoporosis

Generic name	Some FDA-approved formulations as of 2002		Primary emthod of action	Comments
	Treatment	Prevention		
Estrogen	Yes	No	A	Provides relief of menopausal symptoms
Bisphosphonates	Yes	Yes	A	Some formulations approved for men
Selective estrogen receptor modulators	Yes	Yes	A	May provide some protection against breast cancer
Calcitonin	Yes	No	A	Analgesic effect after acute fracture
Fluoride	No	No	F	
Growth hormone	No	No	F	
Parathyroid hormone	Yes	No	F	Approved for men and women at high risk for fracture
Statins	No	No	F	
Anabolic steroids	No	No	F	

A, Antiresorptive; *F,* formation.

FRACTURES AND FALLS

Fractures occur when bones encounter an outside force that exceeds their strength. Fragility fractures occur with minimal trauma from a standing height or less. A small percentage of fragility fractures are spontaneous, meaning that they occur with no apparent force being applied. The most common sites for fractures associated with osteoporosis are the hip, spinal vertebrae, wrist (Colles fracture), ribs, and proximal humerus, but other bones can be affected. Current estimates of fracture in the United States are that approximately 1.5 million osteoporotic fractures occur each year; these include 700,000 vertebral (only one third are clinically diagnosed), 300,000 hip, 250,000 wrist, and 300,000 other fractures. One in two women and one in four men older than age 50 will have an osteoporotic fracture in their remaining lifetime.

Risk factors for fracture include being female, low bone mass, personal history of fracture as an adult, history of fracture in a first-degree relative, current cigarette smoking, and low body weight (<127 lb or 58 kg).

Hip fractures account for 20% of osteoporotic fractures and are the most devastating, both for the patient and in terms of health costs. Some important points about hip fracture include the following:

- The overall 1-year mortality rate following hip fracture is 1 in 5.[1]
- Two to three times as many women as men suffer hip fractures, but the 1-year mortality rate for men is twice as high.
- Two thirds of hip fracture patients never regain their preoperative activity status. One fourth require long-term care.
- A woman's risk of hip fracture is equal to her combined risk of breast, uterine, and ovarian cancer.
- Protective undergarments with side padding, called *hip pads,* have proven effective in preventing hip fracture from a fall in the elderly. Resistance to wearing the garment is the only limitation.

[1]National Institutes of Health Consensus Development Panel on Osteoporosis Prevention, Diagnosis, and Therapy: Osteoporosis prevention, diagnosis, and therapy, *JAMA* 285:785, 2001.

Vertebral fractures are the most common osteoporotic fracture, but only approximately one third are clinically diagnosed. The effects of vertebral fractures have traditionally been underestimated but are beginning to be recognized and quantified. These fractures cause pain, disfigurement, and dysfunction and decrease the quality of life. Recent studies link them to an increased risk of mortality. Vertebroplasty is a minimally invasive procedure for managing acute painful vertebral fractures. This procedure involves injecting bone cement into the fractured vertebra under fluoroscopic guidance (see Fig. 24-28). Balloon kyphoplasty is a minimally invasive procedure that can reduce back pain, as well as restore vertebral body height and spinal alignment. This procedure involves actually reducing the vertebral compression and injecting the cement into this space created within the vertebral body (Fig. 36-5). Fluoroscopic guidance is also used for this procedure.

The presence of even one osteoporotic vertebral fracture significantly increases the risk of future vertebral fractures and progressive curvature of the spine.

Most osteoporotic fractures are caused by falls. Therefore identifying elderly persons at increased risk for falls and instituting fall prevention strategies are important goals. Some risk factors for falling are use of some medications including sedatives, sleep aids, and antidepressants; impaired muscle strength, range of motion, balance, and gait; impaired psychologic functioning including dementia and depression; and environmental hazards including lighting, rugs, furniture, bathroom, and stairs. Fall prevention strategies through a physical therapy program include balance, gait, and strengthening exercises. Addressing psychologic issues, reviewing medication regimens, and counseling patients on correct dosing are other prevention methods. Homes and living areas should be inspected for hazards, and safety measures should be implemented.

Fig. 36-5 Diagram of balloon kyphoplasty.

BONE HEALTH RECOMMENDATIONS

The National Osteoporosis Foundation's Bone Health and Prevention Recommendations are as follows:

- Get your daily recommended amounts of calcium and vitamin D.
- Engage in regular weight-bearing and resistance exercise.
- Avoid smoking and excessive alcohol.
- Talk to your health care provider about bone health.
- Have a bone density test and take medication when appropriate.

Surgeon General's Report on Bone Health

The 2004 Surgeon General's Report on Bone Health and Osteoporosis includes an extensive review of the factors affecting bone health including the health consequences associated with poor bone health.

The report provides a list of recommendations to promote better bone health and health status in general:

- Getting adequate levels of calcium and vitamin D
- Engaging in physical activity
- Reducing hazards in the home that can lead to fractures and falls
- Talking with your doctor about preventative strategies to promote bone health
- Maintaining a healthy weight
- Not smoking
- Limiting alcohol use

Many Americans fail to meet currently recommended guidelines for optimal calcium intake. The National Institute of Health Consensus Conference recommends the following calcium intake: 1000 mg/day for women ages 25 to 50, postmenopausal women on estrogen therapy, and men ages 25 to 65; and 1500 mg/day for postmenopausal women not on estrogen therapy and men older than age 65. Dietary calcium is the best source including yogurt, milk, some cheeses, tofu, salmon, spinach, and broccoli. Dietary shortfall should be met with calcium supplements with the USP designation that supply the appropriate amount of elemental calcium. Be sure to check the number of pills to meet the serving size and whether or not to take with food (Table 36-3).

Adequate intake of vitamin D (at least 400 IU per day) is essential for calcium absorption and bone health. Some calcium supplements and most multivitamins contain vitamin D. Dietary sources are vitamin D–fortified milk and cereals, egg yolks, saltwater fish, and liver (Table 36-4).

Weight-bearing exercise occurs when bones and muscles work against gravity as the feet and legs bear the body's weight. Some examples are weight lifting to improve muscle mass and bone strength, low-impact aerobics, walking or jogging, tennis, dancing, stair climbing, gardening, and household chores.

TABLE 36-3

Daily recommended needs for calcium intake

Your body needs calcium.	
If this is your age,	then you need this much calcium each day (mg).
0-6 months	210
6-12 months	270
1-3 years	500
4-8 years	800
9-18 years	1300
18-50 years	1000
Over 50 years	1200

(Office of the Surgeon General's Report 2004.)
A cup of milk or fortified orange juice has about 300 mg of calcium.

TABLE 36-4

Daily recommended needs for vitamin D intake

You need more vitamin D as you get older.

Multivitamins typically provide 400 IU of vitamin D.

One cup of vitamin D–fortified milk or juice provides 50 IU.

200 IU — Until age 50
400 IU — Age 51–70
600 IU — Over age 70

Office of the Surgeon General's Report 2004.

Physical and Mathematic Principles of Dual Energy X-Ray Absorptiometry

The measurement of bone density requires separation of the x-ray attenuating effects of soft tissue and bone. The mass attenuation coefficients of soft tissue and bone differ and also depend on the energy of the x-ray photons. The use of two different photon energies (dual energy x-ray) optimizes the differentiation of soft tissue and bone. Lunar and Norland use a different method of producing the two energies than Hologic.

Lunar and Norland use a rare-earth, filtered x-ray source. The primary x-ray beam is passed through selected rare-earth filters to produce a spectrum with peaks near 40 and 70 kiloelectron volts (keV), as compared with the usual continuous spectrum with one peak near 50 keV (Fig. 36-6, *A* and *B*). Sophisticated pulse-counting detectors are used to separate and measure the low- and high-energy photons (Fig. 36-7). Calibration must be performed externally by scanning a calibration phantom on a regular basis.

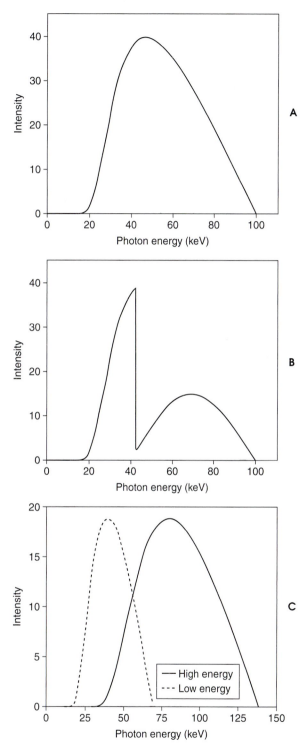

Fig. 36-6 Energy spectra (keV) for x-ray sources used in bone densitometry instruments. **A,** Continuous spectrum from an x-ray tube. **B,** Continuous x-ray spectrum modified by a K-edge filter. **C,** High- and low-energy spectra from a kV-switching system.

(Courtesy Blake G, Wahner H, Fogelman I: *The evaluation of osteoporosis: dual energy x-ray absorptiometry and ultrasound in clinical practice,* London, 1998, Martin Dunitz.)

The Hologic scanners use an energy-switching system that synchronously switches the x-ray potential between 100 and 140 kVp. This produces a primary beam with two photon energies with peaks near 40 and 80 keV (see Fig. 36-6, *C*). The energy-switching system continuously calibrates the beam by passing it through a calibration wheel or drum (Fig. 36-8) containing three sectors for an open-air gap, a soft tissue equivalent, and a bone equivalent. Each sector is divided so that it can differentiate and measure the low- and high-energy photons. This permits the use of a relatively simple current-integrating detector that does not have to separate the photons.

Common physics problems of DXA are as follows:

- Beam hardening in energy-switching systems. With increasing body thickness, a higher proportion of low energy photons are absorbed within the body, shifting the spectral distribution toward high-energy photons.
- Scintillating detector pileup in K-edge filtration systems. A detector can only process one photon at a time and assign it to the high- or low-energy channel. An incoming photon may be missed if the preceding photon has not yet been processed. Digital detectors do not have this problem.
- Crossover in K-edge filtration systems. Some high-energy photons lose energy passing through the body and are counted as low-energy photons by the detector. This is solved by subtracting a fraction of the high-energy counts from the low-energy channel, depending on body thickness.

The low- and high-energy x-rays are attenuated differently within each patient. This produces a unique attenuation pattern at the detector, which is transmitted electronically to the scanner software. Mathematic computations that subtract the soft tissue signals, thereby producing a profile of the bone, are then performed (Fig. 36-9). Proprietary bone edge detection algorithms are next applied, and a two-dimensional area is calculated. The average BMD is calculated for all areas, and finally the BMD is calculated as BMD = BMC ÷ area. Thus the three bone densitometry parameters reported on the DXA printouts are area in centimeters squared (cm^2), BMC in grams (g), and BMD in g/cm^2. BMD is the most widely used parameter because it reduces the effect of body size.

Fig. 36-8 Calibration drum used as internal reference standard in Hologic energy-switching instruments. The different segments represent a bone standard, a soft tissue standard, and an empty segment for air value.

Fig. 36-7 Schematic drawing of a Norland model XR-36 illustrating the principle of operation of a rare-earth filtered system. *A,* High-energy detector. *B,* Low-energy detector. *C,* Laser indicator. *D,* Samarium filter module (one fixed, three selectable). *E,* Ultra-stable 100 kV x-ray source.

BMD can be calculated if BMC and area are known by the equation BMD $\times$ BMC $\div$ area. This equation can be used to determine if a change in BMD is due to a change in BMC, area, or both. A decrease in BMC results in a decrease in BMD; conversely, a decrease in area results in an increase in BMD. If BMC and area move proportionally in the same direction, BMD remains unchanged. Generally a change in a patient's BMD over time should be from a change in BMC, not area. A change in area could be from the technologist not reproducing the baseline positioning or from a change in the software's bone edge detection. Changes in area over time should be investigated and corrected, if possible.

BMD is based on a two-dimensional area, not a three-dimensional volume, making DXA a *projectional*, or *areal*, *technique*. Techniques to estimate *volumetric density* from DXA scans have been developed but have not been shown to have any improved diagnostic sensitivity over traditional areal density. Fig. 36-10 shows the lateral spine areal and estimated volumetric BMDs.

BMD values from scanners made by different manufacturers cannot be directly compared. However, mathematic formulas have been developed for converting BMD from any manufacturer to *standardized BMD* (sBMD) values that can be compared.[1,2] Standardized BMD values are best used for large populations, such as standardizing a reference population database. They must be used with caution for individuals because the sBMD from one manufacturer can vary by 3% to 6% from the sBMD of either of the other manufacturers. For this reason, it is not widely recommended to use sBMD to compare an individual's scans done on different manufacturers' scanners.

[1]Genant HK: Development of formulas for standardized DXA measurements, *J Bone Miner Res* 9:997, 1995.
[2]Genant HK et al: Universal standardization for dual x-ray absorptiometry: patient and phantom cross-calibration results, *J Bone Miner Res* 9:1503, 1994.

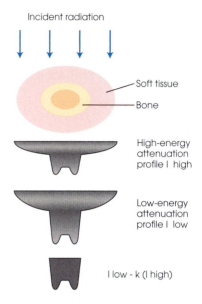

Fig. 36-9 Soft tissue compensation using DXA. By obtaining data at two energies, the soft tissue attenuation can be mathematically eliminated. The remaining attenuation is due to the amount of bone present.

(Courtesy Faulkner KG: *DXA basic science, radiation use and safety, quality assurance,* unpublished certification report, 1996, personal communication, Madison, Wis.)

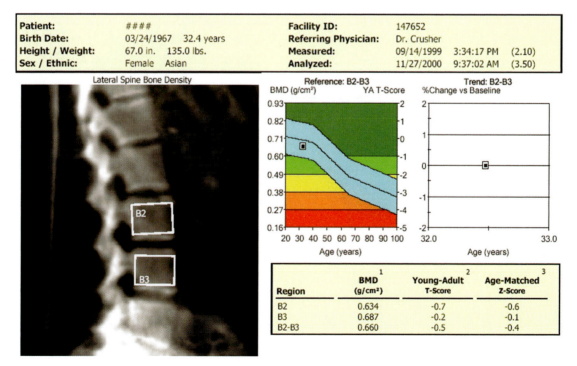

Patient:	####	Facility ID:	147652
Birth Date:	03/24/1967 32.4 years	Referring Physician:	Dr. Crusher
Height / Weight:	67.0 in. 135.0 lbs.	Measured:	09/14/1999 3:34:17 PM (2.10)
Sex / Ethnic:	Female Asian	Analyzed:	11/27/2000 9:37:02 AM (3.50)

Region	BMD[1] (g/cm²)	Young-Adult[2] T-Score	Age-Matched[3] Z-Score
B2	0.634	-0.7	-0.6
B3	0.687	-0.2	-0.1
B2-B3	0.660	-0.5	-0.4

Fig. 36-10 Lateral spine BMD scan.

Pencil-Beam, Array-Beam, and Smart Fan Collimation Techniques

The original DXA scanners employed a pencil-beam system. With this system a circular pinhole x-ray collimator produces a narrow (or pencil-beam) stream of x-ray photons that is received by a single detector. The pencil-beam of x-ray moves in a serpentine (also called *rectilinear* or *raster*) fashion across or along the length of the body (Fig. 36-11). This system has good resolution and reproducibility, but the early scanners had relatively long scan times of 5 to 7 minutes. Newer models have reduced scan times to 1 minute. It should be noted that pencil-beam systems are stable and are still in widespread use, with modern systems incorporating enhancements to improve image quality and achieve shorter scan times.

The array-beam (also called fan-beam) system has a wide "slit" x-ray collimator and a multielement detector (Fig. 36-12). The scanning motion is reduced to only one direction, which greatly reduces scan time and permits supine lateral lumbar spine scans to be performed (Fig. 36-13). The array-beam system introduces geometric magnification and a slight geometric distortion at the outer edges. Consequently, careful centering of the object of interest is necessary to avoid parallax (Fig. 36-14). The software takes into account the known degree of magnification and produces an *estimated* BMC and estimated area.

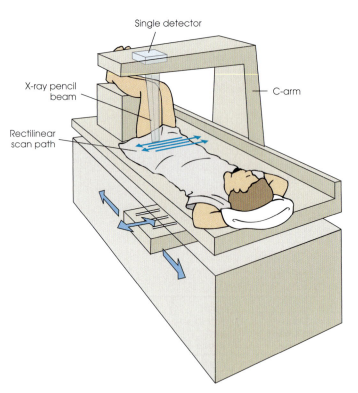

Single detector

X-ray pencil beam

C-arm

Rectilinear scan path

Fig. 36-11 DXA system using a pencil-beam single detector.

Fig. 36-12 DXA system using an array-beam multiple detector.

Fig. 36-13 DXA system using a movable C-arm and array-beam multiple detector to perform a lateral supine lumbar spine scan.

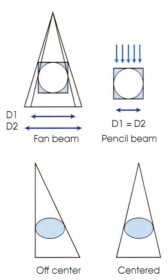

Fig. 36-14 Potential array-beam errors including magnification *(top)* and parallax *(bottom)*. Both area and BMC are influenced by magnification to the same degree, such that the BMD is not significantly affected. Parallax errors can cause changes in BMD by altering the beam path through the object being measured.

(Courtesy Faulkner KG: *DXA basic science, radiation use and safety, quality assurance,* unpublished certification report, 1996, personal communication, Madison, Wis.)

The newest DXA technology is known as a smart fan-beam system, manufactured by GE Lunar. With this system the narrow "slit" x-ray collimator is oriented parallel to the longitudinal axis of the patient and scans in a transverse pattern across the body (Fig. 36-15). This geometry is less sensitive to object position than wide beam technology. Magnification error is reduced, as the maximum offset from the beam is six times smaller than with wide-angle fan beams. The narrow fan-beam system uses acquisition with multiple, overlapping passes over the region of interest (Fig. 36-16). Each smart fan-beam pass overlaps slightly with the previous pass. This acquisition technique allows true object location to be calculated with multiview image reconstruction (MVIR).

MVIR is an imaging technique perfected in CT, in which multiple images are acquired, each with a small overlap. By sliding these overlapping images over one another for a perfect match, the true distance of the object from the detector is determined. Knowing the true object plane assures accurate BMC, area, and soft tissue results. The high efficiency of the CZT (cadmium zinc telluride) detector allows reduced scan time and radiation exposure.

Fig. 36-15 A, Narrow-angle fan beam with smart fan machine, with detail of the beam geometry in **B.**

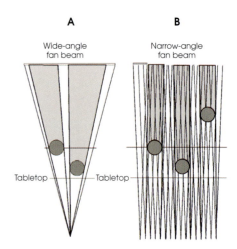

Fig. 36-16 Wide-beam technology in **A** compared with narrow fan beam with multiple, overlapping passes in **B.**

ACCURACY AND PRECISION

Three statistics are particularly important in bone densitometry: mean, standard deviation (SD), and percent coefficient of variation (%CV).

1. The mean is commonly called the average. It is the sum of the data values divided by the number of values.
2. The standard deviation (SD) is a measure of variability that measures the spread of the data values around their mean. It takes into account the average distance of the data values from the mean. The smaller the average distance or the spread, the smaller the SD. This is the goal in bone densitometry—a smaller SD is better. Fig. 36-17 plots two sets of phantom BMD data measured over 6 months. The means are the same (1.005 g/cm²), but the red dataset has an SD that is twice as large as that of the green dataset (0.008 g/cm² vs. 0.004 g/cm²). It is better to have phantom BMD data that look like the green dataset.
3. The %CV is a statistic that allows the comparison of variability between different datasets, whether or not they have the same mean. A smaller %CV means less variability and is preferred in bone densitometry. The %CV is calculated using the following equation:

$$\%CV = (SD/Mean) \times 100$$

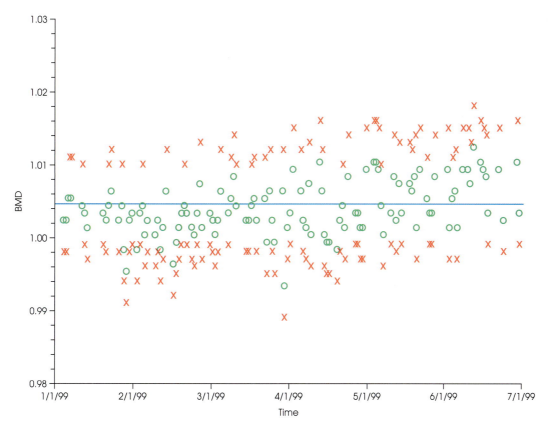

Fig. 36-17 Two datasets of longitudinal phantom BMD (*blue line* is the mean). Green dataset has mean = 1.005 g/cm², SD = 0.004 g/cm², and %CV = 0.35. Red dataset has mean = 1.005 g/cm², SD = 0.008 g/cm², and %CV = 0.81.

In Fig. 39-14 the green dataset has a %CV of 0.35 and the red dataset has a %CV of 0.81. This is the %CV that must be checked on a Hologic spine phantom plot (Fig. 36-18). The red data would not pass the criteria that the %CV should be less than or equal to 0.6. The %CV is also used to express precision.

Bone densitometry differs from diagnostic radiology in that good image quality, which can tolerate variability in technique, is not the ultimate goal. Instead, the goal is accurate and precise quantitative measurement by the scanner software, which requires stable equipment and careful, consistent work from the technologist. Therefore two important performance measures in bone densitometry are *accuracy* and *precision*. Accuracy relates to the ability of the system to measure the true value of an object. Precision relates to the ability of the system to reproduce the same (but not necessarily accurate) results in repeat measurements of the same object. A target may be used to illustrate this point. In Fig. 36-19, *A,* the archer is precise but not accurate. In Fig. 36-19, *B,* the archer is accurate but not precise. Finally, in Fig. 36-19, *C,* the archer is both precise and accurate.

Setup	Reference Values	Plot Statistics
a Lumbar Spine SPINE phantom #4718 System S/N: 45539	Limits: ±1.5% of mean Mean: 1.003 (g/cm²) SD: 0.005 (g/cm²)	Number of Points: 28 Mean: 0.998 (g/cm²) SD: 0.004 (g/cm²) CV: 0.381 %

Fig. 36-18 Hologic spine phantom quality control plot. All plotted BMD points are within the control limits *(dotted lines),* which indicate 1.5% of the mean. The coefficient of variation (CV) (under Plot Statistics) is within acceptable limits at 0.43%.

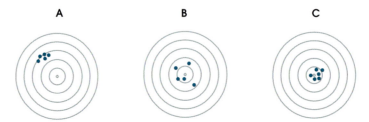

Fig. 36-19 Illustration of accuracy vs. precision, assuming an archer is shooting for the center of the target. **A,** Precise but not accurate. **B,** Accurate but not precise. **C,** Accurate and precise.

In bone densitometry practice, accuracy is most important at baseline when the original diagnosis of osteoporosis is made. Accuracy is determined primarily by the calibration of the scanner, which is set and maintained by the manufacturer. Preventive maintenance once or twice a year is recommended. Precision is followed closely because it is relatively easy to determine and is the most important performance measure in following a patient's BMD over time. Precision can be measured in vitro (in an inanimate object, e.g., phantom) or in vivo (in a live body). Precision is commonly expressed as %CV, and a smaller value indicates better precision.

In vitro precision is the cornerstone of the quality control systems built into the scanners to detect drifts or shifts (variations) in calibration. Each manufacturer provides a unique phantom for this purpose.

In vivo precision has two main aspects in bone densitometry:
1. The variability within a patient that makes it easy or difficult to obtain similar BMD results from several scans on the same patient, on the same day, with repositioning between scans. (Patients with abnormal anatomy, very low bone mass, or thick or thin bodies are known to reflect a larger precision error.)
2. The variability related to the skill of the technologist and how attentive he or she is to obtaining the best possible baseline scan and then reproducing the positioning, scanning parameters, and placement of ROI on all *follow-up scans.*

Each DXA lab must know its in vivo precision. This precision is used to determine the magnitude of change in BMD that must occur over a period of time to be certain that the change is due to a change in the patient's BMD, not to the precision error of the technologist and scanner. Calculating in vivo precision involves performing multiple scans on a number of patients and computing some statistical parameters.[1,2] Although this process is time consuming, it is worth the effort involved. In vitro precision can never be substituted into a formula that requires in vivo precision.

The primary factors affecting precision include the following:
- Reproduction of positioning, acquisition parameters (e.g., mode, speed, current), and ROI placement
- Anatomic variations and pathology and their degeneration over time
- Body habitus (e.g., excessive thickness or thinness)
- Large weight changes over time
- Geometric factors on array scanners
- Stability of scanner calibration and bone edge detection

[1]Bonnick SL: *Bone densitometry in clinical practice: application and interpretation,* Totowa, NJ, 1998, Human Press.
[2]Glüer CC et al: Accurate assessment of precision errors: how to measure the reproducibility of bone densitometry techniques, *Osteoporos Int* 5:262, 1995.

Pencil-beam, array-beam, and smart fan collimation techniques

Z-SCORES AND T-SCORES

A BMD measurement from a patient is most useful when it can be compared statistically with an appropriate sex-matched *reference population*. The three DXA manufacturers have separately collected reference population databases. These reference databases vary because different populations, entrance criteria, and statistical methods were used. To correct this problem, the third National Health and Nutrition Examination Survey (NHANES III) DXA total hip database was adapted to provide a *standardized hip* reference database for all manufacturers. This database is widely used today. All reference databases are separated by gender and provide the BMD mean and SD at each age.

In order to compare a patient's BMD with the reference population BMD, two standardized scores have been developed called the *Z-score* and *T-score* (see Fig. 36-10, *C*). In older adults the Z-score is greater than the T-score.

The Z-score indicates the number of SDs the patient's BMD is from the average BMD for the patient's respective age and sex group. Z-score is used to determine if the measured BMD is reasonable and if evaluation for secondary osteoporosis is warranted. It is calculated using the following:

$$\text{Z-score} = (\text{Measured BMD} - \text{Age-matched mean BMD})/\text{Age-matched SD}$$

The T-score indicates the number of SDs the patient's BMD is from the average BMD of young, normal, sex-matched individuals with peak bone mass. T-score is used to assess fracture risk, diagnose osteoporosis and *osteopenia,* and determine if therapy is recommended. The T-score is calculated using the following:

$$\text{T-score} = (\text{Measured BMD} - \text{Young adult mean BMD})/\text{Young adult SD}$$

The Z-score or T-score, or both, may also be adjusted for ethnicity or weight, or both. It is incorrect to assume that because ethnicity and weight have been entered into the scan biographical information that the standardized scores have been adjusted. Some manufacturers allow an ethnicity to be entered for which there is no reference database; these patients are compared with Caucasians. Some manufacturers adjust for weight and ethnicity on the Z-score but not the T-score. To determine what adjustments have been made, first carefully check the information on the scan printout including footnotes. If a question remains, call the manufacturer's customer service line and ask.

As of November 1, 2003, the International Society of Clinical Densitometry (ISCD) recommends use of a uniform Caucasian (non–race adjusted) female normative database for women of all ethnic groups. A uniform Caucasian (non–race adjusted) male normative database for men of all ethnic groups is being used. All manufacturers' defaults are not adjusted to this recommendation. The technologist needs to be familiar with the defaults of the specific equipment and know how to make adjustments.

Bone mass is normally distributed (i.e., has a bell-shaped curve) in the population, and no one exact cut point exists below which a person has osteoporosis. However, with the widespread availability of DXA and T-scores, there was pressure to declare such a cut point. In 1994 the World Health Organization (WHO) recommended that the classifications presented in Table 36-5 be used in DXA studies of postmenopausal Caucasian women.

Discordance refers to the issue of different T-scores occurring at anatomic sites within a patient, within populations, and between modalities. It makes the diagnosis of osteoporosis more complicated than simply applying a T-score criteria, and the problems are being researched to find more standardized diagnostic criteria. For example, a patient may be found to have a low T-score at the hip but not at the spine, and a QCT scan of the spine is likely to produce a lower T-score than a DXA scan of the spine in the same patient.

The WHO classifications have become widely used in clinical practice. However, applying the T-score criteria designed for DXA to other modalities (e.g., QUS, QCT) has proved to be problematic. The best practice is to apply the T-score criteria only to DXA until ongoing research provides acceptable criteria for other modalities. Importantly, the T-score is one important risk factor for osteoporosis, but the patient's medical history, lifestyle, medications, and other risk factors must also be considered in a complete clinical evaluation. Physicians who interpret bone density scans need to be educated in the complexities of the task.

Large epidemiologic studies have investigated the clinical value of BMD in elderly women and have yielded information on the relationship of BMD and T-scores to fracture risk. A gradient of risk has been observed between BMD and fracture incidence, with lower BMD or T-score conferring increased risk of fracture. For each 1 SD decrease in T-score, the risk for fracture increases 1.5- to 2.5-fold. For example, a woman with a T-score of −2 has roughly twice the risk of fracture compared with a woman with a T-score of −1, all other factors being equal. This information helps clinicians explain the meaning of a bone density test to patients. Patients can then make informed decisions about the level of fracture risk they are willing to accept and whether to begin or continue therapy.

TABLE 36-5

World Health Organization classifications of bone density by T-score

Classification	Criteria
Normal	BMD or BMC T-score of ≥ -1
Low bone mass (osteopenia)	BMD or BMC T-score between -1 and -2.5
Osteoporosis	BMD or BMC T-score of < -2.5
Severe osteoporosis	BMD or BMC T-score of < -2.5 and 1 or more fragility fractures

Data from Kanis JA: World Health Organization (WHO) Study Group: assessment of fracture risk and its application to screening for postmenopausal osteoporosis: a synopsis of the WHO report, *Osteoporos Int* 4:368, 1994.
BMC, Bone mineral content; *BMD,* bone mineral density; *T-score,* the number of standard deviations a BMD is from the average BMD of a young, normal, sex-matched individual with peak bone mass.

Dual Energy X-Ray Absorptiometry Scanning

RADIATION PROTECTION

Radiologic technologists receive extensive instruction in radiation physics, biology, and protection during their professional education. Practicing proper radiation protection and achieving the goal of *ALARA* (*a*s *l*ow *a*s *r*easonably *a*chievable) is relatively simple for DXA. The effective radiation dose in *sieverts* (Sv) for DXA scans is low compared with conventional radiography doses and similar to natural background radiation (Table 36-6). If the positioning or acquisition parameters of a scan are questionable, the scan should be repeated because the risk from the additional radiation dose is negligible compared with the risk of an incorrect medical diagnosis.

Time, distance, and shielding relate to DXA in the following ways:

1. The manufacturer sets the time for the scan based on the array or scan mode appropriate for the thickness of the body part being scanned.
2. The manufacturer sets the distance from the x-ray tube to the patient. This is a fixed distance.
3. Distance is the best form of protection for the technologist. The technologist's console should be at least 3 feet (1 m) from the x-ray source (x-ray tube) scanner for pencil-beam scanners and up to 9 feet (3 m) from heavily used array-beam scanners (array beam produces higher dose than pencil beam). If these distances cannot be accommodated, a mobile radiation shield can be used.

Shielding is built into the scanner via collimation. Additional lead shielding should not be used on DXA patients.

Other important radiation safety points include the following:

- The technologist should wear an individual dosimetry device (film badge, thermoluminescent dosimeter [TLD], or optically stimulated luminescence [OSL] device) at the collar on the side adjacent to the scanner. Another monitor can be placed outside the scan room. A staff member should be charged with understanding and monitoring the dosimetry records and performing any necessary follow-up. A radiation warning sign should be posted and highly visible.

- The technologist should remain in the room during the scan and monitor the acquisition image, allowing the scan to be aborted as soon as the need for repositioning and rescanning is obvious.
- The technologist should have adequate instruction and experience to minimize repositioning and repeated scans. For example, it is important to know how to prepare the patient to eliminate artifacts. However, any questionable scan should be repeated.
- The technologist should follow proper procedures to avoid scanning a pregnant patient and place documentation in the permanent record. If a woman of childbearing age will not sign that she is not pregnant, the 10-Day Rule allows scanning during the first 10 days after the first day of her last menstrual period.
- Patients should be screened at scheduling for problems that require postponement of scanning, such as pregnancy and recent barium, contrast, or nuclear medicine examinations.

The most effective radiation safety practice is a knowledgeable, well-educated, and conscientious DXA technologist. It is essential for DXA technologists to receive instructions from the manufacturer of a specific model of scanner. This might consist of review of videotapes or DVDs, as well as a 1- or 2-day session with a field applications specialist and review of performed scans. Once experience is obtained, a technologist can be certified by the International Society for Clinical Densitometry (ISCD) or test for a certificate of added qualifications by the American Registry of Radiologic Technologists (ARRT), or both. Technologists must obtain continuing education in bone densitometry to meet the qualifications of a current status in this ever-changing field.

TABLE 36-6

Bone densitometry radiation doses compared with other commonly acquired doses

Type of radiation exposure	Effective dose (mSv)
Daily natural background radiation	5-8
Round-trip air flight across the United States	60
Lateral lumbar spine radiograph	700
PA chest radiograph	50
QCT with localizer scan (from scanner offering low kV and mAs; may be up to 10 times higher for other scanners)	60
DXA scan (range allows for different anatomic sites; Lunar EXPERT-XL may be higher)	1-5
SXA scan	≤1
Quantitative ultrasound	0

Data from Kalender WA: Effective dose values in bone mineral measurements by photon absorptiometry and computed tomography, *Osteoporos Int* 2:82, 1992.
DXA, Dual energy x-ray absorptiometry; *kV,* kilovolt; *mAs,* milliampere-seconds; *PA,* posteroanterior; *QCT,* quantitative computed tomography; *SXA,* single energy x-ray absorptiometry.

PATIENT CARE AND EDUCATION[1]

Typical DXA patients are ambulatory outpatients; however, many are frail and at increased risk for fragility fractures. Patient care and safety requires attention to the following points of courtesy and common sense:

- All areas of the laboratory including the front entrance, waiting room, and scan room should be monitored daily and modified for patient safety. Check the location of floor-level cables in the scan room.
- The technologist should maintain professionalism at all times by introducing himself or herself and other staff to the patient and explaining the procedure.
- The technologist needs to remove all external artifacts. Some DXA laboratories have all patients undress and gown. However, it is possible to scan a patient who is wearing loose cotton clothing with no buttons, snaps, or zippers (i.e., "sweats"). If clothing is not removed, the brassiere must be undone, and all hooks and underwires must be removed from the scan field. Considering that shoes should be removed for proper height measurement, a long-handled shoehorn would be a practical aid.
- The technologist should provide a simple explanation of the expected action of the scan-arm, the proximity of the scan-arm to the patient's face and head, the noise of the motor, and the length of time for the scan. This information may reduce the patient's anxiety.

- The technologist must listen to any concerns the patient may have about the procedure and be ready to answer questions about radiation exposure, the length of the examination, and the reporting protocol used by the laboratory.
- Although the scan tables are not more than 3 feet (about 1 m) in height, a steady footstool with a long handle is recommended. All patients should be assisted on and off the table.
- On completion of the examination, the technologist should be sure the scan arm has returned to the home position, clearing the patient's head. The patient should sit upright for several seconds to regain stability before descending from the scanner.

In some institutions it is the responsibility of the DXA technologist to provide education to the patient and the family. Topics may include osteoporosis prevention, proper nutrition, calcium supplementation, weight-bearing exercise, and creating a hazard-free living environment. Many technologists give community educational programs, staff in-service seminars, and participate in health fairs.

PATIENT HISTORY[1]

Each bone density laboratory should develop a patient questionnaire customized for the types of patients referred and the needs of the referring and reporting physicians. Before scanning is performed, identify any information that could postpone or cancel the scan. The questionnaire should be directed at obtaining information in four basic categories:

Sample questions include the following:
1. Scanning criteria:
   - Is there a possibility of pregnancy?
   - Is it impossible for you to lie flat on your back for several minutes?
   - Have you had a nuclear medicine, barium, or contrast x-ray examination performed in the last week?
   - Have you had any previous fractures or surgeries in the hip, spine, abdomen, or forearm areas?
   - Do you have any other medical conditions affecting the bones, such as osteoporosis, curvature of the spine, or arthritis?
2. Patient information. This includes identifying information, referring physician, current standing height and weight, and medical history including medications.
3. Insurance information. Because DXA scans are not universally covered by insurance, it is important to obtain information on the insurance carrier, the need for prior approval, and the information necessary for insurance coding.

In 1998 Congress passed the Bone Mass Measurement Act (BMMA) dealing with reimbursement for Medicare patients. Both central and peripheral technologies are covered. Screening is not covered by Medicare, so a qualified individual must meet at least one of the following requirements:

- Estrogen-deficient woman at clinical risk of osteoporosis
- Individual with hyperparathyroidism
- Individual receiving long-term glucocorticoid (steroid) therapy
- Individual with vertebral abnormalities by radiograph
- Individual being monitored for FDA-approved osteoporosis therapy
4. Reporting information. The type and scope of the report that will be provided determines how much information is necessary about the patient's risk factors for, and history of, low bone mass, fragility fractures, and bone diseases.

[1]Appreciation is extended to JoAnn Caudill, RT (BD), for her work in the preparation of the patient care and education section.

[1]Appreciation is extended to Peg Schmeer, CDT, and Randie Barnett, RT(BD), for their work in the preparation of the patient history section.

REPORTING, CONFIDENTIALITY, RECORD KEEPING, AND SCAN STORAGE

Once the scan has been completed, the following guidelines should be observed:

- The technologist should end the examination by telling the patient when the scan results will be available to the referring physician. If a patient asks for immediate results, the technologist should explain that it is the physician's responsibility to interpret and explain DXA results.
- The technologist should remember that DXA scan results are confidential medical records and should be handled according to the institution's rules for such records. Results should not be discussed with other staff or patients, and printed results, whether on hard copy or a computer screen, should be shielded from inappropriate viewing. Following HIPAA guidelines as of April 2005 must be integrated in the DXA laboratory. Manufacturers have HIPAA-compliant software upgrades available. Manufacturers use privacy tools or HIPAA-secure tools to secure patient confidentiality.
- Complete records must be kept for each patient. If a patient returns in the future for *follow-up* scans, the positioning, acquisition parameters, and placement of the ROIs must be reproduced as closely as possible to the original scans. Thus the technologist should keep a log sheet with the patient's identifying information and date, the file name, and the archive location of each scan. The log should also identify any special information about why particular scans were or were not performed (e.g., the right hip was scanned because the left hip was fractured, or the forearm was not scanned because of the patient's severe arthritis) and any special procedures taken for positioning (e.g., the femur was not fully rotated because of pain) or scan analysis (e.g., the bone edge was manually placed for the radial ultradistal region). The patient questionnaire, log sheet, and complete scan printouts should be stored in an accessible location. All scan archive media must be clearly labeled and accessible.
- The general consensus is that DXA scan results should be kept on file indefinitely because all serial studies are compared with the baseline.

COMPUTER COMPETENCY

DXA scan acquisition, analysis, and archiving is controlled with a personal computer (PC). Therefore DXA technologists must be familiar with the basic PC components and how they work, such as the disk drives (hard, floppy, and optical); keyboard; monitor; printer; and mouse. Newer DXA software runs on the Windows operating system, as opposed to DOS. Technologists working on DOS-based systems must know how to exit to DOS and use basic commands to change paths, check a directory, and copy files to disk. This operating system is becoming obsolete and is not directly supported by the manufacturers.

Windows-based software tends to be more user friendly and requires the use of a mouse to point, click, and drag. Technologists will need to upgrade their computer skills as DXA software and hardware are enhanced to allow communication between scanners and digital imaging systems via multimedia and networking capabilities. This allows a scan to be performed at one location and then be sent electronically to a remote location for reading or review by an interpreting or referring physician.

A technologist must be able to backup, archive, locate, and restore patient scan files. Daily backup and archival is recommended to preserve patient scan files and data. A third copy of data should be stored offsite to ensure retrieval of patient data, as well as to be able to rebuild databases, if there is a computer failure, fire, flood, or theft.

Manufacturers frequently upgrade software versions, and the technologist is responsible for performing this task. Records of upgrades and software installation should be maintained. Current software media should be accessible to service engineers at the time of preventive maintenance and repairs.

Computers consist of software and hardware.[1] Software consists of programs written in code that instruct the computer how to perform tasks. The DXA manufacturer's software controls many aspects of DXA scanning from starting the scan to calculating and reporting the results. Hardware comprises the physical components for central processing, input, output, and storage.

---

[1]Following the introduction of the computer in medicine, the practice and development of radiologic procedures expanded rapidly. In bone densitometry, the computer assisted in major advancements. Due to space considerations in this edition of *Merrill's Atlas,* the "Computer Fundamentals and Applications in Radiology" chapter has been deleted. For those interested in learning more about computer fundamentals, please see Volume 3, Chapter 32 of the eighth or ninth edition of this atlas.

Fig. 36-20 Plot of spine phantom BMD and time (in months). The two arrows show abrupt shifts in BMD. The straight line shows a slow drift downward in BMD. These indicate changes in scanner calibration.

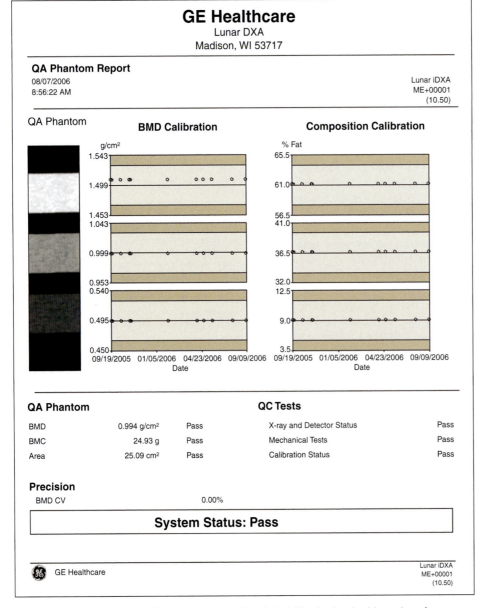

Fig. 36-21 GE Lunar quality assurance results printout. The technologist must perform, as well as review, the data before performing clinical patient scans.

(Courtesy GE Lunar, Madison, Wis.)

DXA SCANNER LONGITUDINAL QUALITY CONTROL

Longitudinal quality control procedures are performed in accordance with the manufacturer's recommendation. Manufacturers' instructions in operator manuals must be followed exactly. These procedures have the common goal of ensuring that patients are scanned on properly functioning equipment with stable calibration. Unstable calibration can take the form of abrupt shifts or slow drifts in BMD, as seen on plots of phantom scan results (Fig. 36-20). These problems make the patient's BMD values too high or too low and prohibit a valid comparison between baseline and follow-up scans.

The procedures use either external or internal instruments to track the calibration of the DXA scanner over time. Lunar and Norland systems necessitate scanning an external calibration block to perform a calibration check. The technologist must observe the procedure; he or she should review the report and note whether the system passed all tests of internal parameters (Fig. 36-21). Hologic systems perform an automatic internal calibration check when the system is turned on.

Manufacturers also provide semi-anthropomorphic and aluminum phantoms for tracking calibration over time. Hologic systems require that the phantom be scanned daily (Fig. 36-22).

When not recommended by the manufacturer, the following procedures are advised by the International Society of Clinical Densitometry (ISCD):

Perform periodic (at least once per week) phantom scans for any DXA system as an independent assessment of system calibration. The BMD is plotted, monitored, and checked with statistical and quality control rules. The quality control rule used to check DXA scanners is modified from Shewhart Control Chart rules. Shewhart rules are a classic method of checking that a quality parameter is stable and within acceptable limits of 3 SDs. For DXA the value of the control limits is modified to *1.5%* of the mean, to provide more uniformity across scanners.

Bone densitometry

The mean and SD are calculated from the first 25 measurements of the parameter. A graph is created displaying the mean and the control limits 1.5 SDs above and below the mean. The parameter measurements are plotted over time and checked for violation of rules, such as one measurement more than 1.5 SDs from the mean. DXA control charts display the mean as the center line with control limits (1.5% of the mean) above and below. This graph is produced automatically by the Hologic software (see Fig. 36-15). For other manufacturers, the graph and plotting must be done by hand. The technologist must verify the phantom BMD after any service is performed on the scanner. When the phantom BMD value falls outside the control limits, the scan should be repeated once; if it fails, service should be called and patients cancelled. If the BMD remains outside the control limits, the manufacturer must be contacted and patients need to be cancelled for the day. No patients should be scanned until the equipment has been repaired and is operating within the known values.

Ten phantom scans should be performed and plotted before and after scanner preventive maintenance, repair, relocation, and software or hardware upgrades. This is to assure that the calibration has not been altered and proper adjustments can be made. These phantoms and values should be reviewed before the service engineer leaves the DXA laboratory. Recalibration adjustments should be made before scanning any patients. The technologist is required to oversee this operation.

Inconsistent phantom scanning, analysis, or interpretation of the results may result in false precision and patient results. The DXA technologist must understand the quality control procedures and follow them consistently. DXA laboratories should have written procedures and documented instructions to ensure consistency among technologists.

The technologist is required to maintain service logs, as well as compliance with government inspections, radiations surveys, and regulatory requirements.

Fig. 36-22 Hologic phantom.

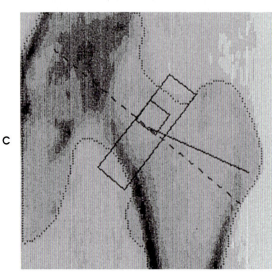

Fig. 36-23 Examples of incorrect and correct follow-up scan positioning. Note the difference in BMD between the scans. **A,** Baseline hip scan. **B,** Incorrectly positioned follow-up scan. Size and shape of lesser trochanter and angle of femoral body do not match baseline. **C,** Correctly positioned follow-up scan.

ANATOMY, POSITIONING, AND ANALYSIS

Radiologic technologists receive extensive instruction in anatomy during their radiology training. DXA scanning requires knowledge of densitometric anatomy. This anatomy relates to properly positioning the patient for scan acquisition. The points presented in this section generally apply to all DXA scanners; however, instruction from the particular scanner's manufacturer is required before operating the scanner. The operator's manual that accompanies the equipment is the referred guideline.

Like all technologies, DXA has operating limits. Accuracy and precision may be impaired if the bone mass is low, the patient is too thick or thin, the anatomy is abnormal, or there have been significant changes in soft tissue between serial scans. The added value of the experienced DXA technologist is recognition and adaptation to abnormal situations. Any anomaly or protocol variation that may compromise the scan results must be noted by the technologist and taken into consideration by the interpreting physician.

DXA calculations are based on soft tissue as well as bone. Adequate amounts of soft tissue are essential for valid results.

Serial scans

DXA is a qualitative instrument used to monitor BMD change over time. True comparison of BMD results require that serial scans be performed on the same scanner that was used for the baseline scans.

Precision is in the hands of the technologist. The less amount of intervention from the technologist and the DXA equipment, the more precise the results will be, reflecting a true biologic change. It is imperative that the patient positioning be exactly the same for both baseline and serial scans. The same scan settings (e.g., field size, mode, or speed and current) and ROI should be placed identically on the images. These steps ensure that scan results are comparable over time. When recommended, the software's *compare feature* should be used. The baseline printouts should be available at the time of the patient's appointment. Documentation of any procedures out of the range of the laboratory's standard operating procedure (SOP) needs to be available when performing serial scans.

Fig. 36-23 shows the comparison of a patient's hip scans from 1995 (Fig. 36-23, *A*) and 2001 and is an example of why follow-up positioning must match baseline if the BMDs are to be compared. The first follow-up scan (Fig. 36-23, *B*) did not reproduce the baseline positioning. The rotation of the femoral neck was different, as indicated by the larger lesser trochanter and the femoral body being more abducted. This resulted in the midline being placed differently by the software and therefore a different angle for the neck ROI. The scan was repeated (Fig. 36-23, *C*) to correctly reproduce the baseline positioning. The difference in total hip BMD between scans A and B is −13% compared with a difference of −10% between scans A and C.

AP (PA) lumbar spine

Spine scans are most appropriate for predicting vertebral fracture risk. Underestimation of fracture risk occurs in patients older than the age of 65 who present with degenerative changes that can artifactually elevate spinal BMD. The following points can help with positioning patients for AP (PA) lumbar spine DXA scans, analyzing the scan results, and evaluating the validity of the scans:

1. Degenerative changes in the spine, such as *osteophytosis,* overlying calcification, and compression fractures (Fig. 36-24) or scoliosis greater than 15 degrees (Fig. 36-25), can falsely elevate the BMD. Artifacts in the vertebral bodies or very dense artifacts in the soft tissue also affect the BMD,

depending on the model of the scanner and version of the software. The interpreting physician should develop policies and protocols for the technologist in these circumstances (e.g., do not include the spine but include another site, such as forearm).

2. The lumbar spine is centered in the scan field. In a patient with scoliosis, L5 may need to be off center so that adequate and relatively equal amounts of soft tissue are on either side of the spine throughout the scan.

3. Some visualization of iliac crests should be acquired in the scan region. This ensures the inclusion of all of L4. The iliac crest is an excellent landmark for consistent placement of the intervertebral markers at baseline and follow-up scanning.

A

Region	Area(cm²)	BMC(g)	BMD(g/cm²)
L1	13.56	10.07	0.743
L2	13.75	11.63	0.846
L3	14.56	11.83	0.812
L4	16.44	14.34	0.872
TOTAL	58.31	47.87	0.821

B

Region	Area(cm²)	BMC(g)	BMD(g/cm²)
L1	11.45	10.88	0.951
L2	12.97	11.72	0.903
L3	14.95	11.80	0.789
L4	16.50	14.35	0.870
TOTAL	55.87	48.75	0.873

Fig. 36-24 Use of Hologic compare feature indicates that L1 bone map and ROI from baseline scan **(A)** no longer fits the follow-up scan **(B)** because of a compression fracture of L1. Both scans should be analyzed to exclude L1 before comparing total BMD. Note the differences in BMD and area measurements.

Fig. 36-25 DXA AP spine scan with scoliosis and scoliosis analysis technique.

Fig. 36-26 Characteristic shapes of L1-L5 and their relationship to the iliac crests as seen on a DXA AP spine scan.

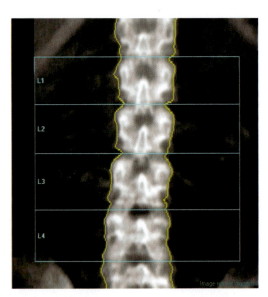

Fig. 39-27 Six lumbar vertebrae. Note that the vertebral labeling is done from the bottom to the top according to the shape of the vertebrae.

4. The AP (PA) spine scan image displays the posterior vertebral elements, which have unique characteristic shapes unlike a general lumbar radiograph. These shapes can be used to differentiate placement of the intervertebral markers. When degenerative disease has obscured the intervertebral spaces, these shapes can aid in determining proper labeling of the vertebral levels. L1, L2, and L3 have a U shape, L4 has an H or X shape and appears to have "feet," and L5 looks like a sideways I or "dog bone" (Fig. 36-26). Another aid is that L3 typically has the widest transverse processes. L1, L2, and L3 are approximately the same height. L4 is a bit taller than the others, while L5 is the shortest in height. The iliac crest usually lies at the level of L4-L5 intervertebral space.

5. A small percentage of patients appear to have four or six lumbar vertebrae rather than five, which is most commonly seen. The vertebrae can be labeled by locating L5 and L4 on the basis of their characteristic shapes and then counting upward (Fig. 36-27). The procedure of counting from the bottom superiorly biases toward a higher BMD and avoids including T12 without a rib, which significantly lowers the BMD. This procedure ensures a conservative diagnosis of low BMD.

6. Only if absolutely necessary should the bone edges be adjusted or the intervertebral markers angled or moved. These techniques should be performed in a fashion that will be easy to reproduce at serial scanning. Documentation of these variations to protocol should be made.

7. Check that the patient is lying straight on the table by observing from the head or foot end of the table. If a patient is lying straight on the table but the spine is not straight on the scan, do not attempt to twist the patient to get the image straight. This unusual positioning will not be reproducible at follow-up. Make a note in the record that the patient was positioned straight on the table.

8. The purpose of the leg-positioning block is to reduce the lordotic curve, open up the intervertebral spaces, and reduce the part-image distance. Consistency in using the same height of the leg-positioning block when a patient returns for serial scans is important. Documentation of the block height should be noted.

9. A checklist for a good AP (PA) spine scan (see Fig. 36-24, *A*) includes the following:
   - The spine is straight and centered in the scan field. Note that patients with scoliosis should have equal amounts of soft tissue on either side of the spine.
   - The scan contains a portion of the iliac crest and half of T12; the last set of ribs is shown, when applicable.
   - The entire scan field is free of external artifacts.
   - The intervertebral markers are properly placed.
   - The vertebral levels are properly labeled.
   - The bone edges are correct.

Proximal femur

The hip scan is perhaps the most important because it is the best predictor of future hip fracture, which is the most devastating of the fragility fractures. Compared with the spine scan, the hip scan is more difficult to perform properly and precisely because of variations in anatomy and the small ROIs. The following points can help in positioning patients for hip DXA scans, analyzing the results, and evaluating the validity of the scans:

1. With the patient in a supine position, the hip should be rotated 15 to 25 degrees medially to place the femoral neck parallel with the tabletop and perpendicular to the x-ray beam. Successful rotation is achieved when the lesser trochanter is diminished in size and only slightly visible (or not visible). A large, pointed lesser trochanter could indicate too little rotation (see Fig. 36-23, *B, C*). However, patient anatomy is not always textbook in quality. Patients can have a prominent lesser trochanter, and proper rotation is achieved when the femoral neck region is free of overlapping ischium and appropriate pelvis separation is visualized. This positioning will allow proper placement of the femoral neck ROI. All scanners come with positioning aids that should be used according to manufacturers' instructions.

2. The shaft of the femur must be straight and parallel to the long axis of the table.

3. A few patients have little or no space between the ischium and femoral neck. In some cases, part of the ischium lies under the femoral neck, elevating the BMC and falsely elevating the femoral neck BMD (Fig. 36-28). This could be caused by the ischium (pelvis) being rotated. The patient should be removed from the table and repositioned. If the problem still exists, slightly overabduct the leg until the ischium and neck are separated. Whatever is performed at baseline must be noted and reproduced at the time of the serial scan.

A

B

Fig. 36-28 A, Despite use of the software tool to "cut out the ischium," bone from the ischium underlies the femoral neck ROI. The BMC will be increased, thereby increasing the BMD. **B,** One year later the same patient was positioned for a follow-up scan. The pelvis is no longer rotated, as indicated by the narrower width of the ischium. Now adequate space exists between the neck and ischium, and there is no ischium beneath the neck ROI. This is an example of poor pelvis positioning in **A;** the patient must be lying flat on the pelvis as in **B.** These two scans *cannot* be compared for rate of bone loss. The scan in **B** should be considered a new baseline and compared with a properly performed follow-up scan in the future.

4. In order to compare proximal femur BMD over time, the positioning must be exactly reproduced and the angle of the neck box ROI must be the same (see Fig. 36-23). Check these points on the baseline, as well as serial scan images:

• The lesser trochanter must be the same size and shape. If not, change the hip rotation. More rotation will make the lesser trochanter appear smaller.

• The femoral shaft must be abducted the same amount. Adjust the abduction or adduction accordingly.

• The neck box ROI is automatically placed perpendicular to the midline, so the midline must be at the same angle in each scan. If it is not, reposition as required. If positioning is not the problem, proper software adjustments must be made according to the manufacturer's guidelines.

5. One manufacturer provides dual-hip software that scans both hips without repositioning. However, scoliosis, diseases that cause unilateral weakness (e.g., polio, stroke), or unilateral osteoarthritis of the hip may cause left-right differences. If arthritis is present, the less affected hip should be scanned because arthritis can cause increased density in the medial hip and shorten-ing of the femoral neck (Fig. 36-29). In cases of unilateral disease, scan the less affected hip. A fractured or replaced hip with orthopedic hardware should not be scanned. Always reporting on the lowest region of interest is important.

6. In older, DOS-based GE Lunar systems, air is a problem in small patients who do not have adequate soft tissue lateral, anterior, or posterior to the proximal femur. For these GE Lunar scans, no air should be present in the ROI because it will cause an incorrect soft tissue reading and thus affect the BMD. Use of tissue equivalent bags properly and consistently is important in obtaining proper analysis.

7. The limits of the technology are taxed by patients who are very thin or thick or have very low bone mass. These problems are revealed by poor bone edge detection or a mottled appearance of the image, or both. Use a fast speed for thin patients and slow speed for thick patients. Some images show the bone edges, and it is obvious when the proper edge cannot be detected. For images that do not show the bone edges, the area values must be checked and compared. A very large *Ward's triangle* area or a very small trochanter area can indicate that the bone edges are not being properly detected. The operator's manual may not adequately cover these problems. The technologist is responsible for recognizing problems and querying the manufacturer's applications department about the best ways to handle such difficulties. If a patient is deemed unsuitable for a DXA hip scan, a physician can suggest alternative scans at other anatomic sites using DXA or other technologies. Newer software and improved technologies are minimizing the incidence of these situations. Accuracy of scan values is questioned in these situations also.

8. A basic checklist for a good DXA hip scan (see Fig. 36-23, *A*) includes the following:

• The lesser trochanter is small and round or barely visible.

• The midline of the femoral body is parallel to the lateral edge of the scan.

• Adequate space is present between the ischium and femoral neck.

• The midline through the femoral neck is reasonably placed, resulting in a reasonable angle for the femoral neck box.

• The proximal, distal, and lateral edges of the scan field are properly located.

• No air is present in the scan field on GE Lunar scans.

Fig. 36-29 Hip arthritis. Note the increased density in the medial hip and the foreshort-ened femoral neck. Technologist's intervention may be required in this situation. Notation of difficulty with positioning and known arthritis should be mentioned on the patient history form.

Proximal forearm

Two important ROIs are present on the DXA forearm scan: the ultradistal region, which is the site of the common Colles fracture, and the one-third (33%) region, which measures an area that is primarily cortical bone near the midforearm (see Table 36-1). Although the ulna is used for length measurement and available for analysis, only the radius results are reported. The following guidelines can aid in positioning, acquisition, and analysis of forearm DXA scans and evaluating the validity of the scans:

1. The nondominant forearm is scanned because it is expected to have slightly lower BMD than the dominant arm. A forearm should not be scanned in patients with a history of wrist fracture, internal hardware, or severe deformity resulting from arthritis. If both forearms are unsuitable for scanning, other anatomic sites should be considered.

2. The same chair should be used for all patients to ensure consistency over time. The chair should have a back but no wheels or arms. Selection of the chairs will vary from manufacturer to manufacturer.

3. At the time of the baseline scan, the forearm should be measured according to the manufacturer's instructions. The ulna is measured from the ulna styloid to the olecranon process. The distal one third of this measurement is used to place the one-third, or 33%, ROI. The baseline measurement should be noted and then used again for follow-up scans to ensure placing the one-third region at the same anatomic point on each scan. Newer equipment and automated software no longer require measurements or storage of that information. The directions for determining the starting and ending locations of the scan must be followed exactly

(Fig. 36-30, *A*). A common problem is that a scan is too short in the proximal direction, which makes it impossible to place the one-third region properly.

4. The forearm must be straight and centered in the scan field (see Fig. 36-30, *A*). Correct use of the appropriate positioning aids must be applied. For Hologic scanners, this is the only scan that requires adequate amounts of air in the scan field. Soft tissue must surround the ulna and radius, and several lines of air must be present on the ulnar side. If the forearm is wide, the scan must be manually set for a wider scan region so that adequate air is included.

5. Motion is a common problem in forearm scan acquisition (see Fig. 36-30, *A*). The patient should be in a comfortable position so that the arm does not move during the scan. The hand and proximal forearm can be secured with straps or tape placed outside the scan field. Avoid unnecessary conversation during the scan to minimize movement.

Fig. 36-30 DXA forearm scans. **A,** This DXA forearm scan demonstrates several positioning and acquisition mistakes: The forearm is not straight or centered in the scan field, and motion has occurred in the proximal radius and ulna. **B,** This scan demonstrates good patient positioning, scan acquisition, and scan analysis.

6. The placement of the ultradistal ROI should be just below the radial end-plate. This placement is easy to reproduce on serial scans. The ultradistal ROI is subject to low BMD, which could create bone edge detection problems. The bone edge should be adjusted if necessary. Baseline and serial scan bone edges must match for proper analysis, comparison, and report of percent change over time.

7. A basic checklist for a good DXA forearm scan (Fig. 36-30, *B*) includes the following:

- The forearm is straight and centered in the scan field.
- Adequate amounts of soft tissue and air are included.
- No motion is present.
- The proximal and distal ends of the scan field are properly placed.
- Bone edges are properly and consistently placed.
- No artifacts are present in the scan field.

Other Bone Densitometry Techniques

CENTRAL (OR AXIAL) SKELETAL MEASUREMENTS

QCT is an established method using cross-sectional CT images from commercial scanners equipped with QCT software and a bone mineral reference standard. QCT has the unique ability to provide separate BMD measurements of trabecular and cortical bone and true volumetric density measurements in grams per cubic centimeter (g/cm^3). QCT of the spine is used to measure the trabecular bone within the vertebral bodies to estimate vertebral fracture risk and age-related bone loss; it is also used for the follow-up of osteoporosis and other metabolic bone diseases and their therapies (Fig. 36-31). Other current uses of QCT involve measuring BMD at the hip and producing high-resolution three-dimensional images to analyze trabecular bone architecture.

Lateral lumbar spine DXA scans can be performed with the patient in the supine position with scanners that have C-arms (see Fig. 36-13). Decubitus lateral scans are obtained with fixed-arm scanners. Lateral spine DXA allows partial removal of the outer cortical bone and thus gives a truer measurement of the inner trabecular bone, which experiences earlier bone loss and is more responsive to therapy (see Fig. 36-10). However, lateral spine DXA is often confounded by superposition of the ribs and iliac crest with the vertebral bodies and has poorer precision than AP spine DXA. Lateral DXA is not widely used in clinical practice.

Vertebral fracture assessment (VFA) is the term that encompasses looking at the spine "morphometrically" in the lateral projection, which means visualizing the shapes of the vertebral bodies of both the lumbar and thoracic spine to determine if there has been some deformity with resultant compression of the vertebral bodies.

Fig. 36-31 Examples of various elements of a QCT examination: *upper left,* lateral scout image of lumbar spine; *upper right,* localizer lines for midvertebral slices through L1 and L2; *lower left,* CT slice showing the calibration phantom below the patient; *lower right,* elliptic ROI positioned in the trabecular bone of the vertebral body.

Dual-energy vertebral assessment (DVA), lateral assessment (LVA), instant vertebral analysis (IVA), and radiologic vertebral assessment (RVA) are synonymous for this process. The manufacturers of bone densitometers have devised their own way of either enhancing the image or improving the scan acquisition and analysis. Images are obtained in both dual-energy acquisition and the single-energy method. Both methods are comparable.

Unlike traditional lateral spine x-rays, VFA has the capability of visualizing both the lumbar and thoracic spine as one continuous image. This aids the interpreting physician in identifying the vertebral level where abnormalities are present. AP views can also be incorporated into a VFA study. For an accurate representation of the vertebral bodies, the patient's spine must be as straight as possible.

The AP view can help identify artifacts and deformities, such as scoliosis. Scoliosis is the one condition that can cause the greatest challenge in VFA and possibly make a study "unreadable." VFA also exposes the patient to about one one-hundredth the radiation dose of just a single lateral x-ray image. VFA is an adjunct to DXA scanning in cases when a patient might not have been x-rayed for vertebral fracture beforehand. General spine x-ray is still the "gold standard" for visualizing abnormalities in the spine.

VFA uses SXA (for image only) or DXA (for image and BMD) lateral scans of the thoracic and lumbar spines from the level of about T4 to L5 (Fig. 36-32). The images are used to determine vertebral shape abnormalities that may indicate vertebral fragility fractures, which are a strong risk factor for future vertebral fractures. The upper right corner of Fig. 36-32 shows the Genant grading system. The three columns on the right show the types of fracture, and the rows show the grades of severity. Seeing a severe fracture is easy, and seeing a moderate fracture is relatively easy, but it is difficult to determine if a mild deformity is normal for the patient or the beginning of a problem.

VFA should be interpreted by a trained physician by viewing the images on the scan monitor (Fig. 36-33).

Fig. 36-32 MXA scan to detect vertebral shape abnormalities. The Genant grading system is in the upper right corner.

(Courtesy Hologic, Inc., Bedford, Mass.)

Fig. 36-33 Dual VFA.

Total body/body composition

Whole-body DXA measures bone mass (i.e., area, BMC, BMD) and *body composition* for the total body and subregions of the body (e.g., arms, legs, trunk). Body composition can be measured as fat and fat-free mass (with or without BMC) in grams or percent body fat (Fig. 36-34). Careful positioning is required to separate the bones of the forearm and lower leg. Obese patients present a problem when not all of the body will fit in the scan field. The ROIs must be carefully placed according to the manufacturer's instructions. Having internal or external artifacts that cannot be removed is not unusual, and the effect of such artifacts depends on size, density, and location. For example, hip joint replacement hardware will have more effect than a woman's thin wedding band. Each DXA laboratory should have written procedures so that all patients are scanned and analyzed consistently. All deviations from normal and artifacts should be noted for the interpreting physician. Whole-body DXA data are useful for studying energy expenditure, energy stores, protein mass, skeletal mineral status, and relative hydration. These measurements have been used in research studies and clinical trials of, among others, osteoporosis therapies, obesity and weight change, fat and lean distribution, and diabetes. Clinically, whole-body scans are used routinely in pediatrics and for body fat analysis in athletes and patients with underweight disorders (e.g., anorexia nervosa).

Total Body Bone Density

COMMENTS: D:\data\desktop.dfb

Reference: Total

BMD (g/cm²)   YA T-Score

Age (years)

Trend: Total

%Change vs Baseline

Age (years)

Region	BMD[1] (g/cm²)	Young-Adult[2] T-Score	Age-Matched[3] Z-Score
Head	2.467	-	-
Arms	1.115	-	-
Legs	1.341	-	-
Trunk	1.012	-	-
Ribs	0.748	-	-
Pelvis	1.277	-	-
Spine	1.186	-	-
Total	1.278	1.9	2.1

A

| Trend: Total | | | Change vs | |
Measured Date	Age (years)	BMD[1] (g/cm²)	Baseline (%)	Baseline (%/yr)
05.14.02	35.1	1.278	0.0	0.0
06.22.00	33.2	1.278	baseline	baseline

Total Body Tissue Quantitation

Composition Reference: Total

Tissue (%Fat)   Centile

Age (years)

Composition Trend: Total

Total Body (%Fat)   Tissue (%Fat) [Gray]

Age (years)

| Trend: Total | | | | | | | | | |
Measured Date	Age (years)	Tissue (%Fat)	Centile[2,3]	T.Mass (kg)	Region (%Fat)	Tissue (g)	Fat (g)	Lean (g)	BMC (g)	Fat Free (g)
05.14.02	35.1	32.3	58	62.9	30.8	59,950	19,346	40,603	2,956	43,559
06.22.00	33.2	32.5	61	63.2	31.0	60,256	19,560	40,697	2,922	43,618

B

| Trend: Fat Distribution | | | | | |
Measured Date	Age (years)	Android (%Fat)	Gynoid (%Fat)	A/G Ratio	Total Body (%Fat)
05.14.02	35.1	24.7	44.5	0.55	32.3
06.22.00	33.2	26.3	45.0	0.58	32.5

Fig. 36-34 A, Hologic DXA whole-body scan with printout of total body composition results. **B,** The percent body fat *(% Fat)* is reported.

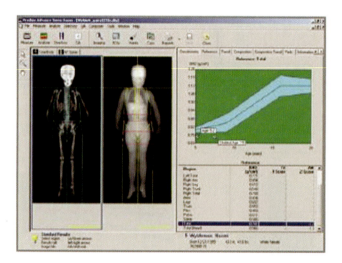

Pediatric DXA is truly in its infancy, but it is possible to make some general statements. The diagnostic capabilities of most scanners start with ages 3 to 5, and some use separate pediatric and adult databases. Experts recommend a whole body scan, as well as spine or hip, or both, and use of BMC to overcome artifacts resulting from bone size. The technologist must carefully ensure that the correct parameters are selected on the machine, such as speed, current, and pixel size. Because pediatric patients have not reached peak bone mass, interpreters only report the Z-score. This compares patients with their physical and chronologic peers. T-scores are not comparable for patients younger than the age of 20 (Fig. 36-35).

In addition to measuring bone mineral, DXA systems have been used for geometric measurements of the hip. The *hip axis length* (HAL), defined as the distance along the femoral neck axis from the base of the greater trochanter to the inner pelvic brim, has been identified as an independent indicator of hip fracture risk. On the basis of results from the Study of Osteoporotic Fractures, each SD increase in HAL (≈6 mm) approximately doubles the risk for hip fracture. At this time HAL is predominantly used as a research tool. It is hoped that future research will define the clinical role of HAL for assessing fracture risk along with other risk factors.

Fig. 36-35 Pediatric BMD and soft tissue assessment.

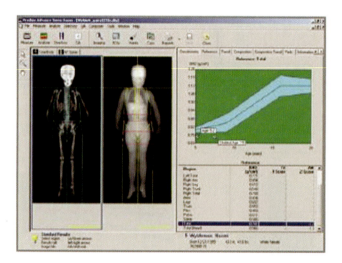

Bone densitometry

PERIPHERAL SKELETAL MEASUREMENTS

Peripheral bone density measurements include scans at the hand, forearm, heel, and tibia. Other skeletal sites are being investigated. The scanners are smaller, some even portable, making the scans more available to the public and less expensive than conventional DXA. Peripheral measurements can predict *overall risk of fragility fracture* to the same degree as measurements at central skeletal sites but are not generally accepted for following skeletal response to therapy.

Radiographic absorptiometry (RA) is a modern adaptation of the early bone density technique. Digital RA uses a hand radiograph that is scanned (digitized) into a computer (Fig. 36-36, *A*). ROIs are placed on the digital image of the metacarpals, and estimated BMD is reported (Fig. 36-36, *B*).

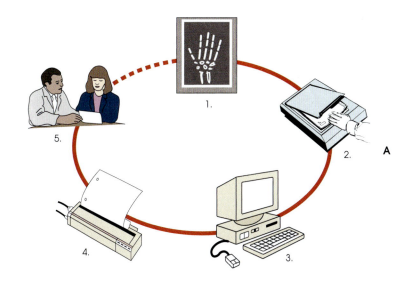

Selected Measurement

Date of recording	1/28/01
Est. BMD	0.480 g/cm²
T-Score	-2.18
Z-Score	-2.51
T-Score (% of H.Y.A)	82
Z-Score (%)	81
Porosity (1-19)	8.2

Fig. 36-36 Pronosco X-posure System for digital BMD estimates. **A,** The five steps of acquiring and digitizing a standard hand x-ray, keying in patient data, receiving a printout, and discussing results with the patient. **B,** A partial report showing the automatically placed ROIs on the metacarpals, estimated BMD, T- and Z-scores, and a unique porosity measurement.

(Courtesy Pronosco A/S, Vedbaek, Denmark.)

Other bone densitometry techniques

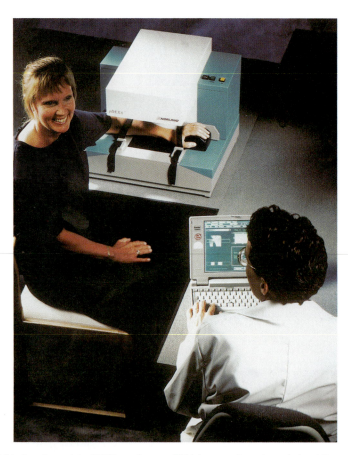

Fig. 36-37 Norland model pDEXA performs pDXA bone mineral analysis of the wrist.

(Courtesy Norland, Inc., Ft. Atkinson, Wis.)

Single energy x-ray absorptiometry (SXA), peripheral dual energy x-ray absorptiometry (pDXA), and peripheral quantitative computed tomography (pQCT) are adaptations of DXA or QCT for measuring the thinner, easier-to-penetrate, peripheral skeletal sites. Most scanners measure the wrist (Fig. 36-37) or the heel.

With *quantitative ultrasound* (QUS) of the heel, ultrasound waves are transmitted laterally through the calcaneus using water, gel, or alcohol (dry system) as a coupling medium (Fig. 36-38). Attenuation increases as the velocity of the ultrasound waves increases, and normal bone attenuates more than osteoporotic bone. These properties of bone and ultrasound signals permit the assessment of the QUS parameters of broadband ultrasound attenuation (BUA) and speed of sound (SOS). BUA, SOS, and proprietary combinations of the two (e.g., stiffness) characterize the mechanical properties of bone relating to elasticity, strength, and consequently fracture risk. QUS measurements at the heel have been found to be good predictors of spine fractures in the elderly when degenerative disease compromises the DXA spine scan. Other measurement sites, some of which are under investigation, include the finger, tibia, iliac crest, vertebral arch and spinous processes, and femoral neck and greater trochanter.

Fig. 36-38 QUS of the heel uses either water as a coupling mechanism *(top)* or a dry system using a gel on the transducers *(bottom)*.

(Courtesy GE Lunar, Madison, Wis.)

Conclusion

The main purpose of bone densitometry is to assist the diagnosis of osteoporosis by detecting low bone mass before fractures occur. Osteoporosis is a preventable, as well as treatable, disease. Patients concerned about their risk of this disease should consult their physicians for a complete evaluation.

DXA scans of the hip and spine are the most widely performed techniques, but simpler, less expensive peripheral scans of the extremities are also available. Technologists performing these scans must be properly trained in scanner quality control, patient scan positioning, acquisition, and analysis. This will ensure accurate and precise bone density results.

Knowledge of the current treatments and expected changes is important for complete technical evaluation of the scan results. History taking and data input are valuable tools for completion of this examination. Technologists are frontline educators to patients, and knowledge in the field is ever changing. The technologist must stay informed with the treatment options and their effects on bone density.

Quality assurance is a key factor in accurate and precise DXA acquisition and analysis. Technology changes frequently, so it is important for the technologist to understand the changes within the industry. The technologist must be able to oversee these applications to properly maintain and update equipment.

Definition of Terms

adult sprue Disease characterized by hypersensitivity to gluten (wheat protein).

anthropomorphic Simulating human form.

ALARA (as low as reasonably achievable) Principle of reducing patient radiation exposure and dose to lowest reasonable amounts.

areal technique See *projectional technique.*

array-beam collimation Dual energy x-ray absorptiometry system that uses a narrow "slit" x-ray collimator and a multielement detector. The motion is in one direction only, which greatly reduces scan time and permits supine lateral spine scans. It introduces a slight geometric distortion at the outer edges, which necessitates careful centering of the object of interest.

biochemical markers Laboratory tests on blood and urine to detect levels of bone formation or resorption.

body composition Results from whole-body scans obtained by dual energy x-ray absorptiometry; reported as lean mass in grams, percent body fat, and bone mineral density of the total body and selected regions of interest.

bone densitometry Art and science of measuring the bone mineral content and density of specific anatomic sites or the whole body.

bone mass General term for the amount of mineral in a bone.

bone mineral content (BMC) Measure of bone mineral in the total area of a region of interest.

bone mineral density (BMD) Measure of bone mineral per unit area of a region of interest.

bone remodeling Process of bone resorption by osteoclasts, followed by bone formation by osteoblasts. The relative rates of resorption and formation determine whether bone mass increases, remains stable, or decreases.

compare feature Software feature of dual energy x-ray absorptiometry that replicates the size and placement of regions of interest from the reference scan to the follow-up scan.

cortical bone Dense, compact outer shell of all bones and the shafts of the long bones; supports weight, resists bending and twisting, and accounts for about 80% of the skeletal mass.

CZT Cadmium zinc telluride, a detector material.

discordance Patient may have T-score indicating osteoporosis at one anatomic site but not at another site or by one modality but not by another.

dual energy x-ray absorptiometry (DXA) Bone density measurement technique using an x-ray source separated into two energies. It has good accuracy and precision and can scan essentially any anatomic site, making it the most versatile of the bone density techniques.

dual photon absorptiometry (DPA) Obsolete method of measuring bone density at the hip or spine using a radioisotope source that produces two sources of photons; replaced by dual energy x-ray absorptiometry.

fragility fractures Nontraumatic fractures resulting from low bone mass, usually at the hip, spinal vertebrae, wrist, proximal humerus, or ribs.

HIPAA The American Health Insurance Portability and Accountability Act of 1996 (HIPAA) is a set of rules to be followed by health plans, doctors, hospitals, and other health care providers. HIPAA took effect on April 14, 2003. In the health care and medical profession, the great challenge that HIPAA has created is the assurance that all patient account handling, billing, and medical records are HIPAA compliant.

hip axis length (HAL) Distance along the femoral neck axis from the base of the greater trochanter to the inner pelvic brim. An independent indicator of hip fracture risk.

hyperparathyroidism Disease caused by excessive secretion of parathyroid hormone (PTH) from one or more parathyroid glands, resulting in excessive calcium in the blood. Affects cortical bone more than trabecular bone.

kyphosis Exaggerated outward curvature of the thoracic spine, also called *dowager's hump.*

longitudinal quality control Manufacturer-defined procedures performed on a regular basis to ensure that patients are scanned on properly functioning equipment with stable calibration. Scanning must be postponed until identified problems are corrected.

mean A statistic commonly called *the average.* The sum of the data values divided by the number of data values.

morphometric x-ray absorptiometry (MXA) Lateral scans of the thoracic and lumbar spine using single or dual x-ray absorptiometry to determine vertebral abnormalities or fractures from the shapes of the vertebrae.

multiview image reconstruction (MVIR) Imaging technique perfected in computed tomography, wherein multiple images are acquired.

osteoblasts Bone-building cells that fill the pits left by resorption with new bone.

osteoclasts Bone-destroying cells that break down and remove old bone, leaving pits.

osteomalacia Bone disorder characterized by variable amounts of uncalcified osteoid matrix.

osteopenia Reduction in bone mass, putting a person at increased risk of developing osteoporosis. By World Health Organization criteria, it is a bone mineral density or bone mineral content T-score between -1 and -2.5.

osteophytosis Form of degenerative joint disease resulting from mechanical stress that increases the measured spinal bone mineral density.

osteoporosis Systemic skeletal disease characterized by low bone mass and deterioration of the bone structure, resulting in decreased mechanical competence of bone and an increase in susceptibility to fracture. By World Health Organization criteria, it is a bone mineral density or bone mineral content T-score of less than −2.5.

overall risk of fragility fracture Risk of suffering an unspecified fragility fracture. The risk for hip fracture specifically is best measured at the hip.

peak bone mass Maximum bone mass, usually achieved between 30 and 35 years of age. Population mean peak bone mass is used as a reference point for the T-score.

pencil-beam collimation Dual energy x-ray absorptiometry system using a circular pinhole x-ray collimator that produces a narrow x-ray stream, which is received by a single detector. Its motion is serpentine (or raster) across or along the length of the body. Modern systems have improved scan time and image quality. Off-centering of the object does not cause geometric distortion.

percent coefficient of variation (%CV) Statistic used to compare standard deviations from different datasets, which may have different means. Also a measure of precision. Calculated as the SD divided by the mean, times 100. A smaller %CV indicates better precision.

peripheral dual energy x-ray absorptiometry (pDXA) Dual energy x-ray absorptiometry system designed to scan only the peripheral skeleton; smaller and simpler to operate than DXA scanners.

peripheral quantitative computed tomography (pQCT) Dedicated QCT system designed to measure bone density on the peripheral skeleton, usually the forearm.

primary osteoporosis Osteoporosis not caused by an underlying disease, classified as Type I or Type II.

projectional (or areal) technique Two-dimensional representation of a three-dimensional object.

quantitative computed tomography (QCT) System for quantitative CT measurements of bone density, allowing true measurement of volume and separation of trabecular and cortical bone; usually measured at spine or forearm, sometimes at hip.

quantitative ultrasound (QUS) Quantitative measurement of bone properties related to mechanical competence using ultrasound. The results are reported in terms of broadband ultrasound attenuation (BUA), speed of sound (SOS), and a nonstandardized proprietary mathematic combination of the two, called the stiffness or Quantitative Ultrasound Index (QUI). It predicts overall or spine fracture risk without using ionizing radiation and is usually measured at the calcaneus.

radiogrammetry Older method of measuring bone loss by comparing the outer diameter and inner medullary diameter of small tubular bones, usually the finger phalanges, or metacarpals.

radiographic absorptiometry (RA) Visual comparison of hand x-ray density with a known standard in the exposure field.

reference population Large, sex-matched, community-based population used to determine the average bone mineral density and standard deviation at each age; used as reference base for T-scores and Z-scores; may also be matched on ethnicity and weight.

regions of interest (ROI) Defined portion of bone density scans where the bone mineral density is calculated; may be placed manually or automatically by computer software.

scintillation counter Counter employing a photomultiplier tube for the detection of radiation.

secondary osteoporosis Osteoporosis caused by an underlying disease.

serial scans Sequential scans, usually performed 12, 18, or 24 months apart, to measure changes in bone density. Scans are best done on the same scanner or on a new scanner calibrated to the original scanner.

Shewhart Control Chart rules Classic quality control rules based on comparing a data value to the mean and standard deviation of a set of similar values.

sieverts (Sv) Measurement of effective radiation dose to a patient. Bone density doses are measured in microsieverts (μSv), which are one one-millionth of one sievert.

single energy x-ray absorptiometry (SXA) Bone density technique for the peripheral skeleton using a single energy x-ray source and an external medium, such as water, to correct for the effects of soft tissue attenuation. Scanners are smaller and simpler to operate than dual energy x-ray absorptiometry scanners.

single photon absorptiometry (SPA) Obsolete method of measuring bone density at the forearm using a single radioisotope source; replaced by single energy x-ray absorptiometry.

smart fan-beam technology Narrow slit x-ray collimator oriented parallel to the longitudinal axis of the patient.

standard deviation (SD) Measure of the variability of the data values about their mean value.

standardized BMD (sBMD) Result of converting bone mineral density values from one manufacturer to values that can be compared with other manufacturers by applying mathematic formulas. Reported in milligrams per centimeter squared (mg/cm^2) to differentiate it from BMD.

subtraction technique Removal of the density attributable to soft tissue so that the remaining density belongs only to bone.

T-score Number of standard deviations the individual's bone mineral density (BMD) is from the average BMD for sex-matched young normal peak bone mass.

trabecular bone Delicate, latticework structure within bones that adds strength without excessive weight; supports compressive loading at the spine, hip, and calcaneus and is also found in the ends of long bones, such as the distal radius.

Type I osteoporosis Primary osteoporosis related to postmenopausal status.

Type II osteoporosis Primary osteoporosis related to aging.

vertebral fracture assessment (VFA) Encompasses looking at the spine "morphometrically" in the lateral projection. Common synonymous terms: DVA (dual-energy vertebral assessment), LVA (lateral vertebral assessment), IVA (instant vertebral assessment, and RVA (radiologic vertebral assessment).

volumetric density Bone mineral density calculated by dividing by the true three-dimensional volume.

Ward's triangle Region on the proximal femur lying on the border of the femoral neck and greater trochanter; has low bone mineral density.

Z-score Number of standard deviations the individual's bone mineral density (BMD) is from the average BMD for sex- and age-matched reference group.

Selected bibliography

Blake G, Wahner H, Fogelman I: *The evaluation of osteoporosis: dual energy x-ray absorptiometry and ultrasound in clinical practice,* London, 1998, Martin Dunitz.

Blunt BA et al: Good clinical practice and audits for dual x-ray absorptiometry and x-ray imaging laboratories and quality assurance centers involved in clinical drug trials, private practice, and research, *J Clin Densitometry* 1:323, 1998.

Bonnick SL: *Bone densitometry in clinical practice: application and interpretation,* Totowa, NJ, 1998, Humana Press.

Bonnick SL, Lewis LA: *Bone densitometry for technologists: application and interpretation,* Totowa, NJ, 2001, Humana Press.

Genant HK, Guglielmi G, Jergas M: *Bone densitometry and osteoporosis,* New York, 1997, Springer-Verlag.

International Society for Clinical Densitometry: *Official positions* (website): www.iscd.org/Visitors/positions/OfficialPositionsText.cfm. Accessed July 20, 2006.

National Institutes of Health Consensus Development Panel on Osteoporosis Prevention, Diagnosis, and Therapy: Osteoporosis prevention, diagnosis, and therapy, *JAMA* 285:785, 2001.

National Osteoporosis Foundation physician's guide, Washington, DC, 1998, National Osteoporosis Foundation.

Rosen CJ: *Osteoporosis: diagnostic and therapeutic principles,* Totowa, NJ, 1997, Humana Press.

Resources for Information and Instruction

American College of Radiology: *ACR standard for the performance of adult dual or single x-ray absorptiometry (DXA/pDXA/SXA).* Contact the Standards & Accreditation Department, American College of Radiology, 1891 Preston White Dr., Reston, VA 22091.

American Registry of Radiologic Technologists: *Provides a postprimary examination leading to a certificate of added qualifications in bone densitometry.* For details see the Examinee Handbook for Bone Densitometry. Contact the American Registry of Radiologic Technologists, 1255 Northland Dr., St. Paul, MN 55120-1155. Internet address: www.arrt.org

American Society of Radiologic Technologists: *Approved elective curriculum in bone densitometry for radiography programs.* Contact the American Society of Radiologic Technologists, 15000 Central Ave. SE, Albuquerque, NM 87123. Internet address: www.asrt.org

International Society for Clinical Densitometry: Certification courses, annual and regional meetings, continuing education, newsletter, *Journal of Clinical Densitometry,* and website with links. Contact International Society for Clinical Densitometry, 2025 M St. NW, Suite 800, Washington, DC 20036. Internet address: www.iscd.org

National Osteoporosis Foundation: Excellent source of osteoporosis information and educational materials for technologists, physicians, and patients. Contact the National Osteoporosis Foundation, 1232 22nd St. NW, Washington, DC 20037-1292. Internet address: www.nof.org

Scanner manufacturers: source for technologist instruction and answers to scanner-specific application questions. Refer to the operator's manual for contact information.

Surgeon General's Report website: www.surgeongeneral.gov

National Osteoporosis Foundation website: www.NOF.org

StrongerBones.org

Mindways.com

37

RADIATION ONCOLOGY

LEILA A. BUSSMAN-YEAKEL

AP pelvic radiograph demonstrating contrast in the bladder and its relationship to the prostate gland.

Principles of Radiation Oncology

Radiation oncology,[*] or *radiation therapy,* is one of three principal modalities used in the treatment of cancer. The others are surgery and chemotherapy. In radiation therapy for malignancies, *tumors* or *lesions* are treated with *cancericidal doses* of ionizing radiation as prescribed by a *radiation oncologist,* a physician specialized in the treatment of malignant disease with radiation. The goals of the treatment are to precisely deliver a cancericidal dose of radiation to the tumor but to limit as much as possible the dose of radiation received by normal, noncancerous tissues. These dual tasks make this form of treatment complex and often challenging. Input from all members of the radiation oncology team is crucial in developing the optimum treatment plan or approach for a patient.

Cancer treatment requires a multidisciplinary approach. First, diagnostic radiologic studies such as radiographs, computed tomographic (CT) scans, magnetic resonance imaging (MRI), positron emission tomography (PET) scans, and/or sonograms are obtained to acquire information about the location and anatomic extent of the tumor. Second, a tissue specimen (*biopsy*) is removed surgically. A *pathologist* then examines the tissue to determine whether the lesion is cancerous. Once cancer is diagnosed, the plan for the best treatment is determined through consultation with various *oncology* specialists (e.g., surgical *oncologist,* radiation oncologist, and/or medical oncologist).

Although radiation oncology may be used as the only method of treatment for malignant disease, a more common approach is to use radiation in conjunction with surgery, chemotherapy, or both. Some cancer patients may be treated only with surgery or chemotherapy; however,

---

*Almost all italicized words on the succeeding pages are defined at the end of the chapter.

approximately 75% of all diagnosed cancer patients are treated with radiation. The choice of treatment can depend on a number of patient variables such as the patient's overall physical and emotional condition, the histologic type of the disease, and the extent and anatomic position of the tumor. If a tumor is small and its margins are well defined, a surgical approach alone may be prescribed. If the disease is *systemic,* a chemotherapeutic approach may be chosen. Most tumors, however, exhibit degrees of size, invasion, and spread and require variations in the treatment approach that in all likelihood will include radiation treatments administered as an adjunct to or in conjunction with surgery or chemotherapy.

Radiation is generally used after surgery when a patient is deemed to be at high risk for tumor recurrence in the *surgical bed.* The risk of recurrence is considered to be increased in the following situations:

- When the surgical margin between normal tissue and cancerous tissue is minimal (less than 2 cm)
- When the margin is positive for cancer, (i.e., when cancerous tissue is not completely removed)
- When the tumor is incompletely resected because of it large size and/or its relationship with normal vital structures
- When the cancer has spread to adjacent lymph nodes

Thus the radiation can be used as definitive (primary) cancer treatment or adjuvant treatment (i.e., in combination with another form of therapy). It can also be used for *palliation.*

Radiation treatments most often are delivered on a daily basis, Monday through Friday, for 2 to 8 weeks. The length of time and the total dose of radiation delivered depend on the type of cancer being treated and the purpose of treatment (*cure* or palliation). Prescribed dosages of radiation can range from 2000 centigray (cGy) for palliation up to 8000 cGy for curative intent (total doses). The delivery of a small amount of radiation per day (180 to 200 cGy) for a certain number

of treatments, instead of one large dose, is termed *fractionation.* Because these smaller doses of radiation are more easily tolerated by normal tissue, fractionation can help minimize the acute toxic effect a patient experiences during treatment, as well as the possible long-term side effects of treatment.

The precision and accuracy necessary to administer high doses of radiation to tumors while not harming normal tissue require the combined effort of all members of the radiation oncology team. Members of this team include the radiation oncologist, a physicist, dosimetrists, radiation therapists, and oncology nurses.

The radiation oncologist prescribes the quantity of radiation and determines the anatomic region(s) to be treated. The *medical physicist* is responsible for calibration and maintenance of the radiation-producing equipment. The physicist also advises the physician about dosage calculations and complex treatment techniques. The *medical dosimetrist* devises a plan for delivering the treatments in a manner to best meet the physician's goals of irradiating the tumor while protecting vital normal structures. The *radiation therapist* is responsible for obtaining radiographs or CT scans that localize the area to be treated, administering the treatments, keeping accurate records of the dose delivered each day, and monitoring the patient's physical and emotional well-being. Educating patients about potential radiation side effects and assisting patients with the management of these side effects are often the responsibilities of the oncology nurse.

The duties and responsibilities of the radiation therapist are more thoroughly described elsewhere in this chapter. In addition, more information is provided about the circumstances in which radiation is used to treat cancer. The steps necessary to prepare a patient for treatment are also described. These steps include (1) simulation, (2) evolution of the optimum treatment plan in dosimetry, and (3) treatment delivery. Current techniques and future trends are also discussed.

Historical Development

Ionizing radiation was originally used to obtain a radiographic image of internal anatomy for diagnostic purposes. The resultant image depended on many variables, including the energy of the beam, the processing techniques, the material on which the image was recorded, and, most importantly, the amount of energy absorbed by the various organs of the body. The transfer of energy from the beam of radiation to the biologic system and the observation of the effects of this interaction became the foundation of radiation oncology.

Two of the most obvious and sometimes immediate biologic effects observed during the early diagnostic procedures were epilation (loss of hair) and erythema (reddening of the skin). Epilation and erythema resulted primarily from the great amount of energy absorbed by the skin during radiographic procedures. These short-term radiation-induced effects afforded radiographic practitioners an opportunity to expand the use of radiation to treat conditions ranging from relatively benign maladies such as hypertrichosis (excessive hair), acne, and boils to grotesque and malignant diseases such as lupus vulgaris and skin cancer.

Ionizing radiation was first applied for the treatment of a more in-depth lesion on Jan. 29, 1896, when Dr. Émile H. Grubbé is reported to have irradiated a woman with carcinoma of the left breast. This event occurred only 3 months after the discovery of x-rays by Dr. W.K. Röntgen (Table 37-1). Although Dr. Grubbé neither expected nor observed any dramatic results from the irradiation, the event is significant simply because it occurred.

The first reported curative treatment using ionizing radiation was performed by Dr. Clarence E. Skinner of New Haven, Connecticut, in January 1902. Dr. Skinner treated a woman who had a diagnosed malignant fibrosarcoma. Over the next 2 years and 3 months the woman received a total of 136 applications of the x-rays. In April 1909, 7 years after initial application of the radiation, the woman was free of disease and considered "cured."

As data were collected, the interest in radiation therapy grew. More sophisticated equipment, a greater understanding of the effects of ionizing radiation, an appreciation for time-dose relationships, and a number of other related medical breakthroughs gave impetus to the interest in radiation therapy that led to the evolution of a distinct medical specialty—radiation oncology.

Cancer

Cancer is a disease process that involves an unregulated, uncontrolled replication of cells; put more simply, the cells do not know when to stop dividing. These abnormal cells grow without regard to normal tissue. They invade adjacent tissues, destroy normal tissue, and create a mass of tumor cells. Cancerous cells can further spread by invading the lymph or blood vessels that drain the area. When tumor cells invade the lymphatic or vascular system, they are transported by that system until they become caught or lodged within a lymph node or an organ such as the liver or lungs, where secondary tumors form. The spread of cancer from the original site to different, remote parts of the body is termed *metastasis*. Once cancer has spread to a distant site via bloodborne metastasis, the patient is considered incurable. Therefore early detection and diagnosis are the keys to curing cancer.

An estimated 1,372,910 persons in the United States were diagnosed with cancer in 2005. This number does not include basal and squamous cell skin cancers, which have high cure rates. These types of cancer are the most common malignant diseases, with more than 1.3 million cases diagnosed in 2000. *The overall lifetime risk for men is 1 in 2 men will develop or die of cancer in their lifetime. For women, the lifetime risk is slightly higher than 1 in 3. Cancer can occur in persons of any age, although the majority of patients are diagnosed after the age of 55 years.*

TABLE 37-1

Significant developments in radiation therapy

Date	Person	Event
1895	W.K. Röntgen	Discovery of x-rays
1896	É. Grubbé	First use of ionizing radiation in treatment of cancer
	A.H. Becquerel	Discovery of radioactive emissions by uranium compounds
1898	M. and P. Curie	Discovery of radium
1902	C.E. Skinner	First documented case of cancer "cure" using ionizing radiation
1906	J. Bergonié and L. Tribondeau	Postulation of first law of radiosensitivity
1932	E.O. Lawrence	Invention of cyclotron
1934	F. Joliot and I. Joliot-Curie	Production of artificial radioactivity
1939	E.O. Lawrence and R.S. Stone	Treatment of cancer patient with neutron beam from cyclotron
1940	D.W. Kerst	Construction of betatron
1951		Installation of first cobalt-60 teletherapy units
1952		Installation of first linear accelerator (Hammersmith Hospital, London)

The most common cancers that occur in the United States are lung, prostate, breast, and colorectal cancer. Prostate cancer is the most common malignancy in men; for women, breast cancer is the most common. In both men and women, the second and third most common cancers are lung and colorectal cancer (Table 37-2).

Cancer is second only to heart disease as the leading cause of death in the United States. Lung cancer is the leading cause of cancer deaths for both men and women. In 2005, an estimated 31% of cancer deaths in men and 27% in women were due to lung cancer. The next most common causes of cancer death are prostate cancer and breast cancer, which respectively account for 10% and 15% of cancer deaths in the United States.

RISK FACTORS
External factors

Many factors can contribute to a person's potential for the development of a *malignancy*. These factors can be external exposure to chemicals, viruses, or radiation within the environment or internal factors such as hormones, genetic mutations, and disorders of the immune system. Cancer commonly is the result of exposure to a *carcinogen,* which is a substance or material that causes cells to undergo malignant transformation and become cancerous. Some of the known carcinogenic agents are listed in Table 37-3. Cigarettes and other tobacco products are the principal cause of cancers of the lung, esophagus, oral cavity/pharynx, and bladder. Cigarette smokers are 10 times more likely to develop lung cancer than are nonsmokers. Occupational exposure to chemicals such as chromium, nickel, or arsenic can also cause lung cancer. A person who smokes and also works with chemical carcinogens is at even greater risk for developing lung cancer than is a nonsmoker. In other words, risk factors can have an additive effect, acting together to initiate or promote the development of cancer.

Another carcinogen is *ionizing radiation.* It was responsible for the development of osteogenic sarcoma in radium-dial painters in the 1920s and 1930s, and it caused the development of skin cancers in pioneer radiologists. Early radiation therapy equipment used in the treatment of cancer often induced a second malignancy in the bone. The low-energy x-rays produced by this equipment were within the photoelectric range of interactions with matter, resulting in a 3:1 preferential absorption in bone compared with soft tissue. Therefore some breast cancer patients who were irradiated developed an osteosarcoma of their ribs after a

15- to 20-year latency period. With the advances in diagnostic and therapeutic equipment and improved knowledge of radiation physics, radiobiology, and radiation safety practices, radiation-induced malignancies have become relatively uncommon, although the potential for their development still exists. In keeping with standard radiation safety guidelines, any dose of radiation, no matter how small, significantly increases the chance of a genetic mutation.

Internal factors

Internal factors are causative factors over which persons have no control. Genetic mutations on individual genes and *chromosomes* have been identified as predisposing factors for the development of cancer. Mutations can be sporadic or hereditary, as in colon cancer. Chromosomal defects have also been identified in other cancers, such as leukemia, Wilms' tumor, retinoblastoma, and breast cancer. Because of their familial pattern of occurrence, breast, ovarian, and colorectal cancer are three major areas currently under study to obtain earlier diagnosis, which increases the cure rate. For example, patients with a family history of breast or ovarian cancer can be tested to see whether they have inherited the altered *BRCA-1* and *BRCA-2* genes. Patients with these altered genes are at a significantly higher risk for developing breast and ovarian cancer. Women identified as carriers of the altered genes can benefit from more intensive and early screening programs in which breast cancer may be diagnosed at a much earlier and thus more curable stage. These patients also have the option of *prophylactic surgery* to remove the breasts or ovaries. Some women, however, still develop cancer in the remaining tissue after surgery.

TABLE 37-2

Top five most common cancers in men and women

Men	Women
1. Prostate	1. Breast
2. Lung and bronchus	2. Lung and bronchus
3. Colon and rectum	3. Colon and rectum
4. Bladder	4. Uterus (endometrium)
5. Melanoma	5. Non-Hodgkin's lymphoma

TABLE 37-3

Carcinogenic agents and the cancers they cause

Carcinogen	Resultant cancer
Cigarette smoking	Cancers of lung, esophagus, bladder, and oral cavity/pharynx
Arsenic, chromium, nickel, hydrocarbons	Lung cancer
Ultraviolet light	Melanoma and nonmelanomatous skin cancers
Benzene	Leukemia
Ionizing radiation	Sarcomas of bone and soft tissue, skin cancer, and leukemia

Familial adenomatous polyposis

Familial adenomatous polyposis (FAP) is a hereditary condition in which the lining of the colon becomes studded with hundreds to thousands of polyps by late adolescence. A mutation in a gene identified as the adenomatous polyposis coli (APC) gene is considered the cause of this abnormal growth of polyps. Virtually all patients with this condition eventually develop colon cancer. Furthermore, they develop cancer at a much earlier age than the normal population. Treatment involves removal of the entire colon and rectum.

Hereditary nonpolyposis colorectal cancer

Hereditary nonpolyposis colorectal cancer (HNPCC) syndrome is a cancer that develops in the proximal colon in the absence of polyps or with fewer than five polyps. It has a familial distribution, occurring in three first-degree relatives in two generations, with at least one person being diagnosed before the age of 50 years. HNPCC has also been associated with the development of cancers of the breast, endometrium, pancreas, and biliary tract.

Familial cancer research

Current research to identify the genes responsible for cancer will assist in detecting cancers at a much earlier stage in high-risk patients. Many institutions have familial cancer programs to provide genetic testing and counseling for persons with strong family histories of cancer. Experts assist in educating persons about their potential risk for developing cancer and the importance of screening and early detection. Genetic testing remains the patient's option, and many patients prefer not to be tested.

TISSUE ORIGINS OF CANCER

Cancers may arise in any human tissue. However, tumors are usually categorized under six general headings according to their tissue of origin (Table 37-4). Ninety percent of cancers arise from *epithelial tissue* and are classified as *carcinomas*. Epithelial tissue lines the free internal and external surfaces of the body. Carcinomas are further subdivided into squamous cell carcinomas and adenocarcinomas based on the type of epithelium from which they arise. For example, a squamous cell carcinoma arises from the surface (squamous) epithelium of a structure. Examples of surface epithelium include the oral cavity, pharynx, bronchus, skin, and cervix. An adenocarcinoma is a cancer that develops in glandular epithelium such as that in the prostate, colon/rectum, lung, breast, or endometrium.

To facilitate the exchange of patient information from one physician to another, a system of classifying tumors based on anatomic and histologic considerations was designed by the International Union Against Cancer and the American Joint Committee for Cancer (AJCC) Staging and End Results Reporting. The AJCC TNM classification (Table 37-5) describes a tumor according to the size of the primary lesion (T), the involvement of the regional lymph nodes (N), and the occurrence of metastasis (M).

TABLE 37-4

Categorization of cancers by tissue of origin

Tissue of origin	Type of tumor
Epithelium	
Surface epithelium	Squamous cell carcinoma
Glandular epithelium	Adenocarcinoma
Connective tissue	
Bone	Osteosarcoma
Fat	Liposarcoma
Lymphoreticular-hematopoietic tissue	
Lymph nodes	Lymphoma
Plasma cells	Multiple myeloma
Blood cells/ bone marrow	Leukemia
Nerve tissue	
Glial tissue	Glioma
Neuroectoderm	Neuroblastoma
Tumors of more than one tissue	
Embryonic kidney	Nephroblastoma
Tumors that do not fit into above categories	
Testis	Seminoma
Thymus	Thymoma

TABLE 37-5

Application of the TNM classification system

Classification	Description of tumor
Stage 0 $T_0N_0M_0$	Occult lesion; no evidence clinically
Stage I $T_1N_0M_0$	Small lesion confined to organ of origin with no evidence of vascular and lymphatic spread or metastasis
Stage II $T_2N_1M_0$	Tumor of less than 5 cm invading surrounding tissue and first-station lymph nodes but no evidence of metastasis
Stage III $T_3N_2M_0$	Extensive lesion greater than 5 cm with fixation to deeper structure and with bone and lymph invasion but no evidence of metastasis
Stage IV $T_4N_3M_1$	More extensive lesion than above or with distant metastasis (M_1)

This is a generalization. Variations of the staging system exist for each tumor site.

Theory

The biologic effectiveness of ionizing radiation in living tissue is dependent partially on the amount of energy that is deposited within the tissue and partially on the condition of the biologic system. The terms used to describe this relationship are *linear energy transfer* (LET) and *relative biologic effectiveness* (RBE).

LET values are expressed in thousands of electron volts deposited per micron of tissue (keV/μm) and will vary depending on the type of radiation being considered. Particles, because of their mass and possible charge, tend to interact more readily with the material through which they are passing and therefore have a greater LET value. For example, a 5-MeV alpha particle has an LET value of 100 keV/mm in tissue; nonparticulate radiations such as 250-kilovolt (peak) (kVp) x-rays and 1.2-MeV gamma rays have much lower LET values: 2.0 and 0.2 keV/mm, respectively.

RBE values are determined by calculating the ratio of the dose from a standard beam of radiation to the dose required of the radiation beam in question to produce a similar biologic effect. The standard beam of radiation is 250-kVp x-rays, and the ratio is set up as follows:

$$RBE = \frac{\text{Standard beam dose to obtain effect}}{\text{Similar effect using beam in question}}$$

As the LET increases, so does the RBE. Some RBE and LET values are listed in Table 37-6.

The effectiveness of ionizing radiation on a biologic system depends not only on the amount of radiation deposited but also on the state of the biologic system. One of the first laws of radiation biology, postulated by Bergonié and Tribondeau, stated in essence that the *radiosensitivity* of a tissue is dependent on the number of *undifferentiated* cells in the tissue, the degree of mitotic activity of the tissue, and the length of time that cells of the tissue remain in active proliferation. Although exceptions exist, the preceding is true in most tissues. The primary target of ionizing radiation is the DNA molecule, and the human cell is most radiosensitive during mitosis. Current research tends to indicate that all cells are equally radiosensitive; however, the manifestation of the radiation injury occurs at different time frames (i.e., acute vs. late effects).

Because tissue cells are composed primarily of water, most of the *ionization* occurs with water molecules. These events are called *indirect effects* and result in the formation of free radicals such as OH, H, and HO_2. These highly reactive free radicals may recombine with no resultant biologic effect, or they may combine with other atoms and molecules to produce biochemical changes that may be deleterious to the cell. The possibility also exists that the radiation may interact with an organic molecule or atom, which may result in the inactivation of the cell; this reaction is called the *direct effect.* Because ionizing radiation is nonspecific (i.e., it interacts with normal cells as readily as with tumor cells), cellular damage will occur in both normal and abnormal tissue. The deleterious effects, however, are greater in the tumor cells because a greater percentage of these cells are undergoing mitosis; tumor cells also tend to be more poorly *differentiated.* In addition, normal cells have a greater capability for repairing sublethal damage than do tumor cells. Thus greater cell damage occurs to tumor cells than to normal cells for any given increment of dose. The effects of the interactions in either normal or tumor cells may be expressed by the following descriptions:

- Loss of reproductive ability
- Metabolic changes
- Cell transformation
- Acceleration of the aging process
- Cell mutation

Certainly the greater the number of interactions that occur, the greater the possibility of cell death.

The preceding information leads to a categorization of tumors according to their radiosensitivity:

- Very radiosensitive
  1. Gonadal germ cell tumors (seminoma of testis, dysgerminoma of ovary)
  2. Lymphoproliferative tumors (Hodgkin's and non-Hodgkin's lymphomas)
  3. Embryonal tumors (Wilms' tumor of the kidney, retinoblastoma)
- Moderately radiosensitive
  1. Epithelial tumors (squamous and basal cell carcinomas of skin)
  2. Glandular tumors (adenocarcinoma of prostate)
- Relatively radioresistant
  1. Mesenchymal tumors (sarcomas of bone and connective tissue)
  2. Nerve tumors (glioma)

Many concepts that originate in the laboratory have little practical application, but some are beginning to influence the selection of treatment modalities and the techniques of radiation oncology. As cellular function and the effects of radiation on the cell are increasingly understood, attention is being focused on the use of drugs, or simply oxygen, to enhance the effectiveness of radiation treatments.

TABLE 37-6

Relative biologic effectiveness (RBE) and linear energy transfer (LET) values for certain forms of radiation

Radiation	RBE	LET
250-kV x-rays	1	2.0
^{60}Co gamma rays	0.85	0.2
14-MeV neutrons	12	75
5-MeV alpha particles	20	100

Technical Aspects

EXTERNAL-BEAM THERAPY AND BRACHYTHERAPY

Two major categories for the application of radiation for cancer treatment are external-beam therapy and brachytherapy. For *external-beam treatment,* the patient lies underneath a machine that emits radiation or generates a beam of x-rays. This technique is also called *teletherapy,* or long-distance treatment. Most cancer patients are treated in this fashion. However, some patients may also be treated with *brachytherapy,* a technique in which the radioactive material is placed within the patient.

The theory behind brachytherapy is to deliver low-intensity radiation over an extended period to a relatively small volume of tissue. The low-intensity isotopes are placed directly into a tissue or cavity depositing radiation only a short distance, covering the tumor area but sparing surrounding normal tissue. This technique allows a higher total dose of radiation to be delivered to the tumor than is achievable with external beam radiation alone. Brachytherapy may be accomplished in any of the following ways:

1. Mould technique—placement of a *radioactive* source or sources on or in close proximity to the lesion
2. Intracavitary implant technique—placement of a radioactive source or sources in a body cavity (i.e., uterine canal and vagina).
3. Interstitial implant technique—placement of a radioactive source or sources directly into the tumor site and adjacent tissue (i.e., sarcoma in a muscle).

The majority of brachytherapy applications tend to be temporary in that the sources are left in the patient until a designated tumor dose has been attained. Two different brachytherapy systems exist. They are *low-dose-rate* (LDR) and *high-dose-rate* (HDR). LDR brachytherapy has been the standard system for many years. A low-activity isotope is used to deliver a dose of radiation at a slow rate of 40 cGy to 500 cGy per hour. This requires that patient to be hospitalized for 3 to 4 days until the desired dose is delivered.

HDR systems are becoming the more standard method of brachytherapy. This system uses a high-activity isotope capable of delivering greater than 1200 cGy per hour. This HDR allows the prescribed dose to be delivered over a period of minutes, allowing this treatment to occur on an outpatient basis. Gynecologic tumors are one of the most common sites to be treated with brachytherapy, LDR or HDR. Classic LDR systems use the isotopes cesium-137 for intracavity applications and iridium-192 for interstitial. HDR systems use a high-activity iridium-192 source.

Permanent implant therapy may also be accomplished. An example of a permanent implant nuclide is iodine-125 seeds. Permanent implant nuclides have *half-lives* of hours or days and are left in the patient essentially forever. The amount and distribution of the radionuclide implanted in this manner depends on the total dose that the radiation oncologist is trying to deliver. Early-stage prostate cancer is commonly treated with this technique. In most cases of brachytherapy implantation, the implant is applied as part of the patient's overall treatment plan and may be preceded by or followed by additional external beam radiation therapy or possibly surgery.

EQUIPMENT

Most radiation oncology departments have available some or all of the following units:

- 120-kVp superficial x-ray unit for treating lesions on or near the surface of the patient
- 250-kVp orthovoltage x-ray unit for moderately superficial tissues
- Cobalt-60 *gamma ray* source with an average energy of 1.25-MeV
- 6-MV to 35-MV *linear accelerator* or *betatron* to serve as a source of high-energy (megavoltage) electrons and x-rays

The dose depositions of these units are compared in Fig. 37-1.

The penetrability, or energy, of an x-ray or gamma ray is totally dependent on its wavelength: the shorter the wavelength, the more penetrating the photon; conversely, the longer the wavelength, the less penetrating the photon. A low-energy beam (120 kVp or less) of radiation tends to deposit all or most of its energy on or near the surface of the patient and thus is suitable for treating lesions on or near the skin surface. In addition, with the low-energy beam a greater amount of absorption or dose deposition takes place in bone than in soft tissue.

A high-energy beam of radiation (1 MeV or greater) tends to deposit its energy throughout the entire volume of tissue irradiated, with a greater amount of dose deposition occurring at or near the entry port than at the exit port. In this energy range, the dose is deposited about equally in soft tissue and bone. The high-energy (megavoltage) beam is most suitable for tumors deep beneath the body surface.

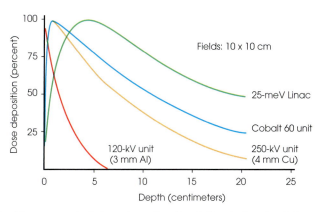

Fig. 37-1 Plot of the percent of dose deposition in relation to the depth in centimeters of tissue for various energies of photon beams.

The *skin-sparing* effect, a phenomenon that occurs as the energy of a beam of radiation is increased, is of value from a therapeutic standpoint. In the superficial and orthovoltage energy range, the maximum dose occurs on the surface of the patient, and deposition of the dose decreases as the beam traverses the patient. As the energy of the beam increases into the megavoltage range, the maximum dose absorbed by the patient occurs at some point below the skin surface. The skin-sparing effect is of importance clinically because the skin is a radiosensitive organ. Excessive dose deposition to the skin can damage the skin, requiring treatments to be stopped and compromising treatment to the underlying tumor. The greater the energy of the beam, the more deeply the maximum dose will be deposited (Fig. 37-2).

Cobalt-60 units

The *cobalt-60* unit was the first skin-sparing machine. It replaced the orthovoltage unit in the early 1950s because of its greater ability to treat tumors located deeper within tissues. ^{60}Co is an artificially produced *isotope* formed in a nuclear *reactor* by the bombardment of stable cobalt-59 with neutrons. ^{60}Co emits two gamma ray beams with an energy of 1.17 and 1.33 MeV. The unit was known as a "workhorse" because it was extremely reliable, mechanically simple, and had little downtime. It was the first radiation therapy unit to rotate 360 degrees around a patient. A machine that rotates around a fixed point, or axis, and maintains the same distance from the source of radiation is called an *isocentric machine*. All modern therapeutic units are isocentric machines. This type of machine allows the patient to remain in one position, lessening the chance for patient movement during treatment. Isocentric capabilities also assist in directing the beam precisely at the tumor while sparing normal structures.

Because ^{60}Co is a radioisotope, it constantly emits radiation as it *decays* in an effort to return to a stable state. It has a half-life of 5.26 years (i.e., its activity is reduced by 50% at the end of 5.26 years). Because the source decays at a rate of 1% per month, the radiation treatment time must be adjusted, resulting in longer treatment times as the source decays.

The use of cobalt units has declined significantly since the 1980s and is rarely used today. This decline has been basically attributed to the introduction of the more sophisticated linear accelerator (linac), which has greater skin-sparing capabilities and more sharply defined radiation *fields*. The radiation beam, or field, from a cobalt unit also has large penumbra, which results in fuzzy field edges, another undesirable feature.

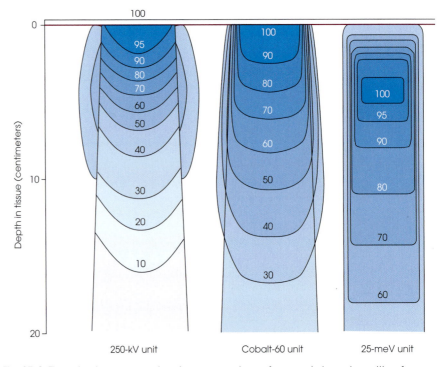

Fig. 37-2 Three isodose curves showing comparison of percent dose deposition from three x-ray units of different energies. As the energy of the beam is increased, the percentage of dose deposited on the surface of the patient decreases.

Linear accelerators

Linacs are the most commonly used machines for cancer treatment. The first linac was developed in 1952 and first used clinically in the United States in 1956. A linac is capable of producing high-energy beams of photons (x-rays) or electrons in the range of 4 million to 35 million volts. These megavoltage photon beams allow a better distribution of dose to deep-seated tumors with better sparing of normal tissues than their earlier counterparts—the orthovoltage or cobalt units.

The photon beam is produced by accelerating a stream of electrons toward a target. When the electrons hit the target, a beam of x-rays is produced. By removing the target, the linac can also produce a beam of electrons of varying energies.

Linacs can now be purchased with a single photon energy or a dual-photon machine with two x-ray beams. Typically a dual-photon energy machine consists of one low-energy (6-MeV) and one high-energy (18-MV) photon beam plus a range of electron energies (Fig. 37-3). The dual-photon energy machine gives the radiation oncologist more options in prescribing radiation treatments. As the energy of the beam increases, so does its penetrating power. Put simply, a lower-energy beam is used to treat tumors in thinner parts of the body, whereas high-energy beams are prescribed for tumors in thicker parts of the body. For example, a brain tumor or a tumor in a limb would most likely be treated with a 6-MeV beam; conversely, a pelvic malignancy would be better treated with an 18-MeV beam. Thus a small oncology center can serve its patients well by purchasing one dual-photon linac for a cost of approximately $1.7 million instead of having to purchase two single-energy 6- and 18-MeV machines for almost $2 million.

Electrons are advantageous over photons in that they are a more superficial form of treatment. Electrons are energy dependent, which means that they deposit their energy within a given depth of tissue and go no deeper, depending on the energy selected. For example, an 18-MeV beam has a total penetration depth of 9 cm. Any structure located deeper than 9 cm would not be appreciably affected. This is important when the radiation oncologist is trying to treat a tumor that overlies a critical structure.

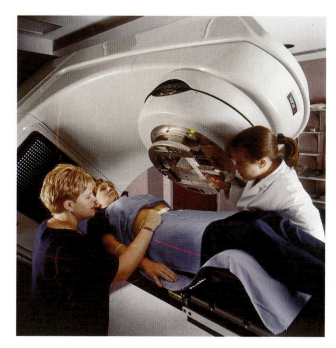

Fig. 37-3 Radiation therapists shown aligning patient and shielding block in preparation for treatment using a modern linear accelerator. X-ray beams of between 6 and 25 million volts may be produced to treat tumors in the body.

Steering system
Radial and transverse steering coils and a real-time feedback system ensure beam symmetry to within ±2% at all gantry angles.

Focal spot size
Even at maximum dose rate, the circular focal spot remains less than 3 mm, held constant by the achromatic bending magnet. Assures optimum image quality for portal imaging.

Standing wave accelerator guide
Guide maintains optimal bunching for different acceleration conditions, providing high dose rates, stable dosimetry and low-stray radiation. Transport system minimizes power and electron source demands.

Energy switch
Patented switch provides energies within the full therapeutic range, at consistently high, stable dose rates, even with low energy x-ray beams. Ensures optimum performance and spectral purity at both energies.

Gridded electron gun
Gun controls dose rate rapidly and accurately. Permits precise beam control for dynamic treatments because gun can be gated. Demountable, for cost-effective replacement.

Achromatic dual-plane bending magnet
Unique design with ±3% energy slits ensures exact replication of the input beam for every treatment. Clinac 2300C/D design enhancements allow wider range of beam energies.

10-port carousel with scattering foils/flattening filters
Extra ports allow future specialized beams to be developed. New electron scattering foils provide homogeneous electron beams at therapeutic depths.

Ion chamber
Two independently sealed chambers, impervious to temperature and pressure changes, monitor beam dosimetry to within 2% for long-term consistency and stability.

Asymmetric jaws
Four independent collimators provide flexible beam definition of symmetric or asymmetric fields.

Fig. 37-4 Dualing asymmetric jaws. Note the four independent collimators.

(Courtesy Varian Associates, Palo Alto, Calif.)

Fig. 37-5 Multileaf collimation system on the treatment head.

As with a diagnostic x-ray machine, the irradiated field of a linac is defined by a light field projected onto the patient's skin. This corresponding square or rectangle equals the length and width setting of the x-ray *collimators.* Today's modern linac is equipped with *dualing asymmetric (independent) jaws;* this allows each of the four collimator blades that define length or width to move independently (Fig. 37-4). For instance, the jaw that defines the superior extent of the field may be 7 cm from the central axis, whereas the inferior region may be at 10 cm. The total length would equal 17 cm, but it is not divided equally as it is in a diagnostic x-ray collimator. This allows the radiation oncologist to design a field that optimally covers the area of interest while sparing normal tissue. Independent collimation can also assist in reducing the total weight of lead shielding blocks normally constructed to protect normal tissues.

Multileaf collimation

Multileaf collimation (MLC) is the newest and most complex beam-defining system. From 45 to 80 individual collimator blades, about ⅜ to ¾ inch (1 to 2 cm) wide, are located within the head of the linac and can be adjusted to shape the radiation field to conform to the target volume (Fig. 37-5). The design of the field is digitized from a radiograph into a computer software program, which is transferred to the treatment room. The MLC machine receives a code that tells it how to position the individual leaves for the treatment field. Before MLC, custom-made lead blocks, or *cerrobend* blocks, were constructed to shape radiation fields and shield normal tissues from the beam of radiation. Heavy cerrobend blocks were placed within the head of the linac for each treatment field. Linacs equipped with the MLC package now receive a custom-designed field at the stroke of a computer keyboard. Today, multileaf collimators can be programmed to move across the radiation field during a treatment to alter the intensity of the radiation beam. Altering the beam intensity across the radiation field allows less dose to be delivered to normal structures/tissues and ensures the tumor or target receives the prescribed dose. This technique is called *intensity modulated radiation therapy* (IMRT).

Steps in Radiation Oncology
SIMULATION

The first step of radiation therapy involves determining the volume of tissue that needs to be encompassed within the radiation field. This is done with a *fluoroscopic simulator* or a *CT simulator.* A fluoroscopic simulator is a diagnostic quality x-ray machine that has the same geometric and physical characteristics as a treatment unit. During simulation, the radiation oncologist uses the patient's radiographic images or the CT or MRI scan to determine the tumor's precise location and to design a treatment volume, or area. The treatment volume often includes the tumor plus a small margin, the draining lymphatics that are at risk for involvement, and a rim of normal tissue to account for patient movement.

With a conventional simulator, the radiation therapist uses fluoroscopy to determine the field dimensions (length and width) and depth of isocenter as specified by the radiation oncologist. The *treatment field* outline and positioning marks are placed on the patient's skin surface (Fig. 37-6). A radiographic image is then obtained of all treatment fields to facilitate treatment planning, multileaf collimator position, or block fabrication, and to document the anatomic regions to be treated. A contour or CT scan would be completed for treatment planning purposes.

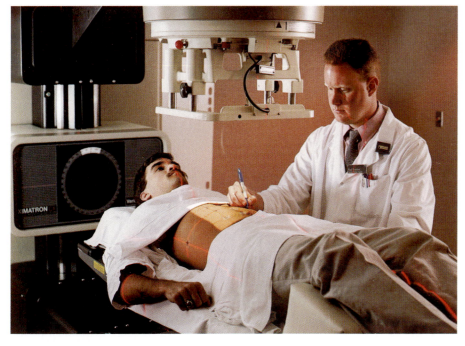

Fig. 37-6 The radiation therapist places skin marks on the patient's skin surface for alignment of the radiation beam during treatment.

Fig. 37-7 CT simulator.

Fig. 37-8 Aquaplast mask.

Today, most centers perform virtual simulations using a CT scanner equipped with radiation oncology software tools (Fig. 37-7). Before CT simulators, the films taken with the conventional simulator were done first to outline and localize areas to be treated. Following the simulation, a CT scan was done with the patient in treatment position. The CT information was then interfaced into the radiation oncology treatment-planning computer for development of the treatment plan. CT simulation combines the two aforementioned steps into one. First, CT images necessary to plan the treatment are obtained; second, a treatment isocenter is selected. Then the traditional marks to be placed on the patient are marked with the unit's sophisticated patient-marking system, and digitally reconstructed images similar to standard simulation radiographs that depict the anatomy are processed. This system enables a more accurate design of treatment fields and facilitates the implementation of three-dimensional (3D) treatment planning.

The main steps of a conventional and CT simulation are important to understand for positive treatment outcomes. The first step of a conventional or CT simulation is to position the patient in a manner that is stable and reproducible for each of the 28 to 40 radiation treatments. Therapists are responsible for constructing immobilization devices to help patients hold their position. It is extremely important for a patient to hold still and maintain the same position. If the patient does not maintain the planned position, critical normal tissues may be irradiated or the tumor may not be irradiated. Immobilization devices greatly assist the therapist in correctly aligning the patient for each treatment, and many patients feel more secure when supported by these devices. Immobilization devices can be constructed for any part of the body but are most important for more mobile parts, such as the head and neck region or the limbs. Many different types of immobilization systems exist. Fig. 37-8 shows a thermoplastic device that secures the head and neck against rotation or flexion/extension. Fig. 37-9 shows a vacuum bag device that may be used to secure upper body or lower extremities.

Contrast material is often administered before or during a simulation to localize the area that needs to be treated or to identify vital normal structures that are to be shielded. For example, a small amount of Gastrografin or Gastroview for CT simulation is injected into the rectum of a patient with rectal cancer to assist in localizing the rectum on the simulation images. In Fig. 37-10, bladder contrast is used to assist in localizing the prostate gland, which lies directly inferior to the bladder. The rectal contrast is used to demonstrate the relationship of the rectum to the prostate to monitor and minimize the dose the rectum receives (Fig. 37-11).

When a CT simulation is performed, a reference isocenter is marked on the patient and a pilot or scout scan is obtained. The radiation oncologist uses the scout or pilot image to determine the superior and inferior extent of the area to be scanned. The CT data are transferred to the virtual simulation computer workstation. From this limited scan, the physician reviews the CT images and uses imaging tools to outline the target volume and critical normal structures. The physician then establishes the actual treatment isocenter. The computer software determines the change in location from the coordinates associated with the reference marks to the newly established treatment isocenter. The radiation therapist adjusts the couch and uses the laser marking system to apply these shifts to mark the treatment isocenter on the patient. The radiation therapist records all details regarding the patient's position in the treatment chart, and the patient is dismissed. The physician creates treatment fields (length and width) electronically with the CT virtual simulation software (Fig. 37-12). The CT simulation data are then transferred to the treatment planning system. In complex cases, the physician communicates preferences for treatment goals to the dosimetrist, who then designs the beam's eye view treatment fields and beam arrangement as part of the 3D planning. A digitally reconstructed radiograph (DRR) for each treatment field is produced. The DRR is analogous to the radiograph taken in the conventional simulator (Fig. 37-13).

Precise measurements and details about the field dimensions, machine position, and patient positioning are recorded in the treatment chart. In some centers the treatment parameters, such as field length, width, couch, and gantry positions, are electronically captured and transferred to the treatment unit. Recording of this information is crucial so that the therapist performing the treatment can precisely reproduce the exact information.

Fig. 37-9 Vacuum bag immobilization device.

Fig. 37-10 AP pelvic radiograph demonstrating contrast in the bladder and its relationship to the prostate gland.

Fig. 37-11 Lateral radiograph demonstrating contrast in the rectum and bladder and their relationship to the prostate gland.

Fig. 37-12 Virtual CT simulation. Note divergent radiation beam lines indicating path of beam. Target volume, kidneys, and spinal cord have been outlined on the CT axial image and reconstructed sagittal and coronal images. Treatment field outline is seen on the DRR and coronal image.

Fig. 37-13 DRR of AP and lateral pelvis. Note outlining treatment field, target, and critical structures.

DOSIMETRY

Dosimetry refers to the measurement of radiation dose, and it demonstrates how the radiation is distributed or *attenuated* throughout the patient's body (absorbing medium). The dosimetrist devises a treatment plan that best fulfills the physician's prescription for the desired dose to the *tumor/target volume* while minimizing the amount of radiation to critical normal structures or tissues.

Each organ of the body has a tolerance dose to radiation that limits the amount it can receive and still function normally. If an organ receives an excess of the tolerance dose, the organ can fail, resulting in a fatal complication. For example, the kidneys are one of the more radiosensitive structures of the body (Table 37-7). A dose in excess of 2500 cGy can result in fatal radiation nephritis. The spinal cord has a higher tolerance dose, but many tumors require even higher doses for treatment to be effective.

Precise localization of dose-limiting structures and their relationship with the target volume is critical for adequate planning. The dosimetrist must devise a plan that delivers a homogeneous dose to the tumor while not exceeding the tolerance dose of a specific organ. This task can be quite challenging. For instance, the radiation oncologist might prescribe 6000 cGy to treat lung cancer located in the mediastinum directly over the spine but must limit the spinal cord dose to 4500 cGy to prevent irreparable damage, which could result in paralysis. The dosimetrist must then devise a plan that enables combined treatment and protection to be accomplished.

The first step in dosimetry is to obtain a contour or CT scan of the patient in treatment position. A *contour* is an outline of the external surface of the patient's body at the level of the central axis (center of treatment field). This is typically performed in the transverse plane, but other planes may be used. Then the tumor volume and critical dose-limiting internal structures are transferred from the simulation radiographs and drawn onto the contour. Today, CT scans from a CT simulator are more commonly used than contours. With CT scanning, the tumor and internal structures and their relationships are directly visible. These images are then interfaced with the treatment-planning computer system for development of the plan. PET scans and MR scans with the patient in treatment position are also sometimes obtained to facilitate the planning process. Fusion of the MR or PET images onto the CT simulation dataset allows a more precise delineation of the tumor volume than what would be seen on CT alone. To obtain an even distribution of radiation to the target volume, radiation is delivered from various angles, all focused on the area of interest. 3D treatment planning allows for the design of a beam that exactly conforms to the shape of the tumor at any plane within the body. The treatment-planning computer can digitally reconstruct the anatomy, which allows the dosimetrist to manipulate the image to view the tumor from any angle or plane. Important critical anatomic structures such as kidneys and spinal cord are also more readily identified. Such a system allows the dosimetrist to plan and design beams that are coplanar and noncoplanar, tightly conforming to the target or tumor volume. This is known as *3D conformal radiotherapy* (3DCRT). The beam's eye view obtained by 3D beams allows higher doses of radiation to be more safely administered by treating the cancer through multiple fields (more than four) on different planes, which reduces the amount of dose that normal tissues receive (Fig. 37-14).

For example, the standard approach for a tumor located in the pelvis, such as rectal cancer, is the use of three fields—PA, right lateral, and left lateral. Using the treatment parameters established in the simulator, the dosimetrist enters this information into the treatment-planning computer, designs beam's eye view conformal fields, and obtains an isodose distribution, which demonstrates how the radiation is being deposited. An *isodose line/curve* is a summation of areas of equal radiation dosage and may be stated as percentages of the total prescribed dose or as actual radiation dosages in *gray* (Gy) units.

TABLE 37-7

Tolerance doses to radiation

Structure	Tolerance dose
Testes	500 cGy
Ovary	500 cGy
Lung (whole lung)	1800 cGy
Kidney (whole organ)	2300 cGy
Liver (whole organ)	3500 cGy
Spinal cord (5 cm³)	4500 cGy

Fig. 37-14 Dosimetry plan showing nine different radiation fields used to treat pancreatic tumor.

The dosimetrist optimizes the plan by eliminating any areas of dose inhomogeneity (e.g., hot spots). A *hot spot* is an area of excessive radiation dose. One method to adjust for hot spots is to add a *wedge filter.* This wedge-shaped device is made of lead and is placed within the radiation beam to preferentially absorb the radiation, altering the shape of the isodose curve (Fig. 37-15). Another method of reducing hot spots is to change the weighting of the radiation beams by, for example, delivering a greater dose of radiation from the anterior field than from the posterior field.

Another major task of the dosimetrist is to monitor the dose that critical structures are receiving and to keep the dose within the established guidelines dictated by the physician. To avoid treating the spinal cord in the aforementioned example, the dosimetrist may angle the entry points of the radiation beams to include the target volume while not irradiating the spinal cord. The resultant fields might be right anterior oblique and left posterior oblique (RAO/LPO) fields. The dosimetrist evaluates the dose distribution after each modifier is added and then looks at different combinations of wedges, beam weighting, beam entry points, and the like, until an acceptable plan is produced. This technique is called *forward planning.* The final plan directs the radiation therapist, who will treat the patient, how to proceed. For the example presented previously (i.e., lung cancer in the mediastinum directly over the spine), the plan might consist of the following:

1. 25 treatments AP and PA fields, RAO and LPO, 30 degrees off vertical
2. Reduce field size to 12 long; do 5 more treatments AP, PA, RAO, and LPO, 30 degrees off vertical

Once the plan is complete, treatment of the patient can commence.

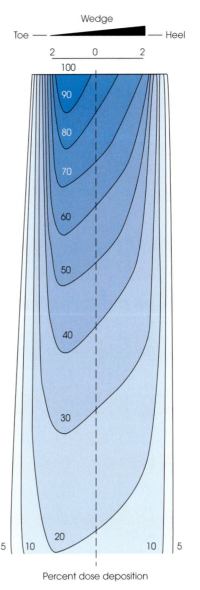

Fig. 37-15 Isodose curve obtained from cobalt-60 unit, with wedge placed between source and absorbing material.

Fig. 37-16 IMRT with dynamic MLC movement. **A,** Start of IMRT treatment. **B,** End of IMRT treatment. Notice shift of MLC position from left to right.

Another type of 3D treatment planning is intensity modulated radiation therapy (IMRT). The planning process begins as previously described, wherein the physician identifies target volume and critical structures. Treatment fields are designed and arranged so the target receives the prescribed dose and the dose to critical structures is limited. However, the optimization of the dose distribution is not done by trying different combinations of wedges or dose weighting as in conventional forward planning. IMRT uses a method called inverse planning. The prescribed dose to the target and the dose limit assigned to each critical structure are entered into the inverse planning system. A sophisticated mathematic algorithm creates a dose distribution that conforms to the target area while sparing critical normal structures. This is achieved by modifying the intensity of radiation within the treatment field. This is accomplished by moving the MLC across the radiation field during a treatment from open to closed position, modulating the intensity of a beam to obtain the desired dose (Fig. 37-16). The plan is computed by dividing the treatment field beam into hundreds of beamlets. Each beamlet can have an intensity from 0% to 100%. The intensity of a beamlet is changed by maintaining the MLC open for a specific amount of time and then closing it.

The IMRT planning process is time-intensive and requires a comprehensive physics quality assurance check of MLC movement and dose verification before treatment is administered for the first time. IMRT has proven to be better at minimizing the dose to normal structures than conventional 3DCRT and has allowed higher doses to be delivered to the target or tumor volume. IMRT was initially used for prostate cancer and cancers of the head and neck region. In prostate cancer treatment, IMRT optimized the dos to the prostate while substantially minimizing the dose to the rectum. When treating a cancer in the head and neck region (e.g., nasopharynx), IMRT significantly reduced the dose to the parotid gland and spinal cord. IMRT is also used in the treatment of brain tumors, gastrointestinal, gynecologic, lung, breast, and soft tissue sarcomas.

TREATMENT

On completion of the planning stage, including simulation and dosimetry, patient treatment can begin. The radiation therapist positions the patient and aligns the skin marks according to what was recorded in the treatment chart at the time of simulation. Accuracy and attention to detail are critical for precise administration of the radiation to the patient. The therapist is responsible for interpreting the radiation oncologist's prescription and calculating the correct monitor units, or timer setting, to achieve a desired dose of radiation for each treatment field. This also involves recording the daily administration of the radiation and the cumulative dose to date.

Precision in positioning the machine, proper selection of treatment field and MLC, accurate placement of cerrobend blocks or wedges, and the implementation of any change in a patient's treatment plan are critical for ensuring optimum treatment. Failure to do any of these may result in an overdose to normal tissue, causing long-term side effects, or underexposure of the tumor, reducing the patient's chance for cure. Today most radiation oncology departments use an electronic radiation oncology medical record and computer verification system that ensures a patient's treatment parameters are correct before treatment may commence. The complexity of 3DCRT and IMRT treatments with the numerous positions of the treatment couch, gantry, or collimator necessitates the use of a verification system. The computer verification system compares the machine settings with the information in the patient's electronic radiation chart. If there is a mismatch between any of the parameters in the electronic chart versus what is being set up for treatment, the therapist will not be able to initiate treatment. When a mismatch occurs, a computer prompt appears, highlighting the areas of disagreement. The therapists must double-check parameters and patient set-up, making corrections before treatment may occur. The verification and record system also records and adds the cumulative radiation doses.

Verification images, called *port films* or *images,* are taken on a weekly basis to ensure accuracy and consistent application of the radiation treatments. These port images are not of diagnostic quality because of the high-energy photon beams of the accelerator, but they are of enough detail to be compared with the simulation radiographs or DRRs to verify accurate alignment of the field and MLC or blocks (Fig. 37-17). The port film is developed and reviewed by the radiation oncologists after the patient is treated. If necessary, the physician will request the therapist to make changes, such as shifting the treatment field superior or anterior, at the next treatment session.

Many linacs are now equipped with electronic portal imaging devices (EPIDs). These retractable imaging devices produce a digital image that is displayed immediately on a computer screen adjacent to the linac computer console. The image can be viewed before treatment and adjustments made before treating the patient, ensuring accurate and precise treatment. Some systems have computer software that compares the simulation image with the EPID image using a registration algorithm. The computer automatically calculates the necessary adjustments (e.g., shift in couch position) to be made. The therapist makes the adjustments and commences with treatment. For example, when this treatment is used in cases of prostate cancer, gold seed markers are injected into the prostate gland before simulation. After the CT simulation is performed, the patient's treatment plan is completed and treatment begins. The therapist positions the patient, aligns the treatment machine, and takes an anterior and lateral EPID image. The images are analyzed, and the computer generates any necessary shifts. These adjustments in couch or collimator position are made before initiating treatment (Fig. 37-18). This process is done daily.

Fig. 37-17 A, AP lung image with cerrobend blocking. **B,** AP pelvis port image with MLC beam shaping.

If the patient has been positioned correctly, why do these changes or errors in treatment field position occur? Patient movement during treatment has always been a major constraint in providing accurate and precise delivery of radiation treatments. Improvements in immobilization devices have been made; however, they do not solve internal organ movement. The prostate may move and be in a different position within the treatment field from day to day due to the filling of the rectum or bladder. Organ movement can also occur due to normal respiration. This can result in a geographic miss of the tumor or irradiation of critical normal structures.

Because movement of internal structures does occur, many technologic innovations are being developed to address this issue. Obtaining daily EPID images before treatment is one method. Another means of ensuring the prostate is in the correct position is with B-mode acquisition technology (BAT). A transabdominal ultrasound is performed before treatment. The ultrasound wand/arm location coordinates are registered to the table and treatment isocenter. Computer algorithms similar to the EPID gold seed compares images and determines whether any shifts are needed. Adjustments in couch position are made, and the treatment is delivered.

Fig. 37-18 Comparison of DRR with EPID image of prostate gold seed markers; green line indicates amount to shift couch.

The process of using images such as EPID or BAT to verify the treatment field position before treatment is known as *image-guided radiation therapy* (IGRT). Two methods of IGRT that are being explored involve the use of a CT scan or an infrared camera system. A CT scan is obtained with the patient in treatment position, immediately before treatment, to verify target, isocenter, and patient position. This has been accomplished by having a CT scanner located in the actual treatment room opposite the linear accelerator, near the foot end of the treatment couch. The scanner can be moved into position to obtain a CT scan with the patient positioned for treatment. Another method that is being investigated is the use of a linear accelerator to obtain a cone beam CT. This is accomplished in one of two ways. One approach is to equip the linac with a kV x-ray tube and panel detector that obtains a cone beam CT when the accelerator gantry rotates a complete 360 degrees. The kV x-ray tube also provides a means of obtaining diagnostic quality images for treatment and patient position verification similar to an image produced by a conventional simulator (Fig. 37-19). Another technique is using the linac's megavoltage beam to acquire a cone beam CT. The cone beam CT is obtained in the same fashion, by rotating the linear accelerator 360 degrees.

Fig. 37-19 A linear accelerator equipped with kV x-ray tube and flat panel detector. The EPID is extended underneath the patient.

The infrared camera is a complex system that detects respiratory motion during simulation and treatment. This is a technique called *respiratory gating*. A reflective marker box is placed on the external surface of the patient's abdomen during simulation. The infrared camera detects the marker box, and a special computer software program connected to the infrared camera monitors the marker box movement (Fig. 37-20). The movement of the reflective marker is correlated with the patient's diaphragm position during the CT simulation. The respiratory cycle is evaluated relative to the treatment target volume and diaphragm movement. A specific portion of the respiratory cycle that has the least amount of motion is selected as the gated interval. This information is saved as a tolerance or standard to use during treatment. When the patient is treated, the reflective marker box is placed on the same place on the abdomen and an infrared camera is used to monitor the movement of the box. Pretreatment portal images (AP and lateral) to verify patient position, isocenter location, and gating interval are obtained with the EPID. Once approved, the therapist initiates treatment. The respiratory-gating computer monitors the marker box movement and automatically turns off the radiation beam if the marker moves out of the acceptable gated interval. Treatment automatically begins again when the marker box returns to the acceptable position. Respiratory gating has been done in a variety of ways. One method is to have patients breathe freely, while another method is to have patients exhale and hold their breath.

Even with all these technologic advancements, the radiation therapist cannot become totally dependent or reliant on the sophisticated equipment. The radiation therapist must still use critical thinking skills to analyze and assess why the couch parameters may need to be adjusted. Does the computer-generated shift make sense? Is the shift or collimator adjustment excessive? The radiation therapist must evaluate all aspects of the patient's set-up and the computer information before automatically implementing such shifts.

The radiation therapist is also responsible for monitoring the patient's physical and emotional well-being. The therapist is generally the only member of the radiation oncology team who sees the patient on a daily basis. The therapist monitors the patient's progress and assists in the management of any side effects. Acting as a liaison between the patient and the physician, the therapist must know when to withhold treatment and when to refer the patient to be seen by the physician or oncology nurse for further evaluation. The daily interaction with the patient is the most rewarding aspect of the therapist's job. Putting the patient at ease and making a cancer diagnosis and subsequent treatment a less traumatic experience is a satisfying aspect of this career. Patients often express their gratitude to the therapists for their care and support.

Fig. 37-20 A, Infrared camera system attached to CT simulator; **B,** reflective marker box.

Clinical Applications

The amount of radiation prescribed depends on the type of tumor and the extent of the disease. The following are brief summaries of radiation therapy treatment techniques used in the management of some of the more common forms of cancer.

LUNG CANCER

Treatment varies by type and stage. Radiation therapy is often used in conjunction with surgery and chemotherapy. A dose of 5000 to 6000 cGy of 10-MeV photons is often applied via a combination of AP, PA, and off-cord oblique fields. The primary tumor plus draining lymphatics are generally included in the treatment volumes (Fig. 37-21).

PROSTATE CANCER

Definitive radiation therapy is a standard treatment for prostate cancer. Surgical removal of the prostate gland is another common approach to the management of this disease. Traditionally, a four-field technique of AP, PA, and right and left lateral ports using a megavoltage beam of 10 MV or more is often used to deliver a dose of 7000 cGy to the prostate gland. Today, a series of six to eight oblique fields delivered with IMRT to a dose of 7600 cGy is a common method of treatment for prostate cancer. Another method of treating limited, early-stage prostate cancer is a brachytherapy procedure known as prostate seed implant (PSI). This involves the permanent implantation of 100 or more seeds of the radioisotope iodine-125 or palladium-103 into the prostate gland. A dose of 145 Gy is delivered with iodine-125 and a dose of 125 Gy is delivered with palladium.

A

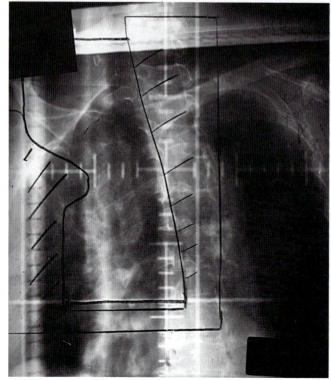

B

Fig. 37-21 A, AP lung-field simulation radiograph. **B,** Off-cord oblique simulation radiograph. The striped lines in **A** and **B** indicate areas to be shielded. **C,** Off-cord oblique port radiograph.

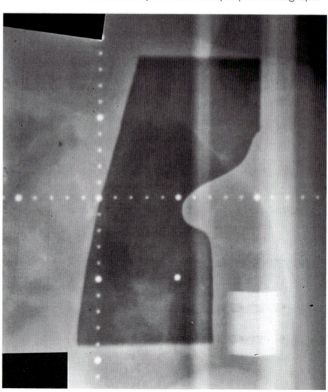

C

HEAD AND NECK CANCERS

A number of approaches may be used, depending on the location, size, and extent of the tumor. A small lesion in the oral cavity may be treated with an intraoral cone to a dose of 6000 cGy in 4 weeks with an orthovoltage beam. Larger lesions may be treated with irradiation through opposing lateral ports from a megavoltage unit, possibly followed by brachytherapy. A lesion in the nasopharynx could be treated with 3DCRT opposed lateral ports and an anterior supraclavicular field or an anterior and series of oblique IMRT fields to a dose of 6000 to 7000 cGy for small lesions or 7000 to 7600 cGy for larger lesions. Many institutions prefer to use IMRT for head and neck cancer sites. IMRT allows a significant reduction in the dose to the parotid gland and spinal cord while allowing a greater dose to be delivered to the target area.

CERVICAL CANCER

Early diagnosed cervical cancers can be treated with either surgery or radiation therapy. A four-field technique of AP, PA, and right and left lateral ports using a megavoltage unit, preferably 10 MV or greater, delivers 4500 to 5000 cGy in 5 weeks to an area of the primary and regional lymph nodes (Fig. 37-22). IMRT is another method of treating cervical cancer. An intracavitary implant is also included in the standard treatment of cervical cancer.

HODGKIN'S DISEASE

The age of the patient and extent of the disease may determine treatment and prognosis for Hodgkin's disease. Today, involved field lymph node irradiation following chemotherapy is more commonly used than the extended field therapy that included the lymphatic chain above and/or below the diaphragm. Treatment consists of 3000 to 4000 cGy delivered through AP-PA fields using a megavoltage unit. Chemotherapy may also be indicated for more advanced cases.

BREAST CANCER

Using two tangential fields to the chest wall or intact breast, megavoltage radiation delivers 5000 cGy in 5 weeks (Fig. 37-23). An electron boost to the site of initial lumpectomy adds an additional 1000 cGy. Irradiation of the axillary, supraclavicular, and internal mammary nodes to a dose of 5000 cGy is indicated for patients with a large primary tumor or node-positive disease. Chemotherapy and/or hormonal therapy is also commonly used for the treatment of breast cancer.

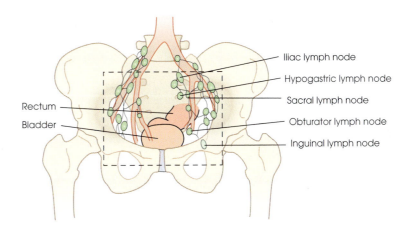

Fig. 37-22 Field used for irradiation of primary tumor and adjacent lymph nodes.

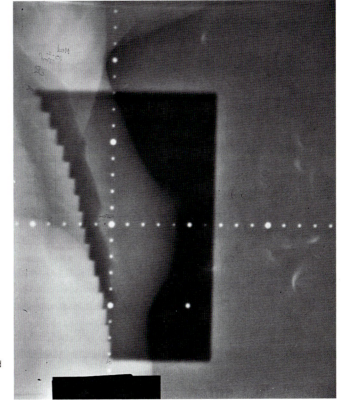

Fig. 37-23 A, Cross section of thorax showing field arrangements to tangentially irradiate the intact breast while sparing the lung (*lines A and B*). **B,** Port image of tangential breast field. Note sparing of lung tissue.

 (labels): Breast / Internal mammary nodes / Pectoral muscle / Lung tissue / Spinal cord

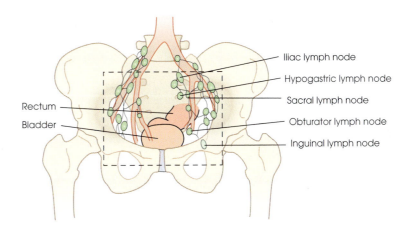 (labels): Iliac lymph node / Hypogastric lymph node / Sacral lymph node / Obturator lymph node / Inguinal lymph node / Rectum / Bladder

LARYNGEAL CANCER

Cancer of the larynx is best treated with megavoltage radiation. Tumors that are confined to the true vocal cord, with normal cord mobility, have a 90% 5-year cure rate; in addition, the voice remains useful. The method of treatment is usually accomplished by using small 5- × 5-cm opposing lateral wedged fields and delivering a dose of 6300 to 6500 cGy over a 6-week period.

SKIN CANCER

Carcinomas of the skin are usually squamous cell or basal cell lesions that may be treated with superficial radiation or surgery. Cure rates tend to run between 80% and 90%, and basal cell lesions less than ⅜ inch (1 cm) in diameter have a cure rate of almost 100%. The method of treatment is usually a single-field approach with attention given to shielding the uninvolved skin and delivering 4000 to 5000 cGy in a 3- to 4-week period.

MEDULLOBLASTOMA

Children with medulloblastoma are usually referred to the radiation oncology department after a biopsy and shunt procedure. The tumor is radiosensitive, and patients who have had treatment of the entire cerebrospinal axis have a 5-year cure rate of greater than 60%. The therapeutic approach tends to be complicated because the entire brain is irradiated with 3600 cGy, the spinal cord receives a dose of between 3500 and 4500 cGy, and the cerebellum receives an additional 1000 cGy (Fig. 37-24). This irradiation is usually accomplished with parallel opposed fields to the cranial vault and an extended single field to the spinal cord. The boost dose of 1000 cGy to the posterior fossa may be given with IMRT to provide better dose optimization to the target and less dose to critical structures. A megavoltage unit is used, with extreme care given to the areas of abutting fields.

C3
C7-T1
S3-S4

Fig. 37-24 Spinal treatment portal for medulloblastoma.

Future Trends

Radiation therapy has entered the electronic age with increased technologic advancement in the areas of dosimetry, simulation, and treatment. Most institutions use computer-interfaced accelerators with treatment verification software packages to ensure accurate treatment. Paperless treatment charting and filmless departments are the standard design of a facility. Intensity-modulated radiation therapy is being used in many facilities to treat a variety of tumor types. Developments will continue to occur in the use of IGRT. Refinements in the application of the linear accelerator cone beam CT and other modalities, such as PET, to verify target, isocenter, and patient position before treatment will occur more routinely. Advancements and implementation of respiratory gating will permit better delineation of 3D conformal target volumes, lessen the chance of a geographic miss of the target volume, and further minimize the dose to normal structures. The use of gating may permit higher doses to be prescribed and result in greater control and cure rates.

Linear accelerators are the most commonly used equipment for treating malignant disease. Recently there has been an increase in the installation of proton facilities worldwide. Proton beams are not a new form of cancer treatment. The first use of a proton beam was in 1954 at the University of California in Berkeley, California; however, due to the complexity, cost, and size of a cyclotron facility, protons were not widely implemented. Proton beams used therapeutically produce beams between 100 and 250 MeV. The use of protons in the treatment of cancer is gaining in popularity once again due to the characteristic properties of the proton beam. Proton beams have minimal scatter and deposit little energy as the beam first traverses tissue. Then as the protons slow down as they reach a certain depth, the majority (80%) of the energy or dose is deposited in tissue and then quickly falls to zero dose within millimeters. This burst of energy deposited at a specific depth is termed the *Bragg peak*. The depth at which this peak deposition of dose occurs can be adjusted by changing the energy of the proton beam and adding beam modifiers. The principal advantage of the proton beam is the sparing of surrounding normal tissues. The proton beam can be precisely controlled to deliver the Bragg peak dose at a prescribed depth. The rapid fall-off of the beam allows treatment of the target while sparing critical structures located within millimeters of the target. Research regarding the effectiveness of protons and dosimetric planning initiatives including intensity-modulated proton therapy are currently being explored. Cost and space constraints are still a major barrier preventing many hospital-based facilities from implementing a proton therapy program.

Conclusion

From a somewhat questionable beginning, radiation therapy has emerged as one of the primary modalities used in the treatment of malignant disease. Radiation therapy departments are currently examining and treating approximately 75% of all newly diagnosed cancer patients. Radiation oncologists and radiation therapists are integral members of the health care team that discusses and selects the appropriate treatment regimens for all cancer patients.

As the factors that initiate cellular change, growth, and spread become better understood, the radiation treatments for cancer will become even more effective. The irradiation techniques presently used may change dramatically based on this new information. In addition, new, more sophisticated radiation-producing equipment is currently under design and may lead to the reevaluation of presently accepted therapeutic techniques and dose levels. Finally, new chemotherapeutic agents are being produced that, when used by themselves or with other drugs, may enhance tumor sensitivity when used in conjunction with irradiation.

Definition of Terms

absorbed dose Amount of ionizing radiation absorbed per unit of mass of irradiated material.

accelerator (particle) Device that accelerates charged subatomic particles to great energies. These particles or rays may be used for direct medical irradiation and basic physical research. Medical units include linear accelerators, betatrons, and cyclotrons.

asymmetric jaws Four independent x-ray collimators that are used to define the radiation treatment field.

attenuation Removal of energy from a beam of ionizing radiation when it traverses matter, accomplished by disposition of energy in matter and by deflection of energy out of the beam.

betatron Electron accelerator that uses magnetic induction to accelerate electrons in circular path; also capable of producing photons.

biopsy Removal of a small piece of tissue for examination under the microscope.

brachytherapy Placement of radioactive nuclide(s) in or on a neoplasm to deliver a cancericidal dose.

cancer Term commonly applied to malignant disease; abnormal growth of cells; neoplasm (new growth) or -*oma* (tumor).

cancericidal dose Dose of radiation that results in the death of cancer cells.

carcinogen Any cancer-producing substance or material, such as nicotine, radiation, or ingested uranium.

carcinoma Cancer that arises from epithelial tissue—either glandular or squamous epithelium.

cerrobend block Beam-shaping device made of a lead alloy that attenuates the x-ray beam, preventing exposure of normal tissue.

chromosome Unit of genetic information that guides cytoplasmic activities of the cell and transmits hereditary information.

cobalt-60 Radioisotope with half-life of 5.26 years, average gamma ray energy of 1.25 MeV (range: 1.17 to 1.33 MeV), and ability to spare skin with buildup depth in tissue of 0.5 cm.

collimator Diaphragm or system of diaphragms made of radiation-absorbing material that defines dimension and direction of beam.

conformal radiation Treatment designed to deliver radiation to the exact target volume as seen on any plane (e.g., transverse, sagittal, vertex views); requires a 3D treatment planning system.

contour Reproduction of an external body shape, typically in the transverse plane at the level of the central axis of the beam; facilitates planning of radiation treatment. Other planes of interest may also be obtained.

cure Usually a 5-year period after completion of treatment during which time the patient exhibits no evidence of disease.

decay or disintegration Transformation of radioactive nucleus, resulting in emission of radiation.

differentiation Acquisition of cellular function/structure that differs from function/structure of original cell type.

direct effect Radiation that interacts with an organic molecule such as DNA, RNA, or a protein molecule. This interaction may inactivate the cell.

dosimetry Measurement of radiation dose in an absorbing medium.

epithelial tissue Cells that line the surfaces of serous and mucous membranes, including the skin.

etiology Study of causes of diseases.

external-beam treatment Delivery of radiation to a patient from a unit such as a linear accelerator in which the radiation enters the patient from the external surface of the body.

field Geometric area defined by collimator or radiotherapy unit at skin surface.

fractionation Division of total planned dose into a number of smaller doses to be given over a longer period. Consideration must be given to biologic effectiveness of smaller doses.

gamma ray Electromagnetic radiation that originates from radioactive nucleus and causes ionization in matter; identical in properties to x-ray.

gray (Gy) International unit for the quantity of radiation received by the patient; previously rad. 1 cGy = 1 rad.

grenz rays X-rays generated at 20 kVp or less.

half-life Time (specific for each radioactive substance) required for radioactive material to decay to half its initial activity; types are biologic and physical.

half-value layer Thickness of attenuating material inserted in beam to reduce beam intensity to half of the original intensity.

high-dose-rate brachytherapy The use of a high-activity radionuclide placed within the body for the treatment of cancer. Delivers more than 1200 cGy per hour.

image-guided radiation therapy (IGRT) The use of images to verify treatment isocenter, target, and patient positioning before initiating radiation treatment.

independent jaws X-ray collimator with four individual blades that can be moved independently of one another (see *asymmetric jaws*).

indirect effect Interaction of radiation with water molecules within the cell; results in the formation of free radicals OH, H, and HO_2, which can damage the cell.

ionization Process in which one or more electrons are added to or removed from atoms, creating ions; can be caused by high temperatures, electrical discharges, or nuclear radiations.

ionizing radiation Energy emitted and transferred through matter that results in the removal of orbital electrons (e.g., x-rays or gamma rays).

intensity-modulated radiation therapy (IMRT) Modification of beam intensity to deliver nonuniform exposure across radiation field.

isocentric Referring to rotation about a fixed point.

isodose line curve Curve or line drawn to connect points of identical amounts of radiation in a given field.

isotope Atoms that have the same atomic number but different mass number.

lesion Morbid change in tissue; mass of abnormal cells.

linear accelerator (linac) Device for accelerating charged particles, such as electrons, to produce high-energy electron or photon beams.

linear energy transfer (LET) Rate at which energy is deposited as it travels through matter.

low-dose-rate brachytherapy The use of a low activity radionuclide placed within the body for the treatment of cancer. Dose is slowly delivered, 40 to 500 cGy per hour, to a small volume of tissue over a period of days.

malignancy Cancerous tumor or lesion.

medical dosimetrist Person responsible for calculation of the proper radiation treatment dose who assists the radiation oncologist in designing individual treatment plans.

medical physicist A specialist in the study of the laws of ionizing radiation and their interactions with matter.

metastasis Transmission of cells or groups of cells from primary tumor to sites elsewhere in body.

multileaf collimator (MLC) Individual collimator rods within the treatment head of the linear accelerator that can slide inward to shape the radiation field.

oncologist Doctor of medicine specializing in the study of tumors.

oncology Study of tumors.

palliation To relieve symptoms; not for cure.

pathologist A specialist in the study of the microscopic nature of disease.

prophylactic surgery Preventive surgical treatment.

radiation oncologist Doctor of medicine specializing in use of ionizing radiation in the treatment of disease.

radiation oncology Medical specialty involving the treatment of cancerous lesions using ionizing radiation.

radiation therapist Person trained to assist and take directions from radiation oncologist in the use of ionizing radiation for the treatment of disease.

radiation therapy Older term used to define medical specialty of treatment with ionizing radiation.

radioactive Pertaining to atoms of elements that undergo spontaneous transformation, resulting in emission of radiation.

radiocurable Susceptibility of neoplastic cells to cure (destruction) by ionizing radiation.

radiosensitivity Responsiveness of cells to radiation.

radium (ra) Radionuclide (atomic number, 88; atomic weight, 226; half-life, 1622 years) used clinically for radiation therapy. In conjunction with its subsequent transformations, radium emits alpha and beta particles and gamma rays. In encapsulated form it is used for various intracavitary radiation therapy applications, such as that for cancer of cervix.

reactor Cubicle in which isotopes are artificially produced.

relative biologic effectiveness (RBE) Compares radiation beams with different LETs and their ability to produce a specific biologic response. Dose in gray from 250 kVp beam of x-rays/dose from another type of radiation to produce the same effect.

simulator A diagnostic x-ray machine that has the same geometric and physical characteristics as a radiation therapy treatment unit.

skin sparing In megavoltage beam therapy, reduced skin injury per centigray (cGy) exposure because electron equilibrium occurs below skin; occurs from ¼ inch to 2 inches (0.6 to 5 cm) deep, depending on energy.

surgical bed Area of excision and adjacent tissues manipulated during surgery.

systemic Throughout the human body.

teletherapy Radiation therapy technique for which source of radiation is at some distance from patient.

treatment field Anatomic area outlined for treatment (e.g., AP or RL pelvis).

tumor/target volume Portion of anatomy that includes tumor and adjacent areas of invasion.

undifferentiation Lack of resemblance of cells to cells of origin.

wedge filter Wedge-shaped beam attenuating device used to preferentially absorb the beam to alter the shape of the isodose curve.

Selected bibliography

American Cancer Society: *Cancer facts and figures 2005,* Atlanta, 2005, American Cancer Society.

Bentel GC: *Radiation therapy planning,* ed 2, New York, 1996, Macmillan.

Bentel GC et al: *Treatment planning and dose calculation in radiation oncology,* ed 3, New York, 1982, Pergamon.

Berson AM et al: Clinical experience using respiratory gated radiation therapy: comparison of free-breathing and breath-hold techniques, *J Radiat Oncol Biol Phys* 60:419, 2004.

Boyer AL: The physics of intensity-modulated radiation therapy, *Phys Today* 55:38, 2002.

Boyer AL, Xing L, Ping X: Beam shaping and intensity modulation. In Van Dyk J, editor: *The modern technology of radiation oncology,* Madison, Wis, 1999, Medical Physics Publishing.

Brenner DJ: Dose, volume, and tumor-control predictions in radiotherapy, *J Radiat Oncol Biol Phys* 26:171, 1993.

Cancer facts and figures—1997, Atlanta, 1997, American Cancer Society.

Cheng J, Chao KS, Low D: Comparison of intensity modulation radiation therapy treatment techniques for nasopharyngeal carcinoma, *J Radiat Oncol Biol Phys* 96:126, 2001.

Coleman A: Treatment procedures. In Washington CM, Leaver DT, editors: *Principles and practices of radiation therapy,* ed 2, St Louis, 2004, Mosby.

Cooper JS et al: *Concepts in cancer care,* Philadelphia, 1983, Lea & Febiger.

Dische S: Radiotherapy in the nineties: increase in cure, decrease in morbidity, *Acta Oncol* 31:501, 1992.

Furlow B: Three-dimensional conformal radiation therapy, *Radiat Therapist* 12:131, 2003.

Gierga DP et al: The correlation between internal and external markers for abdominal tumors: implications for respiratory gating, *J Radiat Oncol Biol Phys* 61:1551, 2005.

Goetein M, Lomax AJ, Pedroni ES: Treating cancer with protons, *Phys Today* 55:45, 2002.

Grabowski CM, Unger JA, Potish RA: Factors predictive of completion of treatment and survival after palliative radiation therapy, *Radiology* 184:329, 1992.

Greenlee RT et al: Cancer statistics 2001, *CA Cancer J Clin* 51:15, 2001.

Hall EJ: *Radiobiology for the radiologist,* ed 4, Philadelphia, 1994, Lippincott-Raven.

Jaffray DA et al: Flat-panel cone-beam computed tomography for image-guided radiation therapy, *J Radiat Oncol Biol Phys* 54:1337, 2002.

Jessup JM et al: Diagnosing colorectal carcinoma: clinical and molecular approaches, *CA Cancer J Clin* 47:70, 1997.

Landis SH et al: Cancer statistics, 1998, *CA Cancer J Clin* 48:6, 1998.

Leaver D: Intensity modulated radiation therapy: part 2, *Radiat Therapist* 12:17, 2003.

Leaver D, Keller R, Uricchio N: Simulation procedures. In Washington CM, Leaver DT, editors: *Principles and practices of radiation therapy,* ed 2, St Louis, 2004, Mosby.

Lipa LA, Mesina CF: Virtual simulation in conjunction with 3-D conformal therapy, *Radiat Therapist* 2:99, 1995.

Marks JE, Armbruster JS: Accreditation of radiation oncology in the US, *Int J Radiat Oncol Biol Phys* 24:863, 1992.

Mell LK, Roeske JC, Mundt AJ: A survey of intensity-modulated radiation therapy use in the United States, *Cancer* 98:204, 2003.

Morgan HM: Quality assurance of computer controlled radiotherapy treatments, *Br J Radiol* 65:409, 1992.

Moss WT et al: *Radiation oncology rationale, technique, and results,* ed 5, St Louis, 1979, Mosby.

Moyer MF: Proton therapy. In Van Dyk J, editor: *The modern technology of radiation oncology,* Madison, Wis, 1999, Medical Physics Publishing.

National Cancer Institute: *Genetic testing for breast cancer risk: it's your choice,* Washington, DC, 1997, National Cancer Institute.

Order SE: Training in systemic radiation therapy, *Int J Radiat Oncol Biol Phys* 24:895, 1992.

Perez CA: Quest for excellence: ultimate goal of the radiation oncologist: ASTRO Gold Medal Address 1992, *Int J Radiat Oncol Biol Phys* 26:567, 1993.

Prado K, Prado C: Dose distributions. In Washington CM, Leaver DT, editors: *Principles and practices of radiation therapy,* ed 2, St Louis, 2004, Mosby.

Rietzel E et al: Four-dimensional image-based treatment planning: target volume segmentation and dose calculation in the presence of respiratory motion, *J Radiat Oncol Biol Phys* 61:1535, 2005.

Roberge SL: Virtual reality: radiation therapy treatment planning of tomorrow, *Radiat Therapist* 2:113, 1996.

Sillanpaa J et al: Integrating respiratory gating into a megavoltage cone-beam CT system, *J Radiat Oncol Biol Phys* 60:197 2004.

Stanton R, Stinson D: *Applied physics for radiation oncology,* Madison, Wis, 1996, Medical Physics.

Travis EL: *Primer of radiobiology,* ed 2, St Louis, 1989, Mosby.

Vlachaki MT et al: IMRT versus conventional 3D CRT on prostate and normal tissue dosimetry using an endorectal balloon for prostate localization, *Med Dosim* 30:69, 2005.

Varmus H, Weinberg R: *Genes and the biology of cancer,* New York, 1993, Scientific American Library.

Wagner LK: Absorbed dose in imaging: why measure it? *Radiology* 178:622, 1991.

Washington CM, Leaver DT: *Principles and practice of radiation therapy: introduction to radiation therapy,* St Louis, 1996, Mosby.

Washington CM, Leaver DT: *Principles and practice of radiation therapy: physics, simulation, and treatment planning,* St Louis, 1996, Mosby.

Washington CM, Leaver DT: *Principles and practice of radiation therapy: practical applications,* St Louis, 1996, Mosby.

INDEX

Page numbers followed by *f* indicate figures; *t*, tables;
b, boxes.

Index

I-5

Index

Index

I-23

Index

Index

Index

Index

Index

I-41

Index

Index

Index

Egas Moniz
(1874-1955)

Schüller
(1874-1957)

Lysholm
(1891-1947)

Albers-Schönberg
(1865-1921)

Béclère, H.
(1880-1937)

Fuchs
(1895-1962)

Waters
(1888-1961)